OXFORD MEDICAL PUBLICATIONS

BLOOD GROUPS AND DISEASES

OXFORD MONOGRAPHS ON MEDICAL GENETICS

BLOOD GROUPS AND DISEASES

A STUDY OF ASSOCIATIONS OF DISEASES WITH BLOOD GROUPS AND OTHER POLYMORPHISMS

A. E. MOURANT
M.A., D.PHIL., D.M. (OXFORD), F.R.C.P. (LONDON), F.R.C.PATH., F.R.S.
Formerly Director, Medical Research Council Serological Population Genetics Laboratory, London
Formerly Honorary Senior Lecturer in Haematology, St. Bartholomew's Hospital, London
Formerly Director, M.R.C. Blood Group Reference Laboratory, London
Sometime Visiting Professor of Serology, Columbia University in the City of New York

ADA C. KOPEĆ
D. ÈS SC. (GENÈVE)
Formerly Statistician, M.R.C. Serological Population Genetics Laboratory, London
Formerly Statistician, Nuffield Blood Group Centre, London

KAZIMIERA DOMANIEWSKA-SOBCZAK
M.PHIL. (WILNO), A.L.A.
Formerly Librarian, M.R.C. Serological Population Genetics Laboratory, London
Formerly Librarian, Nuffield Blood Group Centre, London

WITH AN APPENDIX BY
LARS P. RYDER
AND
ARNE SVEJGAARD

1478
1978

OXFORD
OXFORD UNIVERSITY PRESS
NEW YORK TORONTO

Oxford University Press, Walton Street, Oxford OX2 6DP

OXFORD LONDON GLASGOW
NEW YORK TORONTO MELBOURNE WELLINGTON
KUALA LUMPUR SINGAPORE JAKARTA HONG KONG TOKYO
DELHI BOMBAY CALCUTTA MADRAS KARACHI
IBADAN NAIROBI DAR ES SALAAM CAPE TOWN

British Library Cataloguing in Publication Data

Mourant, Arthur Ernest
Blood groups and diseases – (Oxford monographs on medical genetics).
1. Diseases – Causes and theories of causation – Statistics 2. Blood groups – Statistics
I. Title II. Kopeć, Ada Christina
III. Domaniewska-Sobczak, Kazimiera
IV. Series
616 RB155 77-30711

ISBN 0-19-264170-0

Printed in Great Britain
at the University Press, Oxford
by Vivian Ridler
Printer to the University

CONTENTS

PREFACE

THE subject of this book is the association (or absence of association) between particular blood groups (or other inherited biochemical characteristics) and specific diseases, as shown by a comparison between the frequencies of these characteristics in healthy persons, and in sufferers from the diseases under investigation, drawn from the same populations.

One object of a search for such associations is to try to account, in evolutionary terms, for the wide variations in blood-group frequencies observed between different populations of presumed healthy persons. The principal hypothesis to be tested is that these frequency variations depend, at least in part, upon natural selection related to variations in environmental conditions. Such dependence would exist if, for a given disease, incidence and early mortality or reduced fertility were related to the combined action of the blood group and environmental conditions.

However, the publication of the book has also a more directly medical aim since, where an association is found between a particular blood factor and a disease of hitherto obscure causation, this may lead, and in some cases has led, to a better understanding of the origins of that disease. It may even, in rare cases, serve as an aid to diagnosis.

The term 'blood groups' has been used in the title to avoid a long and complicated phrase, but in deciding upon the scope of the book it has been interpreted with the widest possible connotation, to cover not only the classical blood groups dependent upon the surface antigens of the red cells, but also all other genetic polymorphisms which can be detected by tests upon the blood, and thus to include those due to variants of the plasma proteins, the haemoglobins, the red-cell enzymes, and the histocompatibility antigens. We have also included the ABH secretor and phenylthiocarbamide tasting polymorphisms which do not depend upon blood tests, but which show marked disease associations.

The book is a sequel to the second edition of *The distribution of the human blood groups*, by the same authors. Most of the data for the present work were collected at the same time as those used in the latter, recently published, book. Indeed, many of the papers consulted contained data on blood-group frequencies both in healthy persons and in those suffering from certain diseases. We have, however, included much material published after the tables for the earlier book were compiled but, because we have been working to a much stricter deadline, it has not been possible to achieve the same degree of completeness as was attempted in that book. For the same reason we have included a higher proportion of data quoted at second hand than in that book, though we have tried to quote primary data whenever this was possible without loss of time. For data published before the end of 1970 we have achieved this almost completely.

The bibliographic work has been primarily the responsibility of K. Domaniewska-Sobczak who also, especially in the early stages, carried out a large part of the searching of the literature. The statistical work has been the responsibility of A. C. Kopeć, who extracted nearly all the data from the original publications and also prepared them for electronic computation, or, indeed in a great many cases, did all the computations herself. She then prepared the tables for publication from the computation results. The introduction to the tables, which includes a description of computation methods, is by A. C. Kopeć and A. E. Mourant. The remainder of the text has been written, with much consultation with his co-authors, by A. E. Mourant.

We are greatly indebted to numerous colleagues who have sent us copies of their published papers and, in many cases, of their unpublished results. Many of the latter have since been published, and are quoted here with the appropriate references, but work which, as far as we know, remains unpublished is acknowledged as such in the bibliography. In the earlier stages of the work we received much help, especially on the bibliographical side, from Miss Janina Wasung. We are greatly indebted to Mrs J. Shimell who typed most of the text from our untidy manuscript, and to Mrs M. Makowska who helped with the typing at moments of great urgency.

We are most grateful to Mr B. K. Kelly, Director of the Medical Research Council's Computer Services Centre for writing the programs used in the computations, and for allowing the computations to be carried out at the centre. We are also much indebted to the librarians and staffs of numerous libraries, especially those of the Royal Society of Medicine and St Bartholomew's Hospital Medical College.

The earlier stages of the work were supported by the Medical Research Council, but most of it was carried out in accommodation provided by St Bartholomew's Hospital, with the support of grants from the Wolfson Foundation, the Nuffield Foundation, the World Health Organization, and the Royal Anthropological Institute.

FOREWORD

CONTINUOUS variability is often accepted as a natural phenomenon, but discrete characters, such as those constituting genetic polymorphic systems, excite curiosity and seem to cry out for a meaning. Population geneticists, anthropologists, and medical men all seek to identify factors which keep the morphs in balance, and nowhere has the explanation for the advantage of the heterozygote been sought more assiduously than in these islands. The concept perhaps suits the national genius—with the British love of compromise the golden mean appeals to us so much more than do the extremes.

The trouble with the polymorphic systems is that they now overwhelm the weaker among us by their sheer numbers. In the old days we argued about reciprocal associations between the A and O blood groups and carcinoma of the stomach and duodenal ulcer. Then the secretor character complicated matters a little, but the problem still seemed manageable and we were not submerged by dozens of enzyme polymorphisms, so numerous that they are now in competition for finding a disease.

Dr Mourant and his team have in this book bravely tackled the subject, starting from a consideration of the blood groups and other polymorphic systems, and then via statistical methods they lead us on to a description of the definite (though still ill-understood) associations. Later, the relevance to clinical medicine becomes more obvious, with resistance or susceptibility to infectious diseases, emphysema and trypsin-inhibitor types, phenylthiocarbamide tasting and thyroid disease, and—most important of all—the histocompatibility antigens. These, which were first of importance only in transplantation procedures, have now lit up the whole medical scene with striking findings between tissue antigens and rheumatic disorders, particularly ankylosing spondylitis.

Conferences and workshops on human lymphocyte antigens abound, and it seems as though immunology is taking yet another leap forward and that the pathogenesis of many diseases is a stage nearer solution. It is good that at such an exciting time we have Dr Mourant, who not only has an intimate knowledge of the discipline but is such a master at assessing evidence, marshalling facts, and putting the whole subject in perspective for the clinician.

SIR CYRIL CLARKE, KBE, FRS

1977 *President of the Royal College of Physicians*

1
INTRODUCTION

As is well known, the human ABO blood groups were discovered in 1900 by Landsteiner. From the outset it must have been clear that the blood group was a more or less permanent characteristic of any individual, but the time was not yet ripe for any discussion of its possible hereditary nature, since the fundamental genetical work of Mendel, ignored and forgotten for many years, had been rediscovered only in the same year, and not yet applied to man. But speculation as to the pathological significance of the blood groups soon began, and as early as 1905 Dienst showed that mothers who lacked an A or a B antigen present in their foetus became immunized by that antigen, with a rise of the titre of anti-A or anti-B in their serum. He thus came very near to discovering, 36 years early, the cause of haemolytic disease of the newborn. It appears, however, not to have occurred to him that the antibodies might damage the foetus but, on the other hand, he suggested that the immunization process might tend to cause eclampsia in the mother.

It tends to be forgotten that, simultaneously with the work of Landsteiner, and independently of it, Ehrlich and Morgenroth (1900) discovered blood group antigens and antibodies in goats. It was their observations that led Hirszfeld, who was then in ignorance of Landsteiner's discovery, to begin work on blood groups in dogs. He was already contemplating a study of human blood when he first learned of Landsteiner's work, and began his own life work on the human blood groups. He was responsible, with E. von Dungern (Dungern and Hirszfeld, 1910) for the discovery that the blood groups were inherited as Mendelian characters, and, with his wife (Hirszfeld and Hirszfeld, 1918–19) for the first demonstration that blood group frequencies differed systematically and significantly between different populations. These two discoveries opened the field for a new approach to anthropology, but they also posed the fundamental question of the origin of the differences between populations, in the frequencies of these hereditary factors. Were the differences the result of random genetic drift and founder effects, in small populations which later multiplied and stabilized the original, fortuitous, frequencies, or were they the result of natural selection, arising from differences in fitness between the various blood groups, fitnesses which themselves depended upon locally determined features of the external environment? Most workers now agree that both processes are operative, but their relative importance remains in question.

If, in a certain environment, natural selection is unfavourable to a particular blood group, this must mean that some feature of the environment causes a raised early mortality, or a lowered fertility, in persons of that group. This implies that one or more diseases, caused or exacerbated by that environment, are commoner, or tend to be more severe, in persons of one blood group than of another. If, as we shall later see to be probably the case, blood-group frequencies are stable features of different populations, and if these frequencies are maintained by natural selection, this implies a balance between the selective processes acting against each of the three main genes of the ABO system, which are present in nearly all populations. Thus we may expect certain diseases to attack preferentially persons of one blood group, and other diseases, those of another group. The ideal way of demonstrating this would be by a series of comprehensive blood-group surveys of whole populations, healthy and diseased, but such surveys are possible only in the case of small isolated populations. In larger populations a sampling method must be used and it is possible to determine the blood groups only of limited numbers of healthy and diseased persons. In such surveys a tendency of a given disease to attack persons of a particular blood group will show itself by a higher frequency of that group among the diseased than among the healthy persons.

Before we consider what has been accomplished in this field, however, we must look at certain important earlier developments. From 1900 to 1927 the ABO blood-group system was the only one known. Blood grouping on a large scale as a test for compatibility of blood transfusions began during World War I and, at the end of this, as already mentioned, Hirszfeld and Hirszfeld (1919) first showed the importance of the variations of blood-group frequencies in different populations. It was only after this that meaningful work on blood-group frequencies in diseased persons became possible.

The first authors to realize the possible importance of these findings, and to carry out extensive blood grouping of patients, were Buchanan and Higley (1921) who determined the ABO blood groups of 2446 patients suffering from a wide variety of diseases. They concluded that there was no relationship between blood groups and any disease in which sufficient data were available to justify a conclusion.

With hindsight it is possible to realize that the numbers tested for any one disease were much too small to yield statistically significant results, even for diseases where we now know that associations exist.

Once again it was Hirszfeld (1928) who first attempted a comprehensive treatment of the subject, collecting all available previous data, adding some of his own, and discussing theoretical aspects at length. For most diseases the numbers were still too small to show associations, but he was able to demonstrate them between ABO groups and the responses to certain serodiagnostic tests. He also discussed at length his own previous work (Hirszfeld and Zborowski, 1925) on the effects of ABO-heterospecific pregnancy on the survival and health of the foetus.

It was not until the early 1950s that any further substantial progress was made in the study of associations of blood groups with diseases other than haemolytic disease of the newborn.

In 1927 and 1928 Landsteiner and Levine discovered the M, N, and P groups. These were at once shown to behave as Mendelian characters belonging to two independent systems, MN and P. These were very soon adopted as convenient marker systems by human geneticists, and population studies showed significant frequency variations between populations for both systems. However, neither system appeared to give rise to transfusion incompatibilities, or to any other clinical effects, and therefore very few tests were done on patients.

The case was very different for the Rhesus, or Rh, blood groups, discovered by Landsteiner and Wiener in 1940, using as reagents the sera of rabbits and guinea-pigs immunized with rhesus monkey cells. Anti-Rh antibodies were found not to occur normally in human serum but, also in 1940, Wiener and Peters showed that Rh-negative persons could become immunized to Rh-positive human cells and the resulting anti-Rh antibody would give rise to a reaction if the same person were subsequently transfused with Rh-positive cells. In 1941 Levine and his colleagues (Levine *et al.* 1941*a*, *b*, *c*) showed that Rh antibodies are the cause of the long-known condition of erythroblastosis fetalis, or haemolytic disease of the newborn. A Rhesus-negative mother is liable to become immunized by a Rhesus-positive foetus which has inherited the Rh factor from the father. Subsequent Rh-positive babies will then be born suffering from this condition, which formerly was very often fatal.

The theoretical consequences of this process in terms of natural selection were pointed out independently by Wiener (1942) and Haldane (1942) and are discussed later on page 23. Here then was a disease which was invariably (or almost invariably) associated with a particular blood group. It is, in fact, the most important example known of this type of association, but it has already formed the subject of a vast literature of books and papers, and will therefore be discussed only briefly in this book, and then mainly in relation to interactions between the Rh system and other genetic systems.

An enormous increase in the use of blood transfusion occurred during and soon after World War II; the consequent realization of the clinical importance of immunization both by pregnancy and by transfusion, and a growing interest among geneticists in man as a subject of research, led to a search for new blood-group systems and new antigens within the known systems. This field of research, in which the unquestioned world leaders have been, and continue to be, R. R. Race and Ruth Sanger, has proved fertile beyond all expectations, not merely in the discovery of numerous new genetic systems, and hundreds of new antigens, but in its effects on the whole of human genetic research.

Almost every new antigen discovered (and hence the gene responsible for it) has been shown to vary greatly in frequency from one population to another. This in turn has led, in the last 30 years, to a complete transformation of the subject-matter of physical anthropology, with blood groups and other genetically simple characters first supplementing and then largely replacing anthropometry as the main means of tracing the ancestral relations of human populations.

As already mentioned, the possibility of associations between blood groups and diseases has long interested pathologists, as well as some clinicians. However, with a few exceptions, it is only since 1945 that patients have been blood-grouped in sufficient numbers to make useful statistical studies possible and even then, for some years, the rarity and slightness of associations found tended to discourage further research.

The first association to be overwhelmingly proved, and to convince most waverers, was that shown by Aird, Bentall, and Roberts (1953) to exist between group A and carcinoma of the stomach. The same team continued to find new associations, and were soon joined by that led by C. A. Clarke and R. B. McConnell at Liverpool, who brought the ABH-secretor system, as well as the ABO groups themselves, into their very fruitful investigations.

From then on, more and more research teams joined in the effort, which became world-wide, and more and more blood-group systems were examined for associations. The search for associations with groups outside the ABO system has, however, on the whole, been disappointing and, in the Rh system in particular, little has been found beyond the association with haemolytic disease of the newborn.

The growing interest among geneticists in the potentialities of blood factors for the identification of marker genes on the human chromosomes led, however, to extended searches for identifiable gene products in other parts of the blood than the erythrocyte boundary membrane which carries the blood-group antigens. One of the earliest and most fruitful of such inquiries led to the finding by Pauling in 1949 that persons suffering from hereditary sickle-cell anaemia have a haemoglobin which differs in its physical properties from that present in normal adults. The molecular and population genetics of the abnormal haemoglobins has become a major branch of human genetics and will be described more fully later, but the basic situation must be summarized here as it now represents the classical human example of a balanced polymorphism, a search for which in relation to other polymorphisms has been a major stimulus to workers in the whole field of associations between polymorphisms and diseases. The haemoglobin polymorphism, in the present context, refers only to the β-polypeptide chain of the molecule. Homozygotes for Haemoglobin S, or sickle-cell haemoglobin, have virtually only that type of haemoglobin, and mostly die in infancy of sickle-cell anaemia. Homozygotes for the normal Haemoglobin A, who constitute about 99 per cent of all human beings, are highly susceptible to malignant tertian (falciparum) malaria, and show a high childhood mortality from it in endemic areas. However, A/S heterozygotes, with a mixture of the two haemoglobins, have, as was first clearly shown by Allison (1954, 1973), a considerable resistance to falciparum malaria and also are little inconvenienced by their Haemoglobin S, so that they pass on both genes to the next generation, thus maintaining the polymorphism at an equilibrium level which is related to the degree of malarial endemicity.

The invention of the technique of starch-gel electrophoresis by Smithies (1955) was mainly responsible for opening up the large range of plasma proteins to genetic analysis, though numerous other methods have also been used, and investigation of the system of greatest value in population studies, the Gm system of immunoglobulins, still depends upon laborious agglutination inhibition tests.

The success of starch-gel electrophoresis led to its adoption by numerous workers, but especially by Harris, for the genetic investigation of the red-cell enzymes. Here a very wide range of polymorphisms was revealed, and more are discovered almost monthly, so that by now they possibly outnumber all the other known human polymorphisms.

The plasma-protein and red-cell-enzyme polymorphisms have one great advantage in population studies over the conventional blood groups. We still have only a very imperfect idea of the function of the latter, whereas nearly all the enzymes, whether in the plasma or the red cells, and most of the other plasma proteins, have well-defined functions which ought to supply, and in several cases already do supply, clues as to their possible role in resistance or susceptibility to disease.

Thus we find that the weak or inactive variants of plasma-protease inhibitor predispose to pulmonary emphysema and hepatic cirrhosis, and we may expect to find that the variants of the Gc proteins, which carry vitamin D in the plasma, have some relation to disorders of calcium metabolism. Severe gene-determined deficiencies of certain enzymes, notably glucose-6-phosphate dehydrogenase, are pathogenic in various ways. However, we possess so very much more data on disease relationships with the blood groups, especially of the ABO system, than with the variants in any of the other systems, that on an empirical basis far more relationships are at present known with them than with the theoretically more promising plasma proteins and red-cell enzymes. It must be one of our objects in this book to suggest possible functional explanations for the blood-group associations.

Blood-group workers had long been looking for antigens on the leucocytes and platelets, analogous to those of the red cells. Gradually these emerged, and were looked upon at first as immunological curiosities, difficult to work with. A few were long ago shown to be genetically based.

Then, largely through the work of Dausset, of Cepellini, and of Amos, most of them were shown to be present also in other tissues and to be concerned in the compatibility or incompatibility of tissue and organ grafts. This discovery of a major medical function led to intensive work in numerous laboratories. Techniques of testing have been improved, though they are still very difficult. The genetics of the system are analogous to those of the Rh blood-group system, and of the Gm immunoglobulin groups, but appear to be more complex than either. However, workers on the histocompatibility antigens, as they are now known, have benefited from the early disputes which arose in the investigation of the other systems, and have maintained close contact throughout the world, setting up very rapidly an extensive and efficient system of exchange of antigens and antibodies which rivals those laboriously created over several decades for the erythrocyte and immunoglobulin antigens. One valuable by-product of this organization was the discovery of wide frequency variations between different populations, so that the system has become a most important one in anthropological work.

Suddenly, as recently as about 1973, it began to emerge that these antigens, hitherto for all practical purposes the concern solely of transplantation surgeons, were closely related to a considerable number of important diseases. Particular antigens were found to be closely associated with particular diseases—much more closely than are any diseases to the red-cell groups. Most of the diseases in this category had been regarded, with varying degrees of probability, as having an autoimmune origin, but for most of them the aetiology was far from being understood. The present situation, as regards both immunology and genetics, is one of rapid flux, and new associations are being discovered almost every week. Diseases such as rheumatoid arthritis, psoriasis, and multiple sclerosis, to name only a few out of many, have become the focus of a completely new line of investigation. Such diseases, hitherto of obscure aetiology, and for which no cure, and in some cases no prophylaxis and no reliable palliation, were known, are certainly becoming better understood, and we may hope that in some cases improved methods of prophylaxis and treatment, if not of complete cure, will emerge.

Finally, mention must be made of a disease association with a biochemical polymorphism not so far detectable by a blood test—the association between thyroid diseases and the phenylthiocarbamide taster-non-taster polymorphism. This is probably an enzyme polymorphism and there are suggestions of a balanced polymorphism between thyroid function and the amounts of iodine and of thyroid inhibitors present in the diet. A fuller understanding may lead to improved prophylaxis of the diseases concerned.

I hope that this rapid survey of the field, in the form of a variety of hors-d'œuvres, may whet the appetite for the more solid statistical data presented in subsequent chapters, by suggesting that out of these studies may come a better understanding of the relation of man to his environment, better preventive medicine, and better therapeutics where prevention has failed.

2

THE BLOOD GROUPS AND OTHER POLYMORPHIC SYSTEMS

In this chapter a general account will be given of the genetics, biochemistry, and serology of the ABO and other blood-group systems, and other polymorphic systems, which have been involved in searches for associations with diseases. In some cases, however, it has been found convenient to devote a whole chapter to a particular system, usually because associations with diseases form a large part of our total knowledge of the system. Each such system will, however, be mentioned at least briefly in the present chapter, with a reference if necessary to the one where a full account of it will be found.

Most of our knowledge of associations between genetically polymorphic systems and diseases comes from statistical comparisons between the frequencies of the phenotypes of the system found in patients suffering from the disease, and the frequencies found in the general population from which the patients are drawn. For nearly all the polymorphisms covered in the present book, full descriptions of world distribution, and of population genetics, will be found in a previous book by the present authors (Mourant *et al.*, 1976) to which the present book is to some extent a sequel. A comprehensive account of the genetics and other aspects of the blood groups in the restricted sense will be found in the book of Race and Sanger (1975), while the best general account of most of the other systems is that of Giblett (1969) (which also includes the blood groups).

THE ABO BLOOD GROUPS

The phenotypes known as the ABO blood groups are determined by a system of three allelomorphic genes, *A*, *B*, and *O*. Of these, *A* and *B* each gives rise to a characteristic antigenic (and ultimately biochemical) structure, the A or the B antigen, while the *O* gene behaves as an amorph, not giving rise to any antigen peculiar to itself. These antigens are usually sought on the surface of the red cells, but are in fact found widely distributed elsewhere in the body.

Because of the amorph status of the *O* gene, the genotypes *AA* and *AO* are indistinguishable by any routine tests on the cells of the individual, as are the genotypes *BB* and *BO*.

The standard reagents for the A and B antigens are human sera containing the specific antibodies anti-A and anti-B. Each of these causes the agglutination of red cells carrying the corresponding antigen. All normal human sera contain those antibodies which do not react with the individual's own red cells. Thus the serum of an A person contains anti-B, that of a B person, anti-A. The serum of an O person contains both antibodies, and that of an AB person, neither of them. The relations between genotypes, phenotypes, and antibodies are summarized in Table I.

TABLE I. THE ABO BLOOD GROUPS

BLOOD GROUP (PHENOTYPE)	BLOOD-GROUP SUBSTANCES ON RED CELLS	ANTIBODIES PRESENT IN PLASMA (OR SERUM)	GENOTYPE
O	none	anti-A, anti-B	*OO*
A	A	anti-B	*AO* or *AA*
B	B	anti-A	*BO* or *BB*
AB	A and B	none	*AB*

The anti-A and anti-B antibodies in human serum are still often described as 'naturally occurring', but it is now generally accepted that they are the result of immunization in infancy by substances closely related to the A and B antigens, and derived from the environment through the respiratory or alimentary tracts. It may appear at first sight surprising that these antibodies, the formation of which is stimulated by a variety of environmental antigens, should apparently be so precisely tailored to the blood-group antigens of other human beings. It must, however, be remembered that the normal individual is tolerant of (or does not make antibodies to) antigens forming part of his own body (or at any rate parts which are accessible to plasma antibodies). Thus, for example, any antibody produced in response to an A-like antigen derived from the environment will be so constituted as to react as well as possible with A-like antigens but subject to the restriction of not reacting with the individual's own antigens (which may include substances which are more or less A-like, present in all individuals, whether or not they possess the gene-determined and biochemically sharply defined blood-group A antigen). Such an antibody may also react with non-human A-like substances, such as red-cell antigens of other mammals, but this will not show in tests restricted to human red cells and human plasma or serum. Similar considerations apply to B and anti-B.

This aspect of antigen-antibody relations has been discussed at some length, and is further discussed below, as it may be of considerable importance in determining associations of diseases with ABO blood groups.

The sub-groups of A

Considerable numbers of variants of the A antigen are known, most of which are rare; the B antigen is less variable but several rare variants are known. The most important distinction is between A_1, the commonest antigen, and A_2 which has a frequency of several per cent in most European, African, and West Asiatic populations. Though the distinction has been known for nearly 50 years, its basic nature is still not completely understood, but most of the facts are covered by the following conventional account. Thomsen *et al.* (1930) observed that there were two varieties of the A antigen, A_1 and A_2, allowing the blood groups A and AB to be classified respectively as A_1 and A_2, and as A_1B and A_2B. Both types of antigen react with the ordinary antibody anti-A, but only A_1

reacts with anti-A_1, while A_2 fails to do so. Reaction of antigens is shown, as usual, by agglutination. Anti-A_1 is present in the serum of most B persons together with ordinary anti-A. The latter antibody can be absorbed from a serum containing it, by means of A_2 cells, leaving only anti-A_1 behind, so that the serum becomes a specific anti-A_1 reagent. An excellent anti-A_1 reagent can also be prepared by extracting *Dolichos biflorus* seeds with physiological saline.

The A_1 and A_2 antigens are produced by corresponding allelomorphic genes, so that what we have called the *A* gene is really of two possible kinds, A_1 and A_2. In the genotype A_1A_2 the A_1 gene causes the production of A_1 antigen, and thus the genotypes A_1A_2, A_1O, and A_1A_1 are indistinguishable by methods at present available, since all react both with anti-A and anti-A_1.

As group A_2 is intermediate in several of its properties between A_1 and O, it would be of great interest to know whether this applies to its associations with disease, but unfortunately very few investigators of associations have determined the sub-groups of A in their patients.

THE 'BOMBAY' BLOOD GROUP AND THE H ANTIGEN

The antigen now known as H is present on the red cells of nearly all human bloods, but is present in greatest amount on those of group O. It was long thought to be a product of the *O* gene, but its nature became much clearer as a result of the discovery of the 'Bombay' blood group which lacks this factor (Bhende *et al.*, 1952), and is now known to characterize persons who are homozygous for the *h* gene, the amorph allele of the *H* gene which confers the H antigen on red cells. The *hh* genotype is very rare in all populations, though least so in Indians, especially those living in and around Bombay. The main importance of this system lies in the fact that the H antigen is the substrate upon which the *A* and *B* genes act to produce the A and B antigens. The 'Bombay' type is not known to have any disease associations except for the fact that persons of this type have a strong anti-H antibody which causes difficulties if they need blood transfusion.

THE ABH SECRETOR SYSTEM

It was first shown by Lehrs (1930) and by Putkonen (1930) that some persons do and others do not secrete into their saliva antigens corresponding to their ABO blood group. Schiff and Sasaki (1932) found that the ability to secrete behaved as a simple Mendelian factor, dominant to non-secretion. Group A, B, and AB persons who are secretors secrete the antigens corresponding to their blood groups. Group O persons who are secretors secrete the H substance, as do all other secretors to a somewhat less extent.

The secretor gene is known as *Se*, to distinguish it from *S* of the *MNSs* series. The amorph or non-secretor allele is known as *se*. Bombay-group or *hh* persons have always been found to be non-secretors even if they possess an *Se* gene, apparently since they cannot elaborate, let alone secrete, the H antigen or the A and B antigens which are derived from it.

Another pair of allelic genes that are involved in secretion are the *Y* and *y* of Weiner *et al.* (1957). The action of the *Y* gene is necessary for the normal elaboration of the A antigen on red cells. The extremely rare *yy* persons, if they possess an *Se* gene and an *A* gene, secrete the A antigen normally in their saliva but fail to make it on their red cells. The *Y* gene is not, however, required for the normal production of the H and B red-cell antigens. The *Yy* system is not known to be involved in any disease association, but, like many of these associations, it shows a discrimination between group A on the one hand, and groups B and O on the other. It is for this reason that it is mentioned here.

It was long ago discovered that genetical secretors secrete their blood-group antigens not only in their saliva but in numerous other body fluids, especially those of the gastro-intestinal tract. Since most of the early findings of ABO associations were with diseases of the stomach and intestines, it was realized that the secretor character might also be involved; secretor tests were therefore done and gave some very striking results.

In interpreting disease associations with these two systems it is of value to know the distribution of the ABO antigens in tissue and fluids other than blood, and how far these are dependent upon the secretor status of the individual. A monograph by Hartmann (1931) deals comprehensively with this subject and will be quoted in relation to individual associations. Though originally published so long ago it has not been superseded, and has fortunately been reprinted in 1970 and made widely available.

THE LEWIS SYSTEM OF ANTIGENS

Because of its close serological and biochemical association with the ABO blood groups and with secretion, the Lewis system (Mourant, 1946) must be mentioned here, though it has not been shown conclusively to have any disease associations.

The Lewis antigens are essentially water-soluble antigens present in the saliva and other secretions, and in small quantities in the blood plasma, whence they are taken up by the red cells. They are the products of a pair of allelic genes hitherto known as *Le* and *le*. This notation wrongly implies that, as was believed for many years, *le* is an amorph. This is now known not to be the case, but the notation will be retained here provisionally, so as to avoid burdening the literature with what might prove to be an unacceptable new symbol. The primary product of the *Le* gene is the Le^a antigen, but in the presence of the secretor *Se* gene it is converted into the Le^b antigen. The primary product of the *le* gene is the Le^c antigen (Gunson and Latham, 1972) while the joint product with the *Se* gene is Le^d (Potapov, 1970). Because of the many interconnections between the systems just mentioned, and the weakness of most of the available reagents, the establishment of the Lewis genotype of an individual is a matter of some technical difficulty, so that many of the published data on frequencies in populations must be accepted with some reserve. It is not at all unlikely that the Lewis system does have disease associations but, if so, it will be difficult to establish them conclusively.

The most reliable way to determine the Lewis type of an individual is by means of tests on the saliva, but most published results concern the Le^a reactions of red cells, which are positive in persons who have at least one *Le* gene but are homozygous (*se se*) non-secretors of the ABH antigens. A full and up-to-date account of the serology and genetics of the Lewis system is given by Race and Sanger (1975).

The nature of the antigens

The ABO antigens of the red cells are glycolipids; they are insoluble in water but soluble in alcohol. Most of the work on the biochemistry of the ABO groups has been done on the soluble antigens of saliva and certain other body fluids, which contain glycoproteins in which the antigenic polysaccharide portion is identical chemically and antigenically with that found on the red cell. The polysaccharide chains are, of course, not the immediate gene products. The latter, like all other gene products, are proteins—in this case glycotransferases which catalyse the building up of the antigen groupings.

The A and B antigens are in fact polysaccharide chains of some complexity, and it is only in the last stage of their synthesis that the A or B specificity is conferred.

The initial common substrate is closely related antigenically and biochemically to the capsular polysaccharide of Pneumococcus, Type XIV. Upon this the *H* gene, if present, confers H antigenicity. Two further stages, which interact at the phenotypic level, confer the properties of secretion or non-secretion of the blood-group antigen into the saliva and other fluids, and the Lewis group specificity. Finally, the *A* or *B* gene, if present, converts much of the H substance into A or B substance.

It would be beyond the scope of this book to enter more deeply into this complex situation, and those who wish to pursue the matter further should consult the work of Race and Sanger (1975) and the full bibliography which they give, largely to the work of Morgan and Watkins who have so fully interpreted and confirmed biochemically the work of the blood-group serologists and geneticists.

THE ALKALINE PHOSPHATASES OF THE PLASMA

As will be seen repeatedly in later chapters, the ABO and secretor systems appear to interact in various ways in conferring susceptibility or resistance to particular diseases. Part of this interaction, especially in so far as it affects the diseases of the alimentary tract, may be related to the behaviour of the alkaline phosphatases. A number of such enzymes are found in the human body, each presumably the product of a different gene. Apart, however, from the transient alkaline phosphatases of the foetal part of the placenta, little is known of any possible genetical polymorphism of these enzymes.

It was, however, found by Arfors *et al.* (1963) that when a specimen of human plasma is submitted to electrophoresis, one or two bands giving the reactions of an alkaline phosphatase may be found on the electrophoretogram. One of these is constant in position and intensity, and apparently consists of two overlapping bands due to enzymes from bone and liver. A second band is present only inconstantly, and when present may vary in intensity. It is produced by an enzyme of intestinal origin. The whole pattern was at first ascribed to a single genetic polymorphism, but it was soon shown (Beckman, 1968) that the presence or absence of the intestinal band depends almost entirely on the ABO group and secretor status of the individual. Transfer of the enzyme from the intestine to the plasma is promoted by the secretor factor and suppressed by the A antigen, whether as group A or AB. Beckman (1968) discusses the physiology of the process at some length and suggests that the differential secretion of the enzyme into the plasma may explain the complex relations between the ABO groups, the secretor types, and the incidence of certain gastro-intestinal diseases, especially peptic ulcer (see pp. 29–30).

THE MNSs BLOOD-GROUP SYSTEM

The MN blood groups, discovered by Landsteiner and Levine (1927*a*, *b*) depend upon a pair of allelomorphic genes which behave in nearly all respects as though they determined the antigens M and N respectively. It has, however, recently been shown that the N antigen is a precursor substance, and that the so-called *N* gene is an amorph which leaves the N antigen unchanged, while the *M* gene in the heterozygote converts part of the N antigen into M, and in the homozygote converts nearly but not quite the whole of it.

The S and s antigens (Walsh and Montgomery, 1947; Sanger and Race, 1947; Levine, 1951) are the products of a pair of allelic genes very closely linked to those for M and N. A third allele, which determines the absence of both S and s, and is known as S^u, is not uncommon in Negroids.

The system is one of considerable complexity, involving numerous variants of M and N, and a variety of antigens determined by other closely linked genes. While the system is thus of considerable genetical and anthropological interest, it seldom gives rise to haemolytic disease of the newborn, or to transfusion reactions, and shows few disease associations, so that there is no need to consider its complications in detail.

THE P BLOOD-GROUP SYSTEM

The P blood groups were discovered by Landsteiner and Levine (1927*b*) in the course of the same investigations that defined the MN groups. It was at first thought that only one antigen, P, was involved, determined by a gene *P*, the allele *p* being an amorph, the two genes having each a frequency of about 50 per cent in European populations. Further investigation has disclosed a system of considerable complexity, only one feature of which will be described here. The antigen Tj^a found by Levine *et al.* (1951) was at first regarded as the product of a gene present in nearly all human beings, the extremely rare allele being an amorph, with the homozygotes usually having a strong anti-Tj^a antibody. Sanger (1955) then showed that Tj^a was part of the P system, with three alleles, P_1 (formerly *P*), P_2 (formerly *p*), and the new *p* (formerly regarded as the amorph allele of Tj^a). These relationships are similar to those existing between A_1, A_2, and *O* of the ABO system. P_2 bloods sometimes show anti-P_1 in the plasma, usually with a very low titre, but the rare p bloods always have a high titre of anti-P+anti-P_1. The P_1 antigen is present in hydatid cyst fluid (Cameron and Staveley, 1957) and in a considerable variety of worms, both parasitic and free living. It is likely that the anti-P_1, not infrequently found in the plasma of P_2 individuals and in that of several species of mammals, is a response to worm infestation, but no work appears to have been done on possible associations between the P groups and such infestation.

Women of genotype *pp*, who always have anti-P+anti-P_1 in their plasma, are particularly subject to abortion, apparently resulting from the action of the antibody upon the almost invariably P-positive foetus.

Paroxysmal cold haemoglobinuria is due to the presence in the patient's plasma of a cold-reacting auto-antibody. It was shown by Levine *et al.* (1963) that this usually has anti-P specificity.

THE RHESUS BLOOD GROUPS

From a clinical point of view the Rhesus or Rh system is by far the most important of the blood-group systems other than

ABO. Rh incompatibility is the main cause of haemolytic disease of the newborn, and a major cause of transfusion reactions. As, however, haemolytic disease of the newborn is not being considered in detail in this book, and as the other disease associations of the system are few and relatively unimportant, only a brief account of the system will be given here. The principal antigen of the system, Rh_o or D, was discovered by Landsteiner and Wiener (1940). Subsequently, very numerous other associated antigens were discovered, and considerable controversy arose both as to notation and as to the theoretical interpretation of the uncontroversial observations of geneticists. This is not the place to discuss the controversy and for the purpose of this book the CDE notation of Fisher (Race, 1944) will be used, and its genetical implications of closely linked genes will be assumed. Only the main features of this very complex system will be described. On this basis the principal antigen of the system is known as D, determined by a gene *D*, the allele *d* of which behaves as an amorph. Very closely linked to the *Dd* locus are two other loci each characterized by a pair of major alleles, *Cc* and *Ee* respectively. Each of these four genes gives rise to a correspondingly named antigen.

There are thus eight possible chromosomic combinations of genes, all of which are known to exist, but of which *CDe*, *cDE*, *cDe*, and *cde* are the commonest.

Incompatibility with respect to the D antigen is, as already mentioned, the main cause of haemolytic disease of the newborn, but Cc and Ee incompatibilities are rare causes, as they are also of transfusion reactions. Unlike the antibodies of the ABO system, each of which is universally present in persons lacking the corresponding antigen, antibodies to the Rh antigens are virtually never found except as a result of immunization by pregnancy or transfusion, and reactions appear only at a second exposure to the antigen. This applies also to all the other blood-group systems except the ABO. Very few searches have been made for any other kinds of disease associations of the Rh groups, and nearly all of these are confined to a comparison of the D-positive and D-negative types.

THE DUFFY BLOOD-GROUP SYSTEM

Almost the only other blood-group system which appears to bear any important relation to disease incidence, other than haemolytic disease of the newborn, is the Duffy system. However, the indirect way (p. 21) in which this probable association was discovered suggests that similar unexpected relations may in the future be discovered with other systems. The antigen known as Fy^a was discovered by Cutbush *et al.* (1950) and the Fy^b antigen, the product of its allelic gene, by Ikin *et al.* (1951). The allelic genes Fy^a and Fy^b account for nearly all the phenotypes found in European populations, but it was observed by Sanger *et al.* (1955) that a high proportion of American Negroes are of the phenotype Fy(a− b−). An inspection of the latest tables of Mourant *et al.* (1976) will show that, except in the South African Republic, over 95 per cent of African Negroes are of this type, which represents the homozygote of a third allelic gene, at first regarded as an amorph and so named *Fy*. It is now known that two distinct genes have in the past been confused under this term. One, Fy^x, with a frequency of approximately 1·6 per cent in Europeans, gives a product which is negative with anti-Fy^a but which reacts feebly with anti-Fy^b (Chown *et al.*, 1972). The other, almost universal in Africans, gives a product which completely fails to react with either of these antibodies, but is not a true amorph, for Behzad *et al.* (1973) have shown its product to react specifically with an antibody which they call anti-Fy_4; the gene should presumably be called Fy^4. Miller *et al.* (1975) have, as described on page 21, shown that the homozygote of this type is probably specifically resistant to *vivax* malaria, to which Africans have long been known to be resistant.

THE PLASMA PROTEINS

The blood plasma contains in solution a great variety of proteins, many of which show genetical polymorphism. Unlike the blood groups, these proteins mostly have known functions, for instance as enzymes, or as carriers of simple substances like metals and vitamins. The genetical variants of a particular protein often, and perhaps nearly always, differ quantitatively in their functional activity, thus allowing the possibility of natural selection, which may be the cause of the observed variability of gene frequencies between populations. Only in a few cases have the frequencies of the variants of a particular protein been ascertained in patients suffering from specified diseases.

As in the case of the blood groups, only those systems will be described where possible associations of the polymorphisms have been investigated directly, or where indirect evidence suggests that such associations may exist.

The haptoglobins

The haptoglobins are glycoproteins which combine with any dissolved haemoglobin entering the plasma as a result of the lysis of red cells. This prevents the haemoglobin from being excreted by the kidney, but the share of the haptoglobins in conserving the body's supply of iron is not fully understood. The literature of the biochemistry and genetics of the haptoglobins is extensive and complicated (see Giblett, 1969).

Smithies *et al.* (1962) showed that the complex patterns found on starch-gel electrophoresis could be attributed to three phenotypes, known as Hp 1–1, Hp 2–1, and Hp 2–2, which behaved genetically as though the proteins concerned were the products of two allelomorphic genes, Hp^1 and Hp^2; of the gene products, Hp^1 is more efficient than Hp^2 in removing free haemoglobin from circulating blood. In many populations, but especially among Africans, an absence or a very low level of haptoglobin is found in some individuals. This is in part the result of depletion of haptoglobin through haemolytic anaemia, but a genetical factor is also involved, apparently a variant of the Hp^2 gene, recognizable, however, only in the heterozygote known as Hp 2–1 M. Despite much investigation the relation between genetics and physiology in this system is by no means fully understood. As discussed on page 28, the *Hp* and *ABO* genes appear to interact ante-natally through some form of selection, to affect the frequencies of various combinations of ABO and Hp phenotypes, as shown by numerous family studies.

The transferrins

The transferrins, or siderophilins, are proteins containing 5·5 per cent of carbohydrate, which combine with inorganic iron in the plasma and transfer it to the bone-marrow and other storage organs.

As shown by starch-gel electrophoresis, there is one common gene Tf^C and large numbers of variants, all of which are rare, so that even if they showed disease associations or other selective effects, this would be difficult to prove because of their rarity. The system is, however, mentioned here because of the occurrence in cattle of a well-defined system of balanced polymorphism of the transferrins (Ashton, 1965), and it is therefore possible that such a situation could emerge in a human population having a high frequency of one of the variants.

The Gc groups

The Gc (or group specific component) groups of the plasma are the expression of genetically controlled variants of one of the α-globulins. Their importance, other than as genetical markers, has recently been realized as a result of the discovery by Schanfield *et al.* (1975) that the Gc proteins are the vitamin D carriers of the plasma. They are the products of a system of allelic genes, of which two, Gc^1 and Gc^2, are relatively common. A considerable number of others are known, all of which are everywhere rare, apart from Gc^{Ab} found in the indigenous populations of Australia and New Guinea. As shown by Mourant *et al.* (1976) Gc^1 has in general, though with several exceptions, a high frequency in sunny climates and Gc^2 a relatively high one in dull ones, suggesting that the Gc types are affected by natural selection related to the availability of vitamin D. It is therefore desirable that Gc distribution should be investigated in patients with rickets, which results from vitamin D deficiency, as well as, if possible, in the very rare condition of hyper-vitaminosis-D.

Wendt *et al.* (1968) and Cleve (1973) have summarized work on associations of diseases with Gc types. There are indications that Gc 1-1 may be associated with psoriasis (Jörgensen and Hopfer, 1967) and less probably with carcinoma of the uterus, neurodermatitis, diabetes mellitus, and rheumatoid arthritis. Kitchin *et al.* (1972) suggest an association of the Gc^{Ab} variant with kuru in New Guinea.

The protease inhibitors

Human plasma contains protease inhibitors both in the α_1-globulin and the α_2-globulin fractions. Only the α_1 variety has been found to exhibit electrophoretic polymorphism, and it is the main trypsin inhibitor present in plasma and serum. Only this variety will be further considered here. The history of investigations into its genetics has been summarized by Giblett (1969).

An association between a deficiency of α_1 trypsin inhibitor and pulmonary disease was described by Laurell and Eriksson (1963) and it was only subsequently that this deficiency was found to be hereditary and to form only part of a complex polymorphism at a chromosome locus which has been called *Pi*. At least twenty alleles are now known but all of them but one, Pi^M, are rare in nearly all populations. The product of the gene Pi^S has a somewhat reduced activity, but two alleles, Pi^Z and the very rare Pi^- (or Pi^O) are responsible, in the homozygous state, for most of the severe deficiencies causing pulmonary disease. The Pi^Z gene product has a small but measurable protease inhibitor activity, about 16 per cent of that of Pi^M (Cook, 1975), and the protein itself gives the normal precipitin reaction of the α_1 protease inhibitors. The plasma of Pi^- homozygotes gives no detectable protease inhibitor activity and no precipitin reaction, so that it may represent a gene deletion. The disease associations of the system are further considered on pages 42-3.

The variants of pseudocholinesterase

Red cells contain a cholinesterase which breaks down the acetylcholine produced at nerve endings, especially those controlling voluntary muscles: it thus prevents muscles from going into permanent spasm. Another cholinesterase, now usually called pseudocholinesterase, is present in the plasma; its normal function is uncertain, but the existence of genetically determined variations in its activity came to light as a result of using another acylated choline compound, succinyl choline, as a muscle relaxant in surgical anaesthesia. This substance blocks the action of acetylcholine on voluntary muscles and so produces relaxation. Its effect is usually moderated by, and after some minutes most of it is broken down by, the action of pseudocholinesterase, so that the tone of muscles, including those of respiration, returns to normal. From time to time, however, individuals have been found who remain relaxed and without spontaneous respiration for prolonged periods. This has been found to be due to a deficiency of plasmatic pseudocholinesterase activity. In 1953 Forbat *et al.* showed the condition to be familial. These and other workers further investigated the condition and showed the existence of a series of alleles, several, giving weak enzyme activity, being distinguishable from one another by their interaction with a variety of inhibitors including fluorides.

The common gene giving rise to a normal enzyme is known as E_1^u. The most frequently encountered gene with a product of reduced activity is E_1^a, with a frequency of 1 to 2 per cent in European populations. The gene producing a relatively inactive but fluoride-resistant enzyme is E_1^f, the frequency of which, where ascertained, is usually about 0·5 per cent in Europe. However, in one Greek sample it is as high as 1·61 per cent, and in one from Iceland it is 1·17 per cent with no E_1^a recorded. The last figure is not only the second highest recorded for E_1^f, but the Icelanders are the only population to have E_1^f in the absence of, or with a greater frequency than, E_1^a. It seems possible that this relatively high frequency of E_1^f is due to natural selection in the Icelandic environment, since the volcanic gases of the island contain large amounts of hydrogen fluoride. This has, throughout the ages, led to vast numbers of deaths of sheep from fluoride poisoning, and sometimes to very high human mortality, usually attributed to starvation from the deaths of the animals, but perhaps in part due directly to fluorides.

It would be of interest not only to look for this gene in other fluoride-rich environments but, since fluoride is a frequent enzyme inhibitor, to look also for a possible full strength but fluoride-resistant pseudocholinesterase variant, and for fluoride-resistant variants of other enzymes, in such environments. Such variants, if they exist, are likely to have been missed in the past because no one has looked for them.

The placental alkaline phosphatases

The alkaline phosphatases normally present in plasma have been described on page 6, where their relation to the ABO blood group and secretor systems is discussed. However, in pregnant and recently delivered women, there is found, in addition to the one or two bands normally seen on electrophoresis, a third band or group of bands, nearer the anode than the liver band. This is due to alkaline phosphatases elaborated in the placenta, and determinations are usually performed on placental extracts. It has become clear, especially from twin studies (Arfors *et al.*, 1963; Shreffler, 1965; Robson and Harris, 1967) that each electrophoretic type corresponds to the genotype of the foetus. The phenotypes observed were determined by three common and six rare alleles at an autosomal locus. Two more rare alleles have since been discovered. Besides some minor bands which are not fully explained, the electrophoretic pattern consists of a single band in homozygotes, and of three bands in heterozygotes. The middle band is usually of about twice the intensity of the outer ones, as would be expected if two monomers were involved, combining at random to give the observed dimers, a type of pattern often seen on electrophoresis of genetically determined blood proteins. However, in some of the heterozygotes the outer bands differ from one another in strength, suggesting that some of the primary gene products are either enzymatically less active, less stable, or produced in smaller amounts, than others. The principal alleles are known as Pl^{s_1}; Pl^{f_1} and Pl^{i_1}; giving rise to the gene products S_1, F_1, and I_1 respectively. The possible association of this system with haemolytic disease of the newborn is discussed on page 28.

THE RED-CELL ENZYMES

Inside the boundary membrane of the red cell is a solution, possibly with an elaborate microscopic structure, containing haemoglobin and a variety of other substances, especially enzymes. Haemoglobin and a great many of the enzymes show genetical polymorphism. The enzymes have, of course, precisely known functions and in some cases the products of allelic genes differ quantitatively in functional activity. For each of a considerable number of the enzymes there is at least one allele conferring low or absent activity, and homozygotes for such alleles may suffer from distinct congenital diseases which are not, as such, the subject of this book. Some cases will, however, be discussed where it is a matter of opinion, and perhaps of definition, whether a particular disease is to be regarded as a direct consequence of the genotype or merely associated with it.

Glucose-6-phosphate dehydrogenase

It has long been known that some persons in many Mediterranean countries suffer from favism, a haemolytic anaemia precipitated by consumption of the common horse bean or broad bean, *Vicia faba*. During World War II it was found that some American Negro soldiers suffered from haemolysis when treated with certain antimalarial drugs derived from quinoline, such as primaquine. Investigations by numerous workers finally traced both these conditions, and a number of others such as jaundice among new-born Chinese infants in Singapore, to a deficiency in the red cells, of the enzyme, glucose-6-phosphate dehydrogenase (G6PD). The complicated history of research on the genetics of this enzyme has been reviewed by many authors including Giblett (1969) who gives full references to previous work.

The enzyme (present also in other tissues besides red cells) is an essential catalyst in one of the body's methods of oxidizing glucose, known as the pentose phosphate pathway, since it involves a breakdown from the 6-carbon molecule of glucose to a 5-carbon chain. One of the effects of a deficiency of the enzyme is a tendency of the red cells to haemolyse, especially, as indicated above, in the presence of certain drugs and other substances.

A very large number of variants of G6PD are now known but, in addition to the normal type, only three variants are commonly recognized as being of any importance in population studies. The common type in all populations is known as B+, the B referring to its rate of migration on electrophoresis and the + to its normal enzymic activity. The common abnormal type in the Mediterranean area is B−, migrating at the same speed as the normal but with an activity between 0 and 7 per cent of normal. It is also labile on heating. It is, of course, possible to determine the speed of migration by the standard electrophoretic method only if at least a trace of enzyme activity is present.

In African populations two abnormal types are known, A+ which has normal activity but which migrates faster than the normal, and A− which migrates at the same speed as A+ but has only 8 to 20 per cent of normal activity.

The variants of G6PD are determined by a series of allelomorphic genes on the X chromosome. Thus a male with only one X chromosome can have only one type of enzyme, but a female, having a pair of X chromosomes, can be heterozygous and have genes for two different alleles.

Tests are of three main kinds, screening tests for the presence of enzyme deficiency, precise quantitative tests to measure the degree of deficiency, mainly of use in identifying rare variants, and tests by starch gel electrophoresis, which, provided that blood specimens are fresh so that all the variants retain some enzyme activity, will, in males, and to a large extent also in females, show both the relative electric charge and the activity of any variants present.

Glucose-6-phosphate dehydrogenase deficiency, especially that of the Mediterranean B− type, can, particularly through favism, lead to serious illness with an appreciable mortality. Disease of this kind may be regarded as a simple hereditary disease, and, as such, outside the scope of this book, but variants, both deficient and of normal activity, affect susceptibility to malaria, and this aspect of them is further discussed on page 20.

The acid phosphatases

The acid phosphatase of red cells was first shown to be genetically polymorphic by Hopkinson *et al.* (1963), by means of starch-gel electrophoresis and appropriate staining. The precise function of this enzyme in the red cell is unknown.

Three principal alleles P^a, P^b, and P^c are found in many populations, and a fourth, P^r, is not uncommon in some African peoples, especially the Khoisan. The probable interaction of the acid phosphatases with other genetically determined characters in determining susceptibility to malaria is described on pages 20–1.

THE HAEMOGLOBINS

The study of haemoglobin and its variants has become a major branch of human biochemistry and genetics, and has been of very great importance in population genetics and anthropology. No attempt can be made here to recapitulate the very large amount of information available, and only a brief summary can be given of certain selected aspects of the subject. The general scientific reader is referred to the work of Lehmann and Huntsman (1974) which gives a comprehensive bibliography, while for details of the distribution of the variants in different populations reference should be made to the work of Livingstone (1967). The account given below of the haemoglobins and thalassaemias is a somewhat condensed version of that given in the authors' previous book (Mourant *et al.*, 1976).

The haemoglobin molecule consists of four polypeptide chains, two identical α chains, and two identical β chains, each chain having attached to it one heme group, consisting of an iron atom surrounded by a porphyrin ring which itself contains four pyrrole rings. It is the iron which combines reversibly with oxygen to give haemoglobin its oxygen-carrying power, but the surrounding chains of porphyrin and protein determine the precise conditions under which the iron takes up and gives off oxygen.

The amino-acid sequences in the α and β chains are controlled by genes at separate loci which are not detectably linked, but families yielding potential linkage data are inevitably very rare. The great majority of people everywhere have one type of haemoglobin, normal adult haemoglobin, or Haemoglobin A. About 100 abnormal types are known, of which the majority have abnormal β chains. Most of the abnormal types are extremely rare, and only four of them, Haemoglobins C, D, E, and S, have frequencies which are sufficiently high to be of interest in population studies. These are all the results of substitutions in the β chain of normal adult haemoglobin.

Many substitutions probably occur which do not alter the net electric charge of the whole molecule, but these cannot in general be detected except by very elaborate chemical analysis. Thus the known variants are those in which the net electric charge of the whole molecule differs from that of the normal type, so that they are distinguishable from the latter by the speed with which they move in an electric field. Thus, as with most other classes of blood proteins which show polymorphism, the initial screening for abnormal haemoglobins is carried out by electrophoresis of a solution of the protein; in the case of the haemoglobins such electrophoresis is more simply carried out than for most other proteins. All that is needed for support of the solution is a strip of filter paper, and the colour of the haemoglobin obviates the need for special staining. Once the presence of an abnormal type is established, well-established methods are available for determining its precise type and ultimately, if it is a previously unknown variety, for ascertaining its complete chemical constitution.

Haemoglobin S

Of the abnormal haemoglobins, Haemoglobin S or sickle-cell haemoglobin was the first to be discovered, in 1949 by Pauling *et al.* (1949), who demonstrated that an abnormal haemoglobin was present in the blood of persons showing the sickling phenomenon.

Persons who are homozygous for the Haemoglobin S gene have all their normal adult haemoglobin replaced by the abnormal type. This haemoglobin in the deoxygenated or reduced state has a very low solubility in the internal fluid of the red cell, and is therefore precipitated in the form of angular crystals (strictly, liquid crystals or tactoids) which distort the cells into an angular or sickle shape in which they become unduly susceptible to mechanical damage and destruction. Heterozygotes, with one gene for Haemoglobin S and one for Haemoglobin A, have both types, though more A than S. Each individual molecule detectable by electrophoresis is, however, either A or S; there are no stable molecules with two different types of β chain in them. The mixture of the two haemoglobins also tends to crystallize when in the reduced state, but requires a more complete degree of reduction in order to do so.

Haemoglobin S has been referred to as a variant of normal *adult* haemoglobin. This is because ante-natally, and up to the age of about 6 months, normal human beings have a mixture of two haemoglobins, foetal and adult. The foetal like the adult type has four polypeptide chains to the molecule, but while two are of type α, two are of a type known as γ. The γ polypeptide chain is controlled by a gene at a different locus from that controlling the β chain, and thus is unaffected by the abnormal *S* gene. In normal persons the foetal type is almost completely replaced by the adult type by the age of 6 months. However, in Haemoglobin S homozygotes the foetal type tends to persist in moderate amounts into adult life, partially taking the place of the abnormal adult type.

Despite the persistence of foetal haemoglobin, nearly all Haemoglobin S homozygotes die in infancy of the disease known as sickle-cell anaemia. In advanced communities, and with medical supervision, many are now surviving into adult life and even having children, but the conditions which determine their survival are not fully understood.

Heterozygotes, on the other hand, suffer practically no disabilities under normal environmental conditions, though they react unfavourably to anoxia, as in unpressurized high-flying aircraft, and are somewhat more liable than 'normal' persons to haematuria. However, the sickle-cell phenomenon is easily demonstrated in samples of their blood.

Thus, in a population which has the gene for Haemoglobin S, large numbers of genes of this kind are selectively destroyed in each generation by sickle-cell anaemia, yet the gene persists at high-frequency levels in many such populations. Realization of these facts led to a variety of suggestions as to the genetic mechanism at work. One was that in these populations there was a high frequency of mutation from the β-chain gene for Haemoglobin A to that for S, but this would require a mutation rate many orders of magnitude higher than any other known. The main alternative hypothesis was that the heterozygotes enjoyed some selective advantage over 'normal' persons, perhaps as a result of increased resistance to some disease.

This was the situation when, in 1954, the association of Haemoglobin S with resistance to malaria was discovered, as described in the Introduction and more fully on page 20.

The thalassaemias

The thalassaemias are pathological conditions, but they are due to abnormal single genes, and they are sufficiently frequent in some populations to have considerable significance in population studies. There are two main types of thalassaemia, α-thalassaemia and β-thalassaemia, due respectively to genes which suppress the production of α and of β chains of haemoglobin.

To enable some of their manifestations to be understood, it is necessary to mention yet another type of haemoglobin, present in small amounts in the red cells of normal adults. This is Haemoglobin A_2, with a constitution $\alpha_2\delta_2$. The molecule thus contains two normal α polypeptide chains and two δ chains which are closely similar to, but not identical with, β chains, and are controlled by separate genes. Thus when there is interference with the synthesis of β chains that of δ chains is unaffected, and Haemoglobin A_2 is present in relatively increased amount. However, anything which suppresses the production of α chains will limit the production both of Haemoglobin A and of Haemoglobin A_2. The relative amount of Haemoglobin A_2, as seen on electrophoresis, is thus an important criterion, not only in detecting β-thalassaemia in population screening tests, but also, if thalassaemia is known to be present, in distinguishing one type from the other. The production of foetal haemoglobin, also, is normal or sometimes greatly increased in β-thalassaemia, but is reduced in α-thalassaemia. In both the main varieties of thalassaemia the abnormal gene appears to interfere with the transcription, into an amino-acid sequence, of a gene with normal DNA constitution, coding for an α or a β chain respectively.

β-thalassaemia has been much more fully studied than the

α variety, and is better understood, though it is only in recent years that the distinction between the two varieties (each with subtypes) has become clear.

Heterozygotes for β-thallassaemia (possessing one normal gene for the critical transcription stage and one abnormal one) suffer from a mild anaemia, while homozygotes have a severe anaemia and few of them, without intensive medical care, survive childhood. Death does not take place anything like as early as with sickle-cell anaemia, but the formal genetical situation is almost the same in the two diseases. The population genetics of thalassaemia (but not the molecular genetics) has been understood for a longer period than that of the abnormal haemoglobins, and in the 1940s the problem was already appreciated of accounting for the presence, at very high frequencies in some populations, of a gene which was almost totally lethal in the homozygous state; once again it was the association with malaria that provided the probable solution, as described on pages 19–20.

THE ABILITY TO TASTE PHENYLTHIOCARBAMIDE

In 1931 Fox observed that to some individuals the simple chemical compound, phenylthiocarbamide (PTC), has an intensely bitter taste, while to others it is tasteless. Being a chemist he also showed that a number of other closely related compounds were tasted by the PTC tasters but not by the non-tasters. The ability to taste these substances was shown by Blakeslee and Salmon (1931) and by Snyder (1932) to behave as a Mendelian dominant character.

Harris and Kalmus (1950) showed that the distinction was by no means an absolute one, and that reliable results could be obtained only by the use of solutions of known concentration. They devised a method for ascertaining the lowest concentration which could be tasted by each person. They prepared a saturated solution of PTC in distilled water, and from this a series of twofold dilutions. Starting with the weakest solution, the various dilutions are successively presented to the subject until he claims to be able to taste one. Two glasses of this dilution and two of distilled water are then presented, and he is asked to say which are which. If he answers correctly the dilution is taken to mark his threshold, but if he gives the wrong answer the experiment is repeated with the next stronger solution, and so on.

Nearly every population shows a bimodal distribution of thresholds with a clear-cut intermediate dilution level at which few or no thresholds fall. Those who can taste solutions more dilute than this critical value are classed as tasters, and those whose thresholds fall at higher concentrations, as non-tasters.

The recognition that the substances which define the taster polymorphism are thyroid inhibitors, and that the polymorphism is associated with differences in susceptibility to thyroid diseases, is described on pages 39–41.

EAR-WAX TYPES

Matsunaga (1962) showed that the consistency of ear-wax is under genetical control. Cerumen (ear-wax) may be wet (sticky) or dry (hard); the types are controlled by a pair of allelic genes, that for the wet type expressing itself dominantly in relation to that for the dry. Petrakis *et al.* (1971) summing up his own observations and those of others on the distribution of the alleles, showed that there are wide variations in gene frequencies throughout the world, the dry allele being preponderant in the Mongoloid peoples; in Caucasoids the wet allele usually predominates, and in Negroids the dry allele is almost totally absent. Since the cerumen glands of the ear and the mammary glands are both derived from the apocrine type of sweat glands, attempts have been made, as described on page 14, to show an association between carcinoma of the breast and wax type.

OTHER POLYMORPHISMS

The genetic system controlling inducibility of aryl hydrocarbon hydroxylase, and its probable relation to lung cancer, are described in Chapter 4.

The histocompatibility antigens, which are present on lymphocytes and many kinds of tissue cells, are the products of genes at a complex set of closely linked loci on chromosome 6. Their genetics, and their disease associations, are discussed in Chapter 14. Tables of associations are set out in the Appendix, and they are mentioned in numerous other places listed in the Index.

ASSOCIATION AND LINKAGE

There has in the past been some confusion between two different kinds of relationship between polymorphisms and diseases, linkage and association.

Certain diseases are due to distinct genes with complete or almost complete penetrance. If they bear a relation to a blood-group system or to any other polymorphism, then this must be one of linkage, due to the loci for the disease and for the polymorphism occurring on the same chromosome. Any investigation of such a relationship must take the form of family studies. The first essential is to show that the disease in question is due to a single gene with fully penetrant expression. Until this is established it is not justifiable to ask for numerous blood-group tests. If the tests are done, it is desirable to test patients and their relatives for as many polymorphisms as possible, and there is usually no need to test very large numbers of persons. If linkage is found, it will be with a set of alleles, not with a single phenotype. There is, thus, no functional connection between the disease and a particular gene product, and unless the linkage is very close, the disease is likely to be accompanied by different alleles in different families. Studies of linkage mostly fall outside the scope of this book.

Association, on the other hand, should be sought where a disease, especially one of ill-understood aetiology, is only slightly familial in its incidence. A disease due to a fully penetrant gene cannot be associated with a phenotype of a separate polymorphic system. Association is with one phenotype, or a small number of the phenotypes of a particular polymorphic system, and is a statistical phenomenon; it is important to test, in the first instance, large numbers of unrelated patients, possibly for only one or a few polymorphisms, rather than to try to include numerous polymorphisms.

It is particularly important to avoid the frequent error of using the word 'linkage' when 'association' is meant.

Hitherto the two types of relationship between polymorphisms and diseases have appeared to be completely distinct from one another, but the associations of diseases with the histocompatibility antigens show some features of both. This is because the disease associations, though by no means absolute, are much closer than those of almost any other polymorphism, and this polymorphism is based on a set of four loci, each with numerous alleles, closely linked with one another and with loci controlling other immune phenomena (see pp. 45–7). In some cases there is probably association in the sense described above, a particular histocompatibility antigen causing increased susceptibility to a particular disease. In others it is likely that a specific pathogenic gene is included in the short chromosome section involved, and may thus be truly linked to different histocompatibility alleles in different populations. Thus, while studies of unrelated patients are needed in order to establish the fact of association, much additional information may be obtained by means of family studies.

3

THE NEOPLASTIC DISEASES

THE first association between a blood group and a disease, other than haemolytic disease of the newborn, to be convincingly demonstrated was that found by Aird *et al.* (1953) between carcinoma of the stomach and blood group A; in the subsequent 20 years the investigation of associations with neoplasms has remained one of the most fertile branches of the subject.

It can be said at the outset that cancers in general tend to be associated with group A, and slightly less strongly with group B. It is against this background that all the neoplasms will be considered. This is not a textbook of oncology, and no effort will be made to mention all those numerous forms of cancer which appear in the tables only in small numbers, and with only slight blood-group associations. Those who wish to make a deeper study of any particular group of neoplasms must refer first to the tables, and then if necessary to the bibliography and to the original papers upon which the tables are based. In this chapter we shall mention mainly those cancers which show particularly strong associations with groups A and B, and those which on adequate evidence show little or no such association, or which, on the contrary, are associated with group O. Also, as we are unable to deal, except very superficially, with histological types, the various cancers will be considered in a more-or-less anatomical order. Moreover, most of our sources refer simply to cancer so that we do not here, unless there is a strong reason for it, consider even the major division into carcinomas and sarcomas. Nevertheless, we hope that this rather simple treatment will suffice to guide oncologists to what we think is an important and neglected body of information which only they can fully interpret. Cancer of the lung is given a separate chapter because of the special interest of its apparent association with an enzyme polymorphism.

THE DIGESTIVE TRACT

Cancer of the lip is significantly associated with group A, but not with B. Cancers of the tongue, gum, and cheek are likewise associated with group A; for these diseases taken together the association with A is significant and there is also a non-significant association with B.

Cancers of the nasopharynx show virtually no departure from the control blood-group frequencies. Those of the tonsils, oropharynx, and hypopharynx, which form a natural group, are associated with group B but, apart from a small series of only fifty cases of cancer of the oropharynx, they are associated with group O rather than A.

Cancers of the salivary glands are strongly associated with group A and are also associated with B. On a regrettably small sample of forty-seven they appear also to be associated with the secretor factor. These observations are almost certainly related to the fact that the secretion of these glands contains, in the case of genetical secretors, a considerable concentration of the blood-group antigens characteristic of the individual's ABO group.

Cancer of the oesophagus, of which 2705 cases have been examined, so that precise quantitative data become meaningful, shows highly significant associations both with A and B, the relative incidences A/O and B/O being respectively 1·10 and 1·29; the closer association with B than with A is unusual.

For cancer of the stomach the amount of information is greater than for any other disease, being based on 161 surveys and over 63 000 cases. (There are only 158 sets for B because 3 small sets lack B entirely; see p. 60). The A/O and B/O relative incidences are 1·21 and 1·04. The latter figure is still highly significant on these large numbers. Many investigators have specified which part of the stomach is affected, but there seems to be no definite pattern; there is in fact no systematic histological difference between the cancers of the different parts.

Because of the large number of sets of data the distribution of values of the relative incidence A/O for separate sets well illustrates, as shown in FIGURE 1, what is said on page 61 regarding the nature of heterogeneity as between sets, and the

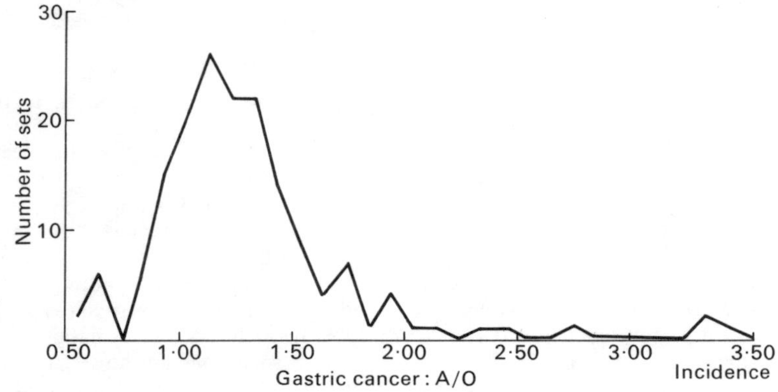

FIGURE 1. The relative incidence of A/O in carcinoma of the stomach. Distribution of values for separate sets of data.

tendency, even among data which are essentially homogeneous, for 'freak' sets to occur, in numbers which are quite small, but nevertheless greater than the laws of probability would predict.

Cases of cancer of the stomach show a small excess of ABH secretors, but, despite the rather large number of cases examined, this is not statistically significant. Nevertheless, it is probable that the associations with blood groups and the secretor factor are once again related to the presence of blood-group antigens in the gastric secretion of persons of the secretor type.

Unfortunately, but not surprisingly, the numbers of cases of cancer of the small intestine investigated are quite inadequate to support any conclusion.

Cancers of the large intestine taken together show an association with A which though highly significant is much lower than for stomach cancer. There is no association with group B. The relative incidences A/O and B/O are respectively 1·08 and 0·99.

'Cancer of the liver', probably a heterogeneous collection of neoplasms, shows a slight association with both groups A and B. Cancers of the gall-bladder and bile ducts, on rather small numbers, have a strong association with groups A and B, as have cancers of the pancreas.

OTHER ORGANS AND TISSUES

Carcinoma of the larynx shows an almost completely normal distribution of blood groups, as does cancer of the lung and bronchus on a total of over 16 000 cases (though, because of the large numbers, the A/O combined relative incidence of 1·055 is formally significant). As already stated, broncho-pulmonary cancer is treated in a separate chapter.

Cancer of the skin, not subdivided, appears, on rather small numbers of cases, to be strongly associated with group O.

Cancer of the breast, on over 12 000 cases, shows a weak but significant association with group A (relative incidence A/O, 1·06) but virtually none with group B. It does, however, on a much smaller sample, show an association, though not a significant one, with non-secretion.

Another blood-group association with cancer of the breast has been proposed by the Boston Collaborative Drug Surveillance Programme (1971). This is one with the ss phenotype of the MNSs blood-group system. Though the total number of patients examined is only 171, the association appears at first examination to be highly significant, the combined relative incidence, ss/SS+Ss, being 1·69, giving a value of χ^2 of 8·83 for difference from unity. However, the same patients were tested also for the phenotypes of five other polymorphic systems in a blind search for associations, and it appears that patients with other diseases were similarly tested. Thus, in relation to the method of ascertainment, and for reasons explained more fully on p. 6, the critical value of a single probability would have to be set considerably lower than the conventional significance limit of five per cent. This result, therefore, may not be significant, though it is sufficiently suggestive to make further tests worth while.

An association has also been suggested with ear-wax type. The gene for the hard ear-wax type (p. 11) has a frequency of over 90 per cent in the Japanese and several other Mongoloid peoples. Japanese women have an exceptionally low frequency of breast cancer. Since, as mentioned on page 11, both the mammary glands and the ear-wax glands are modified apocrine sweat glands, Petrakis *et al.* (1971) considered the possibility that there might be an association between the wet type and carcinoma of the breast. This hypothesis was supported by the examination of a small series of thirty-one Chinese women in California with the disease. Later, however, he and his colleagues (Ing *et al.*, 1973) examined a more adequate series of 246 Chinese women with cancer of the breast in Hong Kong, and found no significant difference in wax types from those present in healthy controls. It might, however, be worth while to repeat the survey on a still larger sample. This could hardly be done on any population other than a Mongoloid one, since in Caucasoids, and especially west Europeans, the frequency of the dry phenotype would be very low in the controls and, if the hypothesis is a true one, it would be still lower in the patients, so that an extremely large sample of the latter would be needed to give any possibility at all of detecting an association.

Cancers of the female reproductive organs tend to show strong associations with group A and slighter ones with group B. Values of the A/O relative incidence showing statistical significance are: Cervix uteri, 1·09; uterus (site unspecified), 1·16; ovary, 1·23; vulva, 1·39. Choriocarcinoma is associated with both groups A and B but because of the special origin and immunological status of this neoplasm it is discussed in Chapter 6. On small numbers, cancers of the uterus (site unspecified) and of the ovary show association with ABH secretion. It should be remembered that (benign) ovarian cysts tend to secrete very large amounts of blood-group antigens.

Cancer of the bladder (both sexes combined) and of the prostate also show marked association with group A, and that of the bladder also with group B. On very small numbers cancer of the prostate is non-significantly associated with secretion, and that of the bladder with non-secretion.

Neoplasms of the brain and nervous system are very consistently, and in some cases strongly, associated with group A, and in most cases also with group B.

Neoplasms of lymphatic and haematopoietic tissue have been on the whole poorly classified in association studies, and have given erratic and in some cases inconsistent results, as may be seen from an inspection of the Tables. However, Hodgkin's disease, one of the few conditions for which more than 1000 cases are reported, is associated with group O. It is now considered possible that this condition is, at least in part, due to a virus infection.

Results for sarcomas include only 219 cases, with no significant blood-group association. Cases reported as 'bone cancers' should presumably be included among sarcomas: the 216 such cases show slight and non-significant association with A but strong association with B (B/O relative incidence, 1·52).

BENIGN NEOPLASMS

Benign neoplasms have mostly been examined only in small numbers. Benign tumours of the salivary glands are associated with groups A and B, but the very large A/O combined relative incidence of 1·56 is mainly due to an aberrant single set of data. Benign tumours of the uterus and ovary are fairly strongly associated with both groups A and B. Mixed salivary adenoma is slightly associated with the secretor status. As already mentioned for malignant salivary gland tumours, these associations are almost certainly related to the blood-group antigen-secretor function of the glands.

Chromophobe adenoma of the pituitary is non-significantly associated with groups O and B.

ANTIGENICITY OF NEOPLASMS

The antigenicity of neoplasms has become a major preoccupation of oncologists, and in this connection, the association of carcinomas, and especially that of the stomach, with group A has received repeated attention, leading to the suggestion that an A-like antigen is present in tumour tissues irrespective of the blood group of the patient. According to Hakomori *et al.* (1967) the biosynthesis of blood-group substances in gastric carcinoma tissue is incomplete and leads to the accumulation in the tissue of a substance immunologically related to blood group A. Hakkinen and Virtanen (1967) extracted a similar substance from the cancer tissue, while Kościelak *et al.* (1971) found an antibody in the blood of a group B patient with cancer of the lung, which was active both against A cells and against cancer cells. The antibody disappeared following pneumonectomy but reappeared when secondary growths developed.

The question of an A-like antigen in neoplasms is further discussed on page 49.

4

CANCER OF THE LUNG

THE group of diseases commonly classed together as cancer of the lung have in recent decades aroused great interest because of their rapidly increasing incidence, particularly in males, and their association with the smoking of tobacco, especially in the form of cigarettes. Most cases of so-called cancer of the lung are bronchogenic carcinomas, histologically classified as squamous-cell carcinoma, adeno-carcinoma, and oat-cell carcinoma.

A great many of the neoplasms included in blood-group surveys are called simply cancer of the lung. There is no doubt that most of these are bronchogenic. Others are described as cancer of the bronchus, but only in relatively few studies is any further classification made. For those described as 'cancer of bronchus' the over-all A/O relative incidence is 1·07, which only just differs significantly from unity. For those listed as 'cancer of lung' the ratio is still lower at 1·03, and the difference from unity is far below the level of significance. The corresponding ratios for B/O are 1·04 and 0·96 respectively, both quite non-significant. Indeed, of all the cancers for which there are large bodies of data, these are among the ones which show the least association with the ABO groups.

In view of the disappointing absence of blood-group associations, it is interesting to find that there is one polymorphism which, on the scanty data so far available, does show an association with lung cancer which is statistically highly significant, and which, if preliminary observations are confirmed, is likely to be of considerable scientific interest and medical importance.

This is the aryl hydrocarbon hydroxylase inducibility polymorphism, which is involved in the metabolism of the well-known polycyclic aryl hydrocarbon carcinogens. The early history of the subject has been reviewed by Kellermann *et al.* (1973*b*). Aryl hydrocarbon hydroxylase is a mixed-function oxidase catalysing the first stage in the oxidation not only of the polycyclic aryl hydrocarbons, but of many other substances as well. The reaction catalysed the formation of an epoxide. The latter, rather than the original hydrocarbon, is thought to be the active carcinogen. Further stages of metabolism, catalysed by other enzymes, lead to the production of relatively harmless substances which are excreted.

Aryl hydrocarbon hydroxylase is an inducible enzyme, showing in experimental animals a marked increase in activity (and presumably in amount) following the administration of various possible substrates. In some but not all strains of mice there is a correlation between the degree of inducibility of this enzyme and the incidence of subcutaneous tumours evoked by administration of 3-methyl cholanthrene, though, in the same strains, no association is found with the incidence of sarcomas caused by 7.12-dimethylbenzanthrene or benzpyrene. Inducibility in mice is under the control of genes at a single locus.

Kellermann *et al.* (1973*b*) have shown that in man also, inducibility is controlled by a pair of alleles at a single locus. These authors used cultured lymphocytes which were induced to proliferate by the use of pokeweed mitogen. While the basal level of enzyme is clearly controlled by the genes, the character which segregates most clearly is the inducibility, the ratio of enzyme activity after induction under specified conditions, to the basal activity. The inducibility among 161 subjects is trimodal, with frequencies of the presumed homozygotes and heterozygotes conforming to the Hardy–Weinberg law. This interpretation is fully borne out by data on 67 families with a total of 165 children. The alleles are named AHH^a and AHH^b, conferring respectively low and high inducibility, with gene frequencies of 0·717 and 0·283. The ethnic groups of the subjects tested (in Houston, Texas) are not stated but they were presumably mostly Whites. It is much to be desired that gene frequencies should be determined separately for Whites, Blacks, and any other ethnic groups which can be studied. The system has, indeed, interesting possibilities in anthropology as well as in oncology.

The same authors, Kellermann *et al.* (1973*a*), have compared a group of 50 patients suffering from bronchogenic carcinoma with a healthy control group of 85 persons and with 46 patients with non-bronchogenic tumours. The control groups do not differ significantly from one another and both are in Hardy–Weinberg equilibrium. The cancer group is not in equilibrium (nor, if association is with phenotypes rather than genes, would it be expected to be so). This group of patients shows a gross relative excess of heterozygotes, and the frequency of the low inducibility homozygote is only 4 per cent, as compared with 45 per cent in the healthy controls. The mere existence of disequilibrium is indeed in itself prima facie evidence for the existence of a selective process. The value of χ^2 for a comparison of low inducibility homozygotes with the rest, in patients and in healthy controls, is 250, corresponding to an infinitesimal probability ($\ll 0{\cdot}01$) that the distribution in the patients is a chance one. Despite this, it is important that many further studies should be made on other groups of patients and controls and, with larger numbers, separation of histological types should be made. The present study has been criticized (*Lancet*, 1974) because the controls were not matched for such variables as age, sex, and smoking history. Such matching is indeed desirable, but probably more important is ethnic composition, as this is the factor which seems most likely to affect substantially the gene frequencies of a group of apparently healthy persons. It would be particularly important in a population, such as that of Texas, of varied ethnic origins. It would be best, if numbers were sufficient, to compare each ethnic group of patients with an ethnically matched control group, and then to combine the results by Woolf's method (1955) or Haldane's method (1955).

It would be particularly interesting to look for evidence of selection, by testing a fairly large number of middle-aged and elderly persons, with a long history of heavy smoking, and free from signs of cancer, to see whether they had a *raised* frequency of the low inducibility homozygote, as compared with the general population, or with a matched group of non-smoking controls (or preferably with both).

A further criticism (Bast *et al.*, 1974) is that the lymphocytes used were induced to proliferate by treatment with pokeweed mitogen, and that the genetic phenomena elicited might be a function of this induced mitosis. The authors recommend the use of monocytes, which can be tested for inducibility without being cultured. It is indeed desirable that comparisons should be made in a limited number of individuals between the inducibility of natural monocytes and of cultured lymphocytes but if, as expected, they show similar properties, then it would appear that the lymphocyte method is the method of choice, for reasons of convenience. It has also not yet been shown whether the polymorphism is one of the hydroxylase enzyme itself, or characterizes an inducing factor, the variants of which act upon a single type of hydroxylase. This could ultimately be ascertained by amino-acid analysis, but if there are variants which differ in electric charge, the differences should be demonstrable by means of gel electrophoresis.

Another desideratum is a repetition of the test on patients suffering from cancers definitely known to be caused by polycyclic hydrocarbons, a causation which has not up to now been convincingly demonstrated in the case of bronchogenic carcinoma. Many other criticisms can be and have been made of the preliminary work so far published, but most of these can probably be met without great difficulty; the results available suggest the possibility of a fundamental advance in knowledge of the aetiology of all chemically induced tumours. Individual, and presumably genetic, factors must be operating to determine why some individuals in a given chemical environment do, and others do not, develop tumours. Such factors may be multiple and very difficult to analyse. It now appears possible, however, that for one group of carcinogens, and for one class of tumours, a single and relatively simple genetic system has a sufficiently large influence to be distinguished from other oncogenic factors by relatively simple means.

According to Rogentine *et al.* (1976) the prognosis in cancer of the lung is associated with certain of the histocompatibility antigens, patients with Aw19 or B5 (or Bw35 which cross-reacts with the latter) having a much more favourable prognosis than those without either antigen.

5

THE INFECTIVE DISEASES

WHEN associations of blood groups with diseases were first sought the expectation was that, if they existed, they would concern mainly the infective diseases, and the relations of the antigens of the infecting organisms with those of the blood groups. It would have been expected, for instance, that if the organism carried an antigen resembling that of blood group A, then group A persons, being unable to make an anti-A antibody, would fare worse than group O persons who already had such an antibody. Damian (1964) has given a valuable critical account of the selective effects of the sharing of similar antigens between parasites and their hosts, which he calls 'molecular mimicry'.

In 1960 Vogel, Pettenkofer, and Helmbold put forward a comprehensive hypothesis which appeared able to account for much of the diversity of world distribution of the ABO blood groups. This was based firstly on historical records of the distribution and severity of recorded epidemics of plague, smallpox, and cholera, secondly on numerous previous discoveries of blood-group-like antigens in bacteria, and thirdly, on their own finding of an H-like antigen in the plague bacillus *Pasteurella pestis* and an A-like one in vaccinia virus (which is closely related to that of smallpox). They found no blood-group-like specificity in the cholera vibrio. From their observations they deduced that group O individuals would have a raised susceptibility to plague, and group A persons to smallpox. Springer and Wiener (1962) published a severe criticism of the immunological work of these authors, and of the deductions made from it, to which Pettenkofer *et al.* (1962) replied.

I am not competent to adjudicate upon a disagreement in the interpretation of microbial immunology tests, but I consider that Pettenkofer and his colleagues then took what was undoubtedly the right attitude from the standpoint of population genetics (and anthropology), by initiating a series of direct observations on patients. They found that A and AB persons tended to have more severe scars from smallpox, and a greater incidence of serious reactions to vaccination, than O and B persons; again, however, other workers disagreed with their results. The detailed results of the work of this group of authors and of others on smallpox will be discussed later in this chapter, under the heading of virus diseases.

BACTERIAL INFECTIONS

Typhoid and paratyphoid infections tend to be associated with a raised group O frequency, but only in the case of paratyphoid does this reach the conventional level of significance. Other intestinal infections show nothing significant. We have been unable to find any data on plague or cholera, which is particularly disappointing in view of the possibility of epidemics of them having had great selective effects in historic times.

Diphtheria, for which data are abundant, shows a complete lack of blood-group association, as do the results of the Schick test for susceptibility.

Haemolytic streptococcal infections, however, give an interesting pattern. Scarlet fever patients show a significantly lowered blood-group A frequency as compared with both O and B, while in the Dick test for susceptibility to the disease, positive reactors have a considerably higher A frequency than negatives. Carriers of haemolytic streptococcus, type A (the type responsible for scarlet fever), show a fairly consistent deficiency of ABH secretors. Haverkorn and Goslings (1969), who examined carriers both for secretor and for ABO blood groups, dividing them only into O and non-O, found no clear blood-group pattern. These results will be discussed further in relation to rheumatic fever (p. 33) and rheumatic heart disease (p. 33). Staphylococcal infections show a somewhat raised frequency of group O.

The tuberculous infections show a puzzling pattern, since pulmonary tuberculosis, on a very large sample, is marked by a raised O frequency. On much smaller samples, tuberculosis of most other sites shows a raised A, yet over 10 000 cases with site unstated, which one would expect to be mostly pulmonary, have a markedly raised A and lowered O. The relatively raised O frequency in haemoptysis conforms to the pattern, further discussed on pages 34–5, shown by every other form of haemorrhage. When all types of tuberculosis are considered together, blood-group associations disappear almost completely.

Sarcoidosis, which may be a special form of reaction to tuberculous infection, shows a raised A frequency.

The pattern for leprosy also is rather puzzling, but the tuberculoid form is associated with a high O level, while all other forms show a raised A, most marked in those described as 'non-lepromatous'.

Syphilis in general is marked by raised A frequencies but the most notable feature, and one that has long been known, is that in treated syphilis a positive Wassermann serological reaction of the serum is on the average much more persistent in A and B than in O persons.

Among a rather mixed group of other bacterial infections, meningitis (presumably mainly meningococcal) is marked by a considerably raised A frequency. A total of 69 cases of rickettsial diseases show nothing of note.

VIRUS INFECTIONS

Poliomyelitis cases taken as a whole show a small deficiency of both A and B as compared with O. When, however, paralytic cases are compared with non-paralytic, there is a significant relative deficiency of both A and B in the former.

The observations on smallpox, already mentioned, are of particular interest because of the former great prevalence of epidemics of this disease. Unfortunately the data show exceptionally large discrepancies between the results of different workers, particularly with regard to the A/O ratio. Most workers divide their cases into fatal and survivors, or into confluent (i.e. severe) and discrete (less severe), so that one might have hoped for valuable data on the problem of natural selection. However, Vogel and Chakravartti (1966) find an extremely high value of the A/O relative incidence for fatal cases in two epidemics, and a very high one for survivors from the same epidemics, both ratios being entirely outside the range found by other workers. The same authors, however, find an A/O relative incidence below unity for cases tested (during epidemics) as survivors from past epidemics. There is also no recognizable regularity in the results of other workers, whether for fatal cases, for surviving cases, or for patients classified by degree of severity. On the whole, however, most workers other than Vogel and Chakravartti find A/O relative incidences below unity. Happily, with the almost complete disappearance of smallpox from the face of the earth, conditions are unlikely ever to recur which would allow the disagreements to be resolved, but the scientist may perhaps be allowed a sigh of regret that he cannot now hope to explain how past smallpox epidemics may have influenced regional blood-group frequencies.

There is also an extreme discrepancy between the results of two sets of observations, each comparing cases of the presence and absence of reaction to smallpox revaccination.

The very high frequency of group A among twenty-six cases of trachoma is almost certainly an accident of sampling.

In dealing with the influenza and associated viruses it must be pointed out that the letters A and B, used to distinguish viral types, imply no relation whatsoever to blood groups A and B.

The majority of investigations of associations of virus infections with the blood groups fall into two classes, the testing of patients suffering from acute infections and those relating the blood groups to titres of antibody in the serum of survivors from past epidemics.

In acute infections McDonald and Zuckerman (1962) found some lowering of the A/O and B/O relative incidences in patients acutely infected with two Influenza A virus strains. In particular, the A/O relative incidence was very significantly lowered, to 0·67 in A_2 virus infection.

Infection with B virus only slightly and quite non-significantly affected the A/O and B/O incidences. With Cocksackie A_2 virus the blood group B/O relative incidence was lowered to 0·48, but on the small numbers available this was not significant. Titrating antibodies in the sera of survivors from past epidemics, Watkin *et al.* (1975) found only a slight and non-significant deficiency of blood group A among strong as compared with weak reactors for each of two different Influenza A strains, while Cuadrado and Davenport (1970) found marked and highly significant deficiencies of blood group A in similar tests. Otter and Schild (1967), classifying antibody results as positive and negative, obtained a similar reduction of the A/O ratio among positive reactors to that found by Cuadrado and Davenport for strong reactors. There is, however, general agreement that both A/O and (in those cases where B tests were done) B/O relative incidences were lower in infected than in non-infected persons, and lower also in those with antibodies or with high titres of antibodies than in those without or with low titres, for all forms of Influenza A. It is nevertheless desirable that further attempts should be made to resolve the marked quantitative differences between the results of different investigators. Influenza B infection, already mentioned, with an A/O relative incidence of 1·01 in infected persons, may be an exception to the general lowering of this ratio in patients, but the total number tested was only sixty-three.

Considering the virus infections as a whole, it is worth noting that, omitting smallpox, regarding which there is considerable disagreement, the over-all relative incidences A/O and B/O are respectively 0·94 and 0·96.

PROTOZOAL INFECTIONS

Malaria

Malaria is the outstanding example of an infection, susceptibility to which is associated with several polymorphisms. There are a number of clinically and pathologically distinct types of malaria, due to infection with different species of the protozoon Plasmodium. We shall be concerned here with only two of these, quartan malaria, a relatively mild disease which is the principal type in temperate regions, caused by the parasite *Plasmodium vivax*, and malignant tertian malaria, the principal type in the tropics but extending into milder climatic regions. It is a much more severe disease, caused by *Plasmodium falciparum*. Rather surprisingly, in view of the importance of the disease, little has been done towards finding an association between malaria and the ABO groups. Such data as exist are mostly rather old, and the authors do not state which type of malaria was involved. Nevertheless, the combined data show a marked excess of A in patients, as compared with O and B. Wood *et al.* (1972), however, claim that Anopheles mosquitoes, which convey malarial infection, tend to bite Group O and B persons in preference to group A ones.

Athreya and Coriell (1967) have suggested that group B confers a selective advantage in relation to malarial infection and that this is why, in the Old World, the distribution of group B tends to correspond with a high degree of malaria endemicity. Wood (1975) using the results of the mosquito-biting experiments, but not the data on association of blood groups with actual infection, as part of her evidence, claims that malaria did not exist in the New World before its discovery by Columbus. It will be seen that the present evidence on possible associations of malaria with the ABO groups is somewhat unsatisfactory, but the problem is one of some importance, and it is to be desired that further surveys should be carried out, with strict attention to the types of parasite and vector. It is also desirable to give some indication of the severity of the infection, preferably by means of parasite counts. This is particularly important in regions where nearly everyone is infected.

The evidence for associations with other polymorphisms is mainly of an epidemiological nature and can perhaps best be understood by following the history of investigations.

The disease of thalassaemia, now known more precisely as β-thalassaemia, had long been known when, in 1944, Valentine and Neel worked out its mode of inheritance, showing that thalassaemia major and minor represented the homozygous and heterozygous forms of this severe anaemia. Thalassaemia major is almost invariably fatal during childhood, while the minor form is only a mildly debilitating disease. It was not until the advent of molecular biology that the precise biochemical aetiology was gradually deciphered, but as soon as the formal genetics were worked out an important problem of population genetics presented itself—how did such a highly lethal gene maintain itself at a moderately high frequency over large parts of the Mediterranean and other regions? It appeared likely that it must carry some hidden benefit, presumably in heterozygotes, to counteract the selective mortality of homozygotes. It was Haldane who, in 1949, first suggested that heterozygotes were more resistant to malarial infection than were normal (i.e. homozygous) non-thalassaemics. Strong support was given to this view when, in 1957, Carcassi *et al.* reported on the distribution of blood groups and of thalassaemia in the villages of the mountainous region of central Sardinia, one which was to become classical in population genetics. In this region there are a number of lowland villages with a recent history of endemic malarial infection, while adjacent highland villages had long been almost completely free from the disease. No significant differences in blood-group frequencies were found between the populations of these two groups of villages, this suggesting that at no very remote period the inhabitants were drawn from the same stock. However, the incidence of thalassaemia was found to be consistently and significantly higher in the lowland than in the highland villages. This was interpreted as being due to a greater resistance to malaria in thalassaemic heterozygotes than in normal persons, postulated by Haldane (1949), so that, by natural selection, acting upon a hitherto uniform population, the sub-populations exposed to malaria developed relatively high frequencies of thalassaemia once the gene for this was introduced to the region. This work was carried out in the light of similar work on haemoglobin variants, described below. It has not yet, however, been possible to show directly, by tests on individual thalassaemic heterozygotes, that they have the postulated improved resistance to malaria.

Sickle-cell haemoglobin

The existence of a hereditary sickle-shaped modification of the red cells, and of an associated, often fatal, anaemia had been known for many years when, in 1949, Pauling *et al.* showed that these phenomena were due to the existence of a molecular variant of haemoglobin which, during electrophoresis, migrates more slowly towards the positive pole than does normal haemoglobin. This work, and genetical investigations by Neel (1949) and by Beet (1949) made it clear that sickle-cell haemoglobin (HbS) and normal adult haemoglobin (HbA) were the products of a pair of allelic genes, heterozygotes having a mixture of the two haemoglobins, and suffering little disability, while homozygotes for Haemoglobin S had virtually only the one type of haemoglobin, and mostly died of anaemia during the first year of life. The genetics of the haemoglobins is more fully described on pages 9–10.

The problem of the maintenance of a high level of a lethal gene in some Negro populations was clearly analogous to that presented by thalassaemia, but even before Haldane's (1949) suggestion of malaria as the selective agent in that disease other minds were moving in the same direction. In 1946 Beet had observed the lower incidence of malaria in sicklers than in non-sicklers, though he was unable in 1947 to confirm this, and in his classic paper (1949) on the genetics of sickling he does not mention malaria.

Meanwhile Brain (1952*b*) had observed that sicklers were less severely affected than non-sicklers by 'malaria and pyrexia of unknown origin', and in another paper (1952*a*) he clearly states the problem of maintenance of the frequency of a lethal gene and suggests that 'the explanation may be that the red cells in sicklers offer a less favourable environment'. He expresses his intention to elaborate this elsewhere, and this he did in his unpublished (1953) M.D. thesis in which he produced evidence, which was just short of statistical significance, for the protective effect given by sickling against malaria. It was, however, Allison (1954) who first published data which showed clearly and at a statistically significant level that sickle-cell heterozygotes were more resistant to malaria than 'normal' homozygotes for HbA. He further showed that this relationship was specifically with malignant tertian malaria, the variety due to *Plasmodium falciparum*. The increased resistance of heterozygotes to malaria has since been demonstrated on a number of occasions by means of parasite counts. Population surveys in Africa and Asia, including comparisons between adjacent and closely related populations, have repeatedly shown a close correlation between the incidence of the *HbS* gene and the current or recent prevalence of falciparum malaria. This situation, as already mentioned on page 2, is the classical example of a balanced polymorphism in man.

Glucose-6-phosphate dehydrogenase deficiency

A hereditary deficiency of the red-cell enzyme glucose-6-phosphate dehydrogenase can, as already mentioned (p. 9), give rise, under certain conditions, to a severe or even fatal haemolytic anaemia. The variants of this enzyme, including some with low activity, are determined by a number of allelic genes on the X chromosome. The deficiency is found mainly in the Mediterranean area and in Africa. It is particularly frequent in Kurdish Jews. It presents a problem analogous to those just mentioned, of accounting for the persistence, in some cases at very high frequency levels, of a gene with harmful effects. The general world distribution of the deficiency once again suggested that it conferred resistance to malaria, and once again investigators turned their attention to Sardinia, where Siniscalco *et al.* (1961) showed that, in the same lowland villages where there had been much malaria, the incidence of the deficiency was high, whereas in the highland villages where there had been little malaria it was low. Numerous other population surveys support the association of high frequencies of the deficiency gene with former or present high incidences of malaria. Moreover, as with sickling but not so far with thalassaemia, it has been possible to show a correlation in individuals between the presence of the deficiency and resistance to malaria (Allison and Clyde, 1961; Harris and Gilles, 1961; Bienzle *et al.*, 1972). The study of Bienzle *et al.*, carried out on Africans, shows that resistance to malaria is associated not only with the relatively common African deficiency gene Gd^{A-} but with the gene Gd^{A+}, which is almost entirely confined to Africa and gives rise to a quantitatively normal enzyme level.

The histocompatibility antigens

Most of the evidence for associations between histocompatibility antigens and diseases is based on the examination of individual patients but, almost inevitably, the now malaria-free inhabitants of the classic Sardinian region have been tested for histocompatibility antigens (Piazza *et al.*, 1973). Three antigens are found to show a highly significant heterogeneity of gene frequency between highland and lowland populations. HL-A1 and W21 are more frequent in the two highland villages investigated, while W5 is more frequent in the lowland villages. The authors tentatively suggest 'HL-A variation may be adaptive and linked (*sic*) to the distribution of malaria'.

Acid phosphatase

Recent investigations into the incidence of the red-cell acid phosphatase variants in Sardinia and Rome concern not malaria but favism, but the work is so intimately connected with that on malaria that it is most conveniently reported here. Favism is a haemolytic anaemia resulting from the eating of the broad bean, *Vicia faba*, by some persons who have a deficiency of glucose-6-phosphate dehydrogenase (G6PD). A group of Italian workers (Bottini *et al.*, 1971; Palmarino *et al.*, 1975) have further investigated the situation in Sardinia, already known to involve former malarial infection, thalassaemia and G6PD deficiency, by taking into account also the red-cell acid phosphatase polymorphism, and treating altitude as a possible independent variable. They also bring into their argument the presence of favism, which is an inconstant manifestation of G6PD deficiency (but do not mention the histocompatibility antigens studied by Piazza *et al.* (1973)).

The earlier paper (Bottini *et al.*, 1971) suggested that in the G6PD-deficient subjects, susceptibility to favism was related to the acid phosphatase type, being highest for the A and CA phenotypes, intermediate for BA and BC, and lowest for B. They mention previous work which showed that thalassaemia gave some protection from favism to the G6PD-deficient persons. The new investigation (Palmarino *et al.*, 1975) reveals an even more complicated situation. The frequency of the P^c allele seems clearly to be positively correlated with altitude. It is also negatively correlated with former malarial incidence, but the authors appear to think that this may be an indirect connection. It would take us too far from malaria susceptibility to consider their evidence in full, but their conclusions are worth complete quotation not only as showing the need for further work on the malarial aspect, but suggesting possibilities that have not hitherto been envisaged in extensive recent work on the physiology of high altitudes. They state:

> It seems reasonable to suggest that while malaria may be the primary environmental factor underlying the distribution of thalassaemia, other ecological variables may be more directly involved in determining the distribution of the G6PD and P^C alleles in Sardinia. Besides the quality of *Vicia faba* used in human alimentation, these variables could include factors such as barometric pressure, partial pressure of O_2 and environmental temperature, as suggested by Ananthakrishnan and Walter (1972) for acid phosphatase. Further complications in the interpretation of the frequency distributions may be due to the varied but high levels of consanguinity which have typified Sardinia (Workman *et al.*, 1975). Since the primary deleterious effect of thalassaemia occurs in the homozygotes, variable consanguinity itself, correlated with altitude, may be an important factor in the pattern of mortality due to thalassaemia. Over all, the data suggest a highly complex interaction among several loci and varied ecological and population characteristics which has led to the current distribution of the erythrocyte polymorphisms in Sardinia. It is clear that considerable (*sic*) more observations, biochemical, clinical, and populational will be required to unravel this complexity.

The same group of workers, Lucarelli *et al.* (1971), in the same Sardinian region, have found a negative correlation between the frequency of the ADA^2 gene of the adenosine deaminase system, and that of the deficiency type gene of the glucose-6-phosphate dehydrogenase system. This suggests that the ADA polymorphism, like the others just mentioned, may be implicated in the complex selective process involved in resistance to malaria (see also p. 51).

The Duffy blood groups

The relationship of the Duffy blood groups to malaria was discovered, not by means of statistical studies but by a brilliant piece of parasitological work on the malaria organism by Miller *et al.* (1975). It has long been known that Africans are mostly of the Duffy blood type Fy(a−b−), the homozygote of what was formerly regarded as the amorph gene *Fy* but is now recognized positively as Fy^4. They are also mostly highly resistant to the malarial parasite *Plasmodium vivax* (the formerly common European type). Miller *et al.*, have now shown, using the closely related monkey parasite, *P. knowlesii*, that the point of attachment and entry into the human red cell is the antigen Fy^a or Fy^b, but that they will not enter cells of type Fy(a−b−).

One may speculate that Africans developed resistance to *P. vivax* by natural selection of the 'amorph' *Fy* gene, biologically an efficient and 'cheap' process. When, however, *P. vivax* had thus almost disappeared from tropical Africa, the much more virulent *P. falciparum* was evolved, to which at first there was no inborn resistance. Thus when the Haemoglobin S gene appeared, possibly introduced from outside Africa, or evolving in some limited focus, the fact that heterozygotes were resistant to *P. falciparum* led to the spread of the new haemoglobin by natural selection. This, however, was a much more 'costly' form of resistance, since it led to the early deaths of nearly all homozygotes.

WORM INFESTATIONS

Several varied diseases caused by worm infestation, notably bilharzial hepatic fibrosis, tape-worm anaemia, and ascariasis, show markedly raised A frequencies.

As such infestations tend to cause allergic reactions, and as allergies in general are characterized by eosinophilia, it is interesting to note that the quite unrelated conditions of allergic dermatosis, and tropical eosinophilia, show high frequencies of blood group A. Damian (1964) gives several examples of the presence of blood-group-like antigens in parasitic worms, and especially of A- and B-like ones in *Ascaris lumbricoides* (see also p. 6).

ARTHROPOD INFESTATIONS

A very small series of cases of pediculosis and scabies shows nothing of interest.

ASSOCIATIONS WITH THE Rh GROUPS

As for most other classes of diseases, the only useful investigations on associations with the Rh groups have been carried out in terms of the Rh(D) positive and negative types only. Very few diseases show any association at the conventional level of significance, and for very few indeed is there a useful body of data contributed by several independent investigators.

Typhoid and paratyphoid infections show highly significant deficiencies of Rh-positives (i.e. excess of Rh-negatives) but these are based on the work of a single investigator (Paciorkiewicz, 1970). Pulmonary tuberculosis, other forms of tuberculosis, and sarcoidosis all show a deficiency of Rh-positives, which for infections of bones and joints, and for those of the genito-urinary system, is statistically significant.

Leprosy, for which, surprisingly, there is an abundance of

data, shows an excess of Rh-positives both for the tuberculoid and the lepromatous forms, though in neither case does this reach a significant level. The various forms of syphilis show, in general, a non-significant deficiency of Rh-positives.

Virus diseases, mostly investigated by Paciorkiewicz (1970), show in general a deficiency of Rh-positives, which is significant for mumps, infectious mononucleosis and viral meningitis. This investigator is to be commended for the wide range of diseases and the large number of cases which he has studied, but as he is almost the only worker to have reported significant deficiencies of Rh-positives in any infectious diseases, it is desirable that independent confirmation should be obtained. It is, however, interesting to see that virus diseases tend, on the present evidence, to attack preferentially the non-antigenic types of both the ABO and the Rh systems, O and Rh-negative respectively.

6

SOME DISORDERS RELATED TO PREGNANCY

THIS chapter is a discussion of a variety of diseases of either the pregnant woman or the foetus, in which the blood groups and other polymorphisms are involved. The connecting link between them is the immunization, actual or potential, of the mother by antigens in the foetus or abnormal conceptus, antigens which it has inherited from the father. The initial discovery from which all the others follow is that made by Dienst (1905) who showed that, in a woman carrying a foetus with an A or a B blood-group antigen which she herself does not possess, the titre of anti-A or anti-B (already, of course, present before pregnancy) becomes raised by immunization to the antigen in question. Dienst further tried to account, not very convincingly, for eclampsia, as being a result of such immunization. Had he concentrated on the foetuses rather than the mothers he might have come across a few cases of haemolytic disease of the newborn among them, and so become the discoverer of the aetiology of this disease.

In 1939 Levine and Stetson, examining the serum of a woman who had given birth to a stillborn foetus, found in it a hitherto unknown haemagglutinin which they correctly attributed to immunization by a factor present in the blood of the foetus, and which it had inherited from the father. Following the discovery of the Rhesus blood-group antigen by Landsteiner and Wiener (1940), and of its immunizing effect by Wiener and Peters (1940), Levine, Katzin, and Burnham (1941) showed that haemolytic disease of the newborn was due to red-cell destruction by an anti-Rhesus antibody passively transferred from the mother. They also showed that the antibody found by Levine and Stetson (1939) was in fact anti-Rh (anti-Rh_0 or anti-D). With the subsequent discovery of the complexity of the Rh blood groups, and the finding of many new independent blood-group systems, it was shown that a great many other antigens could cause maternal immunization, and hence haemolytic disease of the newborn.

The outstanding example of association between blood groups and a disease is in fact that involving haemolytic disease of the newborn, but it has already been the subject of a vast literature of its own, including many thousands of papers and probably over 100 books. Only certain limited aspects of it, therefore, will be considered here.

HAEMOLYTIC DISEASE OF THE NEWBORN AND NATURAL SELECTION

Soon after the discovery of the cause of haemolytic disease of the newborn, Wiener (1942) and Haldane (1942) independently showed that each death from haemolytic disease of the newborn (which, untreated, is a highly fatal disease) causes the destruction of one Rh-positive (*D*) and one Rh-negative (*d*) gene. Hence, in the absence of some form of compensation, whichever gene was initially the commoner in a given population should theoretically alone survive after a number of generations. On this view all the populations of Europe, mostly containing about 40 per cent of *d* genes and 60 per cent of *D*, should be unstable and evolving towards the total elimination of *d*.

One possible explanation for the existing situation seemed to be that the present population of Europe was the result of fairly recent mixing between two main populations, one preponderantly Rh-positive and the other preponderantly Rh-negative. There are many peoples in western Asia as well as in northern Africa which are very largely Rh-positive, but there was then no population known with more than 50 per cent of *d* genes.

Subsequently (Etcheverry, 1945; Mourant, 1947; Chalmers *et al.*, 1948, 1949) it was shown that the Basques of northern Spain and south-western France constitute such a population. Historically, physically, and linguistically they are, indeed, probably the oldest distinct ethnic group at present living in western Europe, and it was suggested by Mourant that they are the relatively unmixed descendants of the late Palaeolithic populations of western Europe who subsequently hybridized with Neolithic newcomers. The population of parts of northern Scotland and the Hebrides, who also are descended from an ancient population group, have likewise a very high *d* frequency, though not as high as the Basques. The hypothesis that there were only two populations taking part in the mixing, and that the mixed population did not compensate in any way for the mortality from haemolytic disease of the newborn, is probably an over-simplified one, but Ammerman and Cavalli-Sforza (1971) support the hypothesis that the Basques do indeed represent the ancient peoples of Europe whom the Neolithic cultivators from the Near East met as they expanded through Europe.

In considering the effect of deaths from haemolytic disease of the newborn it should be pointed out (Li, 1953) that no simple genetical model, either without or with compensation, can account for a balanced polymorphic state such as may have existed before the present stage of effective prophylaxis and treatment of the disease.

ABO BLOOD GROUPS AND ABORTION

As implied in the previous pages, ABO incompatibility between husband and wife, in the sense that the husband possesses an A or a B antigen which is absent in the wife, is a well-recognized cause of haemolytic disease of the newborn, and, as such, has been discussed in numerous works on that disease. Such incompatibility is also, however, as is shown below, an important cause of early abortion, as well, probably, as of infertility. Some of the apparent infertility may, however, result from unrecognized very early abortion.

This chapter is based mainly on published statistical data of many kinds, but the only relevant data which fit into the main tables of this book are those of the ABO groups of women who have had abortions, and a very few records of the ABO groups of aborted foetuses. The three sets of maternal data differ considerably from one another, and when they are combined the only relative incidence to differ significantly from unity is AB/O, with a value of 1·83. However, even this is due entirely to one of the three sets, the other two both showing values below unity, as would be expected if an excess of aborted foetuses had carried an A or a B antigen not present in the mother. Nearly all the data of other kinds discussed below point to such an excess of A and B in aborted foetuses.

THE BLOOD GROUPS OF PARENTS AND LIVING CHILDREN

Hirszfeld and Zborowski (1925) were the first to observe that, in families where the father was of group A and the mother of group O, there was a deficiency of group A offspring whereas when the father was O and the mother A, the numbers of A and O children were as expected from genetical theory in the absence of selection. Waterhouse and Hogben (1947) observed a similar effect, analysing a total of 453 families, and finding a 25 per cent deficiency of A children when the mother was group O.

ABO INCOMPATIBILITY BETWEEN MOTHER AND FOETUS

We have already mentioned the very early work of Dienst (1905) on the effects of ABO incompatibility between a mother and her foetus. Other early investigations are those of Ottenberg (1923), Hirszfeld and Zborowski (1925), and Hirszfeld (1928). The discovery by Levine, Katzin, and Burnham (1941) of Rh isoimmunization as the principal cause of haemolytic disease of the newborn did not immediately lead to the realization that ABO isoimmunization caused what was fundamentally the same disease (in infants born at or near full term)—mainly because both the symptoms and the serology differ markedly from those characterizing the classic Rh disease. The first workers clearly to describe the ABO variety appear to have been Halbrecht (1944) and Polayes (1945).

However, before this, in 1943, Levine had identified ABO incompatibility as a cause of early abortions and stillbirths. From this time onwards numerous workers produced data suggesting, mainly on the grounds of a deficiency of A children, and an excess of abortions, in the families of O women married to A men, that the A foetuses produced by such matings were especially liable to be aborted. Some of the work was criticized on grounds of statistical methodology, and in 1961 Levene and Rosenfield undertook a critical survey of all that had previously been published on the subject, including studies both of full-term haemolytic disease and of early abortion. This paper is recommended to any reader requiring a fuller discussion of early work, especially that on the full-term disease, than can be given here. One aspect of the latter must, however, be mentioned since it (like other more recent work mentioned below) involves the interaction of two genetically independent polymorphisms. Levene and Rosenfield bring together the observations of Zuelzer and Kaplan (1954), Crawford *et al.* (1953), and Wiener *et al.* (1960) who all show that in those cases where the secretor status of infants suffering from ABO haemolytic disease has been ascertained, there is a marked deficiency of ABH non-secretors as compared with the general population. This suggests that the secretion of A or B substance by the foetus plays an important part in the immunization of the mother—presumably via the meconium and the amniotic fluid.

Levene and Rosenfield then give a highly critical and detailed analysis and recalculation of all available published data on the ABO groups of parents and offspring. Most of the information on possible loss of children from maternofoetal incompatibility can be derived from the frequencies of A and O children in A × O matings, comparing those matings where the mother is O with those where she is A. The combined data show a significant deficiency of 25 per cent of A children in the incompatible matings. Other matings, involving B, are less conclusive because of small numbers, but the overall conclusion is that 'there is a loss of between 14 per cent and 32 per cent of all A or B children from matings of an A, B (and presumably AB) father and an O mother, as compared with the reciprocal mating, and that the most likely value for this loss is 25 per cent'.

Published data on total family size are also analysed, and show smaller numbers in incompatible than in compatible matings. The mean deficiency (hard to ascertain because of varying criteria used in obtaining the primary data) is about 0·5 children per family. It will obviously be affected by deliberate compensation for foetal loss or a low rate of conception in matings in which any form of pregnancy limitation is practised.

Relatively few data were available on numbers of abortions in compatible and incompatible matings, but all series show an excess for the incompatible ones. Rather more abundant are the ABO data on matings which have produced two or more abortions. The data are somewhat heterogeneous but show an excess (42·6 per cent, compared with 35 per cent expected) of ABO incompatibility. It has been convenient to quote extensively (above) from the very thorough study of Levene and Rosenfield, incorporating the results of a very large body of previously published data.

Chung and Morton (1961), also, have surveyed the evidence available to them regarding natural selection at the ABO locus. They adversely criticize some previous investigations on both technical and statistical grounds but find, nevertheless, strong evidence for ante-natal and early post-natal selection related to the ABO groups. They, however, regard the reported associations between blood groups and adult disease, which form the main subject of this book, as having at most, second-order selective effects.

Since the publication of these works many further papers on the subject have appeared, nearly all of them reaching similar conclusions. The principal papers consulted are those of Behrman *et al.* (1960), Wren and Vos (1961), Matsunaga (1962), Kircher (1965), Vos and Tovell (1967), Peritz (1967, 1971), Krieg and Kasper (1968), Cohen and Sayre (1968), Cohen (1970), Takano and Miller (1972), and Hiraizumi *et al.* (1973).

Cohen (1970) confirms the observation of most other workers, that there is increased early foetal loss in ABO incompatible matings as compared with ABO compatible ones, but in contrast with most others, finds no evidence that such loss affects the ABO frequencies among the full-term offspring. She does find, on the other hand, that in Rh-incompatible matings, where there is little or no obvious early foetal loss, there is nevertheless a deficiency of Rh-positive (i.e. Rh-incompatible) offspring.

THE BLOOD GROUPS OF ABORTED FOETUSES

The most conclusive evidence that foetuses incompatible with their mothers are more likely to be aborted than compatible ones would be the blood groups of the aborted foetuses themselves, compared with those of their mothers. Unfortunately very few workers have determined the blood groups of such foetuses in this context. Takano and Miller (1972) examined 62 aborted foetuses, but they do not report the actual ABO blood groups, stating only whether they were compatible or incompatible. They found that the number of ABO-incompatible abortuses was significantly greater than expected, but in addition they noted that among the 43 compatible abortuses there were 8 abnormal foetuses (18·6 per cent) while among the 35 incompatible abortuses only 3 were abnormal. Krieg and Kasper (1968) report the blood groups of 61 aborted foetuses and of their mothers. Unlike Takano and Miller, they examined the blood groups only of foetuses for which no other causes of abortion could be found. Having already demonstrated, on a large sample of families, that the abortion rate was significantly higher in ABO matings in which the father was incompatible with respect to the mother than in those in which he was compatible, they found this not to be the case in this very small series in which the foetus was available, but the rate of incompatibility between mother and foetus was 9 per cent higher than expected by chance.

Allen (1964) has grouped twenty-seven products of abortion, together with the blood of the mother in all cases and of the father in fifteen. The abortus specimens were preserved in formalin, and were tested by suspending in a saline serum mixture followed by titration of the centrifuged supernatant. The author claims that this method gives correct results with secretor foetuses but false negative ones with non-secretors. Despite this bias against the detection of incompatibility, there was a marked excess above expectation, of B incompatible foetuses both from white and Negro mothers; A incompatibilities were as expected. The author draws attention to the conclusion, on indirect evidence, by McNeil *et al.* (1954), that B may be more important than A in abortions.

Perhaps the most complete study of spontaneously aborted foetuses is that of Lauritsen *et al.* (1975), who carried out a chromosome analysis of 288 consecutive products of abortion and determined the ABO blood groups of all those, seventy-four in number, where this was at all possible, as well as those of the mothers, and in most cases the fathers. They found that 'there were too many group A and B abortuses among those with normal karyotypes, and too few among those with abnormal karyotypes. Furthermore, the frequencies of maternofetal incompatible pregnancies and of incompatible matings were significantly higher in the group of abortions with karyotypically normal fetuses.'

These investigations of rather small numbers of specimens have been described at some length since the results, on the whole consistent between the various investigations, provide the most direct evidence we possess regarding one of the main ways in which parental blood groups affect those of their surviving offspring.

ABO GROUPS AND INFERTILITY

Several workers have sought evidence of ABO incompatibility in couples whose infertility could not be otherwise explained. If, in the data of Grubb and Sjøstedt (1954–5) one compares reciprocal mating types, e.g. A/O with O/A, then there is a slight, but not significant, excess of compatible matings among couples with involuntary sterility.

Bennett and Walker (1955–6) find childlessness more frequent (but not significantly so) among A and B than among O and AB women, which in no way suggests that incompatibility of the mother (either with the husband's spermatozoa or with very early embryos) is involved. Behrmann *et al.* (1960), on the other hand, find a significant excess of ABO-incompatible couples in 102 persistently sterile matings (87·3 per cent) as compared with 171 fertile couples (38·6 per cent incompatible). They also find, in the case of 7 couples with markedly delayed fertility, that all the 9 children tested were of group O (and hence must have been compatible with the mother). These authors suggest that ABO-related infertility is due to the action of antibodies, in the secretions of the mother's genital tract, on incompatible spermatozoa. It is difficult to explain the marked discrepancies between the results of the different infertility studies, and there is a need for further data.

Kircher (1965) finds an increased proportion of O children in families with more than one child (as would be expected if mothers in ABO incompatible matings became progressively immunized against A or B). He finds that A_2 behaves more like O than like A_1 in this respect. On the other hand, Wren and Vos (1961), studying abortions, find that A_2 behaves like A_1. However, in both cases the numbers of A_2 individuals studied is small.

The papers cited above show, on the whole, very strong evidence that in matings where the husband has an A antigen which the wife does not possess, there is a marked selection against the birth or survival of A (i.e. heterozygous) offspring. The same is probably true of B. It has long been known that some such selection (mostly in fact in the neonatal period) takes place by means of the relatively rare deaths that result from ABO-related haemolytic disease of the newborn. It now appears that a much larger amount of selection takes place at an earlier stage of pregnancy, being manifested by selective abortion of incompatible foetuses, and by a deficiency of heterozygous children possibly due to very early unnoticed abortions. It is still not clear whether total sterility is often due to this cause. More data are needed on the blood groups of aborted foetuses (and on their sex—see 'The sex ratio' below) and of the partners in totally sterile matings. As pointed out by Grubb and Sjøstedt, it is especially desirable to collect data, inevitably a very few at a time, of the groups of partners in situations where a mating has been sterile for at least 5 years and then both partners have had offspring by new partners.

THE SEX RATIO

A further observation, which may reflect selective abortion, is the variation in the sex ratio of the children classified by ABO combinations of mother and child. Allan (1959) has collected and given references for the observations of previous workers as well as those made by himself (Allan, 1958). There is a marked tendency for the sex-ratio (i.e. the ratio of males to females) to be higher in O babies of O mothers than in A babies of A mothers, both in European and in non-European families. Since these mother-child combinations are both ABO-compatible there can be no question of materno-foetal ABO incompatibility being involved. Allan (1972, 1973) has continued to make new observations and to keep his survey of the literature up to date. He has brought to light a highly significant unevennesss in the sex-ratio according to the ABO groups of mothers and offspring, which must be taken into account in any consideration of natural selection affecting these blood groups, but its meaning is at present far from clear. Allan (1973) sums up the matter by saying, 'babies of B mothers . . . have a higher male/female ratio if of the same group as their mother than if of a different group ($P < 0{\cdot}05$), and this is true also for the babies of O mothers ($P < 0{\cdot}05$). In sharp contrast, on the other hand, babies of A mothers have a lower male/female ratio if of the same group as their mother than if of a different group ($P < 0{\cdot}0005$), and this is true also of babies of AB mothers ($P < 0{\cdot}1$).'

INTERACTION BETWEEN THE ABO AND Rh SYSTEMS

Levine, in 1943, in the same paper in which he showed that ABO incompatibility was a cause of abortions and stillbirths, pointed out that, in Rh-negative mothers of infants with haemolytic disease of the newborn, the proportion of ABO incompatible husbands is lower than in the general population. He and others soon interpreted this as a protective effect of ABO incompatibility against Rh immunization, since red cells of a foetus having inherited both the Rh(D) factor and A or B from the father would be destroyed rapidly by the mother's anti-A or anti-B, before they had time to cause Rh immunization. This in turn led to the devising, by Clarke and his colleagues in England and by Levine and his team in America, of the present effective means of prophylaxis against haemolytic disease of the newborn.

One of the most complete studies of the interactions of the Rh and ABO systems is that of Cohen (1970). In her first tables she attempts to avoid using data involving possible interactions between the ABO and Rh systems. Taking only Rh-compatible matings she compares foetal death rates in ABO-compatible and incompatible matings. Early foetal death rates are much higher in ABO-incompatible than in ABO-compatible matings, but late foetal losses are almost completely unaffected by ABO incompatibility as compared with ABO compatibility. Then, taking only ABO-compatible matings she shows the well-known effect of Rh incompatibility on late foetal losses but, rather surprisingly, a similar effect on early foetal losses. However, for early foetal losses the doubly incompatible matings show a lower rate than either of the singly incompatible classes, and close to that of the doubly compatible. It therefore appears that, as regards early foetal deaths, each type of incompatibility protects against the harmful effects of the other. For late foetal deaths the numbers are too small to be meaningful. It must also be stated that, despite the large numbers of matings included in the initial survey, the numbers of deaths are so small that only a few of the results mentioned reach statistical significance. In this clinically and scientifically important field of interaction between systems, there is therefore a need for further extensive surveys.

OTHER BLOOD GROUP SYSTEMS

In addition to the A and B antigens, and the D antigen of the Rh system, many other antigens of the Rh and other systems have, as already mentioned, sometimes caused maternal isoimmunization and haemolytic disease of the newborn. The antigens of the P system do not appear ever to be associated with such disease in the full-term newborn infant, but it has been claimed that isoimmunization to the P antigen (in the modern sense, formerly known as Tj^a) is a cause of abortion. Most of the early examples of anti-P were found in *pp* women who had had an abortion, and it was concluded that the antibody was causing the abortion of heterozygous *Pp* foetuses. When numerous further examples of the antibody were found without a history of abortion, it was questioned whether this was so, but the latest summing-up by Race and Sanger (1975) concludes that anti-P (or possibly its constant companion anti-P^k) is a potent cause of abortion. Vos *et al.* (1964) have found a similar antibody in the serum of P_1-positive women who had previously aborted and were threatened with a second abortion. As the phenomenon is not found in similar circumstances in other regions, Vos *et al.* suggest that an environmental factor may be involved.

Though the finding bears no direct relation to abortion, it is convenient to mention here that the auto-antibody which causes paroxysmal cold haemoglobinuria usually has anti-P specificity (Levine *et al.*, 1963).

TOXAEMIA OF PREGNANCY

The suggestion of Dienst (1905) that isoimmunization to the A or B antigen was a cause of eclampsia at first appeared to be supported by the finding by Pike and Dickins (1954) in women suffering from toxaemias of pregnancy, of a significant excess of group O; subsequent surveys (including that of Hanington (1961)) have failed to confirm this. As in other cases where there is a discrepancy between the results of different surveys, it is desirable that further tests should be done, with particular attention to subtle points in the selection of patients and controls, differences in which may have given rise to the discrepancy.

Jenkins *et al.* (1976) have tentatively suggested an association between pre-eclampsia and a *failure* of the patient to produce antibodies to her husband's HLA antigens, a process which is regarded as normal and presumably protective against foetal HLA antigens of paternal origin. This would suggest a possible role of HLA immunization as a protection against choriocarcinoma. Much work has been done on HLA immunization in this disease, work which has been summed up by Lawler (1976). It is clear that this is an important problem upon which more work is needed but as Lawler states, 'The choice of mate in relation to the HLA system appears not to influence a woman's chance of developing a choriocarcinoma'.

When I started to write the above section on abortion I was firmly convinced that ABO incompatibility between mother and foetus was a major cause of abortion. Having read most of the relevant evidence and criticisms I still regard the hypothesis as valid, but there are certain unexplained apparent discrepancies between the findings of different workers. However, the most direct way of testing the hypothesis is by observing the blood groups of the spontaneously aborted foetuses of parents of known groups, and observations on these are unfortunately few and not fully conclusive. There are obvious difficulties in collecting such data, and it is therefore important that any workers who may have access to such foetuses, even a few, but preferably many, should carry out a cytological examination and the relevant ABO and Rh tests, as a minimum, and make sure that the results get published. We, however, do not know how far other blood groups (or indeed histocompatibility antigens) may be involved, and very full blood testing should be carried out if this is at all possible.

HYDATIDIFORM MOLES AND CHORIOCARCINOMAS

Choriocarcinomas are malignant neoplasms in the maternal tissue, but derived from the trophoblast, the outermost layer of foetal cells forming part of the placenta. They are commonly found in the uterus itself but often elsewhere. They may arise from either an apparently normal full-term pregnancy, from an abortion or from a hydatidiform mole, an abnormal proliferation of the chorionic villi which may or may not be the sole visible product of conception; of these, moles are most particularly liable to undergo malignant change.

Since both hydatidiform moles and choriocarcinomas are, genetically, foetuses or parts of a foetus, they carry genes, and hence antigens, derived from the father as well as the mother. Hence they could be expected to behave as hetero-transplants (as, of course, would normal foetuses), and they therefore have an immunological status quite different from that of any other neoplasms occurring in human beings (though deliberate hetero-transplants of neoplasms are often done in experimental animals). Thus one would expect their fate to depend upon similarities or differences between their blood group, histocompatibility, and other antigens and those of the mother.

There have, unfortunately, been few studies of this relationship, the main ones being that of Bagshawe *et al.* (1971), and recent review articles by Lawler (1976) and Bagshawe (1976), all giving references to previous work. The following account is based on these three papers. The data consist mainly of the ABO groups of women with choriocarcinoma, and of their husbands. The relative incidence of the disease is highly dependent upon the ABO blood groups of both the patient and her husband, but not in the expected manner which would involve the rejection of a potentially malignant conceptus if it carried an A or B antigen not present in the patient (i.e. mother) (and against which she therefore carried an antibody).

If we consider only the blood groups of the patients themselves then, as expected on the above hypothesis, group O women are somewhat more liable than group A women to develop the disease. However, when husband-wife combinations are considered, it is seen that, contrary to expectation, group O women are much more liable to have the disease if their husbands are group A than if they are group O. In the case of group A women, where neither an A nor an O man should father an incompatible conceptus, the risk is much greater if the husband is group O than if he is group A. Combinations involving groups B and AB are too few to enable any conclusions to be reached. It appears, however, that it is the *difference* between the blood groups of husband and wife (and hence presumably between the woman and her conceptus) that causes increased susceptibility to the disease. It has therefore been suggested that some system in the foetus itself detects the difference and is thereby stimulated to undergo malignant change. However, in the few cases where trophoblastic tumours have followed the birth of a normal child, the blood groups of these children (presumably the same as those of the tumours) have shown a normal distribution. Lawler (1976) has therefore suggested that the antigens present in semen and on the spermatozoa (detectable only in ABH secretors) may be in some way involved.

The histocompatibility antigens might have been expected to be even more important than the blood groups in affecting the survival of foreign neoplastic tissue, but, though women with choriocarcinomas are found often to have antibodies against their husband's histocompatibility antigens, this appears to have little effect upon the incidence or progress of the disease.

Though they presumably carry both paternal and maternal genes, both moles and choriocarcinomas are found cytologically to be much more often female than male.

It is clear that the immunological relations of choriocarcinoma are even more important than those of other neoplasms, both in prognosis and, potentially, in prophylaxis and treatment. Much more investigation is needed, and is indeed being carried out. However, in view of the relative rarity of the disease it is important that as many cases as possible of choriocarcinoma as well as of moles should be referred for such investigation, and that the abnormal tissues should be preserved in such a way as not to destroy their immunological properties by fixatives. In due course the ABO groups, secretor status, and histocompatibility antigens of husband, wife, and surviving children should be ascertained. Recent work on spina bifida, described below, makes such investigations even more urgent.

SPINA BIFIDA AND ANENCEPHALY

Spina bifida represents a failure of the membranes and the vertebral arches to close over some part of the spinal cord; anencephaly is a more or less complete failure of the brain to develop. Both geographically and familially they tend to occur together. Anencephalics hardly ever survive birth and never live for more than a few days, so that they do not present an important social problem, but with modern surgery many children with spina bifida survive, and a large proportion of them have severe paralyses and incontinence. The two conditions may be regarded as variants, mainly in severity, of a single disease. Its causes are certainly multiple, but almost entirely unknown. They are partly genetical, but probably mainly environmental, so that an understanding of them might lead to a substantial degree of prevention.

A great many suggestions have been made but none, so far, has survived any prolonged critical testing. The latest suggestion, and one of the most promising, is that of Clarke *et al.* (1975) (who, like several previous workers, use the abbreviation 'ASB' for the pair of related diseases). The authors made a very thorough study of the previous literature, including data of surveys, and previous hypotheses. They then carried out a fresh and extensive survey of cases accessible to them, noting a wide range of possibly relevant features in the environment of the mother, in her obstetric history, and in the history of the family.

From these combined sources they noted that, while the geographical distributions of ASB on the one hand, and of hydatidiform moles and choriocarcinoma on the other, are to a large extent reciprocal, they occur in mothers of similar age groups. All three kinds of conceptus show a marked excess of females. There is a higher frequency of abortions affecting the pregnancy before than that after the one affected by ASB. There is a lack of concordance in occurrence of ASB in twins. The authors had noted the previous suggestion of Knox (1974) regarding the effect of trophoblastic material from the immediately preceding pregnancy.

The hypothesis of Clarke and his colleagues is that ASB arises from an interaction of the early embryo with a residue of pathological trophoblastic material in the uterus, derived from a co-twin or from a previous abnormal pregnancy—an abortion, a stillbirth, or a hydatidiform mole.

This hypothesis will no doubt be modified considerably as

fresh evidence becomes available, but it appears to be one of the most promising yet to be proposed. The authors make various suggestions for further tests, and are no doubt already carrying some of these out. These include blood-grouping tests on parents and offspring. It is rather surprising that there are at present so few data on blood groups of ASB children (Sidana *et al.*, 1970; Coffey, 1974).

It would be of interest to assemble data on blood groups of parents and ASB children, and the sexes of the latter, also on the blood groups of the parents of, and the cytological sexes of, hydatidiform moles and choriocarcinomas, and to see whether these bear any relation to the data, mentioned above, on sex ratios in normal children in relation to their blood groups and those of their parents.

Further suggestions by Clarke *et al.* are: a search for genetic mosaicism (for instance by placental enzyme studies), the following up of series of mothers having had spontaneous and induced abortions, with determination of chorionic gonadotrophin levels in these and, as a control, in women having had normal pregnancies, cytogenetic sex determinations on ASB infants including placentas, and on the hairy patches which tend to cover the spinal defect. With the large amount of investigation now in progress on ASB, the problem of its aetiology must surely soon be solved.

AN INTERACTION BETWEEN THE ABO AND HAPTOGLOBIN SYSTEMS

It was first shown by Ritter and Hinkelmann (1966) and subsequently confirmed by Kirk and his colleagues (Kirk *et al.*, 1970; Kirk, 1971) and by Ananthakrishnan *et al.* (1973) that in matings where the father is incompatible with the mother with respect to the ABO groups, the children show a higher frequency of the Hp^1 gene than do those of families, drawn from the same population, in which the father is ABO-compatible. This was explained as due to deaths from haemolytic disease of the newborn resulting from ABO incompatibility (though mostly unrecognized as such), and related to the fact that the product of the Hp^1 gene is more efficient than that of Hp^2 in removing dissolved haemoglobin from the plasma and conserving the contained iron. Thus in cases where foetuses, or newborn children, are affected by haemolytic disease due to foetal A or B inherited from the father, one who is of type Hp 1–1 should have the best, and one who is Hp 2–2 the worst, chance of survival.

The populations examined by Kirk (1971) included the S-leut subdivision of the Hutterite sect of the United States. Vana and Steinberg (1975) have now examined further families of the S-leut, and also families of the other main subdivision, the L-leut. In both they confirm the tendency towards raised Hp^1 frequencies among the offspring of ABO incompatible matings, but further analysis of the data has shown that the Hp^1 frequencies are intrinsic to the blood groups themselves, irrespective of the type of mating from which they come. They conclude that there is a tendency, which they cannot at present explain, for Hp^1 frequencies to increase with blood group in the order: O, A, B, AB, and indeed in the order of genotypes: *OO*, *AO*, *BO*, *AB*, *AA*, *BB*. This explanation does not, of course, exclude some form of underlying natural selection either of gametes or zygotes.

AN APPARENT INTERACTION BETWEEN THE ABO AND THE PLACENTAL ALKALINE PHOSPHATASE SYSTEMS

Bottini *et al.* (1972), in a single series of observations, have found indications that homozygotes for the placental alkaline phosphatase gene $Pl^{F}{}_{1}$ are protected against haemolytic disease of the newborn resulting from B immunization of the mother, but not from that due to A immunization. It is desirable that similar surveys should be carried out on other populations.

7

PEPTIC ULCERS

VERY soon after the discovery of the association of gastric cancer with blood group A, the original team showed (Aird *et al.*, 1954) that peptic ulceration was strongly associated with group O. This finding was followed up by Clarke *et al.* (1955), who demonstrated that when duodenal and gastric ulcers were classified separately, the former were much more strongly associated with group O than the latter—indeed, it at first appeared that gastric ulceration might not be blood-group associated at all, but subsequent work has shown that it is. The very highly significant A/O and B/O relative incidences for duodenal ulcers are 0·73 and 0·80 respectively, whereas for gastric ulcers both ratios have the value 0·87.

While most workers have classified peptic ulcers only into gastric and duodenal, Johnson (1965) has carried out an elaborate analysis of gastric ulcers as to type and position, and to the presence of other ulcers, in relation to ABO blood-group association. His classification is too long to reproduce here in full, and readers who require the complete details should refer to the original paper. His three main types, to which cases are allocated in the tables, are as follows:

Type 1. Ulcer of the body of the stomach, without abnormality of the duodenum, pylorus, or prepyloric region.

Type 2. Ulcer of the body of the stomach combined with an ulcer or its scar in the duodenum or at the pylorus.

Type 3. Gastric ulcer close to the pylorus. Lesions in this position which were combined with duodenal ulcers, or with a type 2 ulcer proximal to them, were all classified as type 3.

Ulcers of type 1 showed an almost normal ABO distribution while those of types 2 and 3 showed an excess of group O.

In the case of duodenal ulcers Buckwalter *et al.* (1960) and Clarke (1961) investigated the relation of blood groups to ulcers in selected sibships within which some members but not others had ulcers, with particular reference to those sibships which contained both A and O members. They were surprised to find that in the sibships there was no significant association between blood group and ulceration. They did, however, find a just significant association of ulcers with non-secretion within sibships.

These results led Langman and Doll (1965) to suggest that the cause of the apparent association between group O and ulceration was the method of ascertainment, and that it was not the ulceration, but the bleeding often associated with it, that brought patients into hospital, and so led to their being included in a blood-group investigation. Therefore these authors (and subsequently others) investigated the blood groups of a series of ulcer patients classified for bleeding and non-bleeding and in various other ways. The combined results of all investigators showed that for gastric ulcers there is a highly significant association of group O with bleeding as compared with non-bleeding cases, and the non-bleeding ones show no blood-group association, as would be expected if the group-O association were due entirely to the bleeding tendency of the ulcers. While, however, in the case of duodenal ulcers the association between bleeding and group O is even stronger than for gastric ulcers, even the non-bleeding cases show a highly significant association with group O as compared with the general population.

Various surgical operations have been devised to protect the duodenal mucosa from the erosive effects of the acid and proteolytic gastric secretion, which involve the creation of a new entrance or stoma to the small intestine. In most cases ulceration then ceases to occur, but in a small proportion of patients ulceration recurs on the stoma itself. It was suggested (Langman and Doll, 1965) that the patients so affected, having a particularly strong propensity to ulceration, might show an even higher frequency of group O than those affected by simple duodenal ulcers, and this was indeed found to be the case, the frequency of group O being about twice as high in such patients as in the general population—relative incidences being A/O, 0·53; B/O, 0·48. However, numbers are too small to enable any clear conclusion to be reached as regards possible blood-group associations of the bleeding tendency in stomal ulcer patients.

Soon after Aird *et al.* (1953) first showed an association between the ABO blood groups and gastric cancer, Sheppard (1953) drew attention to the fact that the gastric mucosa was one of the tissues affected by the blood-group secretor polymorphism, and suggested that in future investigations in this field the secretor status should be ascertained. This was done in the case of duodenal ulceration by Clarke *et al.* (1956). This and subsequent papers have shown a strong association between non-secretion and both duodenal and gastric ulceration. It might therefore be thought that the actual secretion of blood-group A substance was directly protecting the mucosa from ulceration. However, this simple explanation cannot be upheld, since the relative reduction of the risk of ulceration in A as compared with O persons is as great in non-secretors (who secrete neither A nor H) as it is in secretors.

In contrast with the blood groups, the effect of secretor status on ulceration is, as already mentioned, found within sibships as well as in the general population. As expected from this finding, Langman and Doll (1965) have found in a prospective survey that secretor status (unlike the ABO group) does not significantly affect the tendency of a duodenal ulcer to bleed (since there is no need to call in a bleeding tendency to account for the secretion association in the whole ulcer population, as there is according to them for the blood-group association). There is some disagreement between different authors on this point, clearly related to the smallness of the samples, and the overall result is a small and quite non-significant association between bleeding and non-secretion. For gastric ulcers Langman and Doll themselves find such an association, rather more marked than for duodenal ulcers but still not significant.

The relation between group O and a tendency towards haemorrhage is found in a number of diseases and is further discussed on pages 34–5.

Since the ABO groups and ABH secretion jointly affect the

tendency to peptic ulceration, and also jointly affect the passage into the blood plasma of intestinal alkaline phosphatase (p. 6), it is not unlikely that the phosphatase passage mechanism has some bearing on the aetiology of peptic ulcers. One aspect of this problem has been discussed by Langman *et al.* (1969) in relation to celiac disease.

Duodenal ulceration is the one of the few diseases which (partly because of the very large number of observations) shows a significant association with the Rh groups. The combined relative incidence D+/D− is, however, only 1·11. The corresponding ratio for gastric ulceration is 1·02.

Kaplan *et al.* (1964) have investigated the relation of the taster and non-taster types to gastric and duodenal ulceration. They used 6-n-propylthiouracil (PROP) instead of phenylthiocarbamide (PTC) but this should not appreciably have affected their results. They used the taste-threshold method, with elaborate controls. They found a raised frequency of what they called 'sensitive tasters' among duodenal-ulcer patients as compared with the controls, but since even in the ulcer cases the proportion of sensitive tasters was considerably lower than those found by other workers for 'tasters' among either white or black Americans, it is difficult to interpret their results and the latter do not appear in our tables.

It has been known for some years that there is an association between peptic ulcers and pulmonary emphysema (Hegetschweiler *et al.*, 1960). This was explained when it was shown that trypsin-inhibitor deficiency, besides causing pulmonary emphysema, has a raised frequency among cases of both gastric and duodenal ulcers (Kalliomäki and Seppälä, 1971). André *et al.* (1974) found an approximately trebled frequency of the deficiency in both gastric and duodenal ulcer cases, as compared with controls, the difference being statistically significant in the case of duodenal ulcers. There can thus be little doubt that trypsin inhibitor deficiency is of some aetiological importance in peptic ulceration.

There appears to be a need for a fresh study of duodenal and perhaps also of gastric ulceration, taking into account ABO groups, ABH secretion, trypsin inhibitor types, and PTC tasting, and with special attention paid to the presence or absence of bleeding. Such a study should begin with a survey of unrelated patients, but should if possible be followed by family studies (see p. 51).

8

DIABETES MELLITUS

It has long been realized that diabetes mellitus is a syndrome rather than a disease or, to put it another way, that several diseases of differing aetiology are classed together under the name.

This heterogeneity is reflected in the results of analyses of data relating to the degree of association of one or other of the ABO blood groups with diabetes. There is a highly significant overall association of the condition with blood group A, as compared with O. The data are hardly sufficient to define the status of groups B and AB, and the rest of this discussion will be concerned almost solely with the A/O ratio. The total data show a combined relative A/O incidence of 1·07, with a value of χ^2 of 18·83 which, for one degree of freedom, is highly significant ($P < 0{\cdot}0001$). However, the value of χ^2 for homogeneity is 81 which, even for 42 degrees of freedom, implies a probability of less than 0·0002 that this or a higher degree of heterogeneity could have occurred by chance. It should be noted that the heterogeneity implied is not between individual patients but between the forty-three separate sets of patients included in the analysis. Thus not only is the disease a heterogeneous one, but different clinics, most of them not deliberately selective among diabetes cases, must be attracting or accepting the different variants of the disease in significantly different proportions.

As in all cases where such heterogeneity has been found, we have scrutinized the data further to try to define the relevant variants of the disease which are being merged under the term 'diabetes mellitus'. In this we, as well as those who have produced the individual series of observations, have been guided by previous clinical observations on the varying manifestations of the disease. The main variables used in this further analysis have been sex and age. Far more of the data have been classified by sex than by age. For those series where the relevant breakdown is available, the relative A/O ratio for males as compared with controls is 1·12 ($\chi^2 = 13{\cdot}4$, $P < 0{\cdot}0003$) but for females the ratio is only 1·07 ($\chi^2 = 5{\cdot}31$, $P < 0{\cdot}02$). Comparing males with females the relative incidence A/O is 1·08 ($\chi^2 = 3{\cdot}99$, $P < 0{\cdot}05$, or just significant).

There is not only a strong indication of a higher A/O ratio in males than in females, but the values of χ^2 for homogeneity for the comparisons by sex show a non-significant degree of heterogeneity.

In all the above analyses the four non-European series contribute an undue proportion of the total heterogeneity, which needs further investigation on a variety of large non-European population samples, each anthropologically homogeneous.

For analysis by age the numbers available are smaller than for sex, and different authors specify age in different ways, as can be seen by the descriptions used in the tables. Because of the use of such terms as 'Men and women' and 'Mothers' on the one hand, and 'Juveniles' and 'Children' on the other as the sole description of age groups, we have, in order to bring in the largest possible (though still rather small) numbers, arbitrarily drawn the dividing line at the age of 20.

The children now show a new feature, an A/O relative incidence below unity, of 0·86. The value of χ^2 is only 2·662 which is non-significant ($P =$ approx. 0·10). Adults show a combined relative incidence of 1·10, with a χ^2 value of 14·323, which is highly significant. Unfortunately, with one exception, further discussed below, the published data classified by age do not allow direct comparison within single populations. However, the fall of the relative A/O ratio below unity in juveniles, though non-significant, and the relatively high ratio in the samples consisting solely of adults, taken together, suggest a marked difference. This is fortunately supported by the highly detailed observations of Andersen and Lauritzen (1960), who have most generously made their protocols available to us, showing classification not merely by sex and 5-year age groups, but by the presence or absence of a number of other common manifestations of diabetes mellitus. Their cases with an onset below 10 years of age show an A/O ratio below unity, which steadily rises throughout life so that, as most other workers also find, all the adult ages show an excess of A. Not only the results of Andersen and Lauritzen but all relevant data combined show that the A/O ratio continues to rise at least to the age of 40. This is further discussed below.

Other criteria: the presence or absence of a family history, and the need or lack of need for insulin, do not, on the data at present available, appear to affect the A/O ratio. There is also a disagreement between different series of results as to the correlation, if any, between presence or absence of retinopathy and the A/O ratio.

HISTOCOMPATIBILITY ANTIGENS

Various workers have found a marked association of diabetes mellitus with three of the histocompatibility antigens, HLA-B8, B18, and Bw15. The association is definitely with the juvenile onset type. The increased risks of developing this type of diabetes for individuals carrying the three antigens mentioned are respectively 2·13, 1·72, and 2·11. These figures are very much higher than those for the ABO groups and thus, though tests have included only hundreds of individuals rather than the thousands tested for ABO, the significance of the associations is already overwhelming.

Cudworth and Woodrow (1975) have studied a number of families in which juvenile-onset diabetes is present. In one family three juvenile diabetics and one child with an abnormal glucose tolerance test (also one healthy sib) share the W29.8 haplotype. Two of these, aged 13 and 21 respectively at the time, developed acute-onset diabetes simultaneously after an influenza-like illness; this suggests that the presence of a gene closely linked to the histocompatibility series renders individuals particularly susceptible to a virus infection, one of the manifestations of which is the onset of diabetes mellitus. The authors cite evidence that Coxsackie B_4 virus may be a precipitating factor in acute-onset juvenile diabetes. They point out that some variants of the encephalomyocarditis virus and Coxsackie B virus have been shown experimentally to produce islet-cell damage in mice, and suggest that genes in the chromosomal HL-A region might influence the virus-receptor sites or modify adversely the immune response to certain viruses.

On the basis of rather small numbers of tests, no significant association has been found between diabetes of adult onset and any of the histocompatibility antigens. However, Schernthaner *et al.* (1976) have recently distinguished between an association with HLA-B8 in diabetes of childhood onset and one with HLA-B8, HLA-BW15, and HLA-CW3 in disease of later juvenile onset. This is consistent with the progressive, rather than sudden, increase with age, of the association with group A, and suggests the possible existence of three types of diabetes each with a different range of ages of onset, and pattern of association, or non-association, with the antigens of the ABO and HLA systems.

Diabetes mellitus is also very significantly associated with ABH secretion and with PTC non-tasting, but the data are insufficient to determine whether this is related to age of onset, and further age-based data are needed on these associations.

DIABETES AND NATURAL SELECTION

It has long been realized that diabetes, and especially the type with adult onset, is to a marked extent hereditary, though it clearly is not due to a single fully penetrant gene. Indeed, as we have just seen, the expression of any specific diabetogenic gene is influenced by age, sex, ABO blood group, and ABH secretor and (somewhat doubtfully) PTC tasting types, if not also by other genetic and environmental factors.

It has long been a puzzle, as with certain other strongly hereditary diseases, how this disease could persist at a relatively high frequency in the community despite its high mortality before the introduction of modern therapeutic methods.

Aschner and Post (1956–7) supplied part of the answer when they proved that women with a hereditary tendency to diabetes were on the average more fertile than normal women, and Post and White (1958) further showed that they began to menstruate younger.

Lehmann (1959), however, set these observations in a broader anthropological and evolutionary context by pointing out that in palaeolithic times, when man lived on a low-calorie, low-carbohydrate diet, frank diabetes would rarely develop and thus high fecundity would have maintained the frequency of the gene. Neel (1967), following up the same theme, referred to those with the hereditary diabetic tendency as having a 'thrifty genotype' which would confer a positive advantage upon those possessing it, under conditions of food shortage. Neel was thinking of diabetes of juvenile onset, but if, as suggested earlier in this chapter, juvenile diabetes is the consequence of a virus disease, it might be more appropriate to apply his arguments to the early physiological manifestations of the adult-onset type of disease.

The validity of these arguments appears to be borne out by the observations of Jenkins *et al.* (1974) on the San (Bushmen) of the Kalahari Desert who live on a sparse but by no means starvation diet. These workers found rather low fasting blood-glucose levels but these rose rapidly when a dose of glucose was given, and remained high in a manner which, in Europeans, would have indicated a diabetic tendency.

We may thus suppose that the diabetic diathesis was, and locally still is, advantageous under primitive conditions but, with the availability of an adequate or more than adequate carbohydrate-rich diet, it now gives rise in adult life to frank diabetes mellitus.

9

RHEUMATIC FEVER AND RHEUMATIC HEART DISEASE

THOSE diseases of the circulation which show significant blood-group associations nearly all fall into two distinct categories—rheumatic fever and consequent heart disease on the one hand, and diseases, mostly degenerative, affecting the whole blood-vascular system and the coagulation process on the other. In the context of this book the two categories are so clearly separate as to demand separate chapters, though the present one, on the rheumatic diseases, is somewhat short.

Rheumatic fever is a special immunological response of the whole body to infection by the α-haemolytic streptococcus, usually beginning in the throat but, though the most obvious acute symptoms affect the joints, the organ which is usually the most dangerously affected, both in the acute stage and in the long-term sequelae, is the heart.

In (acute) rheumatic fever A and B frequencies are both raised, the relative incidences being A/O 1·14; B/O, 1·10, only the former being statistically significant. The frequency of non-secretors is significantly raised; the relative incidence sec/non-sec being 0·78.

In rheumatic heart disease relative incidences of both A and B are considerably and significantly raised: A/O, 1·23; B/O, 1·28, but that of secretion is only slightly lowered, to 0·91. All these incidences are based on adequate samples, of one to five thousand individuals. In both diseases frequencies of Rh-negatives are very slightly and non-significantly increased.

It is of interest to compare these observations with the results of tests on other forms and sequelae of streptococcal infection. Chronic infection with α-haemolytic streptococcus shows a markedly raised frequency of group A, but as only 100 patients were tested the results are not significant, while tests on over 3000 cases of scarlet fever, which is due to a particular strain of the α-haemolytic streptococcus, show a lowering of the A/O relative incidence, to 0·88. In each case the B/O ratio is almost unaffected. Individuals positive for the Dick test show a raising of A/O and B/O relative incidences, in each case to 1·46, when compared with negative reactors, who are the ones who remain susceptible to scarlet fever. A not uncommon sequel to scarlet fever is chronic nephritis, or nephrosis. Most, though perhaps not all, cases described as nephrosis, nephritis, chronic nephritis, and nephritis-nephrosis probably come under this heading. On a total of only about 500 cases they show a very slight depression of A and a slight excess of B. They show also non-significantly raised frequencies of secretors, and of Rh-positives. In chronic infections with the α-haemolytic streptococcus the ABH secretor frequency is significantly lowered. Further data on this condition would be of interest.

If we concentrate on the A/O ratio, disregarding for the moment fluctuations of the frequency of B, which are mostly of low statistical significance, owing to the general relative rarity of this blood group, we find a raising of the A frequency in acute rheumatic fever, and even more so in rheumatic heart disease—and also in Dick positive reactors, who have developed an immunity to the streptococcus; while sufferers from scarlet fever, and Dick negative persons, who have not developed an immunity to it, have a lowered A/O ratio.

Thus blood group A would appear to favour the development of both a normal immunological response to the streptococcus, as in the positive Dick reaction, and an abnormal one, as in acute rheumatic fever, while group O persons tend to remain susceptible to acute infection as in scarlet fever. It is difficult to explain this, for if an A-like antigen were present in the bacteria then it would be the O and B persons who would the more readily make antibodies to it. Perhaps it is the higher level of antigen H activity in O than in A individuals which is involved, the A persons more readily making an antibody to an H-like antigen. The secretor relations are even more difficult to explain. The relations of the blood-group and bacterial antigens to those of the affected cardiac, renal, and articular tissues need further investigation. See also 'Diseases of the genito-urinary system (p. 37).

Rheumatoid arthritis has sometimes been thought to bear a relation to rheumatic fever. In rheumatoid arthritis, however, the frequencies of both A and B, especially the former, are markedly and significantly lowered, not as in rheumatic fever but as in scarlet fever, another type of response to the α-haemolytic streptococcus. The data are, however, highly heterogeneous. Rh-positive frequencies are somewhat raised, again a trend opposite to that found in rheumatic fever and heart disease. Rheumatoid arthritis is well known to have an important immunological aspect, shown by the presence of 'rheumatoid factor' in the serum, and the findings just mentioned are likely to bear some relation to this.

Ankylosing spondylitis, which bears some superficial similarity to rheumatoid arthritis, shows only slightly and quite non-significantly raised A/O and B/O ratios. Its autoimmune nature is stressed by its very close association with the histocompatibility antigen HLA-B27. Rather strong associations with this antigen are shown also by Reiter's disease, by arthritis associated with *Yersinia* and *Salmonella* infections, by psoriatic arthropathy, and by juvenile rheumatoid arthritis (Still's disease) (see also p. 46). Adequate ABO and secretor data for all these conditions would be of considerable interest.

10

THROMBOSIS, HAEMORRHAGE, AND OTHER DISORDERS OF THE CIRCULATORY SYSTEM

OF the disorders of the circulatory system, rheumatic fever and heart disease have been considered in the previous chapter. The remaining disorders of this system are mainly cardiovascular degenerative conditions, some of which tend to provoke episodes of thrombosis or haemorrhage.

THROMBOSIS

The decision to bring together consideration of these particular diseases arises from an investigation carried out by the present authors some years ago (Mourant *et al.*, 1971) into the relation of the ABO groups to thrombosis, which led on to a study of vascular conditions in general, and which arose from the then recent discovery of the association of thromboembolic episodes with the use of oral contraceptives.

Slone *et al.* (1969) had observed a deficiency of group O among medical patients with a tendency to thrombosis, who were under treatment with anticoagulants. This led Jick *et al.* (1969) to bring together data on the blood groups of women taking oral contraceptives and suffering from thromboembolism and (separately) pregnant and puerperal women with the same disorder. They also brought together a small number of other cases of thromboembolism. In each case there was a deficiency of group O.

When we became aware of this work, we collected together from the literature all the data which we could find on blood groups in cases of thrombosis of all kinds. At first we classed together coronary thrombosis with cases described by such names as 'coronary occlusion' and 'coronary insufficiency'. We found a highly significant excess of group A among all these cases taken together, but with a quite unacceptable degree of heterogeneity between the sets of cases included. We therefore tried segregating those cases clearly described as coronary thrombosis or cardiac infarction from all other cases of coronary disease. The cases of thrombosis now showed a highly significant and homogeneous excess of A, while the remainder showed an A/O relative incidence which did not significantly exceed unity, and which was statistically homogeneous.

These trends show very clearly in the considerably larger numbers of cases which we have now been able to tabulate. Other miscellaneous cases of thrombosis behave similarly to coronary thrombosis, and in all cases the B/O relative incidence is also very significantly raised, though in most cases not to quite the same level as A/O.

Unfortunately we have not been able to persuade our colleagues to collect many further cases of thrombosis in young women, either taking oral contraceptives or pregnant or puerperal, but the extremely high A/O and B/O relative incidences have been maintained in the new data of Westerholm *et al.* (1971). It is much to be desired that further data should be collected about such women, for they have an obvious relevance to advice on contraception, and the doubled incidence of thrombosis in A and B as compared with O women undergoing normal pregnancy and childbirth needs confirmation on larger numbers if it is to serve as a warning to the obstetrician of possible increased danger.

There are indications also of a particularly high A/O ratio in young as compared with older men suffering from coronary thrombosis. Indeed, it was in their work on coronary heart disease in young adults that Gertler and White (1954) appear to have been the first investigators to notice any association between blood groups and thrombosis. We have, however, been able to find only one subsequent study of myocardial infarction in the young (Ciswicka-Sznajderman *et al.*, 1973). It is much to be desired that fuller data should be collected on this age class, to add to our growing knowledge of the genetics of premature cardiovascular disease, and to guide the clinicians responsible for prophylactic treatment.

In our earlier investigation another source of heterogeneity was found, in that the data for coronary thrombosis in persons not of European or Jewish descent showed, on the whole, particularly high A/O relative incidences. Some authorities consider that such persons have an inborn relative resistance to coronary thrombosis.

The data, as far as they go, thus suggest that the A and B frequencies are particularly high in just those classes of person who do not as a rule suffer from thrombotic episodes, namely women of child-bearing age, young men, and perhaps non-Europeans, and that when members of these classes are exposed to stresses liable to cause thrombosis, the A and B members are especially at risk.

Of other degenerative vascular conditions, hypertension, on the basis of nearly 5000 cases, shows a striking degree of normality of blood group-frequencies.

The marked excess of group O in 180 cases of malignant hypertension needs confirmation on larger numbers. In arteriosclerosis, on the other hand, A and B frequencies are very significantly raised, though to a somewhat less degree than in thrombosis. The observed rise is probably an intrinsic characteristic of arteriosclerosis itself, but may be in part due to limited coronary or other thrombosis, not diagnosed as such, bringing some of the cases to hospital.

HAEMORRHAGE

Langman and Doll (1965) were the first to demonstrate that the observed association of duodenal ulceration with blood group O was due, at least in part, to a specific association of bleeding with group O, explained by the fact that the admission of ulcer cases to hospital is often precipitated by an attack of haemorrhage (see p. 29).

Their work and that of others has shown that, in both duodenal and gastric ulceration, the frequency of group O is higher in those who bleed than in those who do not.

Jick *et al.* (1969) appear to have been the first to suggest that there was a connection between the association of thrombosis with group A and that of haemorrhage with group O, and to relate this to the higher average levels of antihaemophilic globulin in the blood of group A than of group O persons (Preston and Barr, 1964).

We have therefore paid particular attention to possible blood-group associations of haemorrhages of all kinds.

In nearly 2500 cases investigated because of haemorrhage of various kinds (cerebral, gastrointestinal, nasal, related to pregnancy or childbirth, post-operative, haemoptysis, haematuria) the combined A/O relative incidence is 0·75 while the corresponding B/O is 0·80.

In pulmonary tuberculosis (p. 18), comparing haemorrhagic with non-haemorrhagic cases, similar relative frequencies are found to those observed, as discussed on page 29, with peptic ulcers of all kinds (apart from stomal ulcers, where the small number of bleeders (63) give a B/O relative incidence of 1·68, which is almost certainly affected by sampling error).

Secondary anaemia (which results from chronic haemorrhage), menorrhagia, and menopausal metrorrhagia all show depressed A/O incidence, and the first and third of these, depressed B/O also.

A study which emphasizes these relations is that of Ionescu *et al.* (1976) on cerebral strokes. Cases diagnosed as stroke by general practitioners showed blood-group frequencies not differing significantly from the controls, whereas cases brought to post-mortem, and then diagnosed either as cerebral haemorrhage or cerebral thrombosis, showed the expected raised A/O ratio in thrombosis and depressed A/O in haemorrhage. The B/O ratio was slightly depressed in both conditions, but this may have been due to sampling error arising from the small numbers of B patients involved.

Some years ago (Mourant *et al.*, 1971) we stressed the need for further investigations into the relation between the ABO blood groups and the clotting mechanism. With the demonstration, noted in this chapter, of the wide ramifications of the empirical relationship, the need for such investigations has increased with time. Studies should include an exploration of the possible effects of the ABH secretor factor and of the presence or absence in the plasma of intestinal alkaline phosphatase (p. 6). Also, now that a relatively rapid method has been devised (Bartlett *et al.*, 1976) for measuring the amount, as distinct from the clotting activity, of the haemophilia-related factor VIII gene product, it would be of interest, in view of the above-mentioned findings of Preston and Barr (1964), to study both parameters in a series of persons of different blood groups.

11
VARIOUS DISEASES

In this chapter a wide range of diseases will be discussed which either do not show significant associations with any of the ABO groups or, if they do, require only relatively short descriptions. Where any of them show significant associations with other polymorphisms, these also will be mentioned.

ENDOCRINE AND METABOLIC DISEASES

Of the endocrine and metabolic diseases, diabetes and thyroid diseases have chapters to themselves; toxaemia of pregnancy is discussed with disorders related to pregnancy (p. 26). Rickets, which shows no significant ABO association, is further mentioned on page 8, in view of the possibility of its association with the Gc system.

The highly heterogeneous remainder of this group of diseases, pellagra, coeliac disease, haemochromatosis, spasmophilia, and hypogammaglobulinaemia, all show slight and quite non-significant associations with group O. Celiac disease is further discussed in relation to the histocompatibility system. Hypogammaglobulinaemia is due to a specific gene and so would not be expected to show association.

DISEASES OF THE BLOOD AND HAEMATOPOIETIC SYSTEM

Few blood diseases show significant associations with the ABO system. Outstanding among the few that do is pernicious anaemia. The study of this disease was begun very soon after the discovery of the association of group A with carcinoma of the stomach, because the latter is not infrequently an accompaniment of pernicious anaemia. Highly significant associations were found with groups A and B at the expense of O. It is noteworthy that neither in pernicious anaemia nor in stomach cancer is there any significant association with ABH secretion.

Most of the other forms of anaemia show a deficiency of group A and this is most marked in the case of secondary anaemia. Since most cases of this condition are due to haemorrhage this is yet another example of the tendency of group O to be associated with haemorrhages of all kinds (p. 35). It is possible that there is also a haemorrhagic element in the aetiology of many of the other anaemias.

The excess of A and B in idiopathic thrombocytopenic purpura is interesting and it would be desirable to test more cases of this disease.

The large and highly significant excess of A and of B in tropical eosinophilia requires explanation. Though the condition is not associated with worm parasites, it should be noted that infestations with these, which tend to cause eosinophilia, tend likewise to be associated with group A.

MENTAL DISORDERS

Mental disorders show no associations of any apparent importance. Manic-depressive psychosis is just significantly associated with group O and psychopathy with group A. The apparent strong association of schizophrenia with group B is due almost entirely to one of the forty-three sets of data. Senile dementia, post-encephalitic psychosis, and mental retardation all show a deficiency of Rh-negatives, but at least for the first two of these conditions numbers are very small. However, a small proportion of cases of mental retardation are probably sequelae of kernicterus, a manifestation of haemolytic disease of the newborn in Rh-positive children of Rh-negative mothers.

Alcoholism, on the basis of nearly 1400 cases, shows a very close approximation to normal ABO frequencies. There is an apparent excess of non-secretion among the patients but this could, for once, be due to a pharmacogenetic disturbance of the expression of the secretor gene. Overall results for the Rhesus groups show an excess of Rh-negatives, but the two papers on this subject point in completely opposite directions.

DISEASES OF THE NERVOUS SYSTEM AND SENSE ORGANS

In contrast with mental diseases, several non-neoplastic nervous-system and sense-organ diseases show significant ABO group association. The strong association of Huntington's chorea with groups A and B is difficult to explain, as this is a disease due to a single dominantly expressed gene. Since it is present in only a small proportion of all families it is likely that in this case we are dealing with a true population stratification, with the families accessible to the sole investigator having an accidentally raised A and B frequency. This point could be settled by investigating siblings and other close relatives, especially aged ones who have escaped the disease. If, on the other hand, A and B groups tend to precipitate symptoms at an early age in those carrying the corresponding gene, the frequency of A and B in middle-aged relatives without current symptoms should be lowered while that in elderly healthy relatives should be normal.

Multiple sclerosis, on the basis of 2242 cases, shows a marked association with group O at the expense of both A and B. One investigation (Simpson *et al.*, 1965) showed a higher frequency of O in the mild than in the severe cases. There is no overall association with the Rhesus blood groups. However, both for the ABO and Rh systems the data show marked heterogeneity. It is therefore important that further data should be obtained, with particular care paid to the diagnostic criteria of the disease as a whole, and, if possible, to its quantitative and qualitative variations. Multiple sclerosis also shows a strong association with certain of the histocompatibility antigens, and is considered in greater detail in relation to these (p. 52).

Parkinson's disease shows a significant deficiency of A in comparison with both O and B.

Epilepsy, on over 3000 cases, shows no appreciable disturbance of the A/O ratio, but a considerable excess of B, with a relative incidence of 1·22 though with considerable heterogeneity between population samples. Much of the excess of B arises from one paper, that of Gala and Gala (1966) who find a B/O relative incidence of 3·63. If the data from this paper are omitted the B/O relative incidence is diminished, but only to 1·16, which is still significant.

All errors of refraction show an excess of group A and most also in excess of B. In the case of myopia the relative incidences for both A/O and B/O are 2·6. The total number tested is, however, only 519, and there is some disagreement between authors, so that the collection of further data is desirable.

For glaucoma the frequency of A is significantly increased in proportion to B and O. Owing to claims of association of glaucoma with goitre, and with the PTC taster system, this disease is further considered on page 41.

DISEASES OF THE GENITO-URINARY SYSTEM

Non-malignant diseases of the genito-urinary system present few examples of significant ABO association, but numbers tested are in most cases small. Most types of nephritis and nephrosis show a lowered incidence of A. This is of interest since many of these, especially chronic nephritis, are likely to be the result of haemolytic streptococcal infection which tends to be associated with group O (see p. 18).

Urinary calculi and prostatic hypertrophy, on the basis of about 4000 cases of each, show no significant disturbance of ABO frequencies.

Azoospermia, on only fifty cases, shows an extreme deficiency of both A and B. As this may in some cases be an immune condition the finding may be of some prognostic importance and it is desirable that further series of cases should be examined.

Menorrhagia and menopausal metrorrhagia, both on rather small numbers, show a diminution of the A/O relative incidence, such as is found in almost all haemorrhagic conditions (p. 35). Miluničová *et al.* (1969a) find a significantly raised frequency of PTC tasters in menopausal metrorrhagia.

DISEASES OF THE MUSCULO-SKELETAL SYSTEM AND CONNECTIVE TISSUE

Among musculo-skeletal and connective tissue diseases, rheumatoid arthritis and ankylosing spondylitis have been discussed on page 33.

Most other diseases of this system have been tested only in small numbers and show nothing to suggest any important association. However, over 2600 cases of bone fracture show a raised frequency of A and B with both A/O and B/O relative incidences having the value 1·12, which in the case of A/O is significant. This finding has been cited as discrediting the whole effort to find associations of blood groups with diseases, on the assumption that bone fractures are purely of mechanical causation. However, we know that some individuals suffer from an inborn bone fragility, and it is not unlikely that, among normally healthy persons there is a range of strength of the bones which is genetically determined.

CONGENITAL MALFORMATIONS

Most inborn anatomical anomalies tend to run in families but few show any well-defined pattern of inheritance. They are, in general, probably each the product of genes at a number of different loci, acting together with drugs and other external influences to which the pregnant woman is subject.

A surprising number of cases of such anomalies has been examined for ABO blood-group associations, but only four show any significant association.

Pulmonary stenosis shows a just significantly raised A/O ratio, with B/O also somewhat raised. Perhaps, however, these results are an accident of sampling. This appears to be a purely anatomical disturbance which must have arisen at an early stage of pregnancy.

Congenital pyloric stenosis shows a very significant lowering of group A as compared with B and O. This anomaly is thought to be, at least in part, a physiological one, tending to occur in first-born males. The lowered A/O ratio may bear some relation to that found in gastric and duodenal ulcer and in gastritis. The frequency of ABH secretors is raised in pyloric stenosis.

Congenital dislocation of the hip occurs mainly in certain limited areas of Europe, sometimes in well-defined isolates. The doubled frequency of B found among cases, may therefore point to a stratification of the population outside the high-incidence areas. Any further investigation should pay particular attention to the birth places of the parents and more distant ancestors.

The mere twenty cases of xeroderma pigmentosum show a marked and technically 'significant' excess of O, but this is likely to be the result of an accident of sampling. Over 3000 cases of Down's syndrome (mongolism) show blood-group frequencies very near those of the controls. This is not unexpected in a disease due to a single chromosome trisomy.

ALLERGIC DISEASES

It might have been expected, since allergy is an immunological phenomenon, that allergic diseases would tend to show disturbances of blood-group frequencies. It is therefore rather disappointing to find that, apart from asthma and eczema, series of cases of allergic disorders examined for blood groups have been rather few, and the results for allergy as a whole rather inconclusive.

Asthma, on the basis of 1684 cases, shows an A/O relative incidence of 1·13 which is just below the conventional significance level, while the corresponding B/O ratio of 1·47 is highly significant.

For allergic rhinitis (hay fever) the relative incidences for 320 cases are, A/O, 0·94; B/O, 1·26, neither of which is significant. In a series of 435 cases described as 'asthma and/or hay fever', similar values are found. The raised B/O ratio in all these cases is of interest and needs following up in direct immunological investigations of these diseases.

Eczema, on the basis of 883 cases shows no significant departure from control ABO frequencies, nor do urticaria and dermatitis though both of the latter show a somewhat raised B. However, a series of 260 cases of 'dermatosis' shows a greatly raised A and a considerably raised B frequency.

Allergic diseases are further discussed in relation to the histocompatibility system on pages 44–5.

DISEASES OF THE RESPIRATORY SYSTEM

With the exclusion of neoplasms, allergic diseases, and infections with specific organisms, only a few respiratory diseases remain to be discussed here.

One of the first claims for a marked disturbance of ABO frequencies in a disease was made by Struthers in 1951, when he found very significantly raised A and B frequencies in children in Glasgow dying from bronchopneumonia (relative incidences A/O, 2·10; B/O, 2·09). Carter and Heslop (1957), in a similar series of cases, found much lower ratios in a similar series of London cases (A/O, 1·21; B/O, 1·34), but both ratios were nevertheless above unity. It is therefore interesting to see that in respiratory infections in infants Kircher (1968) found ratios of 1·10 and 1·13 respectively.

For 'pneumonia' (presumably mainly lobar pneumonia), on the other hand, the ratios are lower (A/O, 0·91; B/O, 1·11). Pleurisy, however, on only 332 cases, shows non-significantly raised A and B frequencies. Bronchitis shows a slight lowering of both A and B as compared with controls, whereas 242 cases of emphysema show non-significantly raised frequencies. As many cases of pulmonary emphysema are now known to be due mainly to a deficiency of trypsin inhibitor, this condition is further discussed on page 42.

DISEASES OF THE DIGESTIVE SYSTEM

Certain diseases of the digestive system, namely neoplasms, peptic ulcers, and infections with known organisms, are discussed elsewhere. Few diseases of the intestine itself, apart from those just mentioned, show any marked disturbance of ABO frequencies.

The most notable of those which do is gastritis with a significantly raised frequency of A, but with B very slightly depressed (relative incidences A/O, 1·31; B/O, 0·97). These should be compared with gastric ulceration with A/O and B/O relative incidences both 0·87. For gastric cancer on the other hand, the ratios are 1·22 and 1·08 respectively.

Four thousand cases of appendicitis and over 1000 of ulcerative colitis have ABO frequencies very near those of the controls. Ulcerative colitis is further discussed on page 294. In contrast with these diseases of the gut itself, those of the hepatic system show marked blood-group associations. Cirrhosis of the liver, cholelithiasis, cholecystitis, and diseases of the gall-bladder and biliary ducts all show marked and significant excesses of group A and somewhat raised frequencies of group B. Jaundice (unclassified) shows a similar trend. The few cases of pancreatic disease examined, however, show only slight and non-significant differences from the controls.

SKIN DISEASES

Most of the blood-group data for diseases of the skin are based on small numbers of tests. Numbers are further diminished in the case of blood group B because of a failure to record B and AB separately in many cases.

Lupus erythematosus shows a just significant excess of group O. This is well known to be an autoimmune disease (though not known to be associated with any histocompatibility antigen). Psoriasis, on the basis of nearly 2000 tests, also shows a just significant excess of O. This also appears to be an autoimmune disease and it shows associations with a number of histocompatibility antigens.

Acne shows a just significant excess of A. The very considerable excess of O compared with both A and B, in Egyptians with freckles, may be due to population stratification, as Egyptians have higher frequencies of both A and B than most neighbouring populations, and their relatively dark skin should not easily freckle. However, as only seventy persons were tested, the result may be due to sampling error. A marked excess of B in sixty-seven cases of seborrhoeic dermatitis is probably due to sampling error.

12
THE PHENYLTHIOCARBAMIDE TASTING SYSTEM

HISTORY

In 1931 Fox observed that to some individuals the simple chemical compound phenylthiocarbamide (PTC) had an intensely bitter taste, whereas to others it appeared tasteless. Being a chemist he also (Fox, 1932) showed that a number of other closely related compounds were tasted by the PTC tasters but not by the non-tasters.

The ability to taste phenylthiocarbamide was shown by Blakeslee and Salmon (Blakeslee and Salmon, 1931; Blakeslee, 1932) to behave as a dominant Mendelian character. The same was shown by Snyder (1931) for para-ethoxy-phenylthiocarbamide, one of the substances tested by Fox, who mentions it specially as being the thio-analogue of dulcin, an intensely sweet substance which has been used as a sweetening agent: the thio-analogue is, of course, tasted as bitter. Since at this time very few genetical polymorphisms were known in man, this pair of characters was rapidly and extensively applied by geneticists to the study of families and of populations, and such work has been going on ever since, so that we now have a knowledge of the varying frequency of tasters and of the taster gene in large numbers of human populations.

At about the same time as the early work on the taster phenomenon, independent investigations were being done on the inhibition of thyroid function by a variety of substances, both plant products and pure chemical substances. Chesney *et al.* (1928) described investigations of goitre in rabbits fed exclusively on cabbage, but it was not until somewhat later that they (Webster and Chesney, 1930) and others realized that the cabbage diet was the essential cause of the goitre.

In 1931 Suk attributed endemic goitre in man, in Carpatho-Ruthenia, to a cabbage diet. Marine *et al.* (1932) confirmed the work of Chesney (1928), but as late as 1935 Marine, while recognizing the goitrogenic effect of cabbage, attributed it to cyanides and not to derivatives of thiourea. (Thiourea is, of course, the same substance as thiocarbamide, the term mostly used by workers in this field. However, most of the papers from 1932 to 1945 use the word 'thiourea' and it is therefore used here in quoting these particular investigations.)

Hercus and Purves (1936) found turnips and seeds of cabbage-like plants (Brassica) to be goitrogenic, and in 1942 Kennedy showed that in rats allyl thiourea had a similar goitrogenic effect to that of rape seed. In the same year Richter and Clisby found phenylthiourea to be toxic in rats and to cause enlarged thyroids, but they still attributed the goitrogenic effect of cabbage to its content of cyanides. In 1943 Mackenzie and Mackenzie reported on thyroid enlargement in rats caused by a variety both of sulphonamides and of thiourea derivatives.

The general effect of attempting to read the literature of the subject from 1931 to 1943 is somewhat confusing. Part of the difficulties experienced by investigators lay in the varying activity of cabbage, owing to factors summed up, from a number of different authors, by Marine *et al.* (1932) who state, 'It has been shown that there are great seasonal and climatic variations in the goitrogenic activity of cabbage, that drying in a current of air or *in vacuo* causes a loss of the goitrogenic agent, that prolonged steaming does not impair and under certain conditions may increase its goitrogenic power, that boiling for 30 minutes at pH 3·0 (HCl) does not injure it, that the goitrogenic substance may be extracted from cabbage with ether and other ethereal solvents, and that this substance is but slightly extracted by prolonged aqueous leaching'. Subsequent work has shown that when cows consume the offending plants the substance is secreted unchanged in their milk.

Another source of difficulty lay in the fact that, as already mentioned, cabbages and related plants contain thyroid antagonists of two main kinds, thioureas and cyanogen compounds. It is, however, clear from the papers of Astwood and his colleagues (Astwood *et al.*, 1943; Astwood, 1945) that by 1942 they had already fully realized the unique importance of the thioureas, had tested a very large number of them on animals, and had selected thiouracil for therapeutic trial in man, as being the least toxic of the available thioureas in proportion to its thyroid inhibitor effect. In March of that year Astwood began clinical trials with thiourea itself and in September with thiouracil which proved highly effective and safe; it remained for many years the drug of choice in the treatment of hyperthyroidism.

It is interesting to note that the title of the paper by Richter and Clisby (1942) is 'Toxic effects of the bitter tasting phenylthiocarbamide', which suggests that they were aware of the work of Fox. Moreover, among the thiourea derivatives tested for activity on the thyroid by Astwood *et al.* (1943) there were five, in addition to thiourea itself and phenylthiourea, which had previously been tested for the taster phenomenon by Fox. However, the first explicit link between the two series of researches is the observation by Riddell and Wybar (1944) who found, in sixty persons tested, almost complete correspondence in ability to taste phenylthiourea and the thyroid inhibitor drug thiouracil (one partial exception was clearly related to the arbitrary solution strengths used for testing). These authors, however, did not comment upon the large numbers of other related substances that had been shown to behave like PTC in the taste test, and the numerous very similar substances that had been shown to be thyroid repressors.

TASTING AND THYROID DISEASES

These two aspects were more fully brought together by Harris and Kalmus (1949) who reviewed the history of the subject and made many new observations, showing that there is a considerable group of substances, all containing the chemical grouping

$$H-\underset{|}{N}-\underset{|}{C}=S$$

which are repressors of thyroid activity and to which individuals respond similarly either as tasters of all or as non-tasters of all. They mention the importance of the occurrence of such substances in food plants and conclude, 'Differences in taste sensitivity may reflect differences between individuals with respect to these substances. Such metabolic differences could presumably affect the biological fitness of the three genotypes, and hence perhaps lead to a balanced polymorphism.'

They followed this (Harris *et al.*, 1949) by investigating the taster status of persons with nodular non-toxic goitres, in whom they found a lowered frequency of tasters as compared with the normal population. This result was confirmed by Kitchin *et al.* (1959) who also showed a raised frequency of tasters in patients with diffuse toxic goitres. These results, and especially those for non-toxic goitres, have been confirmed repeatedly by subsequent investigators in several different countries.

Considering all the available data, toxic goitre does in fact show a very significant excess of tasters. Non-toxic goitre shows a highly significant excess of non-tasters; the total results are highly heterogeneous but even when we remove two extreme sets of data we still find a highly significant, and now homogeneous, excess of non-tasters. It is, however, not quite certain what is the best criterion for classifying goitres in relation to the taster association. Most toxic goitres are diffuse and a high proportion of non-toxic ones are nodular. However, a few cases are listed as toxic and nodular and some as diffuse or nodular without mention of toxicity. When all the cases described as 'diffuse' are taken together, without reference to toxicity, the relative incidence of tasters rises to 1·24 (from 1·20 for all toxic cases) and all nodular cases give a relative incidence of tasters of 0·55 (as compared with 0·61 for all non-toxic cases).

Endemic goitre shows a small and non-significant excess of non-tasters, and cases classed primarily as hypothyroidism, a very significant excess of the same type: in some sets of data they are said to have goitres. Carcinoma of the thyroid, on rather small numbers, shows a highly significant excess of tasters.

THYROID PHYSIOLOGY AND POPULATION GENETICS

An indication that the taster phenomenon is of importance in relation to the endocrine balance of healthy persons is the finding by Johnston *et al.* (1966) of a tendency to earlier pubertal development in tasters than in non-tasters. The lower incidence of dental caries in tasters than in non-tasters found by Chung *et al.* (1964) is perhaps a related phenomenon.

Widström and Henschen (1963) have further shown that in persons without overt thyroid disease there is a statistical correlation between the level of protein-bound iodine in the serum and the ability to taste PTC, persons with a high iodine level being more frequently tasters than those with a low level. This work appears convincing and is consistent with the observations on goitrous persons, while suggesting that the goitrous cases represent the clinically abnormal extremes of the normal thyroid function range. There have, however, unfortunately been few attempts to confirm these results.

A survey of rather small numbers of persons by Becker *et al.* (1966), directed primarily at investigating a possible relation between glaucoma and thyroid function further discussed below, shows higher protein-bound iodine levels in tasters than in non-tasters, but an extensive unpublished survey of the Irish population, by Tills and Lehmann (1975), shows no significant difference in thyroxine levels between tasters and non-tasters.

One factor to be taken into account in interpreting these results is that the tests have not been the same in all surveys. It is known that under conditions of stress the body economizes iodine by shifting synthesis from the hormone T_3 to T_4. It therefore appears desirable that further surveys should include estimations of both hormones, as well as of total protein-bound iodine, in view of the possibility that other forms of bound iodine may have been involved in the observations of Widström and Henschen.

While the situation demands much further work in order to clarify it, many of the above-mentioned facts would accord with the suggestion by Harris and Kalmus (1949) of a balanced polymorphism related to the amounts of iodine and of thyroid-inhibiting substances in the diet, the frequency of tasters, who fix iodine more efficiently, becoming raised by natural selection to cope at a population level with a low environmental iodine supply or an abundance of thyroid inhibitors, and lowered to meet the opposite conditions.

The occurrence of endemic goitre due to thyroid inhibitors in the diet (presumably in combination with iodine deficiency) has now been observed in several regions, but has been most fully studied in Australia and especially Tasmania, as described by Clements (1955) and Lamp (1963). These writers stress the presence in plants of the cabbage family of other sulphur-containing goitrogenic substances besides derivatives of thiourea, and any population-genetical study of iodine metabolism must, of course, take them into account.

The converse phenomenon, endemic thyrotoxicosis, has recently been described for the first time in Tasmania by Stewart and Vidor (1976) who show that it has arisen from the deliberate addition of iodine to salt or bread as a prophylactic against goitre, together probably with the use of iodine-containing disinfectants in the dairy industry, and of iodine-containing additives to bread to facilitate the 'continuous mix' automated bread-making operation. It would be of interest to know whether the incidence of this form of thyrotoxicosis is related to the taster/non-taster status of individuals. The situation in Tasmania is of course entirely a man-made one but it is just conceivable that it could be paralleled naturally. The most likely place would appear to be the margins of the Atacama Desert, where the residual salt deposits, or 'caliche', consist mainly of sodium nitrate, but with several per cent of sodium iodate. The desert is almost entirely waterless but on its margins nitrate and iodate might get into the groundwater and the streams. There may, however, be other areas with an excess of iodine in the environment.

To revert to the hypothesis of a balanced polymorphism, one set of observations which gives some support to it is that of Cartwright and Sunderland (1967) who have shown that the higher incidence of endemic goitre in Derbyshire than in the geologically similar northern part of Lancashire, is accompanied by a higher incidence of non-tasters in Derbyshire.

The implication of the above hypothesis is that the products of the taster and non-taster genes affect not only the ability to taste phenylthiocarbamide and related substances, but also in some way regulate thyroid function. They must therefore be active both in the tongue (for a direct action on the nerves of taste is most unlikely) but also in the thyroid gland (or, rather improbably, the pituitary). The combination of effects on the tongue and the thyroid is not surprising in view of their embryological association.

As to the precise mode of action of these products, we can at present only speculate, in the hope of finding a testable hypothesis. The gene products are, of necessity, proteins and are likely to be enzymes. In the normal thyroid, several stages can be recognized in the production of functional thyroxine from circulating iodide, each of which can be inhibited, leading to a reduction of thyroxine production and usually to the development of a goitre. Iodide is first taken up selectively as such by the gland, but remains dischargeable by thiocyanate or perchlorate ions. It is then oxidized to 'nascent' elementary iodine by peroxides, through the action of a peroxidase enzyme. This enzyme can be blocked by the substituted thioureas which are oxidized in place of the iodide. The iodine is then taken up by tyrosine to form successively mono- and di-iodotyrosine. Two molecules of the latter condense to form thyroxine, or one molecule of mono-iodotyrosine and one of di-iodotyrosine form tri-iodothyroxine.

The action of a peroxidase enzyme which is blocked by substituted thioureas would seem to point clearly to the point of action of the above-mentioned gene products, perhaps with the non-taster gene giving rise to a somewhat less-active peroxidase than the taster gene.

This simple hypothesis is, however, not consistent with what is known of another genetic system, that responsible for Pendred's syndrome which consists of a combination of congenital deafness and thyroid deficiency with goitre. The pathogenic gene expresses itself recessively, i.e. only in the homozygote (Thould, 1960; Thould and Scowen, 1964). The thyroid takes up iodide normally but peroxidation is partially inhibited and the accumulated iodide remains dischargeable by treatment with perchlorate.

Here again, then, the simplest hypothesis would be that the abnormal gene gives rise to a defective peroxidase. The gene would then, on our previous hypothesis, be an allele of the taster and non-taster genes, and since it gives rise to manifestly defective peroxidation, which the common non-taster gene does not, one would expect it to have non-taster expression. However, according to Thould, sufferers from Pendred's syndrome show almost exactly the same distribution of tasters and non-tasters as the normal population. Thus we are undoubtedly dealing with two non-allelic sets of genes, and it may be that the peroxidation of iodide is more complex than has been supposed, needing at least two enzymes (each subject to genetic variation) acting sequentially.

The subject clearly demands further fundamental biochemical work, in the first place on animal thyroids. If, however, the enzymes in question could be found in the circulating blood, which is unlikely, variants could be sought by the standard methods of electrophoresis; it appears, however, that thyroxine synthesis occurs only in living thyroid cells. Perhaps one day a test will be devised using living cells from tongue scrapings.

However, even in the absence of this fundamental knowledge, further population studies are needed, especially to confirm or refute the relations which have been claimed between the taster/non-taster phenomenon and blood thyroxine levels, growth rates, and the incidence of toxic goitre.

OTHER DISEASES

While the presence of a relation between the taster phenomenon and thyroid function is beyond doubt, whatever may be its explanation, the same cannot be said of the suggested relation of tasting to glaucoma. There are a number of papers, mostly of rather early date, suggesting an association between goitre and glaucoma. Becker and Morton (1964*a*, *b*) have found a raised frequency of non-tasters in primary open-angle glaucoma, and of tasters in angle-closure glaucoma, both in Caucasoids and Negroids.

Becker *et al.* (1966) found low levels of protein-bound iodine in patients with primary open-angle glaucoma, as compared with those having angle-closure glaucoma (no data on healthy persons are included). They also found larger average 24-hour radio-iodine uptakes among angle-closure than among open-angle glaucoma cases. Six out of 38 patients with primary open-angle glaucoma had anti-thyroglobulin antibodies in their plasma, but none of the 21 with angle-closure glaucoma had them. An additional 21 patients with pigmentary glaucoma were tested and 5 had antibodies. None of 30 non-glaucomatous patients had any. However, as the authors state, these observations may simply demonstrate the existence of a general auto-immune process in open-angle glaucoma. They conclude, 'It is clear that the effects of thyroid function on aqueous humour dynamics need further study'.

When the data on the various types of glaucoma are taken together they show a surprising degree of consistency. Primary angle-closure glaucoma, like toxic goitre, is significantly associated with tasting; primary open-angle glaucoma, like non-toxic goitre, even more significantly with non-tasting; while secondary glaucoma (like endemic goitre) shows no overall association with either phenotype. Buphthalmos, on a small sample, is very strongly associated with tasting. The consistency of these results, on rather small numbers, makes it desirable that further observations should be made, perhaps combined with tests for thyroid function. A possible area for a study of these relations is East Greenland, where Alsbirk (1975) has found that in the Eskimos the interior chamber tends to be shallow, and there is a high incidence of angle-closure glaucoma. Unfortunately we possess very few data on the taster phenomenon in Eskimos. While Amerinds have, in general, very high taster frequencies, a situation unfavourable to association studies, this does not appear to be the case with Eskimos.

Other conditions which, on adequate numbers, show a strong association with tasting are tuberculosis and leprosy while, on rather small numbers, there are very strong associations with carcinomas of the breast, cervix and corpus uteri, and ovary, and with menopausal metrorrhagia. The highly significant association of diabetes mellitus with non-tasting is mentioned elsewhere. Apparent associations of cystic fibrosis and schizophrenia with non-tasting may be due to the patients failing to taste PTC, or to report tasting it, for reasons other than being genetic non-tasters.

While it must be admitted that the diagnosis of the taster status of individuals is more liable to systematic error than is that of their laboratory-determined blood factors, the high degrees of association found for the relatively few diseases studied is impressive. The 'combined incidence', or 'relative risk' factors reported are comparable only with those found for alpha$_1$-trypsin inhibitor deficiency, and for the histocompatibility antigens, and should encourage many more observations in this field, as well as further attempts to interpret them biochemically.

13

THE α_1 PROTEASE INHIBITOR SYSTEM

MOST of the polymorphisms found to have disease associations were first discovered in healthy people, and only subsequently were the disease associations found. However, in the case of the α_1 protease inhibitors of the plasma, it was the disease association which revealed the polymorphism. The presence of a protease inhibitor in the α_1 globulin fraction of sera had long been known when Laurell and Eriksson (1963) showed that certain cases of pulmonary disease were characterized by a deficiency of this substance. The genetical basis of the system was largely worked out by Eriksson (1964, 1965) and Fagerhol and Braend (1965), and numerous alleles of the inhibitor have since been recognized. The early history of the investigations has been described by Giblett (1969). Another association of protease inhibitor deficiency, that with liver disease, was first recognized by Sharp *et al.* (1969). The subject developed so rapidly that a comprehensive symposium dealing with it was held at the City of Hope Medical Center, Duarte, California, in 1971. The papers and discussions were published as a volume edited by Dr C. Mittman (1972). A further symposium took place at Bois-Guillaume in 1975 (Martin, 1975), and another in the same year at Bruges (Peeters, 1976). The three sets of proceedings taken together give a comprehensive account of this rapidly developing subject.

About twenty alleles are now recognized, one of which, Pi^{M}, is very much commoner than all the others. Three alleles, Pi^{S}, Pi^{Z}, and Pi^{-} (or Pi^{o}), have gene products with reduced or, in Pi^{-}, absent inhibitory activity; Pi^{Z} and Pi^{-} give rise, in the homozygotes (and presumably in the mutual heterozygotes) to pulmonary emphysema and hepatic cirrhosis. The degree of deficiency is greater for Pi^{Z} than for Pi^{S}, and the former is the more often found in disease associations.

It is likely that all such homozygotes have pathological signs in their lungs and livers, but in a high proportion of cases these do not cause symptoms, or, in the case of emphysema, not until late in life. Liver disease, on the other hand, often becomes manifest, and may even be fatal, in infancy.

The pathogenic importance of the homozygous condition was rapidly recognized by physicians and pathologists, and tests for protease inhibitor level are now regularly performed on cases of pulmonary emphysema, of which homozygous inhibitor deficiency is the main cause in a substantial minority of cases.

It is not, however, clear why the severity of symptoms varies so greatly, so that even among siblings with the same *Pi* genotype one may be severely affected and another symptomatically almost normal. It is possible that genes of other systems are involved, though, especially in elderly persons, lifelong environmental conditions must play a large part.

It has not needed any elaborate statistics to establish the association of homozygous inhibitor deficiency with lung emphysema and liver cirrhosis, but there is considerable doubt about whether, and under what circumstances, heterozygous deficiency is a cause of disease. This is because tests done for clinical purposes are usually limited to quantitative estimations of inhibitor activity, which cannot of themselves establish the genotype.

Non-genetical factors can certainly influence the inhibitor level which, for instance, is raised by infection, which thus tends to mask any moderate genetic deficiency. The amount of inhibitor in the plasma of deficiency heterozygotes is roughly half that in normal persons, but there is some overlap with normals, and the identity of the deficiency gene cannot be established by a quantitative test.

There is little if any quantitative overlap between heterozygous and homozygous deficients but until a considerable number of persons of known genotype have systematically been tested quantitatively it cannot be said with certainty that there is none. Moreover, in those who are homozygous for the deficiency condition it is desirable to establish by electrophoresis which gene or genes are present.

Even a straightforward acid-starch-gel electrophoresis is somewhat more time-consuming than a quantitative test, and even the former may still allow the occasional MZ heterozygote to pass as normal. For an unambiguous genotypic diagnosis it is necessary, in some cases at least, to carry out antigen-antibody crossed electrophoresis. Particular causes of ambiguity in the simple electrophoretic test are disease, pregnancy, and the haptoglobin type 1–1 (which gives overlapping bands) (Fagerhol, in discussion, pp. 152–3, in Mittman, 1972).

It is, moreover, important that attempts should be made to ascertain the part played by protease-inhibitor deficiency states in increasing the susceptibility, of those with an abnormal gene, to other lung diseases than simple emphysema, and to liver diseases in general, as well as to the other diseases mentioned below. The effects of the moderately weak types, MS, MZ, SS, and SZ (as distinct from the severely deficient ZZ, ZO, and OO) in increasing susceptibility to disease need further investigation.

For this purpose it will be necessary to carry out simple electrophoresis on all specimens, and to be prepared to do antigen-antibody crossed electrophoresis in all cases of ambiguity. If a lot of wasted effort is to be avoided such series of tests will need very careful planning. The discovery by Constans and Viau (1975), by a combination of isoelectric focusing and crossed electrophoresis, of a new relatively common allele Pi^{N} in the south-west of France must also serve as a warning since it appears probable that, with less discriminating methods, this has hitherto been confused with the common Pi^{M} gene.

Moreover, the range of organs and tissues sometimes affected extends beyond the lungs and liver. Ward *et al.* (1975) describe the existence of glomerulo-nephritis found *post mortem* in a boy of 9 years who died of liver cirrhosis. These authors also mention other similar cases reported to them by Cox. Cox and Huber (1976), moreover, have shown in a statistical study that the Pi types MZ and SZ are significantly more prevalent in adults with rheumatoid arthritis than in control adults, though similar differences were not found in juvenile rheumatoid arthritis.

The authors suggest that trypsin inhibitor deficiency does not render the occurrence of rheumatoid arthritis more likely, but increases the severity when the disease does occur.

André *et al.* (1974) report a raised incidence of trypsin-inhibitor deficiency, which they attribute to the MZ genotype, in cases both of duodenal and of gastric ulcer, the excess being statistically significant in the case of duodenal ulcer. They mention previous reports of the same association (Kalliomaki *et al.*, 1971) as well as the association of peptic ulcers with pulmonary emphysema (Hegetschweiler *et al.*, 1960). Earlier reports of this association are given by Green and Dundee (1952) and by Latts *et al.* (1956).

These observations suggest that it is desirable to include the Pi types in future statistical studies of possible associations of polymorphisms with many more diseases than the few hitherto shown to be associated with this particular polymorphism.

Burnett *et al.* (1975) have found a raised level of α_1 trypsin inhibitor in the amniotic fluid in cases of severe pre-eclampsia. It would be of interest to examine the molecular types present in the amniotic fluid, and in the plasma of mother and foetus, in such cases.

14

THE HISTOCOMPATIBILITY ANTIGENS

OUR knowledge of the disease associations of the histocompatibility antigens has been one of extremely rapid growth. In 1972, at the time of the Evian symposium, devoted to their anthropological and geographical distribution (Dausset and Colombani, 1973), they were scarcely known to have any such associations. Now, in 1977, as this book goes to press, shortly after the 1976 Paris symposium (Dausset and Svejgaard, 1977), the histocompatibility system has emerged as outstandingly the most important of human polymorphisms in its disease associations.

The whole of the subject-matter of this book is drawn from the work of others, but this is particularly so in the case of the histocompatibility antigens. Nearly all the substance of the present chapter is based on the short but extremely informative monograph of Svejgaard *et al.* (1975). However, though readers will find here constant echoes of that work, we are solely responsible for the use which we have made of it, and for any errors which we have committed in doing so. Moreover, as already stated, we have been able to include full tables of the associations only through the generosity of Lars Ryder and Arne Svejgaard (1976) who have allowed us to reproduce their book *Associations between HLA and disease* as an appendix to this book (see pp. 275–98).

Blood-group workers have known for many years that human sera, especially those of mothers and multiply transfused patients, sometimes contain agglutinins for leucocytes. Dausset (1954) first suggested that the antibodies in such sera were reacting with specific leucocyte antigens, and soon it was shown (Dausset and Brecy, 1957; Dausset, 1958; Payne and Rolfs, 1958) that the antigens concerned were specific and hereditary.

Van Rood partly overcame many of the early technical complications of the tests by the application of computer methods. He also showed (Rood, 1962) that besides occurring in the leucocytes the antigens were present in most tissues of the body, and this opened the way to their recognition as histocompatibility antigens, analogous to those already known in various species of experimental animals. It thus became possible to use the tests for predicting compatibility or incompatibility in human tissue and organ grafting.

I do not have the first-hand knowledge which would enable me to describe in detail the complicated subsequent history of the elucidation of the very complex serology and genetics of this system, or to allot credit for successive discoveries, but must refer readers to the work of Svejgaard *et al.* (1975). The subject has claimed, and continues to claim, the efforts of a large number of brilliant workers, but a remarkable feature of its development has been the way in which workers throughout the world have collaborated by means of frequent international 'workshops'. In this way they have ensured the greatest possible uniformity in defining antigens and antibodies, as well as in the elucidation of the genetics of the former.

This tradition of collaboration and uniformity of notation and presentation has greatly facilitated the preparation by Ryder and Svejgaard of their tables reproduced in the appendix. Similar agreement in the blood-group field would greatly have simplified our task in preparing the other tables of this book.

The histocompatibility antigens, though present, as already mentioned, in most tissues of the body, are most readily identified in lymphocytes. The antisera used in detecting them are mostly derived from the sera of mothers, as these more often contain one or only a few antibodies, whereas the sera of multiply transfused persons are more often polyvalent. The usual tests are based on the microlymphocytotoxicity test of Terasaki and McClelland (1964). The antigens detectable in this way are known as 'serologically detectable' or SD antigens. Other antigens can at present be detected only by 'mixed lymphocyte culture' tests and are known as MLC antigens or sometimes as 'lymphocyte defined' or LD antigens.

The identification of the various antigens has gone in parallel with studies of their inheritance, and it has thus been found that they are dependent upon a set of closely linked genes on a short segment of chromosome No. 6, an arrangement similar to that postulated in Fisher's (Race, 1944) model of the Rh blood group genes, with which most readers will be familiar.

The relations of the genes, as at present understood, are shown diagrammatically in FIGURE 2, reproduced by kind permission from the monograph of Svejgaard *et al.* (1975). The distance of about one centimorgan between loci A and B implies a crossover frequency of 1 per cent per generation. Thus considerably more crossovers have been observed than for the genetically more controversial Rhesus system where few if any have been found. The antigens so far known, coded by the genes at the four loci, are listed in Tables II and III, also reproduced by kind permission from the work of Svejgaard *et al.* (1975). The frequencies there shown for Danes are near those of the British but there are wide variations in other peoples, and non-Europeans have many genes at these loci, not known in Europeans (Dausset and Colombani, 1973).

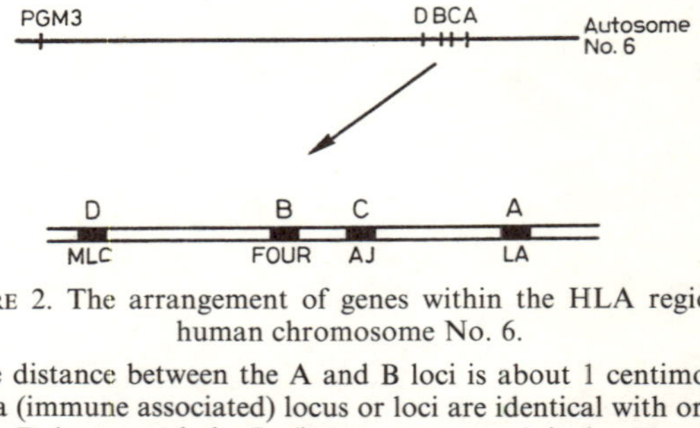

FIGURE 2. The arrangement of genes within the HLA region on human chromosome No. 6.

The distance between the A and B loci is about 1 centimorgan. The Ia (immune associated) locus or loci are identical with or close to the D locus, and the Ir (immune response) loci are probably close to Ia. The loci for Bf and C2 (components of complement) are also close to the B locus. The Chido blood-group locus is close to B or D; the Roger blood-group locus may be identical with B, and the Bg blood-group antigens are probably closely related to those controlled by the *A* and *B* (histocompatibility) genes. (Figure reproduced by permission of the authors and S. Karger, from *The HLA System* (Svejgaard *et al.*, 1975).)

TABLE II. FREQUENCIES OF THE ANTIGENS AND GENES OF THE HLA-A, B, AND C SERIES

A (LA OR 1ST) SERIES			B (FOUR OR 2ND) SERIES			C (AJ OR 3RD) SERIES		
Antigen	Frequency		Antigen	Frequency		Antigen	Frequency	
	Antigen %	Gene		Antigen %	Gene		Antigen %	Gene
HLA-A1	31·1	0·1683	HLA-B5	10·6	0·0545	HLA-Cw1	5·7	0·0287
A2	53·6	0·3228	B7	26·8	0·1419	Cw2	9·7	0·0496
A3	26·9	0·1454	B8	23·7	0·1274	Cw3	35·0	0·1933
A9	17·3	0·0915	B12	25·2	0·1359	Cw4	17·1	0·0897
Aw23	NI		B13	4·27	0·0215	Cw5	NI	
Aw24	NI		B14	4·47	0·0227	T7	33·1	0·182
A10	9·56	0·0489	Bw15	17·9	0·0936	Blank		0·457
Aw25	3·77	0·0190	Bw16	5·39	0·0273			
Aw26	5·85	0·0297	Bw38		0·0138	Total		1·0003
A11	10·1	0·0520	Bw39	2·68	0·0135			
A28	9·96	0·0509	Bw17	7·68	0·0392			
Aw19	18·1	0·0991	B18	7·07	0·0361			
A29	4·5	0·0228	Bw21	3·51	0·0177			
Aw30	NI		Bw22	3·81	0·0192			
Aw31	NI		B27	8·64	0·0440			
Aw32	6·14	0·0312	Bw35	13·1	0·0722			
Aw33	NI		Bw37	1·18	0·0059			
Blank		0·0213	Bw40	17·9	0·0950			
			Bw41	1·37	0·0069			
Total		1·0000	407[x]	0·46	0·0023			
			4A2[x] (TT)	1·17	0·0059			
			Blank		0·0308			
			Total		1·0000			

The data are from Nielsen *et al.* (1975*a*, *b*) and were obtained from investigations of about 400–2000 unrelated Danes. Frequencies of antigens are given as percentages, while those for the corresponding genes are simple frequencies. The *HLA-Aw25* and *Aw26* genes comprise together the *HLA-A10* gene (i.e. an *HLA-A10* gene is either *Aw25* or *Aw26*). A similar relationship exists for *Aw23* and *Aw24* which comprise *A9*, and for *Bw38* and *Bw39* which comprise *Bw16*. In analogy, *Aw19* is made up of *A29*, *Aw30*, *Aw31*, *Aw32*, and *Aw33*. Accordingly, the frequencies of the following genes are not included in the sums: *A10*, *A29*, and *Aw32* of the A series, and *Bw16* of the B series. NI = Not investigated.

Antigen frequencies are calculated by the number of individuals having the antigen divided by the total number of individuals investigated. As there are many heterozygotes (e.g. of the genotype *HLA-A1/A2*), the sum of the antigens from a given series is more than 100% (but can never exceed 200%) because heterozygotes are counted twice (e.g. both for HLA-A1 and A2). *Gene frequencies* indicate the number of genes of a certain type divided by the total number of alleles studied, i.e. twice the number of individuals; as there can be only one gene from a series on one chromosome, the sum of gene frequencies must for one series (locus) be one. The '*blank*' (*null*) genes indicate genes the products of which cannot yet be recognized.

Table reproduced by kind permission of the authors and of Messrs. S. Karger from 'The HLA System' (Svejgaard *et al.*, 1975).

TABLE III. FREQUENCIES OF MLC = HLA-D ANTIGENS

ANTIGEN	NUMBER OF INDIVIDUALS STUDIED	ANTIGEN FREQUENCY %	GENE FREQUENCY
D1	95	19	0·099
D2	157	24	0·128
D3	157	21	0·112
D4	157	17	0·091
D5	34	9	0·045
D6	89	18	0·094
107 (LD-12a)	157	10	0·049
108 (LD-W10a)	157	9	0·046
Sa. 2	34	3	0·015
Blank			0·321
			1·000

Data from Thomsen *et al.* (1975) on unrelated Danes.

Table reproduced by kind permission of the authors and of Messrs. S. Karger from 'The HLA System' (Svejgaard *et al.*, 1975).

The most fully studied antigens are those of the 1st and 2nd series, coded by genes at the A and B loci respectively, and most disease associations have been determined only in terms of antigens of these two series. Antigens coded at the D locus, detectable only by mixed lymphocyte culture (MLC) are a newer discovery and comparatively few associations with them are known.

The total set of genes coded by one of the chromosomes of an individual (analogous to a Rhesus gene complex such as CDe) is known as the haplotype. Any one individual can, of course, possess only two haplotypes (each coded by one of the pair of No. 6 chromosomes) and these, in the absence of the rare phenomenon of crossing-over, are passed on intact upon reproduction.

It is now known that a number of other substances or of functions (which imply substances) related to the body's immunological defence mechanisms are coded at loci on the same chromosome segment. Some of the genes for these, notably the Ir or 'immune response' genes, are postulated mainly on the basis of disease associations and are discussed later. Such genes have, however, been much more firmly established in experimental animals, in which they control the specific functions of T lymphocytes. The Ia or 'immune response associated' antigens similarly interact with B lymphocytes, and there is more direct evidence for the existence of these in man.

Three components of complement have been shown in man to be controlled by genes in the HLA chromosome segment. These are C2, C4, and Properdin factor B. The genes controlling the rather anomalous Bg, Roger, and Chido red-cell blood group antigens are also closely linked to the HLA genes.

LINKAGE DISEQUILIBRIUM

The concept of linkage disequilibrium within a closely linked set of genes is an important one in interpreting associations with diseases. Considering the hypothetical Fisher model of the Rhesus blood-group genes, it would be expected that if crossovers occurred, however rarely, between the separate loci then, for instance, the ratio between the combinations CD and Cd would in the long run be identical with the ratio between the total frequencies of D and d in the population, or about 60/40 in Europeans. In fact CD is very much commoner than Cd (about 40/1). This apparent disequilibrium has been used as an argument for rejecting the model. On the other hand, if the model is accepted, it implies either that there has been insufficient time for equilibrium to be established, since two populations with differing D and d frequencies began to mix, or that the combination CD is in some way greatly favoured by natural selection.

In the HLA system, where crossing-over certainly occurs, the frequencies of many haplotypes differ significantly in frequency from those expected on the hypothesis of free crossing-over uninfluenced by selection. For instance, the combinations A3B7 and A1B8 are much commoner than would be expected with linkage equilibrium. It is also suggested, as discussed below, that disease associations themselves imply linkage disequilibrium.

Most of the associations found between diseases and polymorphisms other than HLA are probably to be explained by the known gene products, such as the blood-group antigens, directly affecting susceptibility to diseases, even if the precise mechanism is in some cases obscure. However, in the HLA system we are dealing with a complex closely linked set of genes, some directly giving rise to the observed histocompatibility antigens, together with others known and yet others suspected of controlling additional immunological activities. Thus, when a disease is found to be associated with a particular histocompatibility antigen, the enhanced susceptibility to the disease may be caused directly by the antigen, or it may be (and perhaps most often is) due to a gene closely linked to that giving rise to the antigen, and in linkage disequilibrium with it. As a rough guide, it is likely that a world-wide association is due to the activity of the histocompatibility antigen itself, whereas if it is relatively local, and especially if the association is with different antigens in different regions or races, the activity of a linked but separate immune response (Ir) gene is indicated.

THE ASSOCIATIONS

The reader who wishes to examine the data for himself will at this point turn to the comprehensive tables of the Appendix. The following pages simply express comments on these data by an outsider familiar mainly with the blood-group associations. They contain some suggestions for more intensive HLA investigations in groups of diseases where associations with other polymorphisms have proved particularly interesting.

The associations have, like those with other polymorphisms, been studied mainly by tests on sets of unrelated patients but, because of the closeness of many associations, family studies have proved more informative than for other polymorphisms.

The classic example of an HLA association is that between ankylosing spondylitis and HLA-B27. Among Europeans, about 90 per cent of patients have the antigen, which is present in only about 9 per cent of the general population.

A similar strong association with B27 is found in American Indians and in Japanese, indicating that this is probably not a case of linkage disequilibrium, but that the antigen itself is in some way increasing susceptibility to the disease. However, the fact that there are 10 per cent of patients who do not have the antigen, and that the majority of people who do have it escape the disease, shows that B27 is not the only possible cause, and that when B27 is present other conditions—perhaps other genes—must interact with the histocompatibility antigen to give rise to the disease.

Several other arthropathies, particularly Reiter's syndrome, but also yersinia and salmonella arthritis and juvenile arthritis (Still's disease), as well as acute anterior uveitis, show strong associations with B27, and psoriatic arthropathy a moderately strong one, which suggests that they all have an important immunological characteristic in common with one another, and probably with the HLA-B27 antigen itself. Ankylosing spondylitis shows no significant ABO blood-group association, while, among the 'rheumatic' diseases, rheumatoid arthritis with a strong group O association, and rheumatic fever and rheumatic heart disease, associated with groups A and B, have shown only slight HLA associations.

An important group of diseases, including several affecting the endocrine system, show moderate associations (relative risk 2 to 10) with HLA-B8. These are dermatitis herpetiformis, chronic autoimmune hepatitis, myasthenia gravis, celiac disease, juvenile diabetes mellitus, Graves' disease (thyrotoxicosis), idiopathic Addison's disease, systemic lupus erythematosus, and Behcet's syndrome. As discussed on page 31, the mechanism in the case of diabetes mellitus may be the facilitation of infection of the islet tissue with a virus. Similar mechanisms might apply in other cases, but in some at least a more directly immunological process seems to be involved; perhaps one or more Ir genes in linkage disequilibrium with B8 are involved.

A considerable number of allergic conditions are showing indications of association with HLA, and in some cases there are grounds for assuming that specific HLA-linked Ir genes are responsible. Some cases at least of sudden death in infancy may fall into this class. The association of the A1B8 haplotype with infantile eczema and hay fever may have some diagnostic and prognostic value.

Psoriasis vulgaris is moderately associated with HLA B13, B17, and Bw37.

As shown elsewhere, neoplastic diseases show some of the most striking associations with the ABO blood groups. Unfortunately relatively few studies have been done on possible HLA associations with malignant disease. The few studies done of carcinoma of the stomach and of the breast show no significant HLA associations. Hodgkin's disease, though clearly malignant, is now thought by some investigators to result from a virus infection. It is one of the few neoplastic conditions which, unlike most neoplasms but like several virus diseases, is associated with blood group O. It is weakly associated with HLA A1, B5, B8, and B18.

Acute lymphatic leukaemia is weakly associated with HLA A2, B8, and B12. The leukaemias, poorly classified in many ABO association studies, show no very clear associations with the HLA antigens.

The ABO and HLA associations of multiple sclerosis are discussed on page 52.

It is anticipated that the fuller publication to be made of the papers presented at the Paris (1976) symposium on HLA and disease (Dausset and Svejgaard, 1977) will considerably clarify the picture with regard to neoplastic diseases as well as many others, but further studies of the incidence of the HLA antigens in various forms of cancer, and possible relations with increase or retrogression of the lesions are much to be desired, especially now that immunological methods are being introduced into therapy.

More information is needed also on HLA associations of infectious diseases generally, of peptic ulcers, and of liver diseases, all of which show interesting ABO associations.

15

SOME CONCLUSIONS

As stated in the Introduction, this book is a sequel to the second edition of *The distribution of the human blood groups* (Mourant *et al.*, 1976) and one of our objects in writing it has been to bring together data which may help to explain the existing very diverse blood-group frequencies, found in different populations. The data contained in the previous book will undoubtedly be subject to extensive analysis by others than ourselves, for instance by the methods described by Bodmer *et al.* (1973), designed to show from their intrinsic characteristics, and without reference to independent evidence, how far they are to be explained by random processes such as genetic drift, how far by stabilizing natural selection, and how far by disruptive selection leading to phenotype and gene frequencies related to varying environmental pressures.

While admitting the importance of the random processes and of stabilizing selection, we have undertaken the present study as an active search for the effects of disruptive selective processes. Since, as we show, there are significant associations between particular phenotypes of certain polymorphisms and particular diseases with an environmental component in their aetiology, then (apart from diseases confined to old age) disruptive selection must be taking place. We have already advanced various hypotheses as to how it is happening. In this chapter we attempt to put forward some general conclusions.

We have, however, tried to cover a field extending far beyond the limits of our own specialized knowledge, and one of our objects in sorting and publishing the data has been to stimulate specialists in the various groups of diseases concerned to draw their own conclusions. Also, by attracting attention to gaps in the data we hope to induce readers to fill them.

INFECTIONS AND NATURAL SELECTION

One of our first tasks must, however, be to admit at least a partial failure to substantiate one of our working hypotheses. In our previous book (Mourant *et al.*, 1976, pp. 176–7), as well as in a number of earlier publications, I had drawn attention to the high O frequencies which occur on islands and highlands around the periphery of Europe, as well as in the deserts of North Africa and Arabia, and I suggested that this was due to ante-natal selection in favour of group O, occurring in all populations, this trend remaining fully effective in isolated populations on highlands and mountains, and in the desert, but being balanced in areas more accessible to epidemic infections, by mortality from diseases relatively unfavourable to group O persons.

It was for this reason that, in addition to studying the blood-group associations of infectious diseases, we have made a special study of published work on ante-natal selection affecting the blood groups (Chapter 6). There can be little doubt that there is a considerable mortality both in early pregnancy by spontaneous abortion, and in late pregnancy and the early days of extra-uterine life, of A and B foetuses carried by group O mothers. There must be some opposing selective effect preventing all populations from becoming entirely of group O, but the other leg of our argument has proved less convincing.

There are, indeed, some well-defined associations of blood groups with particular infections, but more with group A than with group O, and evidence related to the major epidemic infections is rather unsatisfactory. There is considerable disagreement between investigators regarding smallpox associations; malaria seems to be associated with group A; there are no data for cholera or bubonic plague and hardly any for typhus. Influenzal infection, however, seems to be mainly associated with group O and thus favours our hypothesis.

It is noteworthy that, while the bacterial infections have greatly varying associations, there seems to be a general tendency for viral infections to be associated with group O. Though our major hypothesis on the distribution of the ABO groups in Europe has thus not been substantiated (but not convincingly demolished) the detailed associations of the various infections (which are of course shown in their geographical context in the tables) should provide valuable material to epidemiologists who are prepared to study them on a regional basis in conjunction with data on blood-group distribution (Mourant *et al.*, 1976) and with public-health statistics on distribution of infections. However, part of the reason for the failure of the infective diseases to yield as full and convincing a picture as, for instance, the neoplasms, is the relative paucity or absence of data for many immunologically interesting infective conditions.

NEOPLASTIC DISEASES

One of the most striking features of the combined data on associations of diseases with the ABO blood groups is the highly consistent association of carcinomas with group A. There is probably some meaning (or more probably several meanings) in the grading of the association, from a relative A/O incidence, among adequately studied types, of 1·06 for the bronchus and for the body of the uterus to 1·23 for the ovary, or, if we include rarer conditions, to 1·55 for the salivary glands. One possible contributory factor to this variation, suggested to me by Professor A. E. Jones, may have wide implications in the whole study of associations between polymorphisms and diseases. I drew his attention to the fact that, while bronchial carcinoma is significantly associated with group A, the degree of association is less than for most other carcinomas. He said that this would be expected, since there is such a very strong association with cigarette smoking that it probably largely overrides the effects of genetic polymorphisms in general. This would not, however, apply to the association with the aryl-hydrocarbon hydroxylase polymorphism, if it should be substantiated, since this is, by definition, a polymorphism which directly controls the response to a main cigarette-smoke carcinogen.

However, almost as interesting as the associations with group A are the exceptions to it, and in particular, the relative A/O incidence of only 0·90 for Hodgkin's disease, a neoplasm now regarded by some as due to a viral infection. Other low A/O incidences based on moderately adequate data are shown by carcinomas of the larynx, the nasopharynx, and the combined oropharynx, hypopharynx, and tonsils (combined because of the similarity of the neoplasms).

Among the consistently high A/O relative incidences for neoplasms of the nervous system, the value of 0·96 for the aetiologically very different chromophobe adenoma of the pituitary stands out as an exception. The possible meaning of these general trends and of the exceptions is further discussed on page 37.

Since patients suffering from a great many different diseases have been tested for their ABO groups, and those suffering from a considerable variety, for their histocompatibility antigens, it might have been expected that many would have been tested for both systems, but the number is in fact surprisingly small. However, of those which have, and which have shown associations with both systems, a remarkably high proportion are associated with group O; these mostly have a known or suspected autoimmune component in their aetiology. The values of the A/O combined relative incidences for these (irrespective of aetiology) are as follows: ankylosing spondylitis, 1·07; rheumatoid arthritis, 0·73; multiple sclerosis, 0·89; psoriasis, 0·91; juvenile diabetes, 0·91; thyrotoxicosis, 0·89; uveitis, 0·88; coeliac disease, 1·05; pernicious anaemia, 1·25; lupus erythematosus, 0·86; Hodgkin's disease, 0·90; nasopharyngeal carcinoma, 0·91. By no means all these individual ratios differ significantly from unity, but the total picture of excess of O is impressive, especially when compared with the opposite trend in neoplasms as a whole. It is, however, perhaps only fair to include here three diseases which are now being shown to have some form of association with the histocompatibility system, though full statistics are not yet available —these, with their A/O relative incidences, are: eczema, 1·03; asthma, 1·13; and hay fever, 0·94.

Macfarlane Burnet long ago claimed that there is a basic antithesis between those persons whose immune systems are underactive and who tend to tolerate neoplasms, and those with overactive systems who reject nearly all neoplasms, but also tend to react against their own tissues.

We have now seen that most neoplasms are associated with group A, and that in some cases the neoplastic tissue contains an A-like antigen even in patients not of group A. On the other hand, many autoimmune diseases are associated with group O (as well as with HLA antigens).

These observations suggest a more general hypothesis, that in the tissues, both normal and neoplastic, of all persons, there are blood-group-A-like antigens present at a biochemical level at which they are usually inaccessible to the immune system. However, in the course of an auto-immune process, or of the immune response to a growing neoplasm, the antigen may become accessible. Then an A person, who cannot make anti-A, will be more likely than an O person to tolerate the neoplasm, but less likely than an O one to attack his own tissues. If this is true of A, it may be true also of other genetically determined antigens.

As Bodmer *et al.* (1973) have pointed out, random genetic drift will tend to cause frequency variations between populations, of the same order of magnitude for all polymorphisms and, except in the case of small isolates, such variations will be small. On the other hand, natural selection affecting any polymorphism will tend to cause much greater variations. Large variations may thus be taken as evidence in favour of the operation of natural selection.

There is, however, one aspect of the recognition of natural selection, which has not perhaps received adequate attention. This is the question of the size of the population units or topographic 'cells' between which variation becomes important for any polymorphism. I have suggested (Mourant, 1954; Mourant *et al.*, 1976) that the limiting size may serve as a measure of the intensity and speed of the selective process.

It appears likely, for instance, that the worldwide tendency of ABO frequencies to vary as between adjacent countries, and even provinces, is an indication of the operation of natural selection responding to local features of the environment. Such a response may become detectable in periods measured only in centuries, or perhaps in one or two thousand years.

The Rh and MN blood groups, on the other hand, while showing variations between major races, of the same order of magnitude as those of the ABO system, seem to show very much less variation between adjacent countries and provinces.

This point of view was supported by the case of the Haemoglobins A and S (pp. 3 and 10). The frequencies of these almost certainly respond, by natural selection, to the quite local distribution of falciparum malaria, within a few hundred years at most.

These considerations led me to suggest that by suitable mathematical treatment the various polymorphisms could provide us with a series of graduated probes into the past, according to the speed with which they responded to natural selection.

One of the difficulties has, however, been that of making sure that the apparent varying 'cell' sizes of variation are not artefacts. When I first considered this matter (Mourant, 1954) there were already abundant data showing marked local variation in ABO frequencies, for instance within the United Kingdom (Kopeć, 1970) but data for the distribution of the Rh and MN groups tended to be based on population samples covering whole countries, so that local variations, if any, would have been obscured.

Now, however, with the abundance of geographically minutely classified data which have become available for numerous polymorphisms (Mourant *et al.*, 1976) there can be no doubt that, to take the three systems already mentioned, the ABO groups show much more marked local variations than do the MN and Rh groups, when data for the same or comparable population samples are considered for each system.

However, to carry this type of analysis much further, and at the same time to avoid the danger of subjective judgements, requires a new type of mathematical analysis, and I hope that if the problem is not already under consideration by statistical geneticists, this crude statement may provoke them into activity. I feel that some sort of a filter of the data by 'cell-size' may be achieved, somewhat analogous to the computerized analysis of mixed light or sound waves by frequency and wavelength.

Then, by reference to the facts of recorded history and time-based archaeology, it might be possible to transform the initial 'cell-size' scale into a chronological one. Another aspect of such an analysis would be the possibility, in analyses for a particular purpose, to achieve some sort of objective weighting of the polymorphisms, to replace the arbitrary weightings which we have all, however unconsciously, been applying.

It was my co-author, Ada Kopeć, who drew my attention to the probable relation of this problem to that of the varying amount of disease association shown by the various polymorphisms.

There is no doubt that a large number of diseases of many kinds are associated with the ABO system, whereas far fewer are known to be associated with the Rh or MN system. Most of the disparity undoubtedly arises from lack of data about Rh and MN, but there does appear to be a lesser tendency towards association with these systems than with ABO, whereas the ABH secretor and PTC tasting systems seem to be more richly associated with diseases. Here again there is a need for a sophisticated means of analysis to make an objective test of these conclusions. As a practical consideration, anyone analysing such data must be on guard against systematic errors of some of the more difficult tests, in cases where apparently strong associations are all due to the work of one or two authors.

Then, when adequate means are available to analyse on a world scale the data both of frequency distributions among normal populations, and of disease associations, it may become possible to tie both kinds of knowledge, on a similar broad scale, to the epidemiology of the diseases concerned.

I have called this chapter 'Some conclusions', but the subject of the book is one which, after a long slow start, is now advancing rapidly, and these remarks cannot claim to present anything but interim conclusions. Perhaps, rather, they should be called 'Some beginnings'.

The book will serve its purpose if it enables readers to appreciate the present state of research in its field and, more ambitiously, if it becomes a starting-point for new investigations.

New and perhaps very different editions will be needed in the coming years: I hope that I may see the next one at least, and perhaps even participate, with my co-authors, in its preparation.

ADDENDA

CHOLERA

It has been claimed by Vogel *et al.* (1960) that the cholera vibrio carries an H-like antigen (see p. 5), and that the geographical distribution of the *O* gene, when compared with the distribution of past cholera epidemics, suggests that the disease may have been more frequently fatal among persons of group O than among those of other groups. When the tables for this book were being prepared no frequency data for cholera could be found, but Barura and Paguio (1976) have now found higher frequencies of group O and lower ones of group A among cholera patients than in a control population. They have found, however, a similar frequency distribution also in patients with diarrhoea in whom the vibrio could not be detected. This result gives limited support to the hypothesis of Vogel *et al.*, but tests need to be done on much larger samples of patients.

MALARIA

The polymorphisms claimed as associated with the various manifestations of malaria continue to multiply.

Baer *et al.* (1976) state that elliptocytosis which, in Malaya, defines an important polymorphism is associated, in the Temuan, with resistance to malaria. They suggest that Haemoglobin E may also be so associated, but did not find enough examples of the variant to test the hypothesis.

Harrison *et al.* (1976) find associations of malarial parasitism with the acid phosphatase heterozygote, P^aP^b, possibly with the 6-phosphogluconate dehydrogenase type C-A, with Haemoglobin J-Tongariki and, as elsewhere, with glucose-6-phosphate dehydrogenase (G6PD) deficiency. It is notable that Haemoglobin J (unlike Haemoglobin S elsewhere) appears to *increase* susceptibility to malaria. Parasitism was found to be associated with a reported total absence of G6PD activity rather than with mere weak reactions, but it must be borne in mind that the enzyme tests were performed on specimens several days old. Attempts should be made to define more precisely the enzyme variant concerned.

Hepatomegaly and splenomegaly, common manifestations of malarial infection, are associated with the N blood group as compared with MN (the M type is vanishingly rare in New Guinea), and with Haptoglobin type 1–1.

FILARIASIS

Ayres *et al.* (1976) have produced new data on the possible blood group associations of filariasis. They quote the data of Anand (1965) which are included in the tables of this book, but also old data of Franks (1946) and of Nair *et al.* (1959), which are not. The total rather heterogeneous data on 2360 patients show very slight and quite non-significant associations with A and with B.

DUODENAL ULCERATION

Addis and D'Ovidio (1977) have produced strong evidence that, in Sardinia, duodenal ulceration is associated with glucose-6-phosphate dehydrogenase (G6PD) deficiency. Because of the stratification of the Sardinian population for this deficiency, it is important to note that the controls used by authors were duly matched for place of origin. It would, however, have been interesting to know whether the association could be detected separately in the high and in the low enzyme-deficiency areas.

In view of the numerous polymorphic characters, mentioned on pp. 29–30, for which claims of association with duodenal ulcer have been made (including blood group O, ABH non-secretion, Rh-positiveness, α_1-trypsin inhibitor deficiency, and PTC tasting) as well as G6PD deficiency, just mentioned, it would probably now be worth while to undertake a comprehensive genetic survey of a restricted population, such as that of an island, and to try to find out how much of the duodenal-ulcer incidence would be predicted solely from a knowledge of the complete polymorphic type of each individual.

DIABETES MELLITUS AND THE ACETYLATOR SYSTEM

The acetylator system, now claimed to be associated with neuropathy in patients with diabetes mellitus, has not been described in chapter 2 or elsewhere in this book, but a full account of its population genetics, with references, has been given by Mourant *et al.* (1976).

Within the syndrome of diabetes, some patients develop neuropathies in the course of years, while others live many years without doing so. McLaren *et al.* (1977) have shown that those with neuropathy include a significantly lower frequency (42 per cent) of rapid accelerators than is found in patients who have survived for 10 years or more without neuropathy (64 per cent). It is, however, surprising that the frequency in healthy controls (39 per cent) is near to that of the neuropathic patients, whereas diabetics without neuropathy have a higher frequency than the controls. No association was found between age of onset of diabetes and acetylator type.

It is clearly desirable that larger numbers of patients with and without neuropathy should be tested than the total of 130 so far examined. They should be tested also for the other factors mentioned in chapter 8 as having probable associations with diabetes. Tests ought also to be done on patients from the Far East, where the normal frequency of fast acetylators is much higher than among Europeans.

CHRONIC GRANULOMATOUS DISEASE AND THE KELL SYSTEM

Klebanoff and White (1969), followed by Giblett *et al.* (1971), detected a tendency of chronic granulomatous disease to be associated with weakness or absence of the red-cell antigens of the Kell system. These antigens are, of course, inherited by means of autosomal genes, whereas chronic granulomatous disease usually behaves as a sex-linked recessive condition. The anomaly has now been explained by Marsh *et al.* (1975, 1976).

The K_o phenotype, in which the normal antigens of the Kell system are absent, depends upon a recessively expressed gene at the autosomal Kell locus. In this condition, however, one particular antigen, K_x, is present in unusually large amounts both on the red cells and on leucocytes. K_x is now thought to be a basic substrate, from which the genes of the Kell system elaborate the normal Kell antigens. If these are not being elaborated, an excess of K_x accumulates. K_o cells are morphologically normal.

Another type, the McLeod phenotype, has now been recognized in which there is a deficiency of K_x as well as of the other Kell antigens, and the red cells are morphologically abnormal. It is this type which is associated with chronic granulomatous disease.

This disease is characterized by a defect in the bactericidal function of the neutrophil leucocytes. Marsh *et al.* (1975) suggest that boys with the disease lack a membrane glycoprotein which possesses K_x antigenic specificity, and which has a further function in giving rise to the ordinary antigens of the Kell system.

The situation is, however, further complicated by the observation of Marsh *et al.* (1976) that the leucocyte and erythrocyte characters do not invariably accompany one another, and they postulate the existence of four allelic sex-linked genes, X^1k which gives rise to normal cells of both kinds, X^2k which produces abnormalities in both, with type II chronic granulomatous disease; X^3k which affects leucocytes only and causes chronic granulomatous disease, type I; and X^4k which does not affect the leucocytes but gives rise to the McLeod phenotype red cells, with morphological abnormalities. This situation strongly suggests the existence of two pairs of alleles at closely linked loci, those at one locus acting on the leucocytes and at the other on the erythrocytes. This association of leucocyte function with a red-cell antigen system may prove to be an important clue in ascertaining the normal function of the blood groups.

The association may also be of immediate clinical importance since, if transfusion is needed in a patient with the disease, and especially if he is already immunized to one or more antigens of the Kell system, blood of compatible type may be very difficult to obtain. That this is a real danger is shown by the fact that 4 out of 5 cases of chronic granulomatous disease, type II, known to Marsh *et al.* (1976) have required periodic transfusion to correct anaemia.

DEPRESSIVE PSYCHOSIS

Rundle *et al.* (1977) have examined the adenylate kinase types of 24 manic depressives ('bipolar illness') and 72 pure depressives ('unipolar illness'). They find that the depressives have a significantly raised frequency of the AK 2-1 phenotype and the AK^1 gene as compared with controls. This clearly needs confirmation on much larger groups of patients. The authors suggest that the association is due to the known fact that the AK^2 gene product has less enzymic activity than the much commoner AK^1 product and that it thus gives rise to a less effective energy control mechanism in the brain.

MULTIPLE SCLEROSIS

The intestinal variety of alkaline phosphatase, as shown on p. 6, appears in the plasma mainly in persons who are of blood group O or B, and are genetic secretors of the ABH antigens into the saliva and intestinal secretions. Papiha and Roberts (1975) show that the proportion of persons with this phosphatase in the plasma is reduced in multiple sclerosis, and that the reduction is most marked, and is statistically significant, in those of group O. The authors suggest a connection with the previously known association of multiple sclerosis with group O, and a possible connection with the high incidence of the disease in the Orkney Islands where the frequency of non-secretors of ABH is also particularly high. They also draw attention to the previously suspected intestinal factor in the aetiology of multiple sclerosis, and recommend further study of phosphate metabolism in this disease.

Among northern Europeans, who have a relatively high incidence of multiple sclerosis, associations have been established with a number of histocompatibility antigens, but especially with BT 101 coded at the D locus (pp. 44–5). Kurdi *et al.* (1977) have now shown that in a series of Arabs, mostly natives of Jordan, there is no significant association with BT 101 but a highly significant one with BT 102 (which in Northern Europeans is negatively associated with the disease). The authors, accepting the view that the disease is caused by a virus, consider it likely that the syndrome in Arabs is due to a different virus from that affecting Europeans. However, they accept the possible validity of the alternative hypothesis that the disease is due to a gene closely linked but not identical with the HLA gene concerned, in which case we have here an important example of linkage disequilibrium (p. 46) differing markedly between northern Europeans and Arabs.

FAMILIAL BRONCHIECTASIS

Winzeler *et al.* (1974) have described a family in which 4 (out of 8) siblings who had bronchiectasis following whooping cough (pertussis) were shown also to have hereditary α_1-trypsin-inhibitor deficiency. If this association can be confirmed in other families, then it will be desirable that in families with a history of bronchiectasis, or of the other pathological manifestations of the trypsin-inhibitor deficiency, either the deficient individuals or the whole families should receive early immunization against pertussis. In such individuals the risk of lifelong bronchiectasis would, on the above hypothesis, greatly outweigh the very small risk of encephalitis following immunization.

ASSOCIATIONS IN NEW GUINEA

In addition to their study of malaria associations in New Guinea, Harrison *et al.* (1976) have reported a number of associations with other diseases.

Despite the small numbers found of the Rhesus phenotype CCD^{u}ee ($R_1{}^uR_1{}^u$), the latter has been shown to be significantly associated with proteinuria, as is phosphoglucomutase type PGM_1 2–1 (as compared with 1–1). The phosphoglucomutase 2–1 type, and also the Ss type (as compared with ss) of the MNSs system, appear to be associated with parotid enlargement.

The large number of apparent associations found in New Guinea (which include the malaria association described on p. 51) is clearly due to the fact that considerable numbers of persons were tested for numerous polymorphisms, and that the same persons underwent a clinical examination. Such a procedure is of course liable to give rise, purely by chance, to a number of spurious associations, but the method is ideal for discovering genuine new associations. Tests for each apparent association ought therefore to be done on larger numbers in the original population, as well as on other populations.

TABLES OF ASSOCIATIONS BETWEEN POLYMORPHISMS AND DISEASES

CONTENTS OF TABLES

TABLES

INTRODUCTION

CONTROLS

In preparing this book we have extracted from the relevant literature all the numerical data which we have been able to find on the presence or absence of associations between particular blood groups and particular diseases. We have interpreted the term 'blood group' as meaning any hereditary character detectable by tests on the blood (and a few that require other tests) and have included among 'diseases' such conditions as the presence of antibodies to pathogenic organisms. We have tabulated the data, performed appropriate calculations on them, and then tried to explain the results.

The ideal method for demonstrating an association would be, as mentioned in the Introduction, to examine the whole of a 'randomly interbreeding' population for the presence or absence of the genetic character and for the presence or absence of the disease. It is, however, only in rare cases that data approaching this degree of completeness are available, and they constitute a special case which is dealt with on page 60.

In most cases the population examined consists of a number of persons suffering from a particular disease, and these are classified as to the numbers of them possessing each of a given set of characters, such as the four blood groups of the ABO system. In order to find out whether there is an association between the disease and a given character we need to compare the frequency of this character in the sample of diseased persons with its frequency in a healthy population of the same genetic stock. If they differ markedly, and 'significantly' according to accepted criteria, then an association is likely. Conclusions thus depend fundamentally upon the correct choice of a healthy 'control' population for comparison.

The original author if he has an understanding of population genetics will always be the best judge as to what is the best control population and (however much we may have suspected the author's judgement in a small proportion of cases) we have always accepted his choice of controls where these have been given. To have done otherwise would have exposed us to the risk of a much more dangerous form of bias. As might have been expected, a high proportion of observations have been made in large cities where, as is well known, blood-group frequencies may differ from district to district, and this may be the reason why different authors often use different controls for the same city, and why sometimes one author has used diverse controls for separate sets of patients. Often the reasons for such choices are stated.

However, a considerable number of sets of observations on patients are not accompanied by control data. The omission of such observations would have deprived our analysis of much valuable material; we have therefore needed to provide control data from other sources. In doing so we have been guided by the principles set out below, and we have used in nearly all cases data already compiled by ourselves (Kopeć, 1970; Mourant *et al.*, 1976).

The first principle was to match as nearly as possible the geographical location from which the patients were drawn and, in the few cases where the point arose, their ethnic group. However, for many regions or cities we had more than one possible control sample available. If so, we then chose the one for which the date of publication came nearest to that of the data on the patients since, especially in large cities, frequency variations with time have been found to exist, corresponding to the entry or departure of substantial population groups. This point is particularly important in dealing with old data from Europe where wars have led to large movements of peoples. Where more than one sample satisfied the above criteria and appeared to be representative, we have tended to use the largest of these. In a few cases where the choice was small and the available samples differed appreciably we have used their sum.

In some cases data were not available for the precise place specified by the authors and we have had to use controls from the nearest available place. This necessity arose only exceptionally for the ABO groups, but rather more often for the other systems, for which published data are less extensive.

It will be observed that, occasionally, we have used two sets of controls for different samples from the same place. This is the outcome of our working routine. Sheets for computation were prepared from each paper as soon as it reached us, and we chose the best controls then available, those provided by the author, if any, or others selected on the principles just mentioned. When another paper arrived giving data for the same place, the author may have provided other controls, or new and better controls may have become available to us. Needless to say, the frequencies found in the disease sample were never allowed to influence the choice of the control.

In the tables, a single entry in the 'Authors' column means that the author of the observations on patients has provided his own controls. Where there is more than one entry the first is that of the authors of the observations on patients. The other or others refer to the authors whose data we have used as controls. If only names and year are stated, the exact reference will be found in the bibliography of the present book.

If, however, they are followed by the symbol M2, they will be found under the appropriate geographical heading, in the 'Authors' column of the table for the relevant system, of our *The distribution of the human blood groups* (Mourant *et al.*, 1976). If they are followed by M1, they will be found similarly in our *The ABO blood groups* (Mourant *et al.*, 1958) which has been reprinted as an appendix to our 1976 book. In such cases the *names* are those of the authors who performed the tests adopted by us as controls, and who are not in all cases the same as the authors of the papers from which we extracted the data; the reference *number* in the M1 or M2 table will direct the reader to the reference from which we obtained the data. Thus in consulting M1 or M2 the reader should look first at the appropriate table, and not go straight to the bibliography. In both M1 and M2 such second-hand references in the tables are marked with an asterisk. In case of difficulty the names of all first-named authors, whether quoted directly or at second-hand, can be found in the author index of M2, which covers both books.

A second entry is given only when the authors give no controls, and the choice was our own. Where an author quotes controls compiled by another author, no second entry is made. In cases where authors recommend controls from another paper, without actually setting them out, but giving a precise reference, we have extracted them from the paper referred to, but have given no second entry.

COMPARISONS BETWEEN TWO PARTS OF A LIMITED POPULATION SAMPLE

The above account concerns 'controls' in the usual sense of the word, groups of presumably healthy persons taken without selection from the same population as those suffering from the disease under consideration. The designation of the control group depended, however, on an act of judgement independent of the operations, statistical, clinical, and pathological, which designated the group of patients.

The tables, however, contain also comparisons where the question of 'controls' in this sense does not arise. These are comparisons where one population has been divided into two parts according to the presence or absense of a disease, symptom, or reaction to a test. Here the clinical or pathological tests which defined the group of patients automatically and simultaneously defined the 'controls'.

In some such cases the comparison is between two parts of a group of persons, such that the group as a whole, for example a body of soldiers or blood donors, was not selected for any medical reason. Here, if the disease or other condition is a relatively rare one, the situation is the ideal one envisaged on page 59, and should not differ greatly in practice from that where, as in the greater part of the tables, a group of patients is compared with an independent group of controls. In a statistical sense, however, the two kinds of 'control' differ fundamentally in their method of ascertainment.

In other cases the group under examination is more or less evenly divided between presence and absence of the particular disease or reaction, so that the 'control' is not merely automatically designated, but is far from being a true sample of the whole population group under examination.

In yet other cases all the members of the group examined and subdivided suffered from variants of a single disease, and the total disease group will, in many cases, have been compared as a whole with an independent set of controls. This adds a second type of statistical distinction separating the situation from that occurring in the main part of the tables.

However, as already shown, all these types of cases share a single statistical status differing from that of the rest of the entries. They are placed in their proper sequence in the tables, under the heading of the disease or condition concerned, but are printed in italics and, at the end of any series of entries divided by a common criterion, the total numbers for each of the parts are printed.

ARRANGEMENT OF THE TABLES

For each of the systems chosen for full tabulation (see pp. 62–3) we have included in the tables all the data which we could find in the literature, or which were communicated to us unpublished. When the published data have contained some lacuna or ambiguity, we have tried to obtain the missing information from the authors. When we have succeeded, and the data tabulated by us differ in any way from those originally published, the total number tested is followed by the symbol 'a'. When the required information has been unobtainable we have used as much of the data as could be fitted into our scheme.

The names of the diseases are, as far as possible, those used by the authors or, for the many papers published in languages other than English, their English equivalents. For nomenclature as well as for classification we have followed the *Manual of the international statistical classification of diseases, injuries and causes of death* (WHO, 1967). The main groups into which we have subdivided diseases are also the 'subcategories' used in that publication, except that we have added one for all allergies. The same is largely true for the sequence of diseases within each main group. As a consequence of this rule the main group of infective diseases contains only those for which the pathogenic agent is stated, or can be identified with confidence. Other diseases, known only to be infective, but which can be due to any of a variety of organisms, such as 'pneumonia', may therefore be found elsewhere, but their exact location can be found in our index (as well as in the WHO index).

In the tables, the column 'additional information' attempts to provide, in the minimum space, the maximum of information about the disease and the patients. It gives the author's designation of the disease whenever this differs from the 'official' one used by us, and also particulars of any special form of it, too infrequent in our material to deserve a separate class. The column gives also information provided by the authors with regard to the patients, such as ethnic group, sex, or age. Finally an indication (s) is given whenever, in the original paper, the data are further subdivided. The symbol '(s)A' means that they are subdivided by age, '(s)C' chronologically (i.e. the population as listed by us contains two or more series tested at different times), '(s)G', geographically, and '(s)S', by sex. When the further subdivision is according to a genetic system other than the one under consideration, the '(s)' is followed by the accepted designation of that system.

STATISTICAL TREATMENT

The statistical method used here for the analysis of the data is that recommended by Woolf (1954–5). It is summarized here for the benefit of readers who may not have access to the original paper.

Woolf's method makes it possible, first, to compare the frequencies of two characters in two populations (e.g. patients and controls) and then to combine the results for all sets within a series, so as to assess the over-all difference in those frequencies, even when the frequencies of the characters concerned are different in each control population (the differences are usually genetical, but this is irrelevant to the primary statistical treatment).

Let P and p be the numbers in which two characters, such as blood group A and blood group O, are observed among patients suffering from a particular disease, and C and c the corresponding numbers among the presumably healthy controls. Then the two characters are found in the ratio P/p in patients and C/c in controls. Thus the relative incidence is

$$\frac{P}{p}\bigg/\frac{C}{c} = \frac{Pc}{pC} = x.$$

If the two ratios are similar, x will be near unity, but we need to estimate the significance of its difference from unity. For each individual set of data, let:

$$y = \log_e x$$

$$V = \frac{1}{P} + \frac{1}{p} + \frac{1}{C} + \frac{1}{c},$$

its sampling variance and

$$w = \frac{1}{V}, \text{ its weight.}$$

To estimate the difference of x from unity, we estimate the difference of y from zero, and the significance of each such difference is given by

$$\chi_1^2 = wy^2.$$

Then all sets of a series are combined in the following way:

$$Y = \Sigma wy/\Sigma w.$$

This is the weighted mean of the values of y and its anti-logarithm X is the combined estimate of the values of x. The significance of its difference from unity is given by:

$$\chi_1^2 = (\Sigma wy)^2/\Sigma w.$$

If N is the number of sets in a series, their homogeneity is estimated by:

$$\chi_{N-1}^2 = \Sigma wy^2 - (\Sigma wy)^2/\Sigma w.$$

Beneath the line marking the end of a series, the estimated combined relative incidence is entered in the column below the separate relative incidences, and the first of the above combined values of χ^2 in the column below the separate values of χ^2 for the individual sets of data. The second χ^2 (for homogeneity) is in the next line. In the ABO tables, where both the comparisons A/O and B/O are made, there are of course separate values of combined relative incidence and of χ^2 for each comparison.

The basic material of our analysis consisted of observed *numbers*, and only they are quoted in the tables. In a considerable number of cases published data consisted of frequencies. Wherever it was possible to use these to calculate numbers, the latter have been entered in the tables, with the symbol (c) against the total, to show that this has been done.

As already stated, we have included in our tables, for each disease, and each genetic system, all the data available to us, even if a particular character (and blood group B in particular) was absent among the patients, or even in the controls, owing to its rarity in the general population. Such data cannot be analysed by Woolf's method. We have, however, included them in our tables, but their total is excluded from the over-all total for the series and, of course, the number of degrees of freedom of the value of χ^2 for homogeneity will be one (or more) below that for the number of sets actually tabulated.

In the tables for the ABO system, which show both the comparisons A/O and B/O, it has happened occasionally, as just mentioned, that B was absent among the patients, and in other cases the author gave only the totals for A and O, and not for B. Such sets have a blank in the column of the B/O analysis and account for the existence of two overall totals and two numbers of degrees of freedom for the χ^2 for homogeneity.

This defect of Woolf's method does not appear to be generally known and we did not appreciate it until we received the results of the electronic computations done by this method, with blanks in the appropriate places. Though, as we now know, there are various ways of overcoming this problem, it was by then much too late to contemplate recomputing all the data by another method. While the exclusion from analysis of series with no group B among patients will tend to increase the apparent ratio of B/O in the combined data, the numbers of patients concerned are very small, and we have satisfied ourselves that the over-all effects are negligible.

As we now realize, this problem, like so many basic problems of population genetics, was long ago solved by Haldane (1955–6). His correction to the method of Woolf (1954–5) involves the following changes in the equations on page 60. The relative incidence, x, becomes

$$x = \frac{(2P+1)(2c+1)}{(2p+1)(2C+1)}$$

(instead of $x = Pc/pC$).

The value of y, the natural logarithm of x, becomes

$$y = \log_e \frac{(2P+1)(2c+1)}{(2p+1)(2C+1)}$$

V, the sampling variance of y, becomes

$$V = \frac{1}{P+1} + \frac{1}{p+1} + \frac{1}{C+1} + \frac{1}{c+1}$$

$$\left(\text{instead of } V = \frac{1}{P} + \frac{1}{p} + \frac{1}{C} + \frac{1}{c}\right).$$

For the reasoning behind the corrections Haldane's (1955–6) paper should be consulted. The correction is negligible when, as in most of the cases considered by us, the observed number of patients (P and p) are large. It becomes more marked when the numbers are small (say, of the order of 50). Also, the corrected method can be used for the cases where P or p is zero, which we have had to exclude from our computations.

For the other polymorphic systems also, there are rare cases where one phenotype is absent either among the patients or in both patients and controls. In the MN system these all concern New Guinea, where the MM phenotype is everywhere extremely rare. Thus virtually no information is lost by the use of Woolf's method.

In the Rh system all cases of absence of D-negatives but one concern either very small series of patients, or populations where D-negatives are rare or absent in the general population. A borderline case is that of asthma cases in Cagliari (Sardinia, Italy) where there were no D-negatives among 50 patients. If this series had been incorporated by Haldane's method (above) this would slightly have enhanced the overall but non-significant deficiency of D-negatives in this disease.

For the secretor system only one very small series is involved, and for the haptoglobin system all cases of absence of a phenotype concern HpO which is very rare or absent in nearly all populations, and is probably mainly of physiological rather than genetic origin.

In the case of the histocompatibility system small numbers and zeros are common among the data, and Haldane's method has been used by Ryder and Svejgaard (1976) in their booklet on HLA and diseases which has been reproduced as an appendix to the present book.

INTERPRETATION

The question of the meaning of the results tabulated in this book depends not only on the crude values of relative incidences but on whether they are statistically significant. In general the tables set out the relative incidences for each disease for one genetic factor at a time. In these circumstances it is generally accepted as appropriate to set the level of significance at a probability of 1 in 20 (the probability that the same or a greater divergence of the relative incidence from unity would occur by chance) which of course means that one false case of apparent association is likely to turn up in every 20 sets. For one degree of freedom the critical value of χ^2 is 3·841. The question of tests of one population for several characters will be mentioned later.

In examining the data, the method which we have used places any given set of observations in one of four categories. The mean incidence of a character may differ significantly from unity or it may not, and it may do so either homogeneously or not. For the present we shall assume that each disease is itself a homogeneous entity, and shall deal later with the possibility that an apparently single disease may itself be heterogeneous. To enable the reader (and indeed ourselves) to see the data as a whole, we have drawn up summarizing tables showing for each combination of a disease and a genetic character the number of patients, the number of sets of patients, the combined incidence, and the values of χ^2 for difference from unity and for homogeneity. We have not attempted to tabulate separately the four categories mentioned above, as this would have involved undue prejudging of the issues and would in many cases have been misleading.

If an association between a genetic character and a disease is to be claimed, it must be shown that the frequency of the character in patients differs from that in controls, and that the difference is unlikely to be due to chance. For each individual set of data this probability may be derived from the value of χ^2 obtained. In a series of sets it must further be shown that the individual differences are not only too marked but also too regular to be due to chance. The degree of similarity or regularity is shown by the value of χ^2 for 'homogeneity'.

A cursory inspection of the summarized tables shows that heterogeneity is present in many series, whether or not the over-all difference from unity is significant. Does this, in particular, always mean that the individual differences are too erratic to allow valid conclusions to be drawn?

There are many series which show significant mean differences but which are heterogeneous. In some such cases inspection of the individual sets may show that the resultant difference from unity is due to just one or two aberrant sets, while for all the others the differences are small. Then, of course, the over-all difference is not representative and does not indicate association.

The elimination of such series still leaves many, including some which, owing to the large number of sets which they contain, are most informative. Does a significant value of χ^2 for homogeneity necessarily discriminate against the value of the information in them?

The study of homogeneity is, of course, the study of the distribution of the individual incidences, and whether they differ from the mean incidence more than may be due to chance. In any large but heterogeneous series it is particularly instructive to plot that distribution. It will obviously often be found that some incidences are far beyond the admissible range, yet the bulk of them lies within it, and has a distribution near that attributable to chance, i.e. a normal distribution centred on the mean incidence. Thus the required regularity still applies to the bulk of the data. The few sets to which it does not are in most cases to be regarded as freaks, perhaps due to technical errors. Their occasional appearance in greater numbers than the laws of probability would allow must be a warning against the drawing of hasty conclusions from a single set of data.

These comments on heterogeneity apply mainly to those diseases which are not known *a priori* to be in some way heterogeneous, and for which fuller study of the statistical results gives no suggestion of any clinical or pathological heterogeneity. However, one of the most useful results of association studies is to draw attention to statistical heterogeneities which are subsequently shown to be due to heterogeneity of the disease itself. Thus any significant heterogeneity, whether or not the combined relative incidence for a genetical factor differs significantly from unity, should be studied closely to see whether a meaningful classification of the data can be made according to the relative incidences shown by the separate sets of data. At this stage little more can be done than classify the sets of data, but once it is suspected that the dichotomy of the disease is real, then subsequent prospective studies with appropriate classification of individual patients should be even more revealing. The most striking cases of heterogeneity attributable to a known cause are those of bleeding and non-bleeding ulcers, both gastric and duodenal. Examples where we ourselves were led to reclassify data because of their heterogeneity are those of the variants of diabetes mellitus (p. 31), and of coronary insufficiency thrombosis (p. 34).

As already mentioned, most of the studies which we have tabulated have involved the testing of sufferers from a single disease for one or a small number of genetic factors. However, in the case of the HLA antigens patients with a single disease are often examined for approximately twenty factors. In the blood-group field too, more and more studies are being done where patients with one disease are examined for a multiplicity of factors. If the number of factors is 20 and we set the value the probability at 1 in 20 it is likely that there will be an apparently significant association with one of the 20 factors, though the situation is complicated where the factors are not independent of one another. The problem has been discussed by Svejgaard *et al.* (1974) who suggest correcting the limiting P value (conventionally 1/20) by multiplying its denominator by the number of characters investigated. The investigation of possible associations with both the A and the B blood groups falls marginally into the above category but if the investigator is concerned primarily, as we have been, with the single ratio, A/O, then a P value of 1/20 remains appropriate.

CHOICE OF DATA AND RESULTS FOR TABULATION

In planning the tables we have been guided on the one hand by the need to include as much as possible of the basic data, especially the numbers in each phenotype, and on the other hand by the undesirability of burdening the tables with masses of derived information which would seldom if ever be used.

For the ABO system, as for all other systems, we have tabulated all phenotypes, but we have given the relative incidences only for A/O and B/O which carry most of the relevant information. Other relative incidences have been computed, but have not been tabulated because they supply so little additional information. In particular, the AB/O relative incidence supplies little information because of the rarity of AB. We have, however, tabulated a few AB results which apply to very large bodies of data, in Table 1.1 (p. 196).

A very few authors have classified group A into sub-groups A_1 and A_2. The total numbers tested have in most cases been small, and the numbers of A_2 very small, and in some cases control data have not been supplied. We have therefore tabulated the A_1A_2 data only for well-defined diseases for which at least two sets of data and appropriate controls were available.

Of the other blood-group systems, only for the MN and Rh systems have data been tabulated and, as may be seen, the results are most disappointing. For the remaining systems data are even more scarce and, despite a few suggestive associations, it was not thought worth while to prepare tables. From our extensive experience of the ABO system we have come to mistrust apparent associations based on single investigations but such associations are, where appropriate, mentioned in the text.

Data for the ABH secretor factor have, on the other hand, proved highly informative and well worth tabulating. The same is true, within their limited field, of data on PTC tasting.

For blood factors with known functions, such as the plasma proteins and red-cell enzymes, it is probable that future work will show important disease associations, but only the haptoglobin system has yet supplied sufficient data to be worth tabulating.

The highly informative data on the histocompatibility system are shown in the appendix which, as already explained, is a reprint of *Associations between HLA and disease* by Lars P. Ryder and Arne Svejgaard, and is included here by kind permission of the authors.

The protease inhibitor system shows very close associations with certain diseases, but most of the data are in the form of studies of small numbers of clinical cases, and few of them are in a form suitable for standard tabulation.

TABLE 1
THE ABO BLOOD GROUP SYSTEM

INFECTIVE AND PARASITIC DISEASES

BACTERIAL INFECTIONS

TYPHOID FEVER

Place	Additional details	Authors		Number	O	A	B	AB	A/O Relative incidence	A/O χ_1^2 for difference from unity	B/O Relative incidence	B/O χ_1^2 for difference from unity
1. Greece, Athínai		Diamantopoulos 1928	P	127(c)	48	54	20	5	1·2560	1·1998	1·5118	2·1501
			C	1216	537	481	148	50				
2. Poland, Warszawa		Górecki & Kulesza 1949	P	99	38	35	20	6	0·7817	1·0669	0·8672	0·2567
		Hirszfeld 1928 M1	C	2886	954	1124	579	229				
3. Poland, Warszawa	Children	Paciorkiewicz 1970	P	445(c)	151	157	94	43	0·8047	3·4046	0·9781	0·0265
			C	6626(c)	2041	2637	1299	649				
4. Romania, Bucureşti		Mironesco & Stefanov 1926	P	36	5	17	8	6	2·8105	4·0436	3·0097	3·6428
		Dumitrescu 1927 M1	C	1031	348	421	185	77				
5. Peru, Lima		Muñoz-Baratta 1962	P	249(c)	179	53	14	3	0·7519	3·3179	0·4091	10·3601
			C	107938(c)	66058	26013	12629	3238				
				956					0·8670	3·2053	0·9381	0·3884
				χ_4^2 for homogeneity of areas						9·8275		16·0478

PARATYPHOID FEVER

Place	Additional details	Authors		Number	O	A	B	AB	A/O Relative incidence	A/O χ_1^2 for difference from unity	B/O Relative incidence	B/O χ_1^2 for difference from unity
1. Poland, Warszawa	A, B, and C; children	Paciorkiewicz 1970	P	237(c)	97	88	37	15	0·7022	5·5459	0·5993	6·7906
			C	6626(c)	2041	2637	1299	649				

UNSPECIFIED SALMONELLA INFECTIONS

Place	Additional details	Authors		Number	O	A	B	AB	A/O Relative incidence	A/O χ_1^2 for difference from unity	B/O Relative incidence	B/O χ_1^2 for difference from unity
1. U.S.A., New York	Enteric; Negroes	Robinson *et al.* 1971	P	28	12	6	8	2	0·9120	0·0337	1·6227	1·1123
			C	2933	1441	790	592	110				
2. U.S.A., New York	Enteric; Puertoricans	Robinson *et al.* 1971	P	17	9	4	3	1	0·8614	0·0607	1·8507	0·8296
			C	928	533	275	96	24				
3. U.S.A., New York	Enteric; Whites	Robinson *et al.* 1971	P	6	2	4	0	0	2·2353	0·8418		
			C	253	114	102	29	8				
				51					1·0349	0·0094	1·6915	1·9160
				χ_2^2 for homogeneity of areas						0·9268		
				(45) χ_1^2 for homogeneity of areas								0·0259

SHIGELLA FLEXNERI DYSENTERY

Place	Additional details	Authors		Number	O	A	B	AB	A/O Relative incidence	A/O χ_1^2 for difference from unity	B/O Relative incidence	B/O χ_1^2 for difference from unity
1. Germany, Berlin		Kerde *et al.* 1962	P	1050	386	467	140	57	1·0244	0·1174	0·9380	0·4017
			C	21104	7725	9123	2987	1269				

UNSPECIFIED BACILLARY DYSENTERY

Place	Additional details	Authors		Number	O	A	B	AB	A/O Relative incidence	A/O χ_1^2 for difference from unity	B/O Relative incidence	B/O χ_1^2 for difference from unity
1. Poland, Warszawa	Children	Paciorkiewicz 1970	P	124(c)	30	54	26	14	1·3932	2·0855	1·3617	1·3048
			C	6626(c)	2041	2637	1299	649				

ESCHERICHIA COLI INFECTIONS

Place	Additional details	Authors		Number	O	A	B	AB	A/O Relative incidence	A/O χ_1^2 for difference from unity	B/O Relative incidence	B/O χ_1^2 for difference from unity
1. Germany, Heidelberg	Enteritis in infants	Vogel *et al.* 1964	P	396(c)	164	179	39	14	0·9644	0·1110	0·8858	0·4587
			C	34513(c)	13748	15559	3691	1515				
2. Poland, Kraków	Enteritis in infants	Socha *et al.* 1969	P	248	90	72	70	16	0·6691	6·2109	1·2466	1·8123
			C	5698	1840	2200	1148	510				
3. U.S.A., New York	Enteric; Negroes	Robinson *et al.* 1971	P	137	61	34	34	8	1·0167	0·0057	1·3567	1·9314
			C	2933	1441	790	592	110				
4. U.S.A., New York	Enteric; Puertoricans	Robinson *et al.* 1971	P	36	17	10	5	4	1·1401	0·1046	1·6330	0·8870
			C	928	533	275	96	24				
5. U.S.A., New York	Enteric; Whites	Robinson *et al.* 1971	P	10	5	2	3	0	0·4471	0·9020	2·3586	1·2770
			C	253	114	102	29	8				
				827					0·8850	2·2588	1·1603	2·0912
				χ_4^2 for homogeneity of areas						5·0754		4·2752

TABLE 1 **THE ABO BLOOD GROUP SYSTEM** *(cont.)*

Place	Additional details	Authors		Number	O	A	B	AB	A/O Relative incidence	A/O χ_1^2 for difference from unity	B/O Relative incidence	B/O χ_1^2 for difference from unity
INFECTIVE AND PARASITIC DISEASES *(cont.)*												
BACTERIAL INFECTIONS (cont.)												
ENTERITIS IN INFANTS (no evidence of *Escherichia Coli*)												
1. Germany, Heidelberg		Vogel *et al.* 1964	P	1316(c)	495	622	132	67	1·1103	2·9081	0·9933	0·0046
			C	34513(c)	13748	15559	3691	1515				
ENTERITIS IN INFANTS (no mention of pathogenesis)												
1. Austria, Vöcklabruck		Kircher 1964	P	728	322	270	94	42	0·9373	0·4687	1·0290	0·0447
			C	2289	987	883	280	139				
2. Egypt		Khalil 1960	P	143	30	50	38	25	1·5308	3·3626	1·6967	4·6300
			C	10045(c)	3279	3570	2448	748				
				871					1·0051	0·0034	1·1561	1·4973
				χ_1^2 for homogeneity of areas						3·8279		3·1774
GONORRHOEA												
1. Finland		Mustakallio 1937	P	194	73	87	26	8	0·9856	0·0078	0·8065	0·8297
			C	2595	908	1098	401	188				
2. United Kingdom, Newcastle upon Tyne	(s) S	Schofield 1966	P	374	176	156	35	7	1·1355	1·3264	1·0783	0·1647
			C	54579	27008	21082	4981	1508				
3. Japan, Okayama		Ohmichi 1928	P	40	12	12	10	6	0·7107	0·6961	0·9980	0·0000
		After Furuhata 1933 M1	C	6936	1921	2703	1604	708				
				608					1·0650	0·4953	0·9684	0·0541
				χ_2^2 for homogeneity of areas						1·5350		0·9403
BRUCELLOSIS												
1. Peru, Lima		Muñoz-Baratta 1962	P	165(c)	104	37	19	5	0·9034	0·2809	0·9556	0·0331
			C	107938(c)	66058	26013	12629	3238				
WHOOPING COUGH												
1. Poland, Warszawa	Children	Paciorkiewicz 1970	P	684(c)	213	250	138	83	0·9084	0·9643	1·0180	0·0240
			C	6626(c)	2041	2637	1299	649				
2. Romania, Bucureşti		Mironesco & Stefanov 1926	P	14	8	5	0	1	0·5166	1·3207		
		Dumitrescu 1927 M1	C	1031	348	421	185	77				
3. U.S.A., New York		Brody *et al.* 1936	P	109	59	38	2	10	0·8721	0·3884	0·1328	7·7300
			C	1000	478	353	122	47				
				807					0·8905	1·7252	0·9698	0·0792
				χ_2^2 for homogeneity of areas						0·9482		
				(793) χ_1^2 for homogeneity of areas								7·6748
DIPHTHERIA												
1. Denmark	(s) S, A, C	Rosling 1929	P	2034	852	885	218	79	1·0639	0·6095	1·3682	5·3841
			C	1151	508	496	95	52				
2. Poland, Warszawa		Paciorkiewicz 1970	P	672	220	262	126	64	0·9217	0·7193	0·8999	0·8100
			C	6626	2041	2637	1299	649				
3. U.S.A., New York		Brody *et al.* 1936	P	21	12	7	1	1	0·7899	0·2407	0·3265	1·1456
			C	1000	478	353	122	47				
				2727					1·0000	0·0000	1·0682	0·5588
				χ_2^2 for homogeneity of areas						1·5694		6·7809

TABLE 1 THE ABO BLOOD GROUP SYSTEM (*cont.*)

Place	Additional details	Authors		Number	O	A	B	AB	A/O Relative incidence	A/O χ_1^2 for difference from unity	B/O Relative incidence	B/O χ_1^2 for difference from unity
Schick Test for Susceptibility, +/−												
1. Austria, Wien	Children	Nowak 1931–2	+	*169*	*61*	*77*	*29*	*2*	*1·4359*	*2·4754*	*1·4421*	*1·4078*
			−	*215*	*91*	*80*	*30*	*14*				
2. France, Northern		Balgairies 1934	+	*163*	*75*	*66*	*17*	*5*	*0·8067*	*0·9647*	*1·0686*	*0·0339*
			−	*237*	*99*	*108*	*21*	*9*				
3. France, Lille	20/25 years old	Farjot 1933	+	*109*	*52*	*44*	*10*	*3*	*0·8638*	*0·2577*	*1·3462*	*0·3128*
			−	*106*	*49*	*48*	*7*	*2*				
4. Poland	Soldiers	Kaczynsky 1926	+	*455*	*151*	*197*	*82*	*25*	*1·0912*	*0·3839*	*0·8039*	*1·5976*
			−	*696*	*225*	*269*	*152*	*50*				
5. Poland, Warszawa		Hirszfeld *et al.* 1924	+	*95*	*40*	*40*	*10*	*5*	*0·9130*	*0·1030*	*0·8289*	*0·1819*
			−	*156*	*63*	*69*	*19*	*5*				
				991/1410					*1·0342*	*0·1297*	*0·9535*	*0·1371*
				χ_4^2 for homogeneity of areas						*4·0551*		*3·3968*
SCARLET FEVER												
1. Austria, Vöcklabruck	(s) S	Kircher 1969	P	697	312	272	83	30	0·9527	0·2407	0·9858	0·0095
			C	1708	730	668	197	113				
2. Austria, Wien		Nowak 1932	P	232	110	80	30	12	0·7041	3·5633	0·7026	1·8887
			C	384	152	157	59	16				
3. Germany, Düsseldorf	(s) S	Körwer 1932	P	363	145	168	32	18	1·1586	1·2626	1·1481	0·3700
			C	1045(c)	463	463	89	30				
4. Germany, Duisburg-Hamborn		Vossschulte & Ziegler 1935	P	133	59	32	25	17	0·5424	7·1270	2·2043	8·8816
			C	1045(c)	463	463	89	30				
5. Germany, Frankfurt am Main		Fischer 1928–31	P	240	100	107	23	10	1·0173	0·0136	0·8838	0·2573
			C	2000(c)	830	873	216	81				
6. Germany, Köln	Children	Bernecker 1936	P	500	213	223	46	18	0·9871	0·0126	0·8246	1·0092
			C	1100(c)	462	490	121	27				
7. Hungary, Budapest		Kiss & Teveli 1930	P	172	78	59	24	11	0·4197	20·9911	0·3972	13·4184
		Ferró & Gajzágó M1	C	1000	253	456	196	95				
8. Poland, Warszawa	Children	Paciorkiewicz 1970	P	697(c)	242	251	132	72	0·8028	5·3711	0·8570	1·8358
			C	6626(c)	2041	2637	1299	649				
9. Romania, Bucureşti		Mironesco & Stefanov 1926	P	38	6	14	13	5	1·9287	1·7731	4·0757	7·8379
		Dumitrescu 1927 M1	C	1031	348	421	185	77				
10. U.S.A., New York		Brody *et al.* 1936	P	302	137	93	54	18	0·9192	0·3088	1·5443	5·2309
			C	1000	478	353	122	47				
				3374					0·8766	8·9465	1·0317	0·2569
				χ_9^2 for homogeneity of areas						31·7173		40·4825
Dick Test for Susceptibility, +/−												
1. Poland	Soldiers	Kaczynsky 1926	+	*447*	*123*	*197*	*101*	*26*	*1·4601*	*6·9503*	*1·4611*	*4·9912*
			−	*742*	*258*	*283*	*145*	*56*				
CHRONIC INFECTION WITH HAEMOLYTIC STREPTOCOCCUS A												
1. Romania, Timişoara	School-children; (s) ABH secretion	Radivoievici *et al.* 1972	P	100	30	52	13	3	1·4797	1·4549	0·8922	0·0659
			C	100	35	41	17	7				
STAPHYLOCOCCAL INFECTIONS												
1. Austria, Vöcklabruck	Infants; (s) S	Kircher 1968	P	309	144	118	31	16	0·8937	0·7496	0·8001	1·1730
			C	3405	1468	1346	395	196				
2. U.S.A., Iowa	Septicaemia	Buckwalter *et al.* 1964	P	156(c)	76	57	21	2	0·7943	1·7229	1·3178	1·2480
			C	49979	22392	21144	4695	1748				
				465					0·8572	2·1805	0·9817	0·0136
				χ_1^2 for homogeneity of areas						0·2920		2·4074

TABLE 1 **THE ABO BLOOD GROUP SYSTEM** *(cont.)*

Place	Additional details	Authors		Number	O	A	B	AB	A/O Relative incidence	A/O χ_1^2 for difference from unity	B/O Relative incidence	B/O χ_1^2 for difference from unity
INFECTIVE AND PARASITIC DISEASES *(cont.)*												
BACTERIAL INFECTIONS (cont.)												
STAPHYLOCOCCI, CARRIERS/NON-CARRIERS, +/−												
1. United Kingdom	R.A.F. recruits	Zuckermann *et al.* 1964	+	988	468	422	73	25	0·9287	0·6685	0·7743	2·4545
			−	1238	551	535	111	41				
2. United Kingdom, London	Male surgical patients	White & Shooter 1962	+	596	289	232	59	16	0·7495	4·7277	1·0584	0·0621
			−	459	197	211	38	13				
3. Australia, Adelaide		Coulter 1962	+	291	135	127	22	7	0·8771	0·6797	0·5073	6·2099
			−	481	193	207	62	19				
				1875/2178					0·8692	4·2896	0·7779	4·4321
				χ_2^2 for homogeneity of areas						1·7863		4·2944
COCCAL SKIN INFECTIONS												
1. Egypt	(s) S	el-Hefnawi *et al.* 1963	P	100	32	32	28	8	0·9383	0·0636	1·1588	0·3179
			C	5200	1674	1784	1264	478				
TETANUS												
1. Poland, Warszawa	Children	Paciorkiewicz 1970	P	57(c)	23	22	9	3	0·7403	1·0066	0·6148	1·5182
			C	6626(c)	2041	2637	1299	649				
2. United Kingdom, St. Andrews		Alexander 1921	P	25(c)	12	8	4	1	0·8070	0·1510	1·2778	0·1106
			C	50(c)	23	19	6	2				
				82					0·7550	1·1388	0·7238	0·8631
				χ_1^2 for homogeneity of areas						0·0188		0·7657
TUBERCULOSIS												
PULMONARY TUBERCULOSIS												
1. Belgium		Moureau 1935	P	250	120	101	23	6	0·9381	0·2089	1·0762	0·0966
			C	3500(c)	1634	1466	291	109				
2. Czechoslovakia, Praha	Males; (s) A	Miluničová & Dominec 1966	P	106	37	42	16	11	0·9459	0·0541	0·7593	0·7667
		Miluničová & Sottner 1965 M2	C	878	295	354	168	61				
3. Denmark København		Viskum 1973	P	609	287	233	63	26	0·7480	10·3940	0·8183	1·9941
		Andersen 1955 M1	C	14304	5804	6299	1557	644				
4. France, Paris		Dufourt *et al.* 1933	P	100	54	34	10	2	0·6016	4·3533	0·7963	0·3474
			C	400	172	180	40	8				
5. Germany, Berlin		Connerth 1927	P	667(c)	278	263	93	33	0·9077	0·5651	0·7745	2·1826
			C	560(c)	213	222	92	33				
6. Germany, Nordrhein-Westfalen		Schmitt 1928	P	564	241	249	57	17	0·8547	0·8723	0·7422	1·3238
			C	236	91	110	29	6				
7. Germany, Württemberg		Tiedemann 1929–30	P	361	174	139	33	15	0·7446	5·7172	0·8030	1·1411
			C	2058	851	913	201	93				
8. Hungary, Budapest		Holló & Lénard 1926	P	200	62	85	42	11	1·2267	0·7485	1·0237	0·0071
			C	200	68	76	45	11				
9. Italy		de Paoli 1932	P	108	55	34	12	7	0·4895	10·0887	0·6173	2·1558
		Viola 1928–9 M1	C	1669	597	754	211	107				
10. Italy, Cuneo		Gunella 1936	P	330(c)	130	146	40	14	1·1918	0·5684	2·2857	3·5086
		Formentano 1951 M1	C	109	52	49	7	1				
11. Italy, Firenze		Aloigi 1929	P	170(c)	89	67	12	2	0·7887	1·1404	0·5933	1·7483
		Montanari 1929	C	200(c)	88	84	20	8				
12. Italy, Milano		Dossena & Lanzara 1925	P	30	13	13	3	1	1·2821	0·3494	0·8876	0·0310
		Dossena 1924 M1	C	214	100	78	26	10				
13. Italy, Napoli		Valentini 1938	P	808	412	280	76	40	1·0731	0·2721	0·7174	2·8389
			C	417	210	133	54	20				
14. Italy, Roma		Gunella 1936	P	90	45	42	3	0	1·1105	0·1906	0·2458	5·1767
		Siciliano & Mittiga 1953 M1	C	414	188	158	51	17				

TABLE 1 **THE ABO BLOOD GROUP SYSTEM** (*cont.*)

Place	Additional details	Authors		Number	O	A	B	AB	A/O		B/O	
									Relative incidence	χ_1^2 for difference from unity	Relative incidence	χ_1^2 for difference from unity
15. Italy, Trieste		Tagliaferro 1937[b]	P	628	246	260	88	34	1·0711	0·4337	0·8578	1·1526
		Goldstein 1927, 1929 M1	C	1766	681	671	284	129				
16. Poland	(s) S	Promińska 1967	P	935	305	365	188	77	0·9728	0·0917	0·9940	0·0031
			C	2492	795	978	493	226				
17. Spain		Samitier Azparren & Chacon 1958	P	126	61	50	10	5	0·7886	1·5385	0·7882	0·4835
			C	16563(c)	7154	7436	1488	485				
18. United Kingdom, Lancashire		Bradbury 1934/5	P	494	294	154	38	8	0·5612	5·9661	0·5288	2·8426
			C	103	45	42	11	5				
19. United Kingdom, London		Lewis & Woods 1961	P	894	436	348	77	33	0·8661	3·6765	0·9084	0·5549
			C	10000	4578	4219	890	313				
20. United Kingdom, Glasgow		Campbell 1956	P	450	258	133	45	14	0·8593	1·8805	0·8699	0·6942
			C	5898	3177	1906	637	178				
21. N. India, Jaipur		Jain 1970	P	1600	460	308	576	256	0·9903	0·0131	1·2094	6·6654
			C	3799	1300	879	1346	274				
22. N. India, Kanpur		Navani & Narang 1962	P	1000	374	204	300	122	0·7308	6·0793	0·7792	4·6978
			C	820	272	203	280	65				
23. N. India, Lucknow		Nath *et al.* 1963	P	228	77	53	80	18	0·9461	0·0899	0·8514	0·9498
			C	3330(c)	1035	753	1263	279				
24. S. India, Bombay	Mahars	Kothare 1959	P	151	42	35	54	20	1·0040	0·0002	1·1084	0·1737
			C	325	100	83	116	26				
25. S. India, Bombay	Marathas	Kothare 1959	P	284	93	78	86	27	0·9578	0·0529	1·3059	2·0113
			C	534	185	162	131	56				
26. S. India, Bombay	Moslems	Kothare 1959	P	272	102	68	75	27	0·8120	1·1349	0·6730	4·4865
			C	505	162	133	177	33				
27. S. India, Bombay	Occupational castes	Kothare 1959	P	66	23	26	11	6	1·0378	0·0118	0·5151	2·5673
			C	180	56	61	52	11				
28. S. India, Bombay		Shenoy & Daftary 1962	P	360	123	100	112	25	1·0173	0·0108	0·8480	1·0883
			C	760	244	195	262	59				
29. S. India, Gwalior	(s) S, A	Laha & Dutta 1963	P	300	142	47	81	30	0·4558	14·2019	0·4616	19·3295
			C	500	157	114	194	35				
30. S. India, Gwalior		Gupta & Gupta 1966	P	400	130	93	133	44	0·9258	0·2974	0·8736	1·1082
			C	4720	1461	1129	1711	419				
31. Malaya, Singapore	Chinese	Saha & Banerjee 1968	P	1656	660	452	439	105	1·1470	4·5541	1·1587	5·1586
			C	15262	6644	3967	3814	837				
32. Malaya, Singapore	Chinese	Saha 1973	P	2775	1145	706	756	168	1·0327	0·3841	1·1502	7·5041
			C	15262	6644	3967	3814	837				
33. Malaya, Singapore	Indians	Saha & Banerjee 1968	P	116	46	28	30	12	1·1299	0·2533	0·7574	1·3746
			C	5000	1951	1051	1680	318				
34. Malaya, Singapore	Malays	Saha & Banerjee 1968	P	122	48	36	34	4	1·1494	0·3891	0·9311	0·0992
			C	5461	2098	1369	1596	398				
35. Japan, Hirosaki		Oike *et al.* 1962	P	1174	386	363	323	102	0·8991	1·3867	1·1665	2·5998
			C	2087	697	729	500	161				
36. Japan, Sendai	Pleural	Moniwa 1960	P	80	25	26	17	12	0·9042	0·1289	0·9536	0·0228
			C	21199	6769	7786	4827	1817				
37. Japan, Sendai		Moniwa 1960	P	723	252	253	166	52	0·8728	2·2569	0·9238	0·6079
			C	21199	6769	7786	4827	1817				
38. Libya, Cyrenaica	Negro, Mulatto, and white males; (s) A	Fossati 1968	P	3785	1865	1013	608	299	0·9778	0·1690	0·9465	0·7186
			C	4000	1919	1066	661	354				
39. Argentina		Celaya 1939	P	200	128	52	15	5	0·8499	0·5688	0·6901	1·1678
			C	267(c)	159	76	27	5				
40. Colombia, Bogotá		Soriano Lleras 1954	P	642	417	159	50	16	1·1387	1·1482	1·5588	4·5281
			C	943	663	222	51	7				
41. Peru, Lima		Muñoz-Baratta 1962	P	642	446	114	66	16	0·6491	16·8764	0·7740	3·7512
			C	107938	66058	26013	12629	3238				
42. Australia, Sydney	(s) A_1A_2	Kooptzoff & Walsh 1957	P	470	231	191	40	8	0·9659	0·0864	0·6274	5·6338
			C	1123	500	428	138	57				
				24966					0·9311	15·0460	0·9779	1·1040
		χ_{41}^2 for homogeneity of areas								84·1581		104·1899

TABLE 1 **THE ABO BLOOD GROUP SYSTEM** (*cont.*)

Place	Additional details	Authors		Number	O	A	B	AB	A/O Relative incidence	A/O χ_1^2 for difference from unity	B/O Relative incidence	B/O χ_1^2 for difference from unity
INFECTIVE AND PARASITIC DISEASES (*cont.*)												
BACTERIAL INFECTIONS (*cont.*)												
TUBERCULOSIS (*cont.*)												
PULMONARY TUBERCULOSIS, WITH HAEMOPTYSIS												
1. France	(s) S	Dujarric de la Rivière & Kossovitch 1928	P	84	38	29	3	14	0·7594	1·1524	0·2988	3·9279
		Kossovitch 1929 M1	C	962	405	407	107	43				
2. United Kingdom		Weinberger 1943	P	406	193	157	36	20	0·9103	0·7622	1·0172	0·0088
		Dobson & Ikin 1946 M1	C	190177	88782	79334	16280	5781				
3. U.S.S.R., Odessa		Alperin 1926	P	147(c)	57	45	30	15	0·7009	2·0556	0·8177	0·5051
		Alperin M1	C	264	87	98	56	23				
				637					0·8578	2·7747	0·8910	0·6054
					χ_2^2 for homogeneity of areas					1·1955		3·8364
PULMONARY TUBERCULOSIS, WITHOUT HAEMOPTYSIS												
1. France	(s) S	Dujarric de la Rivière & Kossovitch 1928	P	232	75	126	20	11	1·6717	10·0802	1·0093	0·0012
		Kossovitch 1929 M1	C	962	405	407	107	43				
2. United Kingdom		Weinberger 1943	P	594	263	265	47	19	1·1276	1·8977	0·9746	0·0264
		Dobson & Ikin 1946 M1	C	190177	88782	79334	16280	5781				
3. U.S.S.R., Odessa		Alperin 1926	P	320	96	133	64	27	1·2299	1·0805	1·0357	0·0222
		Alperin M1	C	264	87	98	56	23				
				1146					1·2318	8·4706	0·9963	0·0010
					χ_2^2 for homogeneity of areas					4·5878		0·0488
PULMONARY TUBERCULOSIS, WITH/WITHOUT HAEMOPTYSIS												
1. France	(s) S	Dujarric de la Rivière & Kossovitch 1928	With	*84*	*38*	*29*	*3*	*14*	*0·4543*	*7·5851*	*0·2961*	*3·5019*
			Without	*232*	*75*	*126*	*20*	*11*				
2. United Kingdom		Weinberger 1943	With	*406*	*193*	*157*	*36*	*20*	*0·8073*	*2·3970*	*1·0438*	*0·0316*
			Without	*594*	*263*	*265*	*47*	*19*				
3. U.S.S.R., Odessa		Alperin 1926	With	*147*	*57*	*45*	*30*	*15*	*0·5698*	*5·4828*	*0·7895*	*0·7210*
			Without	*320*	*96*	*133*	*64*	*27*				
				637/1146					*0·6883*	*11·4157*	*0·8525*	*0·8299*
					χ_2^2 for homogeneity of areas					*4·0492*		*3·4246*
TUBERCULOUS MENINGITIS												
1. Poland, Warszawa	Children	Paciorkiewicz 1970	P	38	15	15	7	1	0·7740	0·4891	0·7332	0·4568
			C	6626	2041	2637	1299	649				
TUBERCULOSIS OF INTESTINES AND PERITONEUM												
1. Japan, Sendai		Moniwa 1960	P	119	31	44	36	8	1·2340	0·7998	1·6285	3·9379
			C	21199	6769	7786	4827	1817				
2. Peru, Lima	Intestines	Muñoz-Baratta 1962	P	30(c)	17	12	0	1	1·7925	2·3952		
			C	107938(c)	66058	26013	12629	3238				
3. Peru, Lima	Peritoneum	Muñoz-Baratta 1962	P	31(c)	16	10	5	0	1·5871	1·3127	1·6346	0·9195
			C	107938(c)	66058	26013	12629	3238				
				180					1·4101	3·6945	1·6296	4·8574
					χ_2^2 for homogeneity of areas					0·8132		
				(150)	χ_1^2 for homogeneity of areas							0·0000

TABLE 1 **THE ABO BLOOD GROUP SYSTEM** (*cont.*)

Place	Additional details	Authors		Number	O	A	B	AB	A/O Relative incidence	A/O χ^2_1 for difference from unity	B/O Relative incidence	B/O χ^2_1 for difference from unity
Tuberculosis of Bones and Joints												
1. United Kingdom, Glasgow	(s) S	Campbell 1956	P	100	57	26	12	5	0·7603	1·3210	1·0500	0·0232
			C	5898	3177	1906	637	178				
2. N. India, Kanpur		Nand & Yadav 1964	P	600	200	132	222	46	1·1000	0·3506	1·4800	7·2597
			C	500	200	120	150	30				
3. Japan, Sendai		Moniwa 1960	P	186	60	66	39	21	0·9563	0·0622	0·9115	0·2012
			C	21199	6769	7786	4827	1817				
				886					0·9714	0·0735	1·2327	3·5191
				χ^2_2 for homogeneity of areas						1·6603		3·9651
Tuberculosis of Genito-Urinary System												
1. Italy, Milano	Female genital organs	Dossena & Lanzara 1925 Dossena 1924 M1	P	34	13	17	3	1	1·6765	1·6839	0·8876	0·0310
			C	214	100	78	26	10				
2. Italy, Veneto	Kidney	Mobilio & Torchiana 1960	P	174	92	66	9	7	1·0066	0·0014	0·4161	5·8325
			C	1093	536	382	126	49				
3. United Kingdom, Glasgow		Campbell 1956	P	155	84	55	13	3	1·0914	0·2473	0·7719	0·7392
			C	5898	3177	1906	637	178				
4. Japan, Okayama	Urinary	Ohmichi 1928 after Furuhata 1933 M1	P	20	7	9	4	0	0·9137	0·0319	0·6844	0·3651
			C	6936	1921	2703	1604	708				
5. Peru, Lima	Kidney	Muñoz-Baratta 1962	P	53(c)	34	11	7	1	0·8216	0·3209	1·0769	0·0318
			C	107938	66058	26013	12629	3238				
				436					1·0529	0·2226	0·7022	3·6420
				χ^2_4 for homogeneity of areas						2·0628		3·3576
Tuberculosis of Skin												
1. Italy, Trentino	Lupus tuberculosus	Nardelli 1928 Formentano 1951 M1	P	21	12	8	1	0	0·8155	0·1853	0·4757	0·4875
			C	279	137	112	24	6				
2. Poland, Warszawa		Straszyński 1925[a]	P	25	7	13	5	0	1·7250	1·3398	1·3461	0·2553
			C	2613	914	984	485	230				
				48					1·1887	0·2678	1·0553	0·1551
				χ^2_1 for homogeneity of areas						1·2573		0·5877
Tuberculosis of Lymphatic System												
1. Japan, Sendai		Moniwa 1960	P	69	26	23	15	5	0·7691	0·8386	0·8090	0·4257
			C	21199	6769	7786	4827	1817				
Tuberculosis, Sites Unspecified												
1. Austria, Wien		Flamm & Friedrich 1929 Corvin M1	P	38	12	19	6	1	1·2401	0·3394	1·1673	0·0954
			C	10392	3635	4641	1557	559				
2. Finland		Sievers 1929	P	1048(c)	309	470	184	85	1·2004	3·9582	1·2785	4·2935
			C	1711	584	740	272	115				
3. Finland		Mustakallio 1937	P	524	164	242	79	39	1·2203	3·2386	1·0907	0·3375
			C	2595	908	1098	401	188				
4. Finland		Streng & Ryti 1927	P	928	278	413	158	79	1·1639	2·3327	1·1342	0·9677
			C	1383(c)	463	591	232	97				
5. Germany, Berlin		Mertens 1964	P	350	117	159	57	17	1·1507	1·3074	1·2599	2·0107
			C	21104	7725	9123	2987	1269				
6. Germany, München		Lützeler & Dormanns 1929 Kruse M1	P	224	98	99	21	6	0·9976	0·0003	0·9463	0·0451
			C	1300	552	559	125	64				
7. Germany, Nordrhein-Westfalen		Kochs & Wilckens 1928	P	732(c)	297	329	74	32	0·9321	0·2501	0·9048	0·1982
			C	367(c)	138	164	38	27				

TABLE 1 **THE ABO BLOOD GROUP SYSTEM** *(cont.)*

Place	Additional details	Authors		Number	O	A	B	AB	A/O Relative incidence	A/O χ^2_1 for difference from unity	B/O Relative incidence	B/O χ^2_1 for difference from unity
INFECTIVE AND PARASITIC DISEASES *(cont.)*												
BACTERIAL INFECTIONS *(cont.)*												
TUBERCULOSIS *(cont.)*												
TUBERCULOSIS, SITES UNSPECIFIED *(cont.)*												
8. Italy	Non-pulmonary	de Paoli 1932	P	147	59	60	24	4	0·8057	1·2742	1·1363	0·2513
		Viola 1928–9 M1	C	1669	595	751	213	110				
9. Italy		Fochi 1937	P	418(c)	96	261	42	19	2·1649	33·6496	1·5253	4·1534
			C	1381	516	648	148	69				
10. Poland, Silesia		Kallabis 1927	P	515(c)	170	227	77	41	1·8304	18·2696	1·2418	1·3709
			C	555(c)	244	178	89	44				
11. Poland, Upper Silesia	Females	Ernst 1928	P	200	55	84	48	13	1·1908	0·8559	1·4713	3·1487
			C	1003	322	413	191	77				
12. Poland, Warszawa		Swider & Kon 1928	P	600	176	286	94	44	1·5330	13·9710	0·7674	3·3081
		Halber & Mydlarski 1925 M1	C	1518	500	530	348	140				
13. Portugal		Lessa & Alarcão 1947	P	71	33	30	6	2	0·8165	0·6206	0·9179	0·0358
			C	1748	732	815	145	56				
14. Portugal		Lessa & Ruffié 1960	P	357(c)	150	172	26	9	1·0474	0·1550	0·9873	0·0033
			C	3353(c)	1424	1559	250	120				
15. United Kingdom, Lancashire	Non-pulmonary	Bradbury 1934–5	P	29	17	11	1	0	0·6933	0·6855	0·2406	1·7313
			C	103	45	42	11	5				
16. United Kingdom, St. Andrews		Alexander 1921	P	50(c)	25	17	6	2	0·8232	0·1943	0·9200	0·0167
			C	50(c)	23	19	6	2				
17. U.S.S.R., Moscow		Awdiejewa & Grycewicz 1924	P	500(c)	105	203	152	40	1·6069	13·1947	2·0141	25·1405
			C	2200(c)	704	847	506	143				
18. U.S.S.R., Moscow		Poppoff 1927	P	160(c)	50	30	60	20	0·4987	8·6542	1·6696	6·5576
			C	2200(c)	704	847	506	143				
19. Lebanon and Syria		Parr 1929	P	346	119	144	45	38	0·8523	1·4937	0·7898	1·6467
			C	3146(c)	967	1373	463	343				
20. Lebanon and Syria	Armenians	Parr 1929	P	164	46	73	29	16	0·9637	0·0350	1·4242	1·9630
			C	1536(c)	436	718	193	189				
21. N. India, Dibrugarh		Mitra 1933	P	77	27	15	28	7	0·6886	1·1958	1·0800	0·0702
			C	526	176	142	169	39				
22. Republic of South Africa	Bantu	Buckwalter *et al.* 1961	P	939	369	276	214	80	1·1826	3·9399	1·2142	4·5110
			C	7105	3197	2022	1527	359				
23. Republic of South Africa	Coloured	Buckwalter *et al.* 1964	P	127(c)	44	45	31	7	0·9837	0·0045	1·0826	0·0838
			C	352(c)	126	131	82	13				
24. Republic of South Africa	Indians	Buckwalter *et al.* 1961	P	111	42	21	38	10	0·8100	0·6136	1·0130	0·0033
			C	7462	2788	1721	2490	463				
25. U.S.A., Ann Arbor		Raphael *et al.* 1927	P	400	176	161	54	9	1·0448	0·1548	1·1998	1·3090
			C	9600	4243	3715	1085	557				
26. U.S.A., New York		Sasano 1931	P	1000	427	403	124	46	1·0428	0·0968	0·9364	0·1163
			C	370(c)	158	143	49	20				
27. Brazil, São Paulo		Saldanha 1957	P	274	110	112	46	6	1·7880	9·0877	2·7372	12·1822
			C	252	144	82	22	4				
				10329					1·1719	32·8466	1·1923	24·1848
				χ^2_{26} for homogeneity of areas						86·7265		51·3663
SARCOIDOSIS												
1. Denmark, Köbenhavn		Viskum 1973	P	52	21	21	8	2	0·9214	0·0701	1·4201	0·7092
		Andersen 1955 M1	C	14304	5804	6299	1557	644				
2. Germany, Göttingen		Jörgensen 1965	P	518	195	252	50	21	1·3178	5·4486	1·1927	0·8011
			C	961	414	406	89	52				

TABLE 1 **THE ABO BLOOD GROUP SYSTEM** *(cont.)*

Place	Additional details	Authors		Number	O	A	B	AB	A/O Relative incidence	A/O χ_1^2 for difference from unity	B/O Relative incidence	B/O χ_1^2 for difference from unity
3. United Kingdom, London	Lungs or hilar lymph nodes	Citron 1956	P	64	38	22	3	1	0·6298	2·9592	0·3868	2·5001
		Discombe 1954 M1	C	10000	4556	4188	930	326				
4. United Kingdom, London		Cudkowicz 1956	P	32	15	12	3	2	0·8703	0·1283	0·9798	0·0010
		Discombe 1954 M1	C	10000	4556	4188	930	326				
5. United Kingdom, London		Smellie 1956	P	80	34	36	6	4	1·1519	0·3467	0·8645	0·1074
			C	10000	4556	4188	930	326				
6. United Kingdom, London		Lewis & Woods 1961	P	164	65	85	8	6	1·4190	4·4358	0·6331	1·4746
			C	10000	4578	4219	890	313				
				910					1·1865	4·5654	0·9921	0·0001
				χ_5^2 for homogeneity of areas						8·8234		5·5933

LEPROSY

Lepromatous Leprosy

Place	Additional details	Authors		Number	O	A	B	AB	A/O Relative incidence	A/O χ_1^2 for difference from unity	B/O Relative incidence	B/O χ_1^2 for difference from unity
1. Italy, Calabria, Lucania, Puglie		Cerri 1938	P	72	26	28	6	2	0·8983	0·1282	0·6212	0·8991
			C	181	82	71	22	6				
2. Spain, Fontilles		Royo Marti 1947	P	120	63	46	9	2	0·6821	3·1349	0·6762	0·9948
		Alcober Coloma 1944 M1	C	500	213	228	45	14				
3. U.S.S.R., Estonia		Paldrock 1929	P	109	35	45	21	8	1·4714	2·4523	0·9654	0·0140
			C	560(c)	214	187	133	26				
4. U.S.S.R., Latvia	(s) G	Weidemann 1930	P	141(c)	47	55	28	11	0·9142	0·1404	0·8391	0·3797
			C	317(c)	100	128	71	18				
5. N. India, Bankura	(s) A_1A_2	Vogel & Chakravartti 1966[b]	P	472	164	126	150	32	1·0771	0·1790	0·9834	0·0103
			C	403	143	102	133	25				
6. N. India, Calcutta		Lowe 1942	P	200	58	49	78	15	1·3109	1·7396	1·3472	2·6459
			C	1638	571	368	570	129				
7. N. India, Varanasi		Sehgal *et al.* 1966	P	169	59	49	49	12	1·3330	1·6201	0·6501	3·9713
			C	615	191	119	244	61				
8. N. India, Varanasi		Singh & Ojha 1967	P	164	47	54	51	12	1·5697	4·7825	1·1028	0·2216
			C	2583	873	639	859	212				
9. N. India, West Bengal		Vogel *et al.* 1971	P	323	122	80	98	23	0·9193	0·1887	0·8637	0·6526
			C	403	143	102	133	25				
10. S. India, Baroda		Verma & Dongre 1965	P	288	92	74	111	11	1·1135	0·3667	1·1648	0·9039
			C	1000	335	242	347	76				
11. S. India, Guinda		Prasad & Ali 1966	P	782	339	166	227	50	0·7959	3·5866	0·8583	1·9158
			C	1208	473	291	369	75				
12. S. India, Vellore		Hsuen *et al.* 1963	P	258	121	62	68	7	0·9506	0·0814	0·6740	5·4578
			C	1000	397	214	331	58				
13. S. India, Vellore		Povey & Horton 1966	P	382	159	75	129	19	0·8211	1·3241	0·7889	2·6717
			C	755	282	162	260	51				
14. Thailand		Vogel *et al.* 1969	P	335	146	59	101	29	0·8551	0·7365	1·1345	0·6415
			C	715	328	155	200	32				
15. Malaya, Singapore	Chinese	Saha *et al.* 1971	P	338	140	87	93	18	1·0408	0·0839	1·1572	1·1642
			C	15262	6644	3967	3814	837				
16. Philippines, Cebu		Lechat *et al.* 1968	P	250	105	57	73	15	0·9002	0·2732	1·6277	5·9311
			C	429	199	120	85	25				
17. Japan, Oshima		Muneuchi 1934	P	307	82	122	78	25	1·0241	0·0236	1·2366	1·4996
			C	1603	455	661	350	137				
18. Ghana		Yankah 1965	P	196	75	54	58	9	1·7696	6·6756	1·5776	4·5705
			C	400	204	83	100	13				
19. Senegal, Dakar	Mainly Bambara	Languillon *et al.* 1973	P	235	99	68	61	7	1·4907	2·8516	0·8162	0·8368
			C	238	102	47	77	12				
20. Argentina	About 50% Italians	Puente 1927–8	P	155	85	51	12	7	0·8070	1·1058	0·6126	2·0292
		Etcheverry 1949 M1	C	464	230	171	53	10				
21. Brazil	White Brazilians	Beiguelman 1963	P	474(c)	239	176	46	13	0·9738	0·0691	0·9617	0·0568
		Mellone *et al.* 1952 M1	C	12492	6166	4663	1234	429				

TABLE 1 THE ABO BLOOD GROUP SYSTEM (*cont.*)

Place	Additional details	Authors			Number	O	A	B	AB	A/O Relative incidence	A/O χ_1^2 for difference from unity	B/O Relative incidence	B/O χ_1^2 for difference from unity
INFECTIVE AND PARASITIC DISEASES (*cont.*)													
BACTERIAL INFECTIONS (*cont.*)													
LEPROSY (*cont.*)													
LEPROMATOUS LEPROSY (*cont.*)													
22. Brazil	White Brazilians	Beiguelman 1964[a]		P	92	51	35	6	0	0·9075	0·1941	0·5879	1·5074
		Mellone *et al.* 1952	M1	C	12492	6166	4663	1234	429				
23. Brazil	Of Italian origin	Beiguelman 1963		P	580(c)	265	227	59	29	1·0390	0·1637	0·9583	0·0806
		Mellone *et al.* 1952	M1	C	6169	2888	2381	671	229				
24. Brazil	Of Italian origin	Beiguelman 1964[a]		P	124	47	60	8	9	1·5484	4·9388	0·7326	0·6537
		Mellone *et al.* 1952	M1	C	6169	2888	2381	671	229				
25. Brazil	Of Portuguese origin	Beiguelman 1963		P	92(c)	42	45	5	0	1·2232	0·8493	0·6899	0·6007
		Mellone *et al.* 1952	M1	C	2577	1217	1066	210	84				
26. Brazil	Of Spanish origin	Beiguelman 1963		P	100(c)	50	39	8	3	1·0820	0·1302	0·9340	0·0309
		Mellone *et al.* 1952	M1	C	2258	1150	829	197	82				
27. Brazil	Whites of mixed Brazilian, Italian, Portuguese, or Spanish origin	Beiguelman 1963		P	203(c)	99	75	22	7	0·9819	0·0130	1·0628	0·0606
		Mellone *et al.* 1952	M1	C	2119	1033	797	216	73				
28. Brazil	Whites of origin other than Brazilian, Italian, Portuguese, or Spanish	Beiguelman 1963		P	89(c)	32	34	15	8	0·8123	0·6912	1·1165	0·1197
		Mellone *et al.* 1952	M1	C	2742	948	1240	398	156				
29. Brazil	Whites of Iberian origin and nationally mixed	Beiguelman 1964[a]		P	96	37	45	11	3	1·3449	1·7654	1·2661	0·4671
		Mellone *et al.* 1952	M1	C	9696	4348	3932	1021	395				
30. Brazil	Negroes and Mulattos	Beiguelman 1963		P	118(c)	55	42	15	6	1·4240	2·8634	0·7248	1·1917
		Mellone *et al.* 1952	M1	C	3429	1738	932	654	105				
31. Brazil	Negroes and Mulattos	Beiguelman 1964		P	28	14	10	3	1	1·3320	0·4749	0·5695	0·7792
		Mellone *et al.* 1952	M1	C	3429	1738	932	654	105				
32. Brazil, Curitiba	Whites; (s) A_1A_2	Salzano *et al.* 1967		P	224(c)	112	86	19	7	1·0471	0·0353	1·0179	0·0018
				C	120(c)	60	44	10	6				
33. Brazil, Florianopólis	Whites; (s) A_1A_2	Salzano *et al.* 1967		P	168(c)	75	70	18	5	0·7368	1·3840	0·9818	0·0018
				C	119(c)	45	57	11	6				
34. Brazil, Pôrto Alegre	Whites; (s) A_1A_2	Salzano *et al.* 1967		P	329(c)	148	139	31	11	1·0532	0·0979	1·1748	0·3189
				C	333(c)	157	140	28	8				
					8013					1·0330	1·0941	0·9845	0·1864
					χ_{33}^2 for homogeneity of areas						44·0509		41·1867
TUBERCULOID LEPROSY													
1. Italy, Calabria, Lucania, Puglie		Cerri 1938		P	11	7	3	0	1	0·4950	0·9843		
				C	181	82	71	22	6				
2. Spain, Fontilles		Royo Marti 1947		P	62	25	32	4	1	1·1958	0·3980	0·7573	0·2438
		Alcober Coloma 1944 M1		C	500	213	228	45	14				
3. U.S.S.R., Estonia		Paldrock 1929		P	62	22	23	12	5	1·1964	0·3250	0·8776	0·1208
				C	560(c)	214	187	133	26				
4. U.S.S.R., Latvia	(s) G	Weidemann 1930		P	52(c)	21	14	11	6	0·5208	3·1092	0·7378	0·5688
				C	317(c)	100	128	71	18				
5. N. India, Calcutta		Lowe 1942		P	200	63	53	72	12	1·3053	1·8108	1·1449	0·5501
				C	1638	571	368	570	129				

TABLE 1 **THE ABO BLOOD GROUP SYSTEM** *(cont.)*

Place	Additional details	Authors		Number	O	A	B	AB	A/O Relative incidence	A/O χ_1^2 for difference from unity	B/O Relative incidence	B/O χ_1^2 for difference from unity
6. S. India, Baroda		Verma & Acharya 1966	P	177	67	38	59	13	0·7178	2·2967	1·0001	0·0000
			C	1000	343	271	302	84				
7. S. India, Vellore		Povey & Horton 1966	P	431	179	87	145	20	0·8461	1·0427	0·8786	0·8428
			C	755	282	162	260	51				
8. Philippines, Cebu		Lechat *et al.* 1968	P	223	96	59	48	20	1·0192	0·0089	1·1706	0·5176
			C	429	199	120	85	25				
9. Japan, Oshima		Muneuchi 1934	P	112	32	47	26	7	1·0110	0·0021	1·0562	0·0401
			C	1603	455	661	350	137				
10. Ghana		Yankah 1965	P	204	121	33	41	9	0·6703	2·8820	0·6912	2·8673
			C	400	204	83	100	13				
11. Senegal, Dakar	Mainly Bambara	Languillon *et al.* 1973	P	245	96	48	81	20	1·0851	0·1070	1·1177	0·2718
			C	238	102	47	77	12				
12. Madagascar, Emyrne	Hova	Hérivaux 1931	P	78(c)	24	20	26	8	0·7500	0·5108	1·0086	0·0005
			C	112(c)	27	30	29	26				
13. Argentina	About 50% Italians	Puente 1927–8	P	78	32	34	7	5	1·4291	1·7991	0·9493	0·0137
		Etcheverry 1949 M1	C	464	230	171	53	10				
14. Brazil	White Brazilians	Beiguelman 1963	P	135(c)	75	52	6	2	0·9168	0·2290	0·3997	4·6459
		Mellone *et al.* 1952 M1	C	12492	6166	4663	1234	429				
15. Brazil	White Brazilians	Beiguelman 1964[a]	P	92	52	33	6	1	0·8392	0·6160	0·5765	1·6229
		Mellone *et al.* 1952 M1	C	12492	6166	4663	1234	429				
16. Brazil	Of Italian origin	Beiguelman 1963	P	132(c)	69	49	10	4	0·8614	0·6245	0·6238	1·9149
		Mellone *et al.* 1952 M1	C	6169	2888	2381	671	229				
17. Brazil	Of Italian origin	Beiguelman 1964[a]	P	124	63	44	13	4	0·8471	0·6992	0·8881	0·1487
		Mellone *et al.* 1952 M1	C	6169	2888	2381	671	229				
18. Brazil	Of Portuguese origin	Beiguelman 1963	P	27(c)	13	13	1	0	1·1417	0·1128	0·4458	0·6030
		Mellone *et al.* 1952 M1	C	2577	1217	1066	210	84				
19. Brazil	Of Spanish origin	Beiguelman 1963	P	32(c)	17	8	5	2	0·6528	0·9784	1·7169	1·1035
		Mellone *et al.* 1952 M1	C	2258	1150	829	197	82				
20. Brazil	Whites of mixed Brazilian, Italian, Portuguese, or Spanish origin	Beiguelman 1963	P	56(c)	25	22	9	0	1·1406	0·1973	1·7217	1·8835
		Mellone *et al.* 1952 M1	C	2119	1033	797	216	73				
21. Brazil	Whites of origin other than Brazilian, Italian, Portuguese, or Spanish	Beiguelman 1963	P	27(c)	11	9	4	3	0·6255	1·0797	0·8661	0·0599
		Mellone *et al.* 1952 M1	C	2742	948	1240	398	156				
22. Brazil	Whites of Iberian origin and nationally mixed	Beiguelman 1964[a]	P	96	41	35	16	4	0·9440	0·0622	1·6619	2·9287
		Mellone *et al.* 1952 M1	C	9696	4348	3932	1021	395				
23. Brazil	Negroes and Mulattos	Beiguelman 1963	P	62(c)	38	14	8	2	0·6870	1·4176	0·5595	2·1984
		Mellone *et al.* 1952 M1	C	3429	1738	932	654	105				
24. Brazil	Negroes and Mulattos	Beiguelman 1964[a]	P	28	19	6	2	1	0·5889	1·2691	0·2797	2·9254
		Mellone *et al.* 1952 M1	C	3429	1738	932	654	105				
25. Brazil, Curitiba	Whites; (s) A_1A_2	Salzano *et al.* 1967	P	32(c)	17	11	3	1	0·8824	0·0828	1·0588	0·0064
			C	120(c)	60	44	10	6				
26. Brazil, Florianopólis	Whites; (s) A_1A_2	Salzano *et al.* 1967	P	20(c)	7	11	2	0	1·2406	0·1699	1·1688	0·0322
			C	119(c)	45	57	11	6				
27. Brazil, Pôrto Alegre	Whites; (s) A_1A_2	Salzano *et al.* 1967	P	65(c)	27	29	5	4	1·2045	0·4071	1·0384	0·0051
			C	333(c)	157	140	28	8				
				2863					0·9223	2·6033	0·9434	0·9600
					χ^2_{26} for homogeneity of areas					20·6191		
				(2852)	χ^2_{25} for homogeneity of areas							25·1558

TABLE 1 THE ABO BLOOD GROUP SYSTEM (*cont.*)

INFECTIVE AND PARASITIC DISEASES (*cont.*)
BACTERIAL INFECTIONS (*cont.*)
LEPROSY (*cont.*)

Place	Additional details	Authors		Number	O	A	B	AB	A/O Relative incidence	A/O χ^2_1 for difference from unity	B/O Relative incidence	B/O χ^2_1 for difference from unity
Indeterminate Leprosy												
1. Brazil,	Whites;	Salzano *et al.* 1967	P	43(c)	25	17	1	0	0·9273	0·0412	0·2400	1·7608
Curitiba	(s) A_1A_2		C	120(c)	60	44	10	6				
2. Brazil,	Whites;	Salzano *et al.* 1967	P	23(c)	10	9	2	2	0·7105	0·4655	0·8182	0·0565
Florianopólis	(s) A_1A_2		C	119(c)	45	57	11	6				
3. Brazil,	Whites;	Salzano *et al.* 1967	P	27(c)	10	13	4	0	1·4579	0·7462	2·2429	1·6641
Pôrto Alegre	(s) A_1A_2		C	333(c)	157	140	28	8				
				93					1·0043	0·0003	1·1198	0·0616
				χ^2_2 for homogeneity of areas						1·2527		3·4197
Dimorphous Leprosy												
1. Italy, Calabria,		Cerri 1938	P	17	6	7	4	0	1·3474	0·2648	2·4848	1·7467
Lucania, Puglie			C	181	82	71	22	6				
2. Spain,		Royo Marti 1947	P	83	37	40	6	0	1·0100	0·0016	0·7676	0·3172
Fontilles		Alcober Coloma 1944 M1	C	500	213	228	45	14				
3. U.S.S.R.,		Paldrock 1929	P	29	9	13	5	2	1·6530	1·2754	0·8939	0·0389
Estonia			C	560(c)	214	187	133	26				
4. S. India,		Povey & Horton 1966	P	251	102	57	85	7	0·9728	0·0206	0·9038	0·3529
Vellore			C	755	282	162	260	51				
5. Thailand		Vogel *et al.* 1969	P	348	137	81	98	32	1·2511	1·7227	1·1731	0·9980
			C	715	328	155	200	32				
				728					1·1307	1·2939	1·0383	0·1177
				χ^2_4 for homogeneity of areas						4·5790		3·3359
Non-Lepromatous Leprosy												
1. N. India,		Sehgal *et al.* 1966	P	454	144	155	109	46	1·7276	11·0578	0·5925	10·7614
Varanasi			C	615	191	119	244	61				
2. N. India,		Singh & Ojha 1967	P	469	165	139	121	44	1·1509	1·2375	0·7453	5·1957
Varanasi			C	2583	873	639	859	212				
3. N. India,	Mostly	Vogel & Chakravartti 1966[b]	P	459	175	116	140	28	1·4653	2·7771	1·0182	0·0081
Bankura	tuberculoid; (s) S	Chakravartti *et al.* 1966 M2	C	200	84	38	66	12				
4. N. India,		Vogel *et al.* 1971	P	308	117	87	90	14	1·0425	0·0470	0·8271	1·0550
West Bengal			C	403	143	102	133	25				
5. S. India,	151 tubercu-	Verma & Dongre 1965	P	306	85	82	120	19	1·3354	2·6927	1·3629	3·6927
Baroda	loid, 66 dimorphous, 87 indeterminate, 2 neural		C	1000	335	242	347	76				
6. S. India,		Prasad & Ali 1966	P	422	158	99	135	30	1·0185	0·0152	1·0952	0·4459
Guinda			C	1208	473	291	369	75				
7. S. India,	130 tubercu-	Hsuen *et al.* 1963	P	268	136	68	55	9	0·9276	0·1933	0·4850	16·8451
Vellore	loid, 51 dimorphous, 85 indeterminate, 2 neural		C	1000	397	214	331	58				
8. Malaya,	Chinese	Saha *et al.* 1971	P	121	46	33	35	7	1·2015	0·6425	1·3254	1·5649
Singapore			C	15262	6644	3967	3814	837				
				2807					1·1915	8·4992	0·8620	6·5679
				χ^2_7 for homogeneity of areas						10·1636		33·0010

TABLE 1 **THE ABO BLOOD GROUP SYSTEM** (*cont.*)

Place	Additional details	Authors		Number	O	A	B	AB	A/O Relative incidence	A/O χ_1^2 for difference from unity	B/O Relative incidence	B/O χ_1^2 for difference from unity
LEPROSY, UNSPECIFIED TYPES												
1. Greece	239 lepromatous, 55 tuberculoid, 6 dimorphous	Markianos *et al.* 1957	P	300	137	109	41	13	0·9257	0·3455	1·1480	0·5690
			C	6027	2712	2331	707	277				
2. Italy, Cagliari		Pinetti 1931	P	31	16	13	2	0	1·3852	0·7128	0·8040	0·0808
		Benassi & Atzeni 1934 M1	C	499	283	166	44	6				
3. Portugal		Lessa & Ruffié 1960	P	149	67	66	12	4	0·8998	0·3550	1·0202	0·0039
			C	3353	1424	1559	250	120				
4. U.S.S.R.		Kolpakov & Andrusson 1928	P	130	45	50	26	9	0·8741	0·3638	0·7928	0·7624
			C	783	236	300	172	75				
5. U.S.S.R., Astrakhan	Ukrainians	Rudchenko 1930	P	186	46	82	32	26	1·4188	3·1753	1·0123	0·0025
		Besedin 1926 M1	C	1219	390	490	268	71				
6. U.S.S.R., Riga		Weidemann 1930	P	106(c)	42	36	18	10	0·7543	1·4045	0·5704	3·6820
			C	1160(c)	374	425	281	80				
7. U.S.S.R., Talsen		Weidemann 1930	P	100(c)	29	38	26	7	1·1531	0·3083	1·1933	0·3944
			C	1160(c)	374	425	281	80				
8. N. India, Dibrugarh		Mitra 1933	P	14	3	6	3	2	2·4789	1·6073	1·0414	0·0024
			C	526	176	142	169	39				
9. S. India, Gwalior		Gupta & Gupta 1966	P	300	90	75	96	39	1·0784	0·2189	0·9108	0·3828
			C	4720	1461	1129	1711	419				
10. S. India, Pondicherry	(s) S	Valle 1937	P	72	56	11	4	1	0·2679	6·5152	0·0893	13·9680
			C	38	15	11	12	0				
11. Thailand, Northern		Saengudom & Flatz 1967	P	302(c)	121	76	82	23	1·4170	5·2214	1·1405	0·7860
			C	3785(c)	1762	781	1047	195				
12. Thailand, Northern		Vogel *et al.* 1969	P	318	135	60	94	29	1·0027	0·0003	1·1718	1·2845
			C	3785	1762	781	1047	195				
13. Thailand, Central		Vogel *et al.* 1969	P	70	23	16	23	8	1·3475	0·7916	0·9935	0·0005
			C	1255	461	238	464	92				
14. Java, Blora		Malaihollo 1940	P	46	18	15	12	1	1·1905	0·1496	0·8000	0·2346
			C	79	30	21	25	3				
15. Java, Poelogadoeng, Wates		Malaihollo 1940	P	91	37	21	30	3	1·0405	0·0048	0·5946	1·2401
			C	33	11	6	15	1				
16. Japan		Hasegawa 1937	P	1426	378	559	339	150	1·1808	5·9635	1·2490	8·4444
			C	301959	92097	115348	66129	28385				
17. Japan, Okayama		Ohmichi 1928	P	89	30	20	31	8	0·4738	6·6250	1·2376	0·6807
		after Furuhata 1933 M1	C	6936	1921	2703	1604	708				
18. Egypt	(s) S	Ali 1931	P	100	18	44	21	17	1·8154	3·7216	0·9658	0·0100
			C	417	101	136	122	58				
19. Mozambique, Nampula		Spielmann *et al.* 1970	P	126(c)	56	32	31	7	1·2925	0·7890	1·9478	4·5502
			C	171(c)	95	42	27	7				
20. Martinique		Montestrug & Caubet 1948	P	100	53	29	16	2	1·0502	0·0390	0·8553	0·2651
			C	685(c)	357	186	126	16				
21. Venezuela, Colonia Tovar	Creoles	Lechat *et al.* 1967	P	16(c)	10	4	2	0	0·6214	0·5966	1·0235	0·0008
			C	165(c)	87	56	17	5				
22. Venezuela, Colonia Tovar	Germans	Lechat *et al.* 1967	P	54(c)	25	26	3	0	0·9916	0·0007	1·4057	0·2195
			C	178(c)	82	86	7	3				
23. New Guinea, Mount Hagen		Simmons *et al.* 1968	P	94	42	21	25	6	0·6022	3·0338	0·7497	1·0705
		MacLennan *et al.* 1967 M2	C	473	165	137	131	40				
				4220					1·0788	3·5021	1·0852	3·2925
				χ_{22}^2 for homogeneity of areas						38·4401		35·3426

TABLE 1 **THE ABO BLOOD GROUP SYSTEM** *(cont.)*

INFECTIVE AND PARASITIC DISEASES *(cont.)*
BACTERIAL INFECTIONS *(cont.)*

SYPHILIS

CARDIOVASCULAR SYPHILIS

Place	Additional details	Authors		Number	O	A	B	AB	A/O Relative incidence	A/O χ^2_1 for difference from unity	B/O Relative incidence	B/O χ^2_1 for difference from unity
1. United Kingdom, Newcastle upon Tyne	Aortitis and/or aneurysms of aorta; (s) S	Schofield 1966	P	95	42	43	7	3	1·3116	1·5604	0·9037	0·0614
			C	54579	27008	21082	4981	1508				
2. United Kingdom, Newcastle upon Tyne	Aortic incompetence; (s) S	Schofield 1966	P	124	69	46	7	2	0·8541	0·6852	0·5501	2·2669
			C	54579	27008	21082	4981	1508				
				219					1·0293	0·0407	0·7001	1·5689
				χ^2_1 for homogeneity of areas						2·2049		0·7595

CEREBROSPINAL SYPHILIS

Place	Additional details	Authors		Number	O	A	B	AB	A/O Relative incidence	A/O χ^2_1 for difference from unity	B/O Relative incidence	B/O χ^2_1 for difference from unity
1. Germany, Bonn		Klövekorn & Simon 1927	P	24	6	14	4	0	2·1593	2·4301	4·7518	5·5088
			C	760	335	362	47	16				
2. U.S.S.R., Odessa		Perkel & Israelsson 1928	P	317	88	141	72	16	1·5315	8·6060	1·1948	1·1078
		Barinstein 1928 M1	C	2120(c)	736	770	504	110				
				341					1·5741	10·5917	1·2996	2·5573
				χ^2_1 for homogeneity of areas						0·4444		4·0593

TABES DORSALIS

Place	Additional details	Authors		Number	O	A	B	AB	A/O Relative incidence	A/O χ^2_1 for difference from unity	B/O Relative incidence	B/O χ^2_1 for difference from unity
1. Germany, Schleswig-Holstein		Gundel & Tornquist 1929	P	81	28	28	18	7	0·9058	0·1366	2·0426	5·5562
			C	19461	7664	8461	2412	924				
2. U.S.S.R., Odessa		Perkel & Israelsson 1928	P	196	79	59	45	13	0·7139	3·5214	0·8318	0·8870
		Barinstein 1928 M1	C	2120(c)	736	770	504	110				
				277					0·7686	3·1127	1·0832	0·2368
				χ^2_1 for homogeneity of areas						0·5453		6·2064

CEREBROSPINAL SYPHILIS, TABES DORSALIS

Place	Additional details	Authors		Number	O	A	B	AB	A/O Relative incidence	A/O χ^2_1 for difference from unity	B/O Relative incidence	B/O χ^2_1 for difference from unity
1. Austria, Wien		Pilcz 1927	P	29	7	16	1	5	1·8962	1·9419	0·2352	1·8196
		Hoche & Moritsch 1926 M1	C	1000	331	399	201	69				

PROGRESSIVE PARALYSIS

Place	Additional details	Authors		Number	O	A	B	AB	A/O Relative incidence	A/O χ^2_1 for difference from unity	B/O Relative incidence	B/O χ^2_1 for difference from unity
1. Austria, Wien		Pilcz 1927	P	226(c)	83	97	36	10	0·9695	0·0344	0·7143	2·3679
		Hoche & Moritsch 1926 M1	C	1000	331	399	201	69				
2. Czechoslovakia, Praha		Leischner 1936	P	218	66	88	45	19	1·0477	0·0755	1·2142	0·9214
			C	2429	796	1013	447	173				
3. France, Lille		Farjot & Spriet 1934	P	130	50	53	19	8	0·9708	0·0210	1·6174	2·8705
			C	1600(c)	664	725	156	55				
4. Germany, Berlin		Jacobsohn 1926	P	100	33	47	17	3	1·0492	0·0423	1·2219	0·4237
		Schiff 1926	C	1750	593	805	250	102				
5. Germany, Leipzig		Kranz 1942	P	52(c)	14	28	9	1	1·7121	2·6696	1·6403	1·3254
		Christiansen *et al.* 1935 M1	C	4277	1582	1848	620	227				
6. Germany, Schleswig-Holstein		Gundel & Tornquist 1929	P	226	64	85	61	16	1·2030	1·2361	3·0285	37·7053
			C	19461	7664	8461	2412	924				
7. Hungary, Budapest		Somogyi & Angyal 1931	P	191	54	88	39	10	1·2662	1·5810	1·3281	1·5256
			C	1000	331	426	180	63				
8. Italy		Laurà 1938	P	29(c)	16	10	2	1	0·7363	0·4989	0·3468	1·8497
			C	200	86	73	31	10				
9. Italy		Andreani 1954	P	29(c)	15	9	4	1	0·7280	0·5522	1·5539	0·5867
			C	970(c)	472	389	81	28				

TABLE 1 **THE ABO BLOOD GROUP SYSTEM** *(cont.)*

Place	Additional details	Authors		Number	O	A	B	AB	A/O Relative incidence	A/O χ^2_1 for difference from unity	B/O Relative incidence	B/O χ^2_1 for difference from unity
10. Italy, Ancona		Fattovich 1928	P	14	7	4	1	2	0·6439	0·4893	0·6146	0·2060
			C	1500(c)	684	607	159	50				
11. Italy, Milano		Bravetta 1930	P	142(c)	65	59	13	5	1·0212	0·0124	0·8604	0·2260
		Cuboni M1	C	1500	684	608	159	49				
12. Italy, Siena		D'Ormea & Centini 1942	P	27(c)	10	11	4	2	1·1369	0·0859	1·5807	0·5967
		Lecchini 1930 M1	C	8720(c)	3758	3636	951	375				
13. Poland, Lower Silesia		Meyer 1928	P	20(c)	6	10	2	2	1·5467	0·6929	1·2374	0·0661
		Kruse M1	C	600(c)	245	264	66	25				
14. Poland, Wrocław		Ohnsorge 1927	P	100	28	44	18	10	1·5714	2·4837	2·0000	3·4266
		Kathe 1942 M2	C	200	84	84	27	5				
15. U.S.S.R., Kiev		Chominskij & Schustova 1928	P	37	22	7	6	2	0·2674	9·1660	0·4542	2·9075
			C	3840	1254	1492	753	341				
16. U.S.S.R., Odessa		Perkel & Israelsson 1928	P	48	10	16	17	5	1·5294	1·0928	2·4825	5·0984
		Barinstein 1928 M1	C	2120	736	770	504	110				
17. U.S.A., Brooklyn		Herman & Derby 1937	P	273	124	103	31	15	0·9131	0·3894	0·7182	2·3479
			C	1444	609	554	212	69				
18. U.S.A., New York	70 Gentiles, 21 Jews, 4 Negroes	Bunker & Meyers 1927	P	91(c)	36	38	13	4	1·3223	1·4301	1·2198	0·3735
		Tiber M1	C	10000(c)	4560	3640	1350	450				
19. Argentina, Buenos Aires		Espejo Solá 1931	P	38	14	16	6	2	1·5714	1·2023	3·1429	3·5990
			C	127	66	48	9	4				
				1991					1·0686	1·4596	1·3055	13·8502
				χ^2_{18} for homogeneity of areas						22·2964		54·5737

MENTAL DISORDERS DUE TO SYPHILIS

Place	Additional details	Authors		Number	O	A	B	AB	A/O Relative incidence	A/O χ^2_1	B/O Relative incidence	B/O χ^2_1
1. Italy, Vercelli		Giuli 1959	P	35	16	17	1	1	1·1922	0·2448	0·2077	2·3032
			C	1000	432	385	130	53				
2. U.S.A., Iowa	(s) S	Buckwalter *et al.* 1959	P	67	32	30	2	3	0·9928	0·0008	0·2981	2·7564
			C	49979	22392	21144	4695	1748				
				102					1·0563	0·0702	0·2644	4·9782
				χ^2_1 for homogeneity of areas						0·1754		0·0814

TERTIARY SYPHILIS

Place	Additional details	Authors		Number	O	A	B	AB	A/O Relative incidence	A/O χ^2_1	B/O Relative incidence	B/O χ^2_1
1. U.S.S.R., Odessa	Internal organs and syphilids of skin	Perkel & Israelsson 1928	P	160	50	59	41	10	1·1279	0·3657	1·1975	0·6803
		Barinstein 1928 M1	C	2120	736	770	504	110				

TREATED SYPHILIS, WASSERMANN REACTION POSITIVE

Place	Additional details	Authors		Number	O	A	B	AB	A/O Relative incidence	A/O χ^2_1	B/O Relative incidence	B/O χ^2_1
1. Germany, Bonn		Klövekorn & Simon 1927	P	108	50	50	0	8	0·9254	0·1313		
			C	760	335	362	47	16				
2. Germany, München		Poehlmann 1930	P	118	49	43	20	6	0·8666	0·4338	1·8024	4·3258
		Kruse M1	C	1300(c)	552	559	125	64				
3. Poland, Warszawa		Amzel & Halber 1924	P	610	135	258	155	62	1·8029	22·8961	1·6496	13·3753
			C	1518(c)	500	530	348	140				
4. Poland, Warszawa		Straszyński 1925[b]	P	206	48	77	54	27	1·5134	4·5528	1·6164	5·2138
			C	1518(c)	500	530	348	140				
5. U.S.S.R., Leningrad		Schapiro 1929	P	474	107	208	101	57	1·9053	20·8852	1·4802	5·7624
		Zhitnikov 1927 M1	C	1000	345	352	220	83				
6. U.S.S.R., Moscow		Gurevič & Gellermann-Gurevič 1929	P	136	42	52	29	13	1·1035	0·1085	1·1324	0·1259
			C	118	41	46	25	6				
7. U.S.S.R., Odessa		Perkel & Israelsson 1928	P	49	14	20	12	3	1·3655	0·7823	1·2517	0·3188
		Barinstein 1928 M1	C	2120	736	770	504	110				
				1701					1·4855	32·1094	1·5557	27·4198
				χ^2_6 for homogeneity of areas						17·6806		
				(1593) χ^2_5 for homogeneity of areas								1·7022

TABLE 1 **THE ABO BLOOD GROUP SYSTEM** (*cont.*)

Place	Additional details	Authors		Number	O	A	B	AB	A/O Relative incidence	A/O χ_1^2 for difference from unity	B/O Relative incidence	B/O χ_1^2 for difference from unity
INFECTIVE AND PARASITIC DISEASES (*cont.*)												
BACTERIAL INFECTIONS (*cont.*)												
SYPHILIS (*cont.*)												
TREATED SYPHILIS, WASSERMANN REACTION NEGATIVE												
1. Germany, Bonn		Klövekorn & Simon 1927	P	138	74	46	10	8	0·5753	7·4570	0·9632	0·0102
			C	760	335	362	47	16				
2. Germany, München		Poehlmann 1930	P	382	160	170	41	11	1·0492	0·1464	1·1316	0·3777
		Kruse M1	C	1300	552	559	125	64				
3. Poland, Warszawa		Amzel & Halber 1924	P	815	312	286	159	58	0·8648	1·9925	0·7322	6·7615
			C	1518	500	530	348	140				
4. Poland, Warszawa		Straszyński 1925[b]	P	412	142	144	91	35	0·9567	0·1097	0·9208	0·2976
			C	1518	500	530	348	140				
5. U.S.S.R., Leningrad		Schapiro 1929	P	1227	372	469	284	102	1·2357	4·2388	1·1972	2·3792
		Zhitnikov 1927 M1	C	1000	345	352	220	83				
6. U.S.S.R., Moscow		Gurevič & Gellermann-Gurevič 1929	P	171	59	53	42	17	0·8007	0·6029	1·1675	0·2283
			C	118	41	46	25	6				
7. U.S.S.R., Odessa		Perkel & Israelsson 1928	P	32	15	11	5	1	0·7010	0·7876	0·4868	1·9194
		Barinstein 1928 M1	C	2120	736	770	504	110				
				3197					0·9677	0·3779	0·9557	0·4761
				χ_6^2 for homogeneity of areas						14·9570		11·4978
TREATED SYPHILIS, WASSERMANN REACTION POSITIVE/NEGATIVE												
1. Germany, Bonn		Klövekorn & Simon 1927	+	*108*	*50*	*50*	*0*	*8*	*1·6087*	*3·0036*		
			−	*138*	*74*	*46*	*10*	*8*				
2. Germany, München		Poehlmann 1930	+	*118*	*49*	*43*	*20*	*6*	*0·8259*	*0·6555*	*1·5928*	*2·1445*
			−	*382*	*160*	*170*	*41*	*11*				
3. Poland, Warszawa		Amzel & Halber 1924	+	*610*	*135*	*258*	*155*	*62*	*2·0848*	*30·0127*	*2·2530*	*28·2506*
			−	*815*	*312*	*286*	*159*	*58*				
4. Poland, Warszawa		Straszyński 1925[b]	+	*206*	*48*	*77*	*54*	*27*	*1·5819*	*4·3996*	*1·7555*	*5·5188*
			−	*412*	*142*	*144*	*91*	*35*				
5. U.S.S.R., Leningrad		Schapiro 1929	+	*473*	*107*	*208*	*101*	*57*	*1·5419*	*9·8815*	*1·2364*	*1·7691*
			−	*1227*	*372*	*469*	*284*	*102*				
6. U.S.S.R., Moscow		Gurevič & Gellermann-Gurevič 1929	+	*136*	*42*	*52*	*29*	*13*	*1·3783*	*1·3055*	*0·9700*	*0·0094*
			−	*171*	*59*	*53*	*42*	*17*				
7. U.S.S.R., Odessa		Perkel & Israelsson 1928	+	*49*	*14*	*20*	*12*	*3*	*1·9481*	*1·5937*	*2·5714*	*2·1166*
			−	*32*	*15*	*11*	*5*	*1*				
				1700/3177					*1·5960*	*38·6249*	*1·6287*	*29·0075*
				χ_6^2 for homogeneity of areas						*12·2272*		
				1592/3039 χ_5^2 for homogeneity of areas								*10·8016*
SYPHILIS, NOT STATED WHETHER TREATED, WASSERMANN REACTION POSITIVE												
1. Belgium		Moureau 1935	P	250	110	123	12	5	1·2463	2·6188	0·6126	2·4899
			C	3500(c)	1634	1466	291	109				
2. Germany, München		Wiechmann & Paal 1926	P	500(c)	132	288	60	20	2·0571	34·1106	1·7355	8·7666
			C	1100(c)	462	490	121	27				
3. Germany, Schleswig-Holstein		Gundel 1928	P	2665	1057	1144	320	144	0·9804	0·1902	0·9620	0·3260
			C	19461	7664	8461	2412	924				
4. Poland, Warszawa		Amzel & Halber 1924	P	175	48	72	32	23	1·4151	3·1204	0·9579	0·0325
			C	1518	500	530	348	140				
				3590					1·0976	5·4578	1·0061	0·0101
				χ_3^2 for homogeneity of areas						34·5822		11·6049

TABLE 1 **THE ABO BLOOD GROUP SYSTEM** (*cont.*)

Place	Additional details	Authors		Number	O	A	B	AB	A/O Relative incidence	A/O χ_1^2 for difference from unity	B/O Relative incidence	B/O χ_1^2 for difference from unity
SYPHILIS, NOT KNOWN TO ORIGINAL AUTHORS WHETHER TREATED, WASSERMANN REACTION NEGATIVE												
1. Poland, Warszawa		Amzel & Halber 1924	P C	1191 1518	430 500	451 530	212 348	98 140	0·9895	0·0132	0·7084	9·9792
SYPHILIS, NOT STATED WHETHER TREATED, WASSERMANN REACTION POSITIVE/NEGATIVE												
1. Poland, Warszawa		Amzel & Halber 1924	+ —	*175* *1191*	*48* *430*	*72* *451*	*32* *212*	*23* *98*	*1·4302*	*3·2608*	*1·3522*	*1·5398*
SYPHILIS, NOT STATED WHETHER TREATED, WASSERMANN REACTION NOT STATED												
1. Finland		Sievers 1929	P C	635(c) 1711	217 584	253 740	117 272	48 115	0·9201	0·5963	1·1576	1·1554
2. Finland		Mustakallio 1937	P C	591 2595	190 908	250 1098	104 401	47 188	1·0881	0·6323	1·2394	2·4941
3. Finland		Streng & Ryti 1927[a]	P C	519 1383	179 463	207 591	94 232	39 97	0·9060	0·6835	1·0480	0·0969
4. Germany, Bonn		Klövekorn & Simon 1927	P C	110 760	48 335	50 362	10 47	2 16	0·9640	0·0289	1·4849	1·0773
5. Germany, München		Lützeler & Dormanns 1929 Kruse M1	P C	82 1300	33 552	39 559	8 125	2 64	1·1670	0·4006	1·0705	0·0281
6. Germany, Oberhessen		Winter 1930	P C	280 1500(c)	118 582	124 678	27 161	11 79	0·9021	0·5385	0·8271	0·6740
7. Germany, Schleswig-Holstein		Gundel 1928	P C	419 19461	154 7664	189 8461	53 2412	23 924	1·1117	0·9313	1·0935	0·3086
8. Greece, Athínai		Diamantopoulos 1928	P C	98(c) 1216	43 537	36 481	16 148	3 50	0·9347	0·0830	1·3501	0·9548
9. Poland	Cerebrospinal syphilis, progressive paralysis, taboparesis	Wilczkowski 1927	P C	138 2613	47 914	48 984	25 485	18 230	0·9486	0·0629	1·0024	0·0001
10. United Kingdom, Newcastle upon Tyne	Contagious syphilis, neuro-syphilis, benign tertiary syphilis; (s) S	Schofield 1966	P C	1207 54579	603 27008	474 21082	105 4981	25 1508	1·0070	0·0127	0·9442	0·2891
11. United Kingdom, St. Andrews	Active	Alexander 1921	P C	50(c) 50(c)	24 23	18 19	6 6	2 2	0·9079	0·0483	0·9583	0·0043
12. India, Dehra Dun, Rourkela	Mostly 'latent' syphilis; (s) A_1A_2	Seth 1969	P C	132 202	47 74	31 48	46 69	8 11	1·0168	0·0032	1·0496	0·0331
13. N. India, Dibrugarh		Mitra 1933	P C	41 526	17 176	8 142	13 169	3 39	0·5833	1·4788	0·7964	0·3518
14. Malaya, Singapore	Chinese	Saha & Banerjee 1971	P C	687 15262	277 6644	175 3967	191 3814	44 837	1·0581	0·3279	1·2012	3·6287
15. Malaya, Singapore	Indians	Saha & Banerjee 1971	P C	121 5000	39 1951	28 1051	48 1680	6 318	1·3327	1·3134	1·4293	2·6813
16. Malaya, Singapore	Malays	Saha & Banerjee 1971	P C	233 5461	96 2098	50 1369	67 1596	20 398	0·7982	1·6069	0·9174	0·2808
				5343					0·9818	0·0003	1·0911	4·0015
				χ_{15}^2 for homogeneity of areas						8·7482		10·0569
YAWS, PRESENT/ABSENT												
1. Central African Republic	Pygmies; (s) C	Jayakar 1974	Present Absent	*17* *940*	*13* *453*	*3* *267*	*1* *177*	*0* *43*	*0·3915*	*2·1126*	*0·1969*	*2·4343*
2. Congo	Pygmies; (s) C	Jayakar 1974	Present Absent	*97* *322*	*38* *127*	*36* *128*	*16* *52*	*7* *15*	*0·9400*	*0·0549*	*1·0283*	*0·0067*
				114/1262					*0·8289*	*0·5894*	*0·8767*	*0·1654*
				χ_1^2 for homogeneity of areas						*1·5782*		*2·2760*

TABLE 1 **THE ABO BLOOD GROUP SYSTEM** (*cont.*)

Place	Additional details	Authors		Number	O	A	B	AB	A/O Relative incidence	A/O χ_1^2 for difference from unity	B/O Relative incidence	B/O χ_1^2 for difference from unity
INFECTIVE AND PARASITIC DISEASES (*cont.*)												
BACTERIAL INFECTIONS (*cont.*)												
SEPTICAEMIA												
1. Poland, Warszawa	Children	Paciorkiewicz 1970	P	45(c)	14	19	7	5	1·0504	0·0194	0·7856	0·2701
			C	6626(c)	2041	2637	1299	649				
2. Peru, Lima		Muñoz-Baratta 1962	P	41(c)	18	11	8	4	1·5519	1·3181	2·3247	3·9395
			C	107938(c)	65058	26013	12629	3238				
				86					1·2571	0·7763	1·4173	1·2382
				χ_1^2 for homogeneity of areas						0·5612		2·9714
BACTERIAL MENINGITIS												
1. Poland, Warszawa	Children	Paciorkiewicz 1970	P	86(c)	37	26	18	5	0·5439	5·5895	0·7644	0·8611
			C	6626(c)	2041	2637	1299	649				
SEPTIC ANGINA												
1. Poland, Warszawa	Children	Paciorkiewicz 1970	P	322(c)	101	132	66	23	1·0115	0·0072	1·0267	0·0264
			C	6626(c)	2041	2637	1299	649				
LUNG ABSCESSES												
1. Italy, Milano		Mor & Sforza 1960	P	156	79	58	12	7	0·6650	4·2301	0·5682	2·6747
			C	500	202	223	54	21				
IMPETIGO, FOLLICULITIS, FURUNCULOSIS												
1. United Kingdom, Glasgow		MacSween & Syme 1965	P	57	37	16	4					
			C	5898	3177	1906	637	178	0·7208	1·1862		
INFECTIOUS DERMATITIS												
1. United Kingdom, Glasgow		MacSween & Syme 1965	P	58	30	21	7		1·1668	0·2909		
			C	5898	3177	1906	637	178				
RICKETTSIAL INFECTIONS												
BARTONELLOSIS												
1. Peru, Lima		Muñoz-Baratta 1962	P	41(c)	24	10	4	3	1·0581	0·0225	0·8718	0·0645
			C	107938(c)	66058	26013	12629	3238				
TYPHUS												
1. Greece, Athínai		Diamantopoulos 1928	P	28(c)	14	11	3	0	0·8772	0·1033	0·7775	0·1532
			C	1216	537	481	148	50				
VIRAL INFECTIONS												
POLIOMYELITIS												
1. Denmark, Hadersleben	(s) A	Kirchmair & Blixenkrone Møller 1936	P	363	145	147	37	34	0·8914	0·5083	0·8873	0·2263
			C	378	153	174	44	7				
2. France, Bas-Rhin		Grooten & Kossovitch 1930	P	78	23	44	11	0	1·3024	0·9866	1·7302	2·0459
			C	1054	369	542	102	41				
3. Germany, Hannover	(s) S, C	Blotevogel & Blotevogel 1934	P	366	194	127	25	20	0·6245	15·4203	0·5275	8·4067
			C	3500	1449	1519	354	178				
4. Germany, Schwerin	(s) A_1A_2	Kreil 1966	P	317	129	125	43	20	0·9559	0·1158	1·0233	0·0153
			C	2725	1096	1111	357	161				
5. Germany, Westfalen		Hatzky 1933	P	131	50	57	22	2	1·0544	0·0707	1·3275	1·1467
			C	2229(c)	887	959	294	89				
6. Poland, Warszawa	Children	Paciorkiewicz 1970	P	187(c)	64	69	40	14	0·8345	1·0570	0·9820	0·0079
			C	6626(c)	2041	2637	1299	649				

TABLE 1 **THE ABO BLOOD GROUP SYSTEM** *(cont.)*

Place	Additional details	Authors		Number	O	A	B	AB	A/O		B/O	
									Relative incidence	χ_1^2 for difference from unity	Relative incidence	χ_1^2 for difference from unity
7. Switzerland		Fanconi 1945	P	507(c)	189	271	34	13	1·2009	2·4722	0·7861	1·2057
			C	1000(c)	402	480	92	26				
8. U.S.A., San Francisco		Shaw *et al.* 1932	P	100	57	37	6	0	0·6491	2·0502	0·4115	2·6427
			C	100	43	43	11	3				
9. Argentina, Buenos Aires		Dimitri *et al.* 1939	P	22	7	10	0	5	1·6126	0·9391		
			C	15045	6702	5937	1570	836				
10. Argentina, Buenos Aires		Sujoy & Allemand 1943	P	150	65	59	21	5	1·0247	0·0182	1·3791	1·6200
			C	15045	6702	5937	1570	836				
				2221					0·9217	2·3684	0·9357	0·6626
					χ_9^2 for homogeneity of areas					21·2700		
				(2199)	χ_8^2 for homogeneity of areas							16·6546
POLIOMYELITIS, PARALYTIC/ABORTIVE												
1. Denmark		Madsen *et al.* 1936	Paral.	*47*	*22*	*18*	*6*	*1*	*0·8456*	*0·2669*	*1·1913*	*0·1369*
			Abort.	*1071*	*463*	*448*	*106*	*54*				
2. Germany		Kleinschmidt 1939	Paral.	*211(c)*	*97*	*92*	*17*	*5*	*0·6070*	*3·4408*	*0·4674*	*3·1495*
			Abort.	*98(c)*	*32*	*50*	*12*	*4*				
3. Germany, Koblenz		Anders 1956	Paral.	*709*	*301*	*293*	*96*	*19*	*1·1755*	*0·6338*	*1·7010*	*2·5040*
			Abort.	*129*	*64*	*53*	*12*	*0*				
4. Canada, Toronto		Erb *et al.* 1938	Paral.	*427(c)*	*217*	*160*	*42*	*8*	*0·8637*	*0·7532*	*0·6104*	*3·9185*
			Abort.	*276(c)*	*123*	*105*	*39*	*9*				
5. U.S.A., New York		Jungeblut & Smith 1932	Paral.	*444*	*218*	*159*	*39*	*28*	*0·5587*	*5·6562*	*0·3578*	*9·3020*
			Abort.	*107*	*36*	*47*	*18*	*6*				
				1838/1681					*0·8224*	*3·7963*	*0·6991*	*5·5962*
					χ_4^2 for homogeneity of areas					*6·9546*		*13·4146*
SMALLPOX												
1. Greece, Athínai		Diamantopoulos 1928	P	22(c)	9	11	2	0	1·3645	0·4690	0·8063	0·0748
			C	1216	537	481	148	50				
SMALLPOX, SURVIVORS												
1. N. India, Bihar, West Bengal	(s) S, C; survivors from previous outbreaks	Vogel & Chakravartti 1966[a]	P	549	136	154	225	34	0·7607	2·2786	1·3116	2·2872
			C	350	88	131	111	20				
2. N. India, Bihar, West Bengal	(s) 14 vaccinated, 198 unvaccinated; surviving fresh cases	Vogel & Chakravartti 1966[a]	P	212	32	86	73	21	7·1240	59·5492	2·1895	10·8953
			C	428	167	63	174	24				
3. N. India, Calcutta	Unvaccinated	Bhattacharyya *et al.* 1965	P	252	86	68	73	25	1·1169	0·4488	0·8443	1·1022
			C	8821(c)	2986	2114	3002	719				
4. S. India, Bombay		Sukumaran *et al.* 1966	P	334	117	88	89	40	1·3314	3·4681	1·1252	0·4762
		Shenoy & Daftary 1962 M2	C	1834	747	422	505	160				
5. Thailand, Northern		Saengudom & Flatz 1967	P	108	59	18	26	5	0·6883	1·8766	0·7416	1·5694
			C	3785(c)	1762	781	1047	195				
				1455					1·2704	7·9365	1·1035	1·4348
					χ_4^2 for homogeneity of areas					59·6848		14·8955

TABLE 1 THE ABO BLOOD GROUP SYSTEM (*cont.*)

INFECTIVE AND PARASITIC DISEASES (*cont.*)
VIRAL INFECTIONS (*cont.*)
SMALLPOX (*cont.*)

SMALLPOX, FATAL

Place	Additional details	Authors		Number	O	A	B	AB	A/O Relative incidence	A/O χ^2_1 for difference from unity	B/O Relative incidence	B/O χ^2_1 for difference from unity
1. N. India, Bihar, West Bengal	(s) 8 vaccinated, 217 unvaccinated	Vogel & Chakravartti 1966[a]	P	225	34	130	28	33	10·1354	90·9666	0·7904	0·7199
			C	428	167	63	174	24				
2. N. India, Calcutta	Unvaccinated	Bhattacharyya *et al.* 1965	P	118	51	18	35	14	0·4985	6·3784	0·6826	2·9850
			C	8821(c)	2986	2114	3002	719				
3. S. India, Bombay		Sukumaran *et al.* 1966	P	67	25	19	19	4	1·3453	0·9131	1·1242	0·1426
		Shenoy & Daftary 1962 M2	C	1834	747	422	505	160				
				410					2·2697	27·2074	0·8955	0·3804
				χ^2_2 for homogeneity of areas						71·0507		1·7227

SMALLPOX, FATAL/SURVIVORS

Place	Additional details	Authors		Number	O	A	B	AB	A/O Relative incidence	A/O χ^2_1 for difference from unity	B/O Relative incidence	B/O χ^2_1 for difference from unity
1. N. India, Bihar, West Bengal		Vogel & Chakravartti 1966[a]	Fatal	*225*	*34*	*130*	*28*	*33*	*1·4227*	*1·5538*	*0·3610*	*9·4314*
			Survivors	*212*	*32*	*86*	*73*	*21*				
2. N. India, Calcutta		Bhattacharyya *et al.* 1965	Fatal	*118*	*51*	*18*	*35*	*14*	*0·4464*	*6·4105*	*0·8085*	*0·6149*
			Survivors	*252*	*86*	*68*	*73*	*25*				
3. S. India, Bombay		Sukumaran *et al.* 1966	Fatal	*67*	*25*	*19*	*19*	*4*	*1·0105*	*0·0010*	*0·9991*	*0·0000*
			Survivors	*334*	*117*	*88*	*89*	*40*				
				410/798					*0·8955*	*0·3804*	*0·6806*	*4·6771*
				χ^2_2 for homogeneity of areas						*7·5849*		*5·6104*

SMALLPOX, CONFLUENT

Place	Additional details	Authors		Number	O	A	B	AB	A/O Relative incidence	A/O χ^2_1 for difference from unity	B/O Relative incidence	B/O χ^2_1 for difference from unity
1. S. India, Madras	(s) severity	Downie *et al.* 1965	P	94	51	17	22	4	0·6436	2·4683	0·5168	6·6750
			C	27142	10866	5628	9069	1579				
2. Pakistan, Karachi		Helmbold 1963	P	281	100	74	89	18	0·7400	1·4974	0·5790	5·7634
		Moten & Stewart 1956 M1	C	213	54	54	83	22				
				375					0·6965	3·8245	0·5507	12·3275
				χ^2_1 for homogeneity of areas						0·1412		0·1109

SMALLPOX, DISCRETE

Place	Additional details	Authors		Number	O	A	B	AB	A/O Relative incidence	A/O χ^2_1 for difference from unity	B/O Relative incidence	B/O χ^2_1 for difference from unity
1. S. India, Madras	(s) severity	Downie *et al.* 1965	P	236	109	46	69	12	0·8148	1·3457	0·7585	1·7578
			C	27142	10866	5628	9069	1579				
2. Pakistan, Karachi		Helmbold 1963	P	318	148	75	83	12	0·5068	8·0886	0·3649	20·5912
		Moten & Stewart 1956 M1	C	213	54	54	83	22				
				554					0·6890	6·8802	0·6271	13·5355
				χ^2_1 for homogeneity of areas						2·5541		8·8135

SMALLPOX, CONFLUENT/DISCRETE

Place	Additional details	Authors		Number	O	A	B	AB	A/O Relative incidence	A/O χ^2_1 for difference from unity	B/O Relative incidence	B/O χ^2_1 for difference from unity
1. S. India, Madras		Downie *et al.* 1965	P	*94*	*51*	*17*	*22*	*4*	*0·7898*	*0·5090*	*0·6814*	*1·6581*
			C	*236*	*109*	*46*	*69*	*12*				
2. Pakistan, Karachi		Helmbold 1963	P	*281*	*100*	*74*	*89*	*18*	*1·4602*	*3·2870*	*1·5870*	*5·3294*
			C	*318*	*148*	*75*	*83*	*12*				
				375/554					*1·2255*	*1·3268*	*1·2202*	*1·4357*
				χ^2_1 for homogeneity of areas						*2·4692*		*5·5518*

TABLE 1 **THE ABO BLOOD GROUP SYSTEM** (*cont.*)

Place	Additional details	Authors		Number	O	A	B	AB	A/O		B/O	
									Relative incidence	χ_1^2 for difference from unity	Relative incidence	χ_1^2 for difference from unity
REACTIONS TO SMALLPOX VACCINATION												
1. Irish Republic, Dublin	Students	Bourke *et al.* 1965	+	*612*	*308*	*225*	*63*	*16*	*0·9581*	*0·0502*	*0·9091*	*0·1042*
			—	*169*	*80*	*61*	*18*	*10*				
2. U.S.S.R., Moscow	Revaccination of school-children	Komarovich & Rychkov 1966	+	*344*	*82*	*175*	*51*	*36*	*40·1220*	*59·6388*	*0·8009*	*0·8783*
			—	*172*	*94*	*5*	*73*	*0*				
				956/341					*1·6040*	*7·0793*	*0·8416*	*0·8704*
				χ_1^2 for homogeneity of areas						*52·6096*		*0·1121*
CHICKENPOX												
1. Germany, Heidelberg		Hepp *et al.* 1975	P	262	102	126	20	14	1·0915	0·4295	0·7303	1·6465
			C	34513	13748	15559	3691	1515				
2. Germany, Karlsruhe		Hepp *et al.* 1975	P	316	127	143	29	17	1·0639	0·2530	0·8591	0·5345
			C	14544	5986	6335	1591	632				
3. Germany, Mannheim		Hepp *et al.* 1975	P	303	118	142	27	16	1·0633	0·2410	0·8523	0·5571
			C	34513	13748	15559	3691	1515				
4. Poland, Warszawa	Children	Paciorkiewicz 1970	P	371(c)	106	146	79	40	1·0661	0·2385	1·1710	1·0671
			C	6626(c)	2041	2637	1299	649				
5. U.S.A., New York		Brody *et al.* 1935–6	P	38	16	16	4	2	1·3541	0·7073	0·9795	0·0013
			C	1000	478	353	122	47				
				1290					1·0783	1·4298	0·9498	0·2856
				χ_4^2 for homogeneity of areas						0·4395		3·5209
MEASLES												
1. Poland, Warszawa	Children	Paciorkiewicz 1970	P	1836(c)	608	681	369	178	0·8669	5·1216	0·9536	0·4024
			C	6626(c)	2041	2637	1299	649				
2. Romania, Bucureşti		Mironesco & Stefanov 1926; Dumitrescu 1927 M1	P	64	17	35	8	4	1·7018	3·0516	0·8852	0·0774
			C	1031	348	421	185	77				
3. U.S.A., New York		Brody *et al.* 1935–6	P	130	71	41	10	8	0·7819	1·3940	0·5518	2·8417
			C	1000	478	353	122	47				
				2030					0·8820	4·4960	0·9300	1·0069
				χ_2^2 for homogeneity of areas						5·0721		2·3146
INFECTIOUS HEPATITIS												
1. Czechoslovakia, Praha		Veselý 1969[a]	P	440	157	175	72	36	0·7755	3·8460	0·8620	0·7801
			C	1142(c)	359	516	191	76				
2. Germany, Erfurt	Patients under treatment for acute hepatitis	Thieler *et al.* 1966	P	314	109	127	57	21	0·9707	0·0517	1·4064	4·3314
			C	73548	26981	32386	10032	4149				
3. Germany, Erfurt	Pregnant women who have had hepatitis earlier (90% as children)	Thieler *et al.* 1966	P	725	281	324	84	36	0·9606	0·2408	0·8040	3·0515
			C	73548	26981	32386	10032	4149				
4. Poland, Kraków		Sowa 1970	P	500	155	192	106	47	1·2458	2·0948	1·1355	0·5208
			C	500	176	175	106	43				
5. Poland, Warszawa	Children	Paciorkiewicz 1970	P	728(c)	240	292	126	70	0·9417	0·4267	0·8249	2·7734
			C	6626(c)	2041	2637	1299	649				
6. United Kingdom, Region 1	R.A.F. personnel	Zuckerman & McDonald 1963	P	200	79	94	24	3	1·1510	0·8415	1·6519	4·5792
			C	21134	9244	9556	1700	634				
7. United Kingdom, Region 2	R.A.F. personnel	Zuckerman & McDonald 1963	P	124	51	59	9	5	1·3236	2·1364	0·9674	0·0084
			C	20043	9456	8265	1725	597				
8. United Kingdom, Region 3	R.A.F. personnel	Zuckerman & McDonald 1963	P	54	16	26	8	4	2·3223	6·9755	2·3173	3·7295
			C	5931	2994	2095	646	196				
9. Peru, Lima		Muñoz-Baratta 1962	P	83	38	18	18	9	1·2029	0·4165	2·4777	10·0437
			C	107938	66058	26013	12629	3238				
				3168					1·0072	0·0265	1·0266	0·1976
				χ_8^2 for homogeneity of areas						17·0034		29·6204

TABLE 1 **THE ABO BLOOD GROUP SYSTEM** *(cont.)*

Place	Additional details	Authors		Number	O	A	B	AB	A/O Relative incidence	A/O χ_1^2 for difference from unity	B/O Relative incidence	B/O χ_1^2 for difference from unity
INFECTIVE AND PARASITIC DISEASES *(cont.)*												
VIRAL INFECTIONS (cont.)												
SERUM HEPATITIS, RECIPIENTS OF TRANSFUSIONS FOLLOWED/NOT FOLLOWED BY DISEASE												
1. Poland, Lublin		Szmuness *et al.* 1966	With Without	*19* *1161*	*7* *372*	*9* *445*	*2* *243*	*1* *101*	*1·0748*	*0·0201*	*0·4374*	*1·0526*
2. United Kingdom, Liverpool		Lewkonia & Finn 1969	With Without	*45* *51*	*29* *16*	*13* *25*	*2* *8*	*1* *2*	*0·2869*	*7·2886*	*0·1379*	*5·4362*
3. U.S.A., Chicago	89% White	Allen & Sayman 1962	With Without	*188* *3676*	*73* *1588*	*82* *1450*	*23* *466*	*10* *172*	*1·2302*	*1·5772*	*1·0737*	*0·0843*
				252/4888					*1·0464*	*0·0932*	*0·8656*	*0·4088*
				χ_2^2 for homogeneity of areas						*8·7927*		*6·1642*
SERUM HEPATITIS (AUSTRALIA) ANTIGEN, CARRIERS/NON-CARRIERS												
1. U.S.A., New York	Volunteer donors	Szmuness *et al.* 1971	Carriers Non-carriers	*177* *7919*	*78* *3571*	*61* *2893*	*25* *1104*	*13* *351*	*0·9653*	*0·0417*	*1·0367*	*0·0241*
2. U.S.A., New York	Mentally retarded Whites	Szmuness *et al.* 1971	Carriers Non-carriers	*142* *800*	*68* *369*	*51* *306*	*15* *101*	*8* *24*	*0·9044*	*0·2505*	*0·8059*	*0·4954*
3. U.S.A., New York	Mentally retarded Negroes	Szmuness *et al.* 1971	Carriers Non-carriers	*28* *145*	*9* *80*	*13* *37*	*4* *27*	*2* *1*	*3·1231*	*5·6993*	*1·3169*	*0·1845*
				347/8864					*1·0214*	*0·0281*	*0·9701*	*0·0029*
				χ_2^2 for homogeneity of areas						*5·9634*		*0·7011*
MUMPS												
1. Poland, Warszawa	Children	Paciorkiewicz 1970	P C	403(c) 6626(c)	148 2041	154 2637	64 1299	37 649	0·8054	3·3185	0·6794	6·3181
INFECTIOUS MONONUCLEOSIS												
1. Poland, Warszawa	Children	Paciorkiewicz 1970	P C	274(c) 6626(c)	97 2041	101 2637	53 1299	23 649	0·8059	2·2091	0·8585	0·7648
TRACHOMA												
1. Italy, Perugia		Giannantoni 1928	P C	26 32	3 13	20 11	2 5	1 3	7·8788	7·7306	1·7333	0·2725
VIRAL MENINGITIS												
1. Poland, Warszawa	Children	Paciorkiewicz 1970	P C	129(c) 6626(c)	38 2041	51 2637	33 1299	7 649	1·0388	0·0309	1·3645	1·6686
WARTS												
1. United Kingdom, Glasgow	Plantaris and vulgaris	MacSween & Syme 1965	P C	402 5898	231 3177	117 1906	54 637	 178	0·8442	2·0901		
INFECTION WITH ADENOVIRUS												
1. United Kingdom, S. England	R.A.F. personnel	McDonald & Zuckerman 1962	P C	351 21134	134 9244	179 9556	29 1700	9 634	1·2922	4·9552	1·1768	0·6216
2. United Kingdom, N. England, Wales, and S.W. Scotland	R.A.F. personnel	McDonald & Zuckerman 1962	P C	211 20043	86 9456	92 8265	19 1725	14 597	1·2239	1·7967	1·2111	0·5647
3. United Kingdom, exc. England, Wales, and S.W. Scotland	R.A.F. personnel	McDonald & Zuckerman 1962	P C	105 5931	48 2994	43 2095	9 646	5 195	1·2803	1·3594	0·8690	0·1473
				667					1·2687	8·0272	1·1314	0·7057
				χ_2^2 for homogeneity of areas						0·0841		0·6279

TABLE 1 **THE ABO BLOOD GROUP SYSTEM** (*cont.*)

Place	Additional details	Authors		Number	O	A	B	AB	A/O Relative incidence	A/O χ^2_1 for difference from unity	B/O Relative incidence	B/O χ^2_1 for difference from unity
INFECTION WITH COXSACKIE A21 VIRUS												
1. United Kingdom, S. England	R.A.F. personnel	McDonald & Zuckerman 1962	P	52	29	19	3	1	0·6338	2·3817	0·5625	0·8982
			C	21134	9244	9556	1700	634				
2. United Kingdom, N. England, Wales, and S.W. Scotland	R.A.F. personnel	McDonald & Zuckerman 1962	P	58	29	27	2	0	1·0652	0·0556	0·3781	1·7680
			C	20043	9456	8265	1725	597				
3. United Kingdom, exc. England, Wales, and S.W. Scotland	R.A.F. personnel	McDonald & Zuckerman 1962	P	15	9	5	1	0	0·7940	0·1707	0·5150	0·3957
			C	5931	2994	2095	646	196				
				125					0·8372	0·9031	0·4842	2·8832
					χ^2_2 for homogeneity of areas					1·7048		0·1788
'GRIPPE 1918' INFECTION												
1. Greece, Athínai		Diamantopoulos 1928	P	34	23	8	2	1	0·3883	5·1895	0·3155	2·4103
			C	1216	537	481	148	50				
INFLUENZA A_1 VIRUS INFECTION												
1. United Kingdom, S. England	R.A.F. personnel	McDonald & Zuckerman 1962	P	69	33	31	4	1	0·9087	0·1459	0·6591	0·6184
			C	21134	9244	9556	1700	634				
2. United Kingdom, N. England, Wales, and S.W. Scotland	R.A.F. personnel	McDonald & Zuckerman 1962	P	45	22	17	4	2	0·8841	0·1453	0·9967	0·0000
			C	20043	9456	8265	1725	597				
3. United Kingdom, exc. England, Wales, and Scotland	R.A.F. personnel	McDonald & Zuckerman 1962	P	15	8	5	1	1	0·8932	0·0392	0·5793	0·2644
			C	5931	2994	2095	646	196				
				129					0·8987	0·3257	0·7765	0·5007
					χ^2_2 for homogeneity of areas					0·0047		0·3822
INFLUENZA A_2 VIRUS INFECTION												
1. United Kingdom, S. England	R.A.F. personnel	McDonald & Zuckerman 1962	P	313	171	104	31	7	0·5883	17·9505	0·9858	0·0053
			C	21134	9244	9556	1700	634				
2. United Kingdom, N. England, Wales, and S.W. Scotland	R.A.F. personnel	McDonald & Zuckerman 1962	P	316	167	111	32	6	0·7605	4·9259	1·0504	0·0637
			C	20043	9456	8265	1725	597				
3. United Kingdom, exc. England, Wales, and S.W. Scotland	R.A.F. personnel	McDonald & Zuckerman 1962	P	72	46	22	3	1	0·6835	2·1294	0·3023	4·0104
			C	5931	2994	2095	646	196				
				701					0·6715	22·8695	0·9568	0·1070
					χ^2_2 for homogeneity of areas					2·1364		3·9724
INFLUENZA B VIRUS INFECTION												
1. United Kingdom, S. England	R.A.F. personnel	McDonald & Zuckerman 1962	P	32	19	9	2	2	0·4582	3·7147	0·5724	0·5626
			C	21134	9244	9556	1700	634				
2. United Kingdom, N. England, Wales, S.W. Scotland	R.A.F. personnel	McDonald & Zuckerman 1962	P	25	8	14	2	1	2·0022	2·4508	1·3704	0·1587
			C	20043	9456	8265	1725	597				
3. United Kingdom, exc. England, Wales, S.W. Scotland	R.A.F. personnel	McDonald & Zuckerman 1962	P	6	2	4	0	0	2·8582	1·4690		
			C	5931	2994	2095	646	196				
				63					1·0136	0·0023	0·8623	0·0748
					χ^2_2 for homogeneity of areas					7·6322		
				(57)	χ^2_1 for homogeneity of areas							0·6465

TABLE 1 **THE ABO BLOOD GROUP SYSTEM** (*cont.*)

Place	Additional details	Authors		Number	O	A	B	AB	A/O Relative incidence	A/O χ_1^2 for difference from unity	B/O Relative incidence	B/O χ_1^2 for difference from unity
INFECTIVE AND PARASITIC DISEASES (*cont.*)												
VIRAL INFECTIONS (*cont.*)												
INFLUENZA A/SING/57 VIRUS ANTIBODIES: STRONG/WEAK INHIBITION OF HAEMAGGLUTINATION												
1. Iceland		Watkin *et al.* 1975	Strong		*213*	*109*			*0·7871*	*2·6391*		
			Weak		*323*	*210*						
2. Irish Republic		Watkin *et al.* 1975	Strong		*130*	*63*			*0·8427*	*0·9132*		
			Weak		*313*	*180*						
				515/1026					*0·8088*	*3·4676*		
			χ_1^2 for homogeneity of areas							*0·0847*		
INFLUENZA A2/SING/1/57 VIRUS ANTIBODIES: POSITIVE/NEGATIVE INHIBITION OF HAEMAGGLUTINATION												
1. United Kingdom, Sheffield	(s) A	Potter & Schild 1967	+		*234*	*155*			*0·4215*	*16·9162*		
			−		*49*	*77*						
INFLUENZA A/HK/68 VIRUS ANTIBODIES: STRONG/WEAK INHIBITION OF HAEMAGGLUTINATION												
1. Iceland		Watkin *et al.* 1975	Strong		*130*	*66*			*0·8147*	*1·4353*		
			Weak		*406*	*253*						
2. Irish Republic		Watkin *et al.* 1975	Strong		*286*	*155*			*0·9669*	*0·0407*		
			Weak		*157*	*88*						
				637/904					*0·8897*	*0·9602*		
			χ_1^2 for homogeneity of areas							*0·5158*		
INFLUENZA A_1 VIRUS ANTIBODIES: STRONG/WEAK INHIBITION OF HAEMAGGLUTINATION												
1. Argentina, Brazil, Colombia	Recruits; (s) G	Cuadrado & Davenport 1970	Strong	*885*	*556*	*212*	*99*	*18*	*0·4418*	*47·9748*	*0·8812*	*0·4953*
			Weak	*615*	*292*	*252*	*59*	*12*				
INFLUENZA A_2 VIRUS ANTIBODIES: STRONG/WEAK INHIBITION OF HAEMAGGLUTINATION												
1. Argentina, Brazil, Colombia	Recruits; (s) G	Cuadrado & Davenport 1970	Strong	*1057*	*661*	*259*	*115*	*22*	*0·3574*	*67·8538*	*0·7566*	*2·0043*
			Weak	*443*	*187*	*205*	*43*	*8*				
FUNGAL INFECTIONS												
TRICHOPHYTOSIS												
1. Japan, Okayama		Ohmichi 1928	P	28	11	10	6	1	0·6461	0·9949	0·6533	0·7007
			C	6936	1921	2703	1604	708				
FUNGAL INFECTIONS OF SKIN												
1. United Kingdom, Glasgow	Moniliasis, Tinea	MacSween & Syme 1965	P	59	28	19		2	1·1311	0·1701		
			C	5898	3177	1906	637	178				
2. Egypt		el-Hefnawi *et al.* 1963	P	200	64	68	56	12	0·9970	0·0003	1·1588	0·6231
			C	5200	1674	1784	1264	478				
				259					1·0304	0·0384		
			χ_1^2 for homogeneity of areas							0·1319		
PROTOZOAL INFECTIONS												
MALARIA												
1. Italy	Airmen	Mangiacapra 1936	P	522	159	330	21	12	2·1584	49·6088	0·4753	9·2495
		Tranquilli-Leali 1934 M1	C	1830	781	751	217	81				
2. Italy, Sassari		Fiori 1932	P	74	27	30	10	7	2·0920	7·1359	0·9755	0·0043
		Manai & Simula 1929 M1	C	968	482	256	183	47				
3. United Kingdom, S.W. Region		Farr 1960	P	112	52	49	9	2	0·9528	0·0588	0·9186	0·0552
		Roberts 1948	C	120874	53744	53150	10126	3854				

TABLE 1 **THE ABO BLOOD GROUP SYSTEM** *(cont.)*

Place	Additional details	Authors		Number	O	A	B	AB	A/O Relative incidence	A/O χ_1^2 for difference from unity	B/O Relative incidence	B/O χ_1^2 for difference from unity
4. U.S.S.R., Kharkov, Zhdanov		Rubashkin *et al.* 1927 Rubashkin & Derman 1926 M1	P	636(c)	149	207	144	136	0·9789	0·0240	1·1467	0·8077
			C	808	229	325	193	61				
5. U.S.S.R., Uzbekistan	Uzbeks; (s) A; transmitted by anopheles	Minkievich 1925 Sakharov 1933 M2	P	1159(c)	334	386	322	117	1·1684	0·8825	0·9436	0·1223
			C	307	92	91	94	30				
6. U.S.S.R., Voronezh		Lizunova 1925	P	875	240	347	213	75	0·9789	0·0138	1·6024	4·2737
			C	209	65	96	36	12				
7. N. India, Dibrugarh		Mitra 1933	P	265	89	58	96	22	0·8077	1·1067	1·1233	0·4067
			C	526	176	142	169	39				
				3643					1·3092	19·3035	1·0104	0·0600
				χ_6^2 for homogeneity of areas						39·5270		14·8593
MALARIA, PARASITES PRESENT/ABSENT												
1. New Guinea, Karkar Island	(s) S	Harrison *et al.* 1976	Present	*163*	*93*	*39*	*29*	*2*	*0·8314*	*0·7550*	*1·0164*	*0·0045*
			Absent	*641*	*339*	*171*	*104*	*27*				
PROTOZOAL INFECTIONS OTHER THAN MALARIA												
1. N. India, Dibrugarh		Mitra 1933	P	53	24	9	16	4	0·4648	3·5469	0·6943	1·1501
			C	526	176	142	169	39				
WORM INFESTATIONS												
BILHARZIAL HEPATIC FIBROSIS												
1. Egypt		Khattab *et al.* 1968	P	339	39	194	69	37	4·5684	73·5428	2·3640	18·1220
			C	10045	3275	3566	2451	753				
2. Egypt, Alexandria		Sadek *et al.* 1965[a]	P	14	5	3	4	2	0·5187	0·8055	0·9409	0·0082
			C	3720	1142	1321	971	286				
				353					4·0488	65·9812	2·1905	16·4104
				χ_1^2 for homogeneity of areas						8·3671		1·7198
HYDATID CYST												
1. Portugal		Lessa & Ruffié 1960	P	202(c)	80	99	19	4	1·1303	0·6269	1·3528	1·3075
			C	3353(c)	1424	1559	250	120				
2. Peru, Lima		Muñoz-Baratta 1962	P	153(c)	88	34	21	10	0·9811	0·0089	1·2482	0·8322
			C	107938(c)	66058	26013	12629	3238				
				355					1·0727	0·3264	1·2951	2·0895
				χ_1^2 for homogeneity of areas						0·3094		0·0502
TAPE WORM ANAEMIA												
1. Finland		Kaipainen & Vuorinen 1960 Mäkelä *et al.* 1959 M2	P	197(c)	49	86	38	24	1·3716	2·6346	1·6259	4·1514
			C	891	304	389	145	53				
LOIASIS												
1. Nigeria		Ogunba 1970	P	314	161	67	78	8	1·0061	0·0018	1·0709	0·2434
			C	26027	13404	5544	6064	1015				
FILARIASIS												
1. S. India, Rourkela		Anand 1965	P	603	206	147	206	44	0·9438	0·1297	1·0186	0·0155
			C	487	164	124	161	38				
ASCARIASIS												
1. Japan, Sendai		Moniwa 1960	P	74	20	31	18	5	1·3475	1·0780	1·2621	0·5116
			C	21199	6769	7786	4827	1817				

TABLE 1 **THE ABO BLOOD GROUP SYSTEM** *(cont.)*

Place	Additional details	Authors		Number	O	A	B	AB	A/O Relative incidence	A/O χ_1^2 for difference from unity	B/O Relative incidence	B/O χ_1^2 for difference from unity
INFECTIVE AND PARASITIC DISEASES *(cont.)*												
WORM INFESTATIONS *(cont.)*												
HELMINTHIASIS												
1. Finland		Mustakallio 1937	P	94	31	37	23	3	0·9870	0·0028	1·6800	3·3926
			C	2595	908	1098	401	188				
2. N. India, Dibrugarh		Mitra 1933	P	112	36	27	31	18	0·9296	0·0688	0·8968	0·1657
			C	526	176	142	169	39				
				206					0·9612	0·0457	1·2079	0·9479
				χ_1^2 for homogeneity of areas						0·0259		2·6104
ARTHROPOD INFESTATIONS												
PEDICULOSIS, SCABIES												
1. United Kingdom, Glasgow		MacSween & Syme 1965	P	30	15	11		4	1·2224	0·2545		
			C	5898	3177	1906	637	178				
NEOPLASMS												
MALIGNANT NEOPLASMS												
MALIGNANT NEOPLASMS OF LIP												
1. Norway		Hartmann & Stavem 1964	P	569	201	308	37	23	1·2106	4·3629	0·8372	0·9726
			C	31491	12189	15429	2680	1193				
2. N. India, Kanpur		Tyagi *et al.* 1965	P	11	5	1	2	3	0·2919	1·2621	0·3486	1·5846
			C	6000	1985	1360	2278	377				
				580					1·1987	3·9526	0·8054	1·5101
				χ_1^2 for homogeneity of areas						1·6724		1·0473
MALIGNANT NEOPLASMS OF TONGUE												
1. Germany, Berlin		Kaiser-Meinhardt 1962	P	20	5	13	2	0	2·3582	2·6547	1·0359	0·0018
		Hoffbauer 1961	C	15824	5959	6570	2301	994				
2. Norway		Hartmann & Stavem 1964	P	160	56	87	15	2	1·2214	1·3561	1·2658	0·6537
			C	31491	12197	15514	2581	1199				
3. N. India, Agra		Mital & Gupta 1969	P	76	21	15	30	10	0·8805	0·1410	1·0158	0·0030
			C	14468	4063	3296	5714	1395				
4. N. India, Kanpur		Tyagi *et al.* 1965	P	90	23	27	37	3	1·7134	3·5467	1·4018	1·5966
			C	6000	1985	1360	2278	377				
5. S. India, Bhopal	(s) S	Ghooi *et al.* 1970	P	58	18	8	22	10	1·0159	0·0010	2·3467	4·4957
			C	100	48	21	25	6				
				404					1·2799	3·8044	1·3298	3·7092
				χ_4^2 for homogeneity of areas						3·8951		3·0415
MALIGNANT NEOPLASMS OF GUM												
1. N. India, Agra		Mital & Gupta 1969	P	36	8	10	17	1	1·5409	0·8288	1·5110	0·9248
			C	14468	4063	3296	5714	1395				
2. N. India, Kanpur		Tyagi *et al.* 1965	P	27	10	5	12	0	0·7298	0·3294	1·0457	0·0108
			C	6000	1985	1360	2278	377				
				63					1·1191	0·0981	1·2569	0·5675
				χ_1^2 for homogeneity of areas						1·0606		0·3680

TABLE 1 **THE ABO BLOOD GROUP SYSTEM** (*cont.*)

Place	Additional details	Authors		Number	O	A	B	AB	A/O Relative incidence	A/O χ_1^2 for difference from unity	B/O Relative incidence	B/O χ_1^2 for difference from unity
MALIGNANT NEOPLASMS OF BUCCAL MUCOSA												
1. N. India, Agra		Mital & Gupta 1969	P	299	99	80	101	19	0·9961	0·0007	0·7254	5·0452
			C	14468	4063	3296	5714	1395				
2. S. India, Bombay	Male Marathas	Jayant 1971	P	102(c)	29	31	34	8	1·0846	0·0891	1·4883	2·1940
			C	858(c)	278	274	219	87				
				401					1·0165	0·0152	0·8502	1·6554
				χ_1^2 for homogeneity of areas						0·0746		5·5838
MALIGNANT NEOPLASMS OF CHEEK												
1. N. India, Kanpur		Tyagi *et al.* 1965	P	113	33	36	34	10	1·5922	3·6474	0·8978	0·1917
			C	6000	1985	1360	2278	377				
2. S. India, Bhopal	(s) S	Ghooi *et al.* 1970	P	221	66	48	105	2	1·6623	2·4732	3·0545	14·5817
			C	100	48	21	25	6				
				334					1·6171	6·1075	1·4923	4·5161
				χ_1^2 for homogeneity of areas						0·0131		10·2573
MALIGNANT NEOPLASMS OF BUCCAL CAVITY												
1. France, Paris		Huguenin & Delage 1933	P	38(c)	18	15	5	0	0·7165	0·8399	1·3105	0·2552
		Dujarric de la Rivière *et al.* 1927 M1	C	465	184	214	39	28				
2. Germany, Berlin		Kaiser-Meinhardt 1962	P	57	14	27	10	6	1·7492	2·8742	1·8498	2·1992
		Hoffbauer 1961	C	15824	5959	6570	2301	994				
3. N. India, Agra	Other than mucosa, tongue, and gum	Mital & Gupta 1969	P	20	6	5	8	1	1·0273	0·0020	0·9481	0·0097
			C	14468	4063	3296	5714	1395				
4. N. India, Kanpur	Palate	Tyagi *et al.* 1965	P	10	1	4	3	2	5·8382	2·4881	2·6141	0·6921
			C	6000	1985	1360	2278	377				
5. S. India, Bombay	Except mucosa; male Marathas	Jayant 1971	P	75(c)	27	21	19	8	0·7891	0·6103	0·8933	0·1302
			C	858(c)	278	274	219	87				
				200					1·0503	0·0749	1·1791	0·6431
				χ_4^2 for homogeneity of areas						6·7396		2·6433
MALIGNANT NEOPLASMS OF NASOPHARYNX												
1. Germany, Berlin		Kaiser-Meinhardt 1962	P	18	10	4	2	2	0·3628	2·9345	0·5179	0·7206
		Hoffbauer 1961	C	15824	5959	6570	2301	994				
2. Malaya, Singapore	Chinese	Seow *et al.* 1964	P	232	92	63	63	14	1·1469	0·6919	1·1929	1·1457
			C	15262	6644	3967	3814	837				
3. Kenya	Kamba	Clifford 1970	P	38	27	4	5	2	0·2527	6·4960	0·4648	2·4219
			C	1327	650	381	259	37				
4. Kenya	Kikuyu	Clifford 1970	P	108	58	26	22	2	0·8170	0·7162	0·8773	0·2667
			C	4217	2063	1132	892	130				
5. Kenya	Kisii	Clifford 1970	P	9	4	3	2	0	1·4212	0·2113	0·9242	0·0083
			C	4700	2181	1151	1180	188				
6. Kenya	Luhya	Clifford 1970	P	25	16	3	3	3	0·3236	3·1982	0·4043	2·0595
			C	2772	1298	752	602	120				
7. Kenya	Luo	Clifford 1970	P	32	13	10	9	0	1·4887	0·8854	1·6289	1·2514
			C	3105	1527	789	649	140				
8. Kenya	Nandi	Clifford 1970	P	21	10	5	4	2	0·7206	0·3070	1·5077	0·3768
			C	105	49	34	13	9				
				483					0·9082	0·6791	1·0190	0·0246
				χ_7^2 for homogeneity of areas						14·7613		8·2262

TABLE 1 **THE ABO BLOOD GROUP SYSTEM** (*cont.*)

Place	Additional details	Authors		Number	O	A	B	AB	A/O Relative incidence	A/O χ^2_1 for difference from unity	B/O Relative incidence	B/O χ^2_1 for difference from unity
NEOPLASMS (*cont.*)												
MALIGNANT NEOPLASMS (*cont.*)												
MALIGNANT NEOPLASMS OF OROPHARYNX												
1. Italy, Milano		Manzini 1960	P	28	11	9	8	0	0·7865	0·2848	2·8006	4·8843
		Visconti *et al.* 1961	C	9607	3974	4134	1032	467				
2. S. India, Bombay	Male Marathas	Jayant 1971	P	50(c)	10	19	14	7	1·9277	2·6945	1·7772	1·8411
			C	858(c)	278	274	219	87				
				78					1·2981	0·7617	2·1824	6·2002
		χ^2_1 for homogeneity of areas								2·2176		0·5252
MALIGNANT NEOPLASMS OF HYPOPHARYNX												
1. United Kingdom, Liverpool	(s) S	Stell & Kell 1970	P	105	62	33	10	0	0·6898	2·9392	0·8885	0·1188
		Kopeć 1956 M1	C	9301	4633	3575	841	252				
2. S. India, Bombay	Male Marathas	Jayant 1971	P	93	23	22	35	13	0·9705	0·0093	1·9317	5·4043
			C	858	278	274	219	87				
				198					0·7715	2·1337	1·4096	2·4728
		χ^2_1 for homogeneity of areas								0·8148		3·0503
MALIGNANT NEOPLASMS OF PHARYNX, PART UNSPECIFIED												
1. France, Paris		Huguenin & Delage 1933	P	24(c)	12	6	6	0	0·4299	2·7398	2·3590	2·6205
		Dujarric de la Rivière *et al.* 1927 M1	C	465	184	214	39	28				
MALIGNANT NEOPLASMS OF TONSILS												
1. Germany, Berlin		Kaiser-Meinhardt 1962	P	28	8	9	7	4	1·0204	0·0017	2·2660	2·4926
		Hoffbauer 1961	C	15824	5959	6570	2301	994				
2. N. India, Kanpur		Tyagi *et al.* 1965	P	12	6	3	2	1	0·7298	0·1980	0·2905	2·2894
			C	6000	1985	1360	2278	377				
				40					0·9164	0·0474	1·2572	0·2736
		χ^2_1 for homogeneity of areas								0·1523		4·5085
MALIGNANT NEOPLASMS OF BUCCAL CAVITY, LARYNX*												
1. Italy, Trieste		Tagliaferro 1937[a]	P	46	14	28	4	0	2·0268	4·5329	0·6851	0·4381
		Goldstein 1927, 1929 M1	C	1766	681	672	284	129				
MALIGNANT NEOPLASMS OF SALIVARY GLANDS												
1. United Kingdom, Manchester	Acinic-cell	Garrett *et al.* 1971	P	11(a)	8	3	0	0	0·4371	1·4849		
			C	1554	746	640	130	38				
2. United Kingdom, Manchester	Adenoid cystic	Garrett *et al.* 1971	P	32(a)	11	19	2	0	2·0134	3·3441	1·0434	0·0030
			C	1554	746	640	130	38				
3. United Kingdom, Manchester	Muco-epidermoid	Garrett *et al.* 1971	P	8(a)	2	5	1	0	2·9141	1·6274	2·8692	0·7362
			C	1554	746	640	130	38				
4. United Kingdom, Manchester	Other than in 1, 2, and 3	Garrett *et al.* 1971	P	34(a)	17	11	4	2	0·7542	0·5212	1·3502	0·2837
			C	1554	746	640	130	38				
5. United Kingdom, Glasgow		Cameron 1958	P	35	5	29	1	0	9·6677	21·8738	0·9975	0·0000
			C	5898	3177	1906	637	178				
6. S. India, Bhopal	(s) S	Ghooi *et al.* 1970	P	23	6	6	11	0	2·2857	1·7009	3·5200	4·9739
			C	100	48	21	25	6				
7. U.S.A., New York	Parotid	Osborne & De George 1962	P	202	74	95	26	7	1·4249	5·0004	1·1209	0·2410
			C	4738	2029	1828	636	245				
8. U.S.A., New York	Submaxillary	Osborne & De George 1962	P	48	15	20	8	5	1·4799	1·3055	1·7015	1·4581
			C	4738	2029	1828	636	245				
				393					1·5547	16·1503	1·3740	3·3422
		χ^2_7 for homogeneity of areas								19·2231		
		χ^2_5 for homogeneity of areas		(382)								4·3538

* For larynx alone, see p. 106.

TABLE 1 **THE ABO BLOOD GROUP SYSTEM** (*cont.*)

Place	Additional details	Authors		Number	O	A	B	AB	A/O Relative incidence	A/O χ_1^2 for difference from unity	B/O Relative incidence	B/O χ_1^2 for difference from unity
MALIGNANT NEOPLASMS OF OESOPHAGUS												
1. France, Haut-Languedoc		Larrouy 1960	P	129	59	59	10	1	1·0223	0·0140	1·2937	0·5468
			C	4367	2015	1971	264	117				
2. Germany, Berlin	(s) S	Schröder 1955	P	120	48	47	17	8	0·8507	0·6147	0·9094	0·1121
		Pettenkofer *et al.* 1957 M1	C	12000	4437	5107	1728	728				
3. Italy, Milano		Mor & Sforza 1960	P	70	26	31	11	2	1·0800	0·0739	1·5826	1·3789
			C	500	202	223	54	21				
4. Italy, Milano		Visconti *et al.* 1961[a]	P	148	54	70	15	9	1·2461	1·4541	1·0697	0·0525
			C	9607(c)	3974	4134	1032	467				
5. Italy, Perugia		Benda & Gambelunghe 1962	P	196	76	94	20	6	1·2511	2·0538	1·0631	0·0577
		Benda & Menghini 1957	C	7356	3163	3127	783	283				
6. Norway		Hartmann & Stavem 1964	P	178	75	72	21	10	0·7518	2·9744	1·2611	0·8764
			C	31491	12120	15477	2691	1203				
7. Poland, Warszawa		Kosiński *et al.* 1959	P	27	8	12	6	1	1·4464	0·6498	1·4320	0·4392
			C	4270	1537	1594	805	334				
8. United Kingdom, Birmingham	Squamous	Aird *et al.* 1960	P	69	28	33	7	1	1·3306	1·2274	1·5176	0·9661
			C	9590	4559	4038	751	242				
9. United Kingdom, Bristol	Squamous	Aird *et al.* 1960	P	26	10	13	2	1	1·2368	0·2521	1·0500	0·0039
			C	1989	861	905	164	59				
10. United Kingdom, Bristol	Squamous	Beasley 1964	P	98	32	41	16	9	1·2190	0·6770	2·6250	9·2208
			C	1989	861	905	164	59				
11. United Kingdom, Leeds	Squamous	Aird *et al.* 1960	P	37	15	16	3	3	1·2253	0·3178	1·1518	0·0497
			C	6260	2966	2582	515	197				
12. United Kingdom, Liverpool	Squamous	Aird *et al.* 1960	P	145	68	64	10	3	1·2397	1·4942	0·8240	0·3222
			C	8202	4124	3131	736	211				
13. United Kingdom, London	Squamous	Aird *et al.* 1960	P	137	58	61	15	3	1·1412	0·5118	1·3303	0·9555
			C	10000	4578	4219	890	313				
14. United Kingdom, Leytonstone		Walther *et al.* 1956	P	20	8	10	1	1	1·3074	0·3167	0·8412	0·0264
			C	2325	1070	1023	159	73				
15. United Kingdom, Manchester	Squamous	Aird *et al.* 1960	P	51	27	20	3	1	0·8571	0·2704	0·5828	0·7821
			C	5431	2570	2221	490	150				
16. United Kingdom, Newcastle upon Tyne	Squamous	Aird *et al.* 1960	P	24	12	8	3	1	0·8577	0·1125	1·2700	0·1361
			C	4032	1971	1532	388	141				
17. United Kingdom, Sheffield	Squamous	Aird *et al.* 1960	P	21	7	10	4	0	1·5356	0·7540	3·2399	3·4853
			C	4002	1837	1709	324	132				
18. United Kingdom, Glasgow	Squamous	Aird *et al.* 1960	P	52	25	18	8	1	1·1868	0·3043	1·5112	1·0222
			C	5928	3150	1911	667	200				
19. United Kingdom, Glamorgan I	Squamous	Beasley 1964	P	76	35	32	6	3	1·1179	0·2031	0·7620	0·3721
			C	3514	1658	1356	373	127				
20. United Kingdom, Glamorgan II and Monmouth	Squamous	Beasley 1964	P	98	49	36	11	2	0·7511	1·6649	1·0957	0·0732
			C	4570	2011	1967	412	180				
21. United Kingdom, Cardiff	Squamous	Aird *et al.* 1960	P	48	24	17	5	2	0·7996	0·4729	0·9763	0·0023
			C	874	403	357	86	28				

TABLE 1 **THE ABO BLOOD GROUP SYSTEM** (*cont.*)

Place	Additional details	Authors		Number	O	A	B	AB	A/O		B/O	
									Relative incidence	χ_1^2 for difference from unity	Relative incidence	χ_1^2 for difference from unity
NEOPLASMS (*cont.*)												
MALIGNANT NEOPLASMS (*cont.*)												
MALIGNANT NEOPLASMS OF OESOPHAGUS (*cont.*)												
22. United Kingdom, Belfast		Macafee 1967[b]	P	61(c)	24	27	8	2	1·8742	5·0032	1·9387	2·6227
			C	28566	15715	9433	2702	716				
23. N. India, Kanpur		Tyagi *et al.* 1965	P	16	2	3	6	5	2·1893	0·7357	2·6141	1·3831
			C	6000	1985	1360	2278	377				
24. S. India, Bhopal	(s) S	Ghooi *et al.* 1970	P	55	24	6	19	6	0·5714	1·1315	1·5200	1·1301
			C	100	48	21	25	6				
25. Japan, Niigata		Hirose & Honma 1962	P	133	43	53	29	8	0·9878	0·0035	0·8570	0·4082
			C	12253	3624	4522	2852	1255				
26. Japan, Sendai		Moniwa 1960	P	157	42	53	45	17	1·0971	0·1998	1·5025	3·5732
			C	21199	6769	7786	4827	1817				
27. Republic of South Africa	Bantu	Buckwalter *et al.* 1961	P	112	41	33	32	6	1·2726	1·0470	1·6341	4·2600
			C	7105	3197	2022	1527	359				
28. Republic of South Africa	Coloured	Buckwalter *et al.* 1964	P	27(c)	11	9	7	0	0·7870	0·2638	0·9778	0·0020
			C	352(c)	126	131	82	13				
29. Republic of South Africa	Whites	Buckwalter *et al.* 1961	P	21	6	13	1	1	2·4495	3·2849	0·6446	0·1650
			C	6431	2893	2559	748	231				
30. U.S.A., Iowa		Buckwalter *et al.* 1964	P	232(c)	92	100	31	9	1·1511	0·9448	1·6071	5·1875
			C	49979	22392	21144	4695	1748				
31. Peru, Lima		Muñoz-Baratta 1962	P	75(c)	41	22	10	2	1·3626	1·3696	1·2758	0·4765
			C	107938	66058	26013	12629	3238				
				2705					1·0994	4·6547	1·2876	16·1100
				χ_{30}^2 for homogeneity of areas						25·7427		23·9797
MALIGNANT NEOPLASMS OF STOMACH												
CARDIA												
1. Germany, Berlin		Berndt 1966	P	166	64	70	23	9	0·9482	0·0914	0·8656	0·3412
			C	4752	1739	2006	722	285				
2. Finland, Helsinki and S. Saimaa	(s) S	Turunen & Pasila 1957	P	306	101	132	55	18	1·0214	0·0191	1·1417	0·4588
		Mäkelä *et al.* 1959 M2	C	891	304	389	145	53				
3. Italy, Genova		Cappellini & Guffanti 1956	P	26	10	14	0	2	1·3863	0·5995		
		Macaggi & Gibelli 1933 M1	C	726	304	307	91	24				
		Canepa 1950 M1										
4. Netherlands, Amsterdam		Wayjen 1960	P	118(c)	46	57	12	3	1·2714	1·4602	1·3039	0·6663
			C	23643	10491	10225	2099	828				
5. United Kingdom, London		Doll *et al.* 1960	P	133	49	65	15	4	1·4394	3·6599	1·5746	2·3315
			C	10000	4578	4219	890	313				
6. Japan, Niigata		Hirose & Honma 1962	P	346	126	135	56	29	0·8587	1·4659	0·5647	12·3567
			C	12253	3624	4522	2852	1255				
7. Japan, Tokyo	(s) S	Uetake *et al.* 1958	P	200	55	79	39	27	1·1844	0·9267	1·0013	0·0000
			C	77625	24165	29305	17113	7042				
				1295					1·0584	0·7386	0·9016	1·3331
				χ_6^2 for homogeneity of areas						7·4841		
				(1269) χ_5^2 for homogeneity of areas								14·8215
FUNDUS												
1. Italy, Milano		Visconti *et al.* 1961[b]	P	104	50	34	12	8	0·6540	3·6132	0·9244	0·0591
			C	9607	3975	4133	1032	467				

TABLE 1 **THE ABO BLOOD GROUP SYSTEM** *(cont.)*

Place	Additional details	Authors		Number	O	A	B	AB	A/O Relative incidence	A/O χ^2_1 for difference from unity	B/O Relative incidence	B/O χ^2_1 for difference from unity
ADITUS, FUNDUS												
1. Bulgaria, Sofia		Mazhdrakov & Grancharov 1960	P	52	19	22	9	2	0·8408	0·3055	0·9441	0·0201
		Zographov 1962	C	15422	4953	6821	2485	1163				
CORPUS												
1. Bulgaria, Sofia		Mazhdrakov & Grancharov 1960	P	78	20	40	12	6	1·4523	1·8478	1·1959	0·2389
		Zographov 1962	C	15422	4953	6821	2485	1163				
2. Germany, Berlin		Berndt 1966	P	225	66	115	33	11	1·5105	6·8261	1·2043	0·7288
			C	4752	1739	2006	722	285				
3. Italy, Genova		Cappellini & Guffanti 1956	P	110	62	37	11	0	0·5909	5·5674	0·5927	2·2553
		Macaggi & Gibelli 1933 M1; Canepa 1950 M1	C	726	304	307	91	24				
4. Italy, Milano		Visconti *et al.* 1961[b]	P	113	50	46	16	1	0·8848	0·3545	1·2326	0·5222
			C	9607	3975	4133	1032	467				
5. United Kingdom, London		Doll *et al.* 1960	P	280	119	132	23	6	1·2036	2·0902	0·9942	0·0006
			C	10000	4578	4219	890	313				
6. Japan, Niigata		Hirose & Honma 1962	P	1033	295	443	171	124	1·2035	5·5958	0·7366	9·4771
			C	12253	3624	4522	2852	1255				
7. Japan, Tokyo	(s) S	Uetake *et al.* 1958	P	440	133	176	91	40	1·0912	0·5738	0·9662	0·0637
			C	77625	24165	29305	17113	7042				
8. Chile, Santiago		Dooner & Aguayo 1960	P	21	16	5	0	0	0·6350	0·7822		
		Sandoval 1941 M1	C	4200	2483	1222	382	113				
				2300					1·1455	7·3818	0·8759	3·9121
					χ^2_7 for homogeneity of areas					16·2560		
				(2279)	χ^2_6 for homogeneity of areas							9·3746
CARDIA, CORPUS												
1. United Kingdom, Liverpool	(s) S	Haddock & McConnell 1956	P	220	85	109	19	7	1·6047	10·5315	1·1603	0·3391
		McConnell 1966	C	15377	7527	6015	1450	385				
ANTRUM												
1. Germany, Berlin		Berndt 1966	P	344	125	158	43	18	1·0958	0·5430	0·8286	1·0649
			C	4752	1739	2006	722	285				
2. Italy, Milano		Visconti *et al.* 1961[b]	P	436	174	202	38	22	1·1165	1·0858	0·8412	0·8986
			C	9607	3975	4133	1032	467				
3. United Kingdom, London		Doll *et al.* 1960	P	300	132	125	30	13	1·0275	0·0461	1·1691	0·5774
			C	10000	4578	4219	890	313				
				1080					1·0840	1·4107	0·9181	0·6119
					χ^2_2 for homogeneity of areas					0·2641		1·9290
PREPYLORIC												
1. Netherlands, Amsterdam		Wayjen 1960	P	90	33	47	7	3	1·4613	2·7792	1·0602	0·0197
			C	23643	10491	10225	2099	828				

TABLE 1 **THE ABO BLOOD GROUP SYSTEM** (*cont.*)

Place	Additional details	Authors		Number	O	A	B	AB	A/O Relative incidence	A/O χ_1^2 for difference from unity	B/O Relative incidence	B/O χ_1^2 for difference from unity
NEOPLASMS (*cont.*)												
MALIGNANT NEOPLASMS (*cont.*)												
MALIGNANT NEOPLASMS OF STOMACH (*cont.*)												
PYLORUS												
1. Bulgaria, Sofia		Mazhdrakov & Grancharov 1960	P	122	35	65	15	7	1·3485	2·0182	0·8542	0·2591
		Zographov 1962	C	15422	4953	6821	2485	1163				
2. Finland, Helsinki and S. Saimaa	(s) S	Turunen & Pasila 1957	P	599	167	282	94	56	1·3196	4·9973	1·1801	1·0227
		Mäkelä *et al.* 1959 M2	C	891	304	389	145	53				
3. Japan, Niigata		Hirose & Honma 1962	P	2130	635	909	411	175	1·1472	5·9469	0·8224	8·2448
			C	12253	3624	4522	2852	1255				
				2851					1·1841	11·5021	0·8669	5·3785
				χ_2^2 for homogeneity of areas						1·4603		4·1481
ANTRUM, PYLORUS												
1. Italy, Genova		Cappellini & Guffanti 1956	P	144	58	76	6	4	1·2975	1·8363	0·3456	5·6963
		Macaggi & Gibelli 1933 M1; Canepa 1950 M1	C	726	304	307	91	24				
2. United Kingdom, Liverpool	(s) S	Haddock & McConnell 1956	P	223	118	87	17	1	0·9226	0·3200	0·7479	1·2392
		McConnell 1966	C	15377	7527	6015	1450	385				
3. Japan, Tokyo	(s) S	Uetake *et al.* 1958	P	1367	379	573	269	146	1·2467	10·9030	1·0022	1·0008
			C	77625	24165	29305	17113	7042				
				1734					1·1909	9·1756	0·9483	0·4930
				χ_2^2 for homogeneity of areas						3·8837		6·4432
CARDIA, ANTRUM, PYLORUS												
1. Chile, Santiago		Dooner & Aguayo 1960	P	49	31	15	3	0	0·9832	0·0029	0·6290	0·5830
		Sandoval 1941 M1	C	4200	2483	1222	382	113				
PARTS SPECIFIED BY EXCLUSION												
1. Netherlands, Amsterdam	Other than cardia and prepyloric	Wayjen 1960	P	293	109	157	16	11	1·4778	9·6940	0·7337	1·3276
			C	23543	10491	10225	2099	828				
2. United Kingdom, London	Whole body or site uncertain	Doll *et al.* 1960	P	144	62	70	7	5	1·2251	1·3352	0·5808	1·8419
			C	10000	4578	4219	890	313				
3. Japan, Tokyo	Other than cardia, corpus, antrum, and pylorus, (s) S	Uetake *et al.* 1958	P	72	21	30	16	5	1·1780	0·3312	1·0759	0·0485
			C	77625	24165	29305	17113	7042				
PART UNSPECIFIED												
1. Austria, Wien	(s) S, Rh_D	Speiser 1956	P	1146	415	505	143	83	0·9992	0·0001	0·9316	0·4814
			C	10000	3631	4422	1343	604				
2. Austria, Wien	(s) A_1A_2	Weiser 1957	P	635(c)	216	308	76	35	1·1709	2·9698	0·9513	0·1326
			C	10000	3631	4422	1343	604				
3. Bulgaria		Zographov 1962	P	141	38	78	19	6	1·4905	4·0342	0·9966	0·0001
			C	15422	4953	6821	2485	1163				
4. Czechoslovakia		Vahala *et al.* 1970	P	122	35	64	15	8	1·2687	1·1573	0·8033	0·4646
		Kout 1959 M2	C	1142	358	516	191	77				
5. Denmark, København	(s) C	Køster *et al.* 1955	P	413	141	212	44	16	1·3854	8·7561	1·1632	0·7463
			C	14304	5804	6299	1557	644				

TABLE 1 **THE ABO BLOOD GROUP SYSTEM** (*cont.*)

Place	Additional details	Authors		Number	O	A	B	AB	A/O		B/O	
									Relative incidence	χ_1^2 for difference from unity	Relative incidence	χ_1^2 for difference from unity
6. Denmark,		Jordal 1956	P	385	148	195	31	11	1·2140	3·0791	0·7808	1·5372
København			C	14304	5804	6299	1557	644				
7. Denmark,	(s) S, A	Mosbech 1958	P	1764	673	854	172	65	1·1692	8·1806	0·9527	0·2895
København			C	14304	5804	6299	1557	644				
8. Denmark,		Blegvad 1960[b]	P	61	23	27	6	5	1·0817	0·0762	0·9724	0·0037
København		Andersen 1955 M1	C	14304	5804	6299	1557	644				
9. Finland,	(s) S	Turunen & Pasila 1957	P	85	25	38	16	6	1·1879	0·4106	1·3418	0·7671
Helsinki and S. Saimaa		Mäkelä *et al.* 1959 M2	C	891	304	389	145	53				
10. France, Colmar		Lobstein & Voegtlin 1959	P	110	40	57	9	4	1·1869	0·6765	0·9559	0·0147
			C	5570	2188	2627	515	240				
11. France, Haut-		Larrouy 1960	P	182	73	85	16	8	1·1904	1·1475	1·6729	3·2897
Languedoc			C	4367	2015	1971	264	117				
12. France,		Lobstein & Voegtlin 1959	P	239	88	120	22	9	1·1925	1·5191	1·2658	0·9398
Mulhouse			C	6423	2648	3028	523	224				
13. France, Paris		Khérumian & Moullec	P	1457	590	700	111	56	1·1882	9·4568	0·9709	0·0811
		1959	C	207588	91414	91276	17714	7184				
14. Germany, Berlin		Hirschfeld & Hittmair	P	18	8	8	1	1	0·9561	0·0079	0·2876	1·3662
		1926	C	750	283	296	123	48				
15. Germany,	(s) S	Schröder 1955	P	293	92	138	44	19	1·3032	3·7835	1·2280	1·2266
Berlin		Pettenkofer 1957 M1	C	12000	4437	5107	1728	728				
16. Germany, Berlin		Berndt 1966	P	160	50	67	34	9	1·1616	0·6237	1·6378	4·7384
			C	4752	1739	2006	722	285				
17. Germany, Berlin		Berndt & Pietschker 1966	P	895(c)	305	410	133	47	1·2014	5·5609	1·0949	0·7201
		Schmauss *et al.* 1968	C	15154	5642	6313	2247	952				
18. Germany, Berlin		Scholz 1963	P	500	154	233	76	37	1·5650	16·6968	1·7783	14·7723
			C	3960	1654	1599	459	248				
19. Germany, Bonn		Schreiber *et al.* 1959	P	311	104	165	29	13	1·4543	6·2689	1·0095	0·0015
			C	706	286	312	79	29				
20. Germany,		Seifert 1964	P	1000	375	416	159	50	0·9647	0·2503	0·9960	0·0017
Dresden			C	50000	18370	21125	7820	2685				
21. Germany,		Berg *et al.* 1967	P	46	18	19	5	4	0·6830	1·0917	0·7971	0·1637
Erlangen, Nürnberg			C	193	66	102	23	2				
22. Germany,		Ludwig 1964	P	650	214	305	86	45	1·1530	2·4320	1·1339	0·9233
Greifswald			C	13100	4760	5884	1687	769				
23. Germany, Jena		Seyffert 1963	P	716	247	341	91	37	1·1502	2·7766	0·9909	0·0055
			C	73548	26981	32386	10032	4149				
24. Germany,		Gedicke & Wellhöner	P	514	193	234	58	29	1·0831	0·5781	0·7810	2·4040
Leipzig		1961	C	3174	1198	1341	461	174				
25. Germany,		Breitfeld 1963	P	1279	420	600	183	76	1·2956	13·3076	1·2637	5·5461
Leipzig			C	5000	1920	2117	662	301				
26. Germany,		Borschell 1961	P	200	69	97	24	10	1·1669	0·7444	0·8662	0·2954
Marburg			C	696	254	306	102	34				
27. Germany,		Völter *et al.* 1970	P	722	282	339	70	31	1·1690	3·6832	0·9404	0·2083
Tübingen		Dick *et al.* 1962	C	39031	16283	16745	4298	1705				
28. Hungary		Szabolcs 1960	P	749	196	371	117	65	1·4863	19·5476	1·1222	0·9481
			C	23000	7567	9637	4025	1771				
29. Hungary		István & Széll 1961	P	569	148	288	77	56	1·5280	17·1737	0·9781	0·0243
			C	23000	7567	9637	4025	1771				
30. Hungary,		Weitzner 1925	P	11	4	3	2	2	0·6184	0·3927	1·1369	0·0217
Budapest			C	1000	357	433	157	53				
31. Hungary,		Bárdosi *et al.* 1965	P	233(c)	62	114	35	22	1·2141	1·2446	0·9919	0·0012
Budapest		Backhausz *et al.* 1950 M1	C	1041	311	471	177	82				
32. Hungary,		Bajusz & Hoffman 1965	P	372	93	182	62	35	1·4501	7·8307	1·1968	1·1081
Szeged			C	3972(c)	1253	1691	698	330				

TABLE 1 THE ABO BLOOD GROUP SYSTEM (*cont.*)

NEOPLASMS (*cont.*)
MALIGNANT NEOPLASMS (*cont.*)
MALIGNANT NEOPLASMS OF STOMACH (*cont.*)
Part Unspecified (*cont.*)

Place	Additional details	Authors		Number	O	A	B	AB	A/O Relative incidence	A/O χ_1^2 for difference from unity	B/O Relative incidence	B/O χ_1^2 for difference from unity
33. Iceland		Bjarnason *et al.* 1973	P	323	169	113	32	9	1·1723	1·6893	0·9794	0·0115
			C	26716	14783	8432	2858	643				
34. Italy		Balestra & Mattioli 1958	P	810	316	421	49	24	1·3855	13·0419	0·5581	11·5464
		Tranquilli-Leali 1934 M1	C	1830	781	751	217	81				
35. Italy		Lang 1959	P	832	390	320	85	37	1·0460	0·3485	0·9267	0·3974
			C	42735	20426	16023	4804	1482				
36. Italy, Aquila		Curtoni & Morgante 1964	P	170(c)	74	72	18	6	1·2214	1·4329	1·2053	0·4951
			C	8920(c)	4321	3442	872	285				
37. Italy, Campania		Pollara & Melina 1957	P	300	117	142	33	8	1·4408	6·5018	0·8757	0·3661
			C	1000	444	374	143	39				
38. Italy, Emilia		Spada & Sarra 1958	P	667	281	315	51	20	1·3839	12·8402	1·1157	0·4295
			C	3034	1500	1215	244	75				
39. Italy, Forli		Maltoni & Canali 1956	P	265	92	136	26	11	1·7251	13·7463	1·4978	2·7555
			C	1350	636	545	120	49				
40. Italy, Genova		Cappellini & Guffanti	P	449	187	202	46	14	1·0697	0·2692	0·8218	0·9315
		1956	C	726	304	307	91	24				
		Macaggi & Gibelli 1933 M1										
		Canepa 1950 M1										
41. Italy, Genova		Spandonari &	P	89	31	47	4	7	1·5976	4·0397	0·5188	1·5156
		Carboneschi 1957	C	5893	2569	2438	639	247				
		Calzia 1967 M2										
42. Italy, Lombardia		Ninni & Bedarida 1959	P	897	347	458	72	20	1·2964	5·5023	1·0226	0·0131
			C	640	276	281	56	27				
43. Italy, Milano	(s) S	Beolchini *et al.* 1958[b]	P	678	262	327	63	26	1·2799	6·8518	1·0294	0·0336
			C	2346	1006	981	235	124				
44. Italy, Milano		Mangani 1957	P	75	22	44	8	1	1·9226	6·2219	1·4003	0·6603
		Visconti *et al.* 1961	C	9607	3974	4134	1032	467				
45. Italy, Milano		Rotelli & Corippo 1959	P	314	120	146	38	10	1·0052	0·0017	1·1733	0·7059
			C	8000	3090	3740	834	336				
46. Italy, Milano		Camerini Riviera 1960	P	271	88	143	30	10	1·6664	12·8025	1·4594	2·8609
			C	2346	1006	981	235	124				
47. Italy, Milano		Mor & Sforza 1960	P	470	174	226	52	18	1·1765	1·3481	1·1179	0·2565
			C	500	202	223	54	21				
48. Italy, Milano	(s) S	Visconti *et al.* 1961[b]	P	680	270	304	88	18	1·0823	0·8375	1·2551	3·1694
			C	9607	3974	4134	1032	467				
49. Italy, Napoli		Martella 1938	P	32	11	11	9	1	1·2275	0·2260	2·7525	4·8812
		Sanguigno & Aghina 1954 M1	C	1200	545	444	162	49				
50. Italy, Napoli	Males	Cocchia *et al.* 1963	P	188	78	86	14	10	1·3497	2·2419	0·9103	0·0696
			C	300	142	116	28	14				
51. Italy, Napoli		Spena & Grippo 1964	P	156	50	89	9	8	2·0542	15·5089	0·8397	0·2230
			C	2147	989	857	212	89				
52. Italy, Palermo		Carlo & Ridulfo 1958	P	187	63	97	22	5	2·1094	17·7020	0·9657	0·0175
			C	980(c)	448	327	162	43				
53. Italy, Pavia		Prosser 1957	P	303	106	165	26	6	1·2861	3·9351	0·9088	0·1851
			C	8000	3090	3740	834	336				
54. Italy, Perugia		Benda & Menghini 1957	P	442	188	194	50	10	1·0438	0·1654	1·0744	0·1912
			C	7356	3163	3127	783	283				
55. Italy, Perugia		Benda & Gambelunghe	P	1012	400	482	96	34	1·2189	7·5182	0·9695	0·0661
		1962	C	7356	3163	3127	783	283				
		Benda & Menghini 1957										
56. Italy, Siena	(s) S	Prior & Vegni 1957	P	143	68	62	10	3	1·0485	0·0632	0·5204	3·4254
			C	1025	460	400	130	35				

TABLE 1 **THE ABO BLOOD GROUP SYSTEM** (*cont.*)

Place	Additional details	Authors		Number	O	A	B	AB	A/O Relative incidence	A/O χ_1^2 for difference from unity	B/O Relative incidence	B/O χ_1^2 for difference from unity
57. Italy, Torino		Cavalli *et al.* 1964	P	507	191	240	56	20	1·3665	8·5701	1·3119	2·6066
			C	2360	1056	971	236	97				
58. Italy, Verona	(s) S	Bonzanini 1961	P	110	51	47	9	3	0·9651	0·0302	0·8596	0·1719
			C	5500	2460	2349	505	186				
59. Norway		Hartmann & Stavem 1964	P	546	215	276	39	16	1·0680	0·5147	0·8780	0·5509
			C	31491	12613	15160	2606	1112				
60. Poland, Katowice		Machalski *et al.* 1968	P	190	48	94	33	15	1·6311	7·2574	1·3103	1·3649
			C	3606(c)	1216	1460	638	292				
61. Poland, Kraków		Socha 1960	P	2148	545	1001	421	181	1·5016	55·3880	1·2257	9·3636
			C	37766	12151	14863	7658	3094				
62. Poland, Kraków		Oszacki *et al.* 1965	P	404	110	171	92	31	1·1970	2·0174	1·3122	3·4276
		Socha 1966 M2	C	5201	1627	2113	1037	424				
63. Poland, Lower Silesia		Sagan *et al.* 1957	P	71	21	35	6	9	1·4430	1·7137	0·4932	2·2960
			C	2397(c)	813	939	471	174				
64. Poland, Lublin		Spruch & Dacka 1968	P	319	94	134	60	31	1·2839	2·7321	1·1846	0·8324
			C	1150	399	443	215	93				
65. Poland, Poznań		Wojtowicz *et al.* 1960	P	473	143	203	81	46	1·3376	6·7039	1·0253	0·0306
			C	7951	2773	2943	1532	703				
66. Poland, Poznań		Woszczyk 1966	P	528	185	215	67	61	1·0950	0·7662	0·6555	8·3556
			C	7951	2773	2943	1532	703				
67. Poland, Warszawa		Kosiński *et al.* 1959	P	155	42	83	19	11	1·9055	11·1944	0·8637	0·2739
			C	4270	1537	1594	805	334				
68. Poland, Warszawa		Czaplicki *et al.* 1964	P	83	22	40	19	2	1·7532	4·3940	1·6490	2·5019
			C	4270	1537	1594	805	334				
69. Romania, Sibiu		Coroianu *et al.* 1958	P	43	11	28	2	2	2·3554	5·7350	0·3739	1·6322
			C	3850(c)	1425	1540	693	192				
70. Spain, Barcelona		Vilardell & Jori-Solé 1961	P	166	78	77	9	2	0·8506	1·0087	0·5924	2·2040
		Picazo Guillén 1958 M2	C	31864	13112	15217	2554	981				
71. Sweden		Eklund 1965	P	352	130	170	33	19	1·0731	0·3654	0·9519	0·0638
			C	131659(c)	50702	61788	13521	5648				
72. Sweden, Göteborg	(s) S	Lewin 1960	P	497	166	245	67	19	1·3933	9·9020	1·7787	13·9697
			C	4645	1939	2054	440	212				
73. Sweden, Göteborg		Beckman & Eklund 1961	P	800(c)	266	418	84	32	1·3881	15·1886	1·3518	4·9735
			C	5038	2029	2297	474	238				
74. Sweden, Malmö		Beckman & Eklund 1961	P	800(c)	322	348	87	43	0·9044	0·9100	1·0777	0·1967
			C	922	359	429	90	44				
75. Sweden, Stockholm		Beckman & Eklund 1961	P	1000(c)	351	506	97	46	1·0505	0·4090	0·9540	0·1383
			C	4357	1550	2127	449	231				
76. Switzerland, Basel		Holländer *et al.* 1953	P	704(c)	255	374	53	22	1·3557	12·1586	0·9587	0·0689
			C	4518(c)	1882	2036	408	192				
77. Switzerland, Basel		Moor-Jankowski *et al.* 1961	P	445	166	237	28	14	1·3181	6·0900	0·6202	4·8257
			C	2076	842	912	229	93				
78. United Kingdom, Birmingham		Aird *et al.* 1953	P	100	37	57	3	3	1·7506	3·5919	1·3514	0·1270
			C	100	50	44	3	3				
79. United Kingdom, Leeds		Aird *et al.* 1953	P	217	92	104	16	5	1·3253	1·8988	1·1826	0·1877
			C	217	102	87	15	13				
80. United Kingdom, Liverpool		Aird *et al.* 1953	P	217	85	97	27	8	1·4331	3·0141	2·0180	4·2174
			C	217	108	86	17	6				
81. United Kingdom, Liverpool	(s) S	McConnell 1966	P	288	119	129	28	12	1·3565	5·6509	1·2214	0·8902
			C	15377	7527	6015	1450	385				
82. United Kingdom, London		Aird *et al.* 1953	P	1340	578	617	106	39	1·1601	3·2657	0·9462	0·1441
			C	1340	614	565	119	42				
83. United Kingdom, London, Leytonstone	(s) A_1A_2	Walther *et al.* 1956	P	97	32	55	4	6	1·7977	6·6999	0·8412	0·1037
			C	2325	1070	1023	159	73				

TABLE 1 **THE ABO BLOOD GROUP SYSTEM** (*cont.*)

Place	Additional details	Authors		Number	O	A	B	AB	A/O Relative incidence	A/O χ_1^2 for difference from unity	B/O Relative incidence	B/O χ_1^2 for difference from unity
NEOPLASMS (*cont.*)												
MALIGNANT NEOPLASMS (*cont.*)												
MALIGNANT NEOPLASMS OF STOMACH (*cont.*)												
PART UNSPECIFIED (*cont.*)												
84. United Kingdom, Manchester		Aird *et al.* 1953	P	771	343	349	49	30	1·3865	9·1618	1·0442	0·0424
			C	771	402	295	55	19				
85. United Kingdom, Newcastle upon Tyne		Aird *et al.* 1953	P	101	44	44	12	1	1·4324	1·4138	1·8068	1·4002
			C	101	53	37	8	3				
86. United Kingdom, Scotland		Aird *et al.* 1953	P	478	245	174	46	13	1·1547	1·0212	0·8449	0·5962
			C	478	252	155	56	15				
87. United Kingdom, Glasgow		Wallace 1954	P	299	159	104	30	6	1·0142	0·0119	0·8898	0·3315
			C	7418	3853	2485	817	263				
88. United Kingdom, Glamorgan I		Beasley 1960[a]	P	345	152	157	29	7	1·2629	3·8137	0·8481	0·6124
			C	3514	1658	1356	373	127				
89. United Kingdom, Glamorgan II and Monmouth		Beasley 1960[a]	P	401	159	193	36	13	1·2410	3·7364	1·1051	0·2702
			C	4570	2011	1967	412	180				
90. United Kingdom, Newport (Mon.)		Beasley 1960[b]	P	518	228	236	38	16	1·0481	0·1620	0·8956	0·2616
			C	907	403	398	75	31				
91. United Kingdom, Belfast		Macafee 1967[b]	P	481(c)	228	189	56	8	1·3810	10·5825	1·4285	5·6086
			C	28566	15715	9433	2702	716				
92. U.S.S.R., Moscow	(s) S	Chudina 1963	P	930	310	359	186	75	1·0993	1·3244	0·9954	0·0022
			C	7500	2598	2737	1566	599				
93. Israel	Ashkenazi Jews	Birnbaum & Menczel 1959	P	112(c)	43	37	24	8	0·7987	0·9086	1·4856	2·0882
			C	946(c)	362	390	136	58				
94. S. India, Bhopal	(s) S	Ghooi *et al.* 1970	P	91	18	27	42	4	3·4286	9·4270	4·4800	16·0405
			C	100	48	21	25	6				
95. N. Vietnam		Nguyen Duong Quang *et al.* 1962	P	379	154	75	116	34	1·1111	0·5313	1·1873	1·8480
			C	6750	3080	1350	1954	366				
96. Malaya, Singapore	Chinese	Yeoh 1960	P	200(c)	63	70	54	13	1·9303	11·9030	1·4329	3·2006
			C	1000(c)	443	255	265	37				
97. Philippines, Santo Tomas		Tan 1962	P	100	30	39	25	6	2·4218	10·9621	1·4922	1·8759
			C	500	231	124	129	16				
98. Japan		Inada 1934	P	198	64	82	42	10	1·0565	0·1085	0·9214	0·1698
			C	91440	28290	34307	20150	8693				
99. Japan	(s) ABH secretion	Desai & Creger 1964[a]	P	210	62	74	47	27	0·9625	0·0222	0·8423	0·3699
			C	171	50	62	45	14				
100. Japan, Niigata	Diffuse form	Hirose & Honma 1962	P	138	18	76	38	6	3·3838	21·4697	2·6826	11·8045
			C	12253	3624	4522	2852	1255				
101. Japan, Niigata		Hirose & Honma 1962	P	1139	301	328	378	132	0·8733	2·6722	1·5957	33·1206
			C	12253	3624	4522	2852	1255				
102. Japan, Sendai		Segi *et al.* 1957[b]	P	1385	412	571	296	106	1·1010	2·1568	1·0051	0·0044
			C	530046	161461	203255	115416	49914				
103. Japan, Sendai		Moniwa 1960	P	1671	499	670	358	144	1·1673	6·3433	1·0061	0·0071
			C	21199	6769	7786	4827	1817				
104. Egypt, Alexandria		Sadek *et al.* 1965[a]	P	31	8	16	5	2	1·7290	1·5851	0·7351	0·2898
			C	3720	1142	1321	971	286				
105. Republic of South Africa	Bantu	Buckwalter *et al.* 1961	P	96	36	40	16	4	1·7568	5·9255	0·9305	0·0568
			C	7105	3197	2022	1527	359				
106. Republic of South Africa	Coloured	Buckwalter *et al.* 1964	P	56(c)	19	24	10	3	1·2149	0·3450	0·8087	0·2609
			C	352(c)	126	131	82	13				
107. Republic of South Africa	Indians	Buckwalter *et al.* 1961	P	18	6	7	5	0	1·8900	1·3052	0·9331	0·0131
			C	7462	2788	1721	2490	463				
108. Republic of South Africa	Whites	Buckwalter *et al.* 1961	P	156	66	66	21	3	1·1305	0·4849	1·2306	0·6681
			C	6431	2893	2559	748	231				

TABLE 1 THE ABO BLOOD GROUP SYSTEM (*cont.*)

Place	Additional details	Authors		Number	O	A	B	AB	A/O Relative incidence	A/O χ_1^2 for difference from unity	B/O Relative incidence	B/O χ_1^2 for difference from unity
109. U.S.A., Boston		Hoskins *et al.* 1965	P	207(c)	100	72	22	13	0·9014	0·4311	0·9192	0·1223
			C	4222(c)	1993	1592	477	160				
110. U.S.A., Boston		Hoskins *et al.* 1965	P	130(c)	64	44	18	4	0·9988	0·0000	1·1452	0·2515
			C	5236(c)	2602	1791	639	204				
111. U.S.A.,		Desai & Creger 1964[a]	P	97	44	33	13	7	0·6696	1·7693	1·0552	0·0151
California			C	123	50	56	14	3				
112. U.S.A.,		Eisenberg *et al.* 1958	P	241	93	107	32	9	1·2473	2·4217	1·2878	1·5176
Connecticut			C	75904	33174	30601	8864	3265				
113. U.S.A.,		Eisenberg *et al.* 1958	P	195	87	78	24	6	0·9719	0·0332	1·0324	0·0191
Connecticut			C	75904	33174	30601	8864	3265				
114. U.S.A.,		Eisenberg *et al.* 1958	P	200	69	98	27	6	1·5397	7·5233	1·4645	2·8166
Connecticut			C	75904	33174	30601	8864	3265				
115. U.S.A.,		Eisenberg *et al.* 1958	P	256	95	118	28	15	1·3465	4·6439	1·1031	0·2075
Connecticut			C	75904	33174	30601	8864	3265				
116. U.S.A.,		Glass *et al.* 1962	P	25	11	13	0	1	1·3118	0·4361		
Iowa City and New York		Osborne & De George 1963	C	4738	2029	1828	636	245				
117. U.S.A., Iowa	(s) $A_1 A_2$, ABH secretion, S	Newman *et al.* 1961	P	118	43	61	10	4	1·5599	4·5574	0·9092	0·0686
			C	1261	563	512	144	42				
118. U.S.A., Iowa		Buckwalter *et al.* 1964	P	1158(c)	498	518	109	33	1·1016	2·3211	1·0439	0·1613
			C	49979	22392	21144	4695	1748				
119. U.S.A., Iowa	Negroes	Buckwalter *et al.* 1958	P	90(c)	40	31	17	2	1·4364	2·2566	1·0384	0·0168
			C	6722(c)	3301	1781	1351	289				
120. U.S.A.,		Hogg & Pack 1957	P	237	81	103	33	20	1·3894	4·8218	1·3279	1·8519
New York City			C	12917(c)	5531	5062	1697	627				
121. Mexico		Lisker *et al.* 1964	P	203	107	74	21	1	1·3399	3·6287	1·3047	1·2020
			C	6843	4022	2076	605	140				
122. Argentina		Estevez 1963	P	132	55	68	6	3	1·6994	8·4946	0·6634	0·9080
			C	21715	11165	8123	1836	591				
123. Argentina,		Canonico & Stagnara 1955	P	100	40	45	12	3	1·3774	2·1637	1·3973	1·0291
Buenos Aires			C	29250	13889	11344	2982	1035				
124. Argentina,		Muller 1955	P	81	29	42	9	1	1·7732	5·6128	1·4455	0·9297
Buenos Aires			C	29250	13889	11344	2982	1035				
125. Brazil,		Leite & Goffi 1958	P	98	34	54	5	5	1·9610	8·9803	0·6937	0·5666
São Paulo			C	1818	868	703	184	63				
126. Brazil,		Ribeiro 1963	P	100	35	53	8	4	1·6890	5·6666	0·8436	0·1855
São Paulo			C	4567	2030	1820	550	167				
127. Chile,		Jackson *et al.* 1959	P	168	96	53	15	4	0·9903	0·0030	1·0238	0·0067
Valparaiso			C	2500	1435	800	219	46				
128. Peru, Lima		Muñoz-Baratta 1962	P	307(c)	194	74	28	11	0·9686	0·0542	0·7549	1·9292
			C	107938(c)	66058	26013	12629	3238				
129. New Zealand,		Cotter *et al.* 1961	P	377	148	188	32	9	1·4704	11·9437	1·1417	0·4495
Auckland			C	12428	5856	5059	1109	404				
				53155					1·2228	369·4846	1·0780	23·6766
					χ_{28}^2 for homogeneity of areas					273·1223		
				(53130)	χ_{27}^2 for homogeneity of areas							215·4786

MALIGNANT NEOPLASMS OF SMALL INTESTINE

Place	Additional details	Authors		Number	O	A	B	AB	A/O Relative incidence	A/O χ_1^2 for difference from unity	B/O Relative incidence	B/O χ_1^2 for difference from unity
1. Peru, Lima		Muñoz-Baratta 1962	P	62(c)	29	14	10	9	1·2259	0·3916	1·8037	2·5851
			C	107938(c)	66058	26013	12629	3238				

TABLE 1 **THE ABO BLOOD GROUP SYSTEM** (*cont.*)

Place	Additional details	Authors		Number	O	A	B	AB	A/O Relative incidence	A/O χ^2_1 for difference from unity	B/O Relative incidence	B/O χ^2_1 for difference from unity
NEOPLASMS (*cont.*)												
MALIGNANT NEOPLASMS (*cont.*)												
MALIGNANT NEOPLASMS OF COLON												
1. Austria, Wien	(s) Rh_D, S	Speiser 1958[a]	P	204	67	99	25	13	1·2611	1·7896	1·0534	0·0414
			C	1000	367	430	130	73				
2. Denmark, København		Jordal 1956	P	284	128	110	33	13	0·7918	3·1607	0·9610	0·0406
			C	14304	5804	6299	1557	644				
3. France, Haut-Languedoc		Larrouy 1960	P	264	98	137	23	6	1·4292	6·8901	1·7913	5·8626
			C	4367	2015	1971	264	117				
4. Italy, Milano		Rotelli & Corippo 1959	P	118	52	54	10	2	0·8580	0·6119	0·7125	0·9515
			C	8000	3090	3740	834	336				
5. Italy, Napoli		Martella 1938	P	12	4	3	4	1	0·9206	0·0116	3·3642	2·8973
		Sanguigno & Aghina 1954 M1	C	1200	545	444	162	49				
6. Poland, Warszawa		Czaplicki *et al.* 1964	P	37	15	15	5	2	0·9642	0·0099	0·6364	0·7603
			C	4270	1537	1594	805	334				
7. Switzerland, Basel	(s) S	Moor-Jankowski *et al.* 1961	P	203	79	89	22	13	1·0401	0·0591	1·0239	0·0088
			C	2076	842	912	229	93				
8. United Kingdom, Belfast		Macafee 1967[b]	P	366(c)	169	150	35	12	1·4787	11·9959	1·2045	0·9914
			C	28566	15715	9433	2702	716				
9. Israel	Ashkenazi Jews	Birnbaum & Menczel 1959	P	96(c)	35	38	16	7	1·0078	0·0010	1·2168	0·3805
			C	946(c)	362	390	136	58				
10. S. India, Bhopal		Ghooi *et al.* 1970	P	31	12	6	12	1	1·1429	0·0560	1·9200	1·8705
			C	100	48	21	25	6				
11. Peru, Lima		Muñoz-Baratta 1962	P	38	20	13	2	3	1·6506	1·9780	0·5231	0·7634
			C	107938	66058	26013	12629	3238				
				1653					1·1512	6·4386	1·1372	2·1938
				χ^2_{10} for homogeneity of areas						20·1251		12·3745
MALIGNANT NEOPLASMS OF RECTUM												
1. Austria, Wien	(s) Rh_D, S	Speiser 1958[a]	P	891	302	389	132	68	1·0994	0·8208	1·2339	2·0740
			C	1000	367	430	130	73				
2. Denmark, København		Jordal 1956	P	715	278	349	59	29	1·1567	3·1208	0·7911	2·5699
			C	14304	5804	6299	1557	644				
3. Germany, Berlin	(s) S	Schröder 1955	P	243	101	91	36	15	0·7828	2·8142	0·9152	0·2039
		Pettenkofer 1957 M1	C	12000	4437	5107	1728	728				
4. Italy, Milano		Mangani 1957	P	15	5	9	1	0	1·7303	0·9648	0·7702	0·0568
		Visconti *et al.* 1961	C	9607	3974	4134	1032	467				
5. Switzerland, Basel	(s) S	Moor-Jankowski *et al.* 1961	P	252	101	124	20	7	1·1335	0·7753	0·7281	1·5384
			C	2076	842	912	229	93				
6. United Kingdom, Belfast		Macafee 1967[b]	P	254(c)	147	82	20	5	0·9293	0·2807	0·7913	0·9573
			C	28566	15715	9433	2702	716				
7. S. India, Bhopal		Ghooi *et al.* 1970	P	54	28	10	16	0	0·8163	0·2017	1·0971	0·0540
			C	100	48	21	25	6				
8. Japan, Sendai		Moniwa 1960	P	224	62	88	56	18	1·2340	1·5916	1·2666	1·6266
			C	21199	6769	7786	4827	1817				
9. Peru, Lima		Muñoz-Baratta 1962	P	37(c)	23	8	5	1	0·8833	0·0914	1·1371	0·0678
			C	107938	66058	26013	12629	3238				
				2685					1·0675	1·8667	0·9766	0·1081
				χ^2_8 for homogeneity of areas						8·7948		9·0406

TABLE 1 THE ABO BLOOD GROUP SYSTEM (*cont.*)

Place	Additional details	Authors		Number	O	A	B	AB	A/O Relative incidence	A/O χ_1^2 for difference from unity	B/O Relative incidence	B/O χ_1^2 for difference from unity
MALIGNANT NEOPLASMS OF COLON, RECTUM												
1. Germany,		Brockmüller 1962	P	425	180	197	30	18	1·0642	0·3606	0·6314	5·3953
Tübingen			C	39031	16283	16745	4298	1705				
2. Italy, Milano		Mor & Sforza 1960	P	168	71	65	24	8	0·8293	0·9007	1·2645	0·6951
			C	500	202	223	54	21				
3. Italy, Milano		Visconti *et al.* 1961[a]	P	489	196	220	44	29	1·0790	0·5702	0·8645	0·7303
			C	9607(c)	3974	4134	1032	467				
4. Italy, Napoli		Spena & Grippo 1964	P	102	44	46	9	3	1·2065	0·7554	0·9542	0·0157
			C	2147	989	857	212	89				
5. Italy, Verona	(s) S	Bonzanini 1961	P	70	25	37	6	2	1·5499	2·8298	1·1691	0·1168
			C	5500	2460	2349	505	186				
6. United	(s) S	Aird *et al.* 1954	P	520	237	227	40	16	0·9925	0·0044	0·8223	0·9101
Kingdom, Birmingham			C	1033	458	442	94	39				
7. United	(s) S	Aird *et al.* 1954	P	1514	665	676	128	45	1·1030	2·7971	0·9901	0·0093
Kingdom, London			C	10000	4578	4219	890	313				
8. United	(s) S	Aird *et al.* 1954	P	359	163	152	37	7	1·1195	0·9656	1·3055	2·0510
Kingdom, Manchester			C	9370	4532	3775	788	275				
9. United	(s) S	Aird *et al.* 1954	P	206	99	79	20	8	1·0008	0·0000	1·0090	0·0013
Kingdom, Newcastle upon Tyne			C	13572	6598	5261	1321	392				
10. Japan, Niigata		Hirose & Honma 1962	P	1216	344	497	253	122	1·1579	3·9666	0·9345	0·6121
			C	12253	3624	4522	2852	1255				
11. U.S.A., Iowa		Buckwalter *et al.* 1958	P	256(c)	119	103	24	10	0·9532	0·1218	1·0269	0·0135
			C	6313(c)	2892	2626	568	227				
				5325					1·0852	6·5481	0·9521	0·9656
				χ_{10}^2 for homogeneity of areas						6·7240		9·5849
MALIGNANT NEOPLASMS OF LARGE INTESTINE												
1. Czechoslovakia		Vahala *et al.* 1970	P	280	88	124	51	17	0·9776	0·0212	1·0863	0·1756
		Kout 1959 M2	C	1142	358	516	191	77				
2. United Kingdom,	(s) A_1A_2	Walther *et al.* 1956	P	185	81	80	17	7	1·0330	0·0395	1·4124	1·5207
London, Leytonstone			C	2325	1070	1023	159	73				
3. N. India,		Tyagi *et al.* 1965	P	35	15	4	13	3	0·3892	2·8009	0·7552	0·5455
Kanpur			C	6000	1985	1360	2278	377				
4. Japan, Sendai		Moniwa 1960	P	107	38	34	22	13	0·7779	1·1267	0·8119	0·6022
			C	21199	6769	7786	4827	1817				
				607					0·9306	0·5161	1·0290	0·0485
				χ_3^2 for homogeneity of areas						3·4722		2·7955
MALIGNANT NEOPLASMS OF ANUS, RECTUM												
1. Italy, Napoli		Martella 1938	P	17	8	7	2	0	1·0740	0·0188	0·8410	0·0473
		Sanguigno & Aghina 1954 M1	C	1200	545	444	162	49				
MALIGNANT NEOPLASMS OF INTESTINAL TRACT												
1. Hungary,		Major 1960	P	356	88	163	74	31	1·5479	9·1045	1·5079	5·5943
Nyiregyáza			C	1603	529	633	295	146				
2. Iceland		Bjarnason *et al.* 1973	P	108	57	32	13	6	0·9843	0·0051	1·1797	0·2878
			C	26716	14783	8432	2858	643				
3. Italy, Perugia		Benda & Gambelunghe 1962	P	420	188	180	40	12	0·9685	0·0892	0·8595	0·7185
		Benda & Menghini 1957	C	7356	3163	3127	783	283				

TABLE 1 **THE ABO BLOOD GROUP SYSTEM** (*cont.*)

NEOPLASMS (*cont.*)
MALIGNANT NEOPLASMS (*cont.*)
MALIGNANT NEOPLASMS OF INTESTINAL TRACT (*cont.*)

Place	Additional details	Authors		Number	O	A	B	AB	A/O Relative incidence	A/O χ^2_1 for difference from unity	B/O Relative incidence	B/O χ^2_1 for difference from unity
4. Italy, Torino		Cavalli *et al.* 1964	P	214	78	113	19	4	1·5755	8·7393	1·0900	0·1051
			C	2360	1056	971	236	97				
5. Italy, Trieste		Tagliaferro 1937[a]	P	52	18	26	4	4	1·4638	1·4971	0·5329	1·2760
		Goldstein 1927, 1929 M1	C	1766	681	672	284	129				
6. Poland, Warszawa		Kosiński *et al.* 1959	P	70	26	28	13	3	1·0384	0·0188	0·9547	0·0184
			C	4270	1537	1594	805	334				
				1220					1·2061	7·7551	1·0978	0·8779
				χ^2_5 for homogeneity of areas						11·6989		7·1321

MALIGNANT NEOPLASMS OF OESOPHAGUS, INTESTINAL TRACT

Place	Additional details	Authors		Number	O	A	B	AB	A/O Relative incidence	A/O χ^2_1 for difference from unity	B/O Relative incidence	B/O χ^2_1 for difference from unity
1. Bulgaria		Zographov 1962	P	29	11	12	6	0	0·7922	0·3110	1·0872	0·0271
			C	15422	4953	6821	2485	1163				
2. Argentina	Whites	Estevez 1963	P	209(c)	98	94	13	4	1·3184	3·6287	0·8067	0·5258
			C	21715(c)	11165	8123	1836	591				
				238					1·2481	2·6133	0·8701	0·2955
				χ^2_1 for homogeneity of areas						1·3264		0·2574

MALIGNANT NEOPLASMS OF GASTRO-INTESTINAL TRACT

Place	Additional details	Authors		Number	O	A	B	AB	A/O Relative incidence	A/O χ^2_1 for difference from unity	B/O Relative incidence	B/O χ^2_1 for difference from unity
1. Egypt, Cairo		Awny & Kamel 1959	P	98	33	39	23	3	1·3379	1·4215	1·1576	0·2735
			C	1588	583	515	351	139				
2. U.S.A., Rochester		Mayo & Fergeson 1953	P	935(c)	434	375	88	38	0·9042	1·0644	1·1406	0·6092
		Tinney & Watkins 1941	C	1000	450	430	80	40				
				1033					0·9544	0·2658	1·1451	0·8807
				χ^2_1 for homogeneity of areas						2·2201		0·0021

MALIGNANT NEOPLASMS OF LIVER

Place	Additional details	Authors		Number	O	A	B	AB	A/O Relative incidence	A/O χ^2_1 for difference from unity	B/O Relative incidence	B/O χ^2_1 for difference from unity
1. France, Haut-Languedoc		Larrouy 1960	P	16	8	5	3	0	0·6390	0·6154	2·8622	2·3904
			C	4367	2015	1971	264	117				
2. Malaya, Singapore	Chinese	Chew *et al.* 1973	P	214	85	67	50	12	1·3251	2·9250	1·0278	0·0234
			C	15279	6664	3964	3814	837				
3. Senegal, Dakar		Sankalé *et al.* 1968	P	120(c)	72	23	22	3	0·7226	1·8219	0·6585	2·9152
			C	11363(c)	5825	2575	2703	260				
4. Peru, Lima		Muñoz-Baratta 1962	P	44(c)	17	10	12	5	1·4938	1·0137	3·6922	11·9945
			C	107938(c)	66058	26013	12629	3238				
				394					1·0979	0·5543	1·0981	0·4988
				χ^2_3 for homogeneity of areas						5·8217		16·8248

MALIGNANT NEOPLASMS OF LIVER, BILE DUCTS

Place	Additional details	Authors		Number	O	A	B	AB	A/O Relative incidence	A/O χ^2_1 for difference from unity	B/O Relative incidence	B/O χ^2_1 for difference from unity
1. Italy, Milano		Visconti *et al.* 1961[a]	P	200	83	87	23	7	1·0076	0·0024	1·0671	0·0743
			C	9607(c)	3974	4134	1032	467				
2. Japan, Sendai		Moniwa 1960	P	66	19	21	17	9	0·9609	0·0158	1·2547	0·4605
			C	21199	6769	7786	4827	1817				
				266					0·9984	0·0001	1·1269	0·3791
				χ^2_1 for homogeneity of areas						0·0181		0·1556

TABLE 1 **THE ABO BLOOD GROUP SYSTEM** *(cont.)*

Place	Additional details	Authors		Number	O	A	B	AB	A/O Relative incidence	A/O χ^2_1 for difference from unity	B/O Relative incidence	B/O χ^2_1 for difference from unity
MALIGNANT NEOPLASMS OF GALL-BLADDER												
1. Austria, Wien	(s) S, Rh_D	Speiser 1958[a]	P	54	20	25	7	2	1·0669	0·0441	0·9881	0·0007
			C	1000	367	430	130	73				
2. Germany, Berlin		Schmauss *et al.* 1968	P	100	34	46	16	4	1·2091	0·7005	1·1816	0·3009
			C	15154	5642	6313	2247	952				
				154					1·1571	0·6376	1·1173	0·1935
				χ^2_1 for homogeneity of areas						0·1069		0·1082
MALIGNANT NEOPLASMS OF BILE DUCTS												
1. Poland, Warszawa		Kosiński *et al.* 1959	P	60	20	19	11	10	0·9160	0·0740	1·0501	0·0168
			C	4270	1537	1594	805	334				
2. Peru, Lima		Muñoz-Baratta 1962	P	34(c)	10	10	9	5	2·5394	4·3414	4·7076	11·3631
			C	107938(c)	66058	26013	12629	3238				
				94					1·2980	0·9950	1·9234	5·0218
				χ^2_1 for homogeneity of areas						3·4204		6·3581
MALIGNANT NEOPLASMS OF GALL-BLADDER, BILE DUCTS												
1. United Kingdom, London, Leytonstone	(s) A_1A_2	Walther *et al.* 1956	P	18	10	5	2	1	0·5230	1·3918	1·3459	0·1453
			C	2325	1070	1023	159	73				
MALIGNANT NEOPLASMS OF PANCREAS												
1. France, Haut-Languedoc		Larrouy 1960	P	31	19	9	1	2	0·4843	3·1917	0·4017	0·7870
			C	4367	2015	1971	264	117				
2. United Kingdom, Birmingham		Aird *et al.* 1960	P	53	24	22	6	1	1·0349	0·0135	1·5176	0·8291
			C	9590	4559	4038	751	242				
3. United Kingdom, Bristol		Aird *et al.* 1960	P	54	21	26	5	2	1·1779	0·3034	1·2500	0·1954
			C	1989	861	905	164	59				
4. United Kingdom, Leeds		Aird *et al.* 1960	P	22	11	8	3	0	0·8354	0·1492	1·5707	0·4780
			C	6260	2966	2582	515	197				
5. United Kingdom, Liverpool		Aird *et al.* 1960	P	133	58	67	4	4	1·5215	5·3826	0·3864	3·3626
			C	8202	4124	3131	736	211				
6. United Kingdom, London		Aird *et al.* 1960	P	109	39	56	10	4	1·5581	4·4741	1·3189	0·6035
			C	10000	4578	4219	890	313				
7. United Kingdom, London, Leytonstone		Walther *et al.* 1956	P	13	4	8	0	1	2·0919	1·4453		
			C	2325	1070	1023	159	73				
8. United Kingdom, Manchester		Aird *et al.* 1960	P	78	43	30	2	3	0·8073	0·7978	0·2439	3·7862
			C	5431	2570	2221	490	150				
9. United Kingdom, Newcastle upon Tyne		Aird *et al.* 1960	P	40	17	18	5	0	1·3622	0·8271	1·4941	0·6155
			C	4032	1971	1532	388	141				
10. United Kingdom, Sheffield		Aird *et al.* 1960	P	26	5	18	3	0	3·8696	7·1334	3·4019	2·7915
			C	4002	1837	1709	324	132				
11. United Kingdom, Glasgow		Aird *et al.* 1960	P	62	37	19	5	1	0·8465	0·3452	0·6382	0·8814
			C	5928	3150	1911	667	200				
12. United Kingdom, Cardiff		Aird *et al.* 1960	P	43	17	21	4	1	1·3945	0·9896	1·1026	0·0295
			C	874	403	357	86	28				
13. United Kingdom, Belfast		Macafee 1964[a]	P	119(a)	56	36	23	4	1·0710	0·1026	2·3887	12·2753
			C	28566	15715	9433	2702	716				
14. Japan, Sendai		Moniwa 1960	P	65	20	29	11	5	1·2606	0·6328	0·7713	0·4775
			C	21199	6769	7786	4827	1817				
15. U.S.A., Iowa		Buckwalter *et al.* 1964	P	525(c)	216	223	62	24	1·0933	0·8651	1·3690	4·6932
			C	49979	22392	21144	4695	1748				
16. Peru, Lima		Muñoz-Baratta 1962	P	21(c)	12	6	1	2	1·2697	0·2280	0·4359	0·6364
			C	107938	66058	26013	12629	3238				
				1394					1·1572	6·1144	1·2841	6·9039
				χ^2_{15} for homogeneity of areas						20·7671		
				(1381) χ^2_{14} for homogeneity of areas								25·5382

TABLE 1 **THE ABO BLOOD GROUP SYSTEM** (*cont.*)

Place	Additional details	Authors		Number	O	A	B	AB	A/O Relative incidence	A/O χ_1^2 for difference from unity	B/O Relative incidence	B/O χ_1^2 for difference from unity
NEOPLASMS (*cont.*)												
MALIGNANT NEOPLASMS (*cont.*)												
MALIGNANT NEOPLASMS OF LIVER, GALL-BLADDER, BILE DUCTS, PANCREAS												
1. Iceland		Bjarnason *et al.* 1973	P	119	56	40	14	9	1·2523	1·1758	1·2931	0·7367
			C	26716	14783	8432	2858	643				
MALIGNANT NEOPLASMS OF THYROID GLAND												
1. Czechoslovakia	(s) S	Miluničová & Hájek 1966	P	150	56	60	21	13	0·7434	2·2407	0·7029	1·6911
		Kout 1959 M2	C	1142	358	516	191	77				
2. Japan, Sendai		Moniwa 1960	P	54	11	24	13	6	1·8968	3·0849	1·6573	1·5174
			C	21199	6769	7786	4827	1817				
				204					0·9204	0·2269	0·9124	0·1644
					χ_1^2 for homogeneity of areas					5·0987		3·0441
MALIGNANT NEOPLASMS OF LARYNX												
1. France, Haut-Languedoc		Larrouy 1960	P	36	20	16	0	0	0·8179	0·3562		
			C	4367	2015	1971	264	117				
2. Germany, Berlin		Kaiser-Meinhardt 1962	P	324	131	128	49	16	0·8862	0·9252	0·9687	0·0353
		Hoffbauer 1961	C	15824	5959	6570	2301	994				
3. Italy, Milano		Manzini 1960	P	305	119	151	27	8	1·2198	2·5436	0·8737	0·3907
		Visconti *et al.* 1961	C	9607	3974	4134	1032	467				
4. Italy, Milano		Visconti *et al.* 1961[a]	P	121	51	52	16	2	0·9801	0·0102	1·2081	0·4288
			C	9607	3974	4134	1032	467				
5. Italy, Pavia		Negri *et al.* 1959	P	123	52	57	12	2	0·9056	0·2629	0·8550	0·2357
			C	8000	3090	3740	834	336				
6. Italy, Roma		Celestino & Silvagni 1964	P	429	210	163	49	7	0·8668	1·8362	0·9124	0·3270
			C	20051	8966	8029	2293	763				
7. United Kingdom, Liverpool	(s) S	Stell & Kell 1970	P	129	60	58	9	2	1·2527	1·4759	0·8263	0·2817
		Kopeć 1956 M1	C	9301	4633	3575	841	252				
8. N. India, Kanpur		Tyagi *et al.* 1965	P	42	16	11	13	2	1·0034	0·0001	0·7080	0·8495
			C	6000	1985	1360	2278	377				
9. S. India, Bhopal	(s) S	Ghooi *et al.* 1970	P	21	4	7	8	2	4·0000	4·1660	3·8400	4·1536
			C	100	48	21	25	6				
10. Argentina, Buenos Aires		Muller 1955	P	81	41	31	7	2	0·9257	0·1048	0·7952	0·3132
			C	29250	13889	11344	2982	1035				
				1611					0·9916	0·0584	0·9375	0·5818
					χ_9^2 for homogeneity of areas					11·6227		
				(1575)	χ_8^2 for homogeneity of areas							6·4337
MALIGNANT NEOPLASMS OF BRONCHUS												
1. Austria, Wien	(s) Rh_D, S	Speiser 1958[a]	P	2640	913	1180	388	159	1·1031	1·3764	1·1997	2·3534
			C	1000	367	430	130	73				
2. Denmark, København	Danes	Viskum 1973	P	466	193	208	46	19	0·9930	0·0047	0·8885	0·5043
		Andersen 1955 M1	C	14304	5804	6299	1557	644				
3. Germany, Berlin	(s) S	Schröder 1955	P	384	145	163	58	18	0·9767	0·0415	1·0271	0·0286
		Pettenkofer *et al.* 1957 M1	C	12000	4437	5107	1728	728				
4. Germany, Berlin		Berndt 1966	P	2040(c)	749	873	292	126	1·0104	0·0302	0·9390	0·5896
			C	4752(c)	1739	2006	722	285				
5. Germany, Bonn		Geisler & Saraf 1965	P	567(c)	192	304	53	18	1·5569	12·8773	0·9580	0·0469
		Prokop *et al.* 1961	C	706	295	300	85	26				
6. Germany, Tübingen		Brockmüller 1962	P	207	78	96	19	14	1·1968	1·3819	0·9228	0·0981
			C	39031	16283	16745	4298	1705				

TABLE 1 **THE ABO BLOOD GROUP SYSTEM** *(cont.)*

Place	Additional details	Authors		Number	O	A	B	AB	A/O Relative incidence	A/O χ_1^2 for difference from unity	B/O Relative incidence	B/O χ_1^2 for difference from unity
7. United Kingdom, Birmingham	(s) S	Aird *et al.* 1954	P	274	128	110	30	6	0·8905	0·6302	1·1420	0·3265
			C	1033	458	442	94	39				
8. United Kingdom, London	(s) S	Aird *et al.* 1954	P	384	166	162	43	13	1·0589	0·2593	1·3324	2·6900
			C	10000	4578	4219	890	313				
9. United Kingdom, London		Lewis & Woods 1961	P	697	306	304	63	24	1·0780	0·8044	1·0590	0·1605
			C	10000	4578	4219	890	313				
10. United Kingdom, London, Leytonstone		Walther *et al.* 1956	P	184	79	87	13	5	1·1519	0·7669	1·1074	0·1075
			C	2325	1070	1023	159	73				
11. United Kingdom, Manchester	(s) S	Aird *et al.* 1954	P	340	160	140	34	6	1·0505	0·1746	1·2221	1·0832
			C	9370	4532	3775	788	275				
				8183					1·0668	4·5329	1·0412	0·7727
				χ_{10}^2 for homogeneity of areas						13·8145		7·2160

MALIGNANT NEOPLASMS OF LUNG

Place	Additional details	Authors		Number	O	A	B	AB	A/O Relative incidence	A/O χ_1^2 for difference from unity	B/O Relative incidence	B/O χ_1^2 for difference from unity
1. Czechoslovakia, Praha		Jakoubková & Májský 1965	P	63	20	25	9	9	0·8672	0·2141	0·8435	0·1714
			C	1142	358	516	191	77				
2. France, Haut-Languedoc		Larrouy 1960	P	117	42	59	15	1	1·4361	3·1369	2·7259	10·6122
			C	4367	2015	1971	264	117				
3. Italy, Campania		Pollara & Melina 1957	P	300	128	124	36	12	1·1501	0·9397	0·8733	0·4097
			C	1000	444	374	143	39				
4. Italy, Genova		Cappellini & Guffanti 1956	P	248	124	84	36	4	0·6708	6·0125	0·9699	0·0187
		Macaggi & Gibelli 1933 M1; Canepa 1950 M1	C	726	304	307	91	24				
5. Italy, Milano		Mangani 1957	P	32	19	11	1	1	0·5565	2·3843	0·2027	2·4176
		Visconti *et al.* 1961	C	9607	3974	4134	1032	467				
6. Italy, Milano		Mor & Sforza 1960	P	354	138	160	38	18	1·0502	0·1048	1·0301	0·0154
			C	500	202	223	54	21				
7. Italy, Milano		Visconti *et al.* 1961[a]	P	806	347	357	73	29	0·9890	0·0198	0·8101	2·4913
			C	9607	3974	4134	1032	467				
8. Italy, Milano	(s) Rh_D	Orlandi & Tosi 1962	P	300	84	173	33	10	1·9798	25·6616	1·5128	3·9460
		Visconti *et al.* 1961	C	9607	3974	4134	1032	467				
9. Italy, Napoli		Jovino & Musella 1958	P	101	51	30	16	4	0·7220	1·8598	1·0554	0·0323
			C	1200	545	444	162	49				
10. Italy, Napoli		Percesepe *et al.* 1959	P	90	39	40	8	3	1·6510	4·1536	0·9179	0·0429
			C	500	264	164	59	13				
11. Italy, Napoli		Spena & Grippo 1964	P	184	75	94	10	5	1·4464	5·2088	0·6220	1·8934
			C	2147	989	857	212	89				
12. United Kingdom, Liverpool Region		McConnell *et al.* 1955	P	939	458	377	69	35	0·9516	0·4386	0·7802	3·2622
			C	5956	2807	2428	542	179				
13. United Kingdom, Liverpool		McConnell *et al.* 1954	P	777	379	312	55	31	0·9753	0·0603	0·8618	0·6281
			C	1000	481	406	81	32				
14. United Kingdom, Swansea		Ashley 1969	P	2019	910	833	203	73	1·0629	1·3374	1·0448	0·2628
			C	9652	4482	3860	957	353				
15. United Kingdom, Belfast		Macafee 1962	P	167	99	55	11	2	0·9255	0·2105	0·6462	1·8791
			C	28566	15715	9433	2702	716				
16. N. India, Kanpur		Tyagi *et al.* 1965	P	14	5	3	5	1	0·8757	0·0329	0·8714	0·0473
			C	6000	1985	1360	2278	377				
17. Japan, Niigata		Hirose & Honma 1962	P	103	34	47	20	2	1·1078	0·2049	0·7475	1·0585
			C	12253	3624	4522	2852	1255				

TABLE 1 **THE ABO BLOOD GROUP SYSTEM** (*cont.*)

Place	Additional details	Authors		Number	O	A	B	AB	A/O Relative incidence	A/O χ_1^2 for difference from unity	B/O Relative incidence	B/O χ_1^2 for difference from unity
NEOPLASMS (*cont.*)												
MALIGNANT NEOPLASMS (*cont.*)												
MALIGNANT NEOPLASMS OF LUNG (*cont.*)												
18. U.S.A., Boston	(s) ABH secretion	Krant *et al.* 1968	P	61	35	19	4	3	0·6780	1·6933	0·4226	2·5130
		Dublin *et al.* 1964	C	605	281	225	76	23				
19. U.S.A., Iowa		Buckwalter *et al.* 1964	P	538(c)	268	198	52	20	0·7824	6·7849	0·9254	0·2589
			C	49979	22392	21144	4695	1748				
20. U.S.A., Salt Lake City		McNeil *et al.* 1965	P	87	34	42	7	4	1·4746	2·4525	0·8143	0·2210
			C	578	265	222	67	24				
21. Argentina	Whites	Estevez 1963	P	92(c)	48	30	10	4	0·8591	0·4244	1·2669	0·4608
			C	21715(c)	11165	8123	1836	591				
22. Peru, Lima		Muñoz-Baratta 1962	P	31(c)	14	11	4	2	1·9953	2·9384	1·4945	0·5021
			C	107938(c)	66058	26013	12629	3238				
23. Australia, Sydney		Rennie & Haber 1961	P	218	107	90	18	3	1·0718	0·2334	0·8476	0·4186
		Walsh 1947 M1	C	30000	14672	11514	2912	902				
24. New Zealand, Auckland		Cotter *et al.* 1961	P	263(c)	123	105	28	7	0·9942	0·0019	1·1900	0·6750
			C	13493(c)	6367	5467	1218	441				
				7904					1·0271	1·0105	0·9560	1·0661
					χ_{23}^2 for homogeneity of areas					65·4986		33·1720
MALIGNANT NEOPLASMS OF BRONCHUS, LUNG												
1. Italy, Torino		Cavalli *et al.* 1964	P	327	113	170	36	8	1·6361	14·5066	1·4255	3·0064
			C	2360	1056	971	236	97				
MALIGNANT NEOPLASMS OF RESPIRATORY SYSTEM												
1. Iceland		Bjarnason *et al.* 1973	P	141	65	48	19	9	1·2947	1·8321	1·5120	2·4974
			C	26716	14783	8432	2858	643				
MALIGNANT NEOPLASMS OF BONE												
1. Germany, Berlin	Osteosarcoma	Hirschfeld & Hittmair 1926	P	13	6	2	4	1	0·3187	1·9413	1·5339	0·4273
			C	750	283	296	123	48				
2. Portugal		Lessa & Ruffié 1960	P	45(c)	26	16	3	0	0·5621	3·2439	0·6572	0·4679
			C	3353(c)	1424	1559	250	120				
3. Japan, Sendai		Moniwa 1960	P	89	23	41	19	6	1·5498	2·8166	1·1584	0·2242
			C	21199	6769	7786	4827	1817				
4. Peru, Lima	Osteosarcoma	Muñoz-Baratta 1962	P	69	28	18	14	9	1·6325	2·6302	2·6153	8·6189
			C	107938	66058	26013	12629	3238				
				216					1·1287	0·5411	1·5225	4·3603
					χ_3^2 for homogeneity of areas					10·0909		5·3781
MALIGNANT NEOPLASMS OF SKIN												
1. France, Paris	Facial	Huguenin & Delage 1933	P	62(c)	32	23	6	1	0·6180	2·7304	0·8846	0·0656
		Dujarric de la Rivière *et al.* 1927 M1	C	465	184	214	39	28				
2. Germany, Göttingen	Malignant melanomas	Jörgensen & Lal 1972	P	164	74	70	14	6	0·8304	0·9965	0·7274	0·9861
			C	694	273	311	71	39				
3. Italy, Foggia	Epithelioma	Altobella 1967/8	P	140	80	30	20	10	0·4746	10·8996	0·6592	2·4555
			C	1000	443	350	168	39				
4. United Kingdom, London, Leytonstone	Epithelioma and rodent ulcer (s) A_1A_2	Walther *et al.* 1956	P	20	8	6	3	3	0·7845	0·2007	2·5236	1·8406
			C	2325	1070	1023	159	73				
5. United Kingdom, Glasgow	Rodent ulcer, Bowen's disease, squamous cell carcinoma	MacSween & Syme 1965	P	43	27	11	5		0·6791	1·1630		
			C	5898	3177	1906	637	178				
				429					0·6617	12·1785	0·7803	1·8698
					χ_4^2 for homogeneity of areas					3·8117		
				(386)	χ_3^2 for homogeneity of areas							3·4780

TABLE 1 THE ABO BLOOD GROUP SYSTEM (*cont.*)

Place	Additional details	Authors		Number	O	A	B	AB	A/O Relative incidence	A/O χ_1^2 for difference from unity	B/O Relative incidence	B/O χ_1^2 for difference from unity
MALIGNANT NEOPLASMS OF BREAST												
1. Austria, Wien	(s) Rh_D	Speiser 1958[b]	P	573	199	270	83	21	1·1580	1·5617	1·1775	0·9708
			C	1000	367	430	130	73				
2. Belgium, Liège		Otto-Servais *et al.* 1959	P	100	41	48	10	1	1·2530	1·1068	1·4319	1·0158
			C	6000	2771	2589	472	168				
3. Bulgaria		Zographov 1962	P	302	96	133	50	23	1·0060	0·0020	1·0381	0·0451
			C	15422	4953	6821	2485	1163				
4. Czechoslovakia, Praha		Jakoubková & Májský 1965	P	76	27	31	15	76	0·7966	0·6987	1·0413	0·0147
			C	1142	358	516	191	77				
5. Denmark, København		Thomsen 1931–2	P	223(c)	92	97	20	14	1·1018	0·3136	0·8006	0·6105
			C	533(c)	232	222	63	16				
6. France, Haut-Languedoc		Larrouy 1960	P	77	28	45	3	1	1·6430	4·1830	0·8178	0·1084
			C	4367	2015	1971	264	117				
7. France, Paris		Huguenin & Delage 1933	P	41(c)	26	6	9	0	0·1984	12·1537	1·6331	1·3318
		Dujarric de la Rivière *et al.* 1927 M1	C	465	184	214	39	28				
8. Germany, Berlin		Hirschfeld & Hittmair 1926	P	26	5	13	6	2	2·4858	2·9214	2·7610	2·7262
			C	750	283	296	123	48				
9. Germany, Berlin		Schröder 1955	P	278	104	126	37	11	1·0526	0·1462	0·9135	0·2185
		Pettenkofer *et al.* 1957 M1	C	12000	4437	5107	1728	728				
10. Germany, Berlin		Wehle 1957	P	292	109	126	36	21	0·9788	0·0264	0·8542	0·6641
			C	21104	7725	9123	2987	1269				
11. Germany, Freiburg	Females	Preisler *et al.* 1959	P	100	43	47	7	3	1·0603	0·0751	0·6662	0·9755
			C	4017	1686	1738	412	181				
12. Germany, Tübingen		Völter *et al.* 1970	P	401	150	187	49	15	1·2123	3·0534	1·2376	1·6601
		Dick *et al.* 1962	C	39031	16283	16745	4298	1705				
13. Iceland		Bjarnason *et al.* 1973	P	105	56	34	13	2	1·0644	0·0822	1·2008	0·3516
			C	26716	14783	8432	2858	643				
14. Italy, Firenze		Cutrera & Leoni 1959	P	200	76	106	16	2	1·5760	9·0242	0·9782	0·0063
			C	13633	6259	5539	1347	488				
15. Italy, Milano		Rotelli & Corippo 1959	P	108	42	52	10	4	1·0229	0·0118	0·8822	0·1255
			C	8000	3090	3740	834	336				
16. Italy, Milano		Mor & Sforza 1960	P	88	33	39	15	1	1·0705	0·0710	1·7003	2·3396
			C	500	202	223	54	21				
17. Italy, Milano		Visconti *et al.* 1961[a]	P	344	140	151	43	10	1·0368	0·0917	1·1827	0·8908
			C	9607	3974	4134	1032	467				
18. Italy, Napoli	Females; contains 30% cancer other than breast	Cocchia *et al.* 1963	P	112	56	42	12	2	0·9181	0·1273	1·0867	0·0481
			C	300	142	116	28	14				
19. Italy, Napoli		Spena & Grippo 1964	P	183	86	72	15	10	0·9662	0·0428	0·8137	0·5060
			C	2147	989	857	212	89				
20. Italy, Perugia		Benda & Gambelunghe 1962	P	184	76	92	10	6	1·2245	1·6627	0·5315	3·4808
		Benda & Menghini 1957	C	7356	3163	3127	783	283				
21. Italy, Torino		Cavalli *et al.* 1964	P	395	173	164	42	16	1·0310	0·0671	1·0863	0·1971
			C	2360	1056	971	236	97				
22. Italy, Verona	Females	Bonzanini 1961	P	112	47	58	4	3	1·2924	1·6715	0·4146	2·8329
			C	5500	2460	2349	505	186				
23. Norway		Hartmann & Stavem 1964	P	1600	605	830	109	56	1·0589	1·0918	0·8143	3·7394
			C	31491	12036	15593	2663	1199				
24. Poland, Gdańsk	Females	Domaradzka-Woźniak 1964	P	352	102	135	87	28	1·1623	1·2795	1·4410	6·0772
			C	12125	4058	4621	2402	1044				
25. Poland, Lower Silesia		Sagan *et al.* 1957	P	56	24	23	5	4	0·8297	0·3984	0·3596	4·2691
			C	2397	813	939	471	174				
26. Portugal		Lessa & Ruffié 1960	P	64(c)	22	36	4	2	1·4947	2·1659	1·0356	0·0041
			C	3353(c)	1424	1559	250	120				

TABLE 1 **THE ABO BLOOD GROUP SYSTEM** (*cont.*)

Place	Additional details	Authors		Number	O	A	B	AB	A/O Relative incidence	A/O χ^2_1 for difference from unity	B/O Relative incidence	B/O χ^2_1 for difference from unity
NEOPLASMS (*cont.*)												
MALIGNANT NEOPLASMS (*cont.*)												
MALIGNANT NEOPLASMS OF BREAST (*cont.*)												
27. United Kingdom, Birmingham	Females	Aird *et al.* 1954	P	502	232	219	40	11	0·9781	0·0367	0·8401	0·7209
			C	1033	458	442	94	39				
28. United Kingdom, London	Females	Aird *et al.* 1954	P	85	34	35	11	5	1·1170	0·2095	1·6642	2·1323
			C	10000	4578	4219	890	313				
29. United Kingdom, London, Leytonstone	Females; (s) A_1A_2	Walther *et al.* 1956	P	137	54	64	16	3	1·2396	1·2799	1·9939	5·3972
			C	2325	1070	1023	159	73				
30. United Kingdom, Manchester	Females	Aird *et al.* 1954	P	325	155	124	34	12	0·9604	0·1087	1·2616	1·4454
			C	9370	4532	3775	788	275				
31. United Kingdom, Newcastle upon Tyne	Females	Aird *et al.* 1954	P	105	48	39	17	1	1·0190	0·0076	1·7690	4·0383
			C	13572	6598	5261	1321	392				
32. United Kingdom, Sheffield		Green & Dunsford 1954	P	121	53	61	6	1	1·2243	1·1285	0·6317	1·1175
		Kopeć 1970	C	4435	2020	1899	362	154				
33. United Kingdom, Belfast		Macafee 1962	P	382	199	136	41	6	1·1385	1·3417	1·1983	1·0962
			C	28566	15715	9433	2702	716				
34. N. India, Calcutta		Mitra *et al.* 1962	P	84	29	18	30	7	0·7732	0·7105	0·9852	0·0031
			C	2273	740	594	777	162				
35. N. India, Kanpur	Females	Tyagi *et al.* 1965	P	87	30	15	36	6	0·7298	0·9802	1·0457	0·0321
			C	6000	1985	1360	2278	377				
36. S. India, Bhopal		Ghooi *et al.* 1970	P	212	66	56	76	14	1·9394	4·3242	2·2109	7·0616
			C	100	48	21	25	6				
37. S. India, Bombay	Parsee females	Jayant 1971	P	115(c)	45	26	37	7	0·8745	0·2822	0·9645	0·0252
			C	2282(c)	834	551	711	186				
38. S. India, Gwalior		Majupuria *et al.* 1966	P	130	56	33	28	13	0·6836	1·9828	0·3816	12·5710
			C	300	87	75	114	24				
39. Philippine Islands	Filipinos	Esquivel 1960	P	371(c)	179	100	77	15	1·0044	0·0012	0·9975	0·0000
			C	235952(c)	114067	63443	49189	9253				
40. Japan, Niigata		Hirose & Honma 1962	P	1013	274	410	230	99	1·1992	5·0105	1·0666	0·4825
			C	12253	3624	4522	2852	1255				
41. Japan, Sendai		Moniwa 1960	P	167	59	56	34	18	0·8252	1·0525	0·8081	0·9716
			C	21199	6769	7786	4827	1817				
42. Egypt, Alexandria		Sadek *et al.* 1965[a]	P	20	6	10	3	1	1·4408	0·4971	0·5881	0·5616
			C	3720	1142	1321	971	286				
43. U.S.A., Boston	(s) ABH secretion	Krant *et al.* 1968	P	47	27	15	3	2	0·6938	1·1961	0·4108	2·0445
		Dublin *et al.* 1964	C	605	281	225	76	23				
44. U.S.A., Connecticut	Females	Goldenberg & Hayes 1958	P	1000(c)	447	413	111	29	1·0019	0·0008	0·9275	0·4978
			C	75904(c)	33170	30589	8881	3264				
45. U.S.A., Iowa		Buckwalter & Knowler 1958	P	866	370	383	81	32	1·0962	1·5617	1·0441	0·1217
			C	49979	22392	21144	4695	1748				
46. Peru, Lima		Muñoz-Baratta 1962	P	29(c)	17	6	4	2	0·8963	0·0532	1·2307	0·1395
			C	107938(c)	66058	26013	12629	3238				
				12190					1·0736	11·3362	1·0243	0·5890
				χ^2_{45} for homogeneity of areas						54·4588		75·1499

TABLE 1 **THE ABO BLOOD GROUP SYSTEM** (*cont.*)

Place	Additional details	Authors		Number	O	A	B	AB	A/O Relative incidence	A/O χ_1^2 for difference from unity	B/O Relative incidence	B/O χ_1^2 for difference from unity
MALIGNANT NEOPLASMS OF CERVIX UTERI												
1. Belgium, Gent		Derom & Thiéry 1964	P	345	166	142	27	10	0·9672	0·0635	0·8325	0·6011
			C	1025	476	421	93	35				
2. Czechoslovakia		Matoušek 1935	P	58	22	27	8	1	0·9644	0·0155	0·6475	1·0856
		Leischner 1936 M1	C	2429	796	1013	447	173				
3. Czechoslovakia		Miluničová *et al.* 1969[a]	P	85	29	35	13	8	0·8373	0·4649	0·8402	0·2537
		Kout 1959 M2	C	1142	358	516	191	77				
4. France, Haut-Languedoc		Larrouy 1960	P	240	108	95	24	13	0·8993	0·5423	1·6961	5·0562
			C	4367	2015	1971	264	117				
5. Germany, Berlin		Hoffbauer 1961	P	375	132	173	45	25	1·1887	2·1853	0·8829	0·5105
			C	15824	5959	6570	2301	994				
6. Germany, Berlin		Mosler 1961	P	233	73	116	35	9	1·2740	2·5344	1·2459	1·1007
			C	6128	2188	2729	842	369				
7. Germany, Berlin		Mosler & Wehle 1961	P	1197	421	508	191	77	1·0615	0·6998	1·1121	1·2577
			C	6885	2537	2884	1035	429				
8. Germany, Bonn		Prokop *et al.* 1961	P	442	151	221	51	19	1·4392	7·4173	1·1722	0·6099
			C	706	295	300	85	26				
9. Germany, Erfurt		Schuberth 1961	P	176	53	85	29	9	1·3393	2·7762	1·5100	3·1702
			C	45105	16630	19914	6026	2535				
10. Germany, Frankfurt am Main		Schwenzer 1961	P	133	60	47	16	10	0·7050	3·0288	0·9600	0·0196
			C	2000	792	880	220	108				
11. Germany, Freiburg		Preisler *et al.* 1959	P	762	297	370	61	34	1·2085	4·9557	0·8405	1·3255
			C	4017	1686	1738	412	181				
12. Germany, Heidelberg		Helmbold *et al.* 1958	P	360	116	182	41	21	1·4804	10·3357	1·3285	2·3110
			C	6117	2507	2657	667	286				
13. Germany, Heidelberg		Krah *et al.* 1961	P	1087	384	555	91	57	1·2771	13·1674	0·8827	1·1173
			C	34513	13748	15559	3691	1515				
14. Germany, Halle an der Saale		Mazur & Alex 1961	P	806	258	384	110	54	1·2002	4·4731	1·0719	0·3248
			C	5321	1878	2329	747	367				
15. Germany, Karl-Marx Stadt		Scheffler 1961	P	607	244	262	75	26	1·0472	0·2620	0·8806	0·9072
			C	25080	9967	10220	3479	1414				
16. Germany, Leipzig		Zuber & Andreas 1961	P	1267	450	558	167	92	1·0476	0·3802	0·9428	0·3038
			C	3021	1100	1302	433	186				
17. Hungary, Budapest		Weitzner 1925	P	36	4	16	5	11	3·2979	4·4833	2·8424	2·3766
			C	1000	357	433	157	53				
18. Italy, Brindisi		Perretti & Putignano 1967	P	200	60	96	32	12	1·4439	4·4541	1·0251	0·0116
			C	1812	592	656	308	256				
19. Italy, Milano		Beolchini *et al.* 1958[a]	P	205	81	100	23	1	1·2660	2·2842	1·2156	0·6239
			C	2346	1006	981	235	124				
20. Italy, Milano		Dambrosio 1965	P	541	223	254	60	4	1·1002	1·0477	1·0509	0·1126
		Garibaldi & Gianotti 1964 M2	C	16952	7081	7331	1813	727				
21. Italy, Pisa		Baisi 1959	P	150	63	72	9	6	1·2680	1·7666	0·5732	2·3452
			C	2203	983	886	245	89				
22. Italy, Torino		Cagliero 1961	P	633	276	265	68	24	0·9661	0·1134	0·9870	0·0065
			C	1500	645	641	161	53				
23. Italy, Varese	(s) Rh_D	Carrera 1963	P	40	17	20	1	2	1·2824	0·5444	0·2068	2·3226
			C	1002	436	400	124	42				
24. Norway		Bergsjö & Kolstad 1962[a]	P	745	272	384	65	24	1·0670	0·6147	1·1066	0·4920
		Heistø 1956 M1	C	8292	3135	4148	677	332				
25. Poland, Gdańsk		Domaradzka-Woźniak 1964	P	1465	478	604	272	111	1·1096	2·5709	0·9613	0·2416
			C	12125	4058	4621	2402	1044				
26. Poland, Warszawa		Mogielnicki & Tarłowska 1964	P	1207	364	496	242	105	1·2385	7·1002	1·0327	0·1133
			C	3409	1137	1251	732	289				

TABLE 1 **THE ABO BLOOD GROUP SYSTEM** (*cont.*)

Place	Additional details	Authors		Number	O	A	B	AB	A/O Relative incidence	A/O χ_1^2 for difference from unity	B/O Relative incidence	B/O χ_1^2 for difference from unity
NEOPLASMS (*cont.*)												
MALIGNANT NEOPLASMS (*cont.*)												
MALIGNANT NEOPLASMS OF CERVIX UTERI (*cont.*)												
27. N. India,		Gupta 1968	P	208	49	77	69	13	2·3384	19·9130	1·2943	1·7937
Bikaner			C	2622	875	588	952	207				
28. N. India,		Mitra *et al.* 1962	P	521	172	114	204	31	0·8257	2·0817	1·1296	1·1115
Calcutta			C	2273	740	594	777	162				
29. N. India,		Tyagi *et al.* 1965	P	300	92	60	116	32	0·9519	0·0845	1·0987	0·4336
Kanpur			C	6000	1985	1360	2278	377				
30. N. India,		Tyagi *et al.* 1967	P	556	150	121	222	63	1·1718	1·4386	1·2240	3·1286
Kanpur			C	3022	966	665	1168	223				
31. S. India,		Ghooi *et al.* 1970	P	117	34	42	35	6	2·8235	8·8550	1·9765	3·9068
Bhopal			C	100	48	21	25	6				
32. S. India,	Marathas	Jayant 1971	P	243(c)	85	75	64	19	0·8952	0·3787	0·9558	0·0575
Bombay			C	858(c)	278	274	219	87				
33. S. India,		Majupuria & Gupta 1966	P	150	30	66	48	6	2·5520	11·9726	1·2211	0·5359
Gwalior			C	300	87	75	114	24				
34. Japan, Sendai		Segi *et al.* 1957[a]	P	1534	446	640	304	144	1·1399	4·3805	0·9536	0·3976
			C	530046	161461	203255	115416	49914				
35. Japan, Sendai		Moniwa 1960	P	832	255	318	181	78	1·0842	0·8895	0·9954	0·0022
			C	21199	6769	7786	4827	1817				
36. U.S.A.,		Janus *et al.* 1967	P	1028	473	399	122	34	0·9145	1·7066	0·9653	0·1192
Connecticut			C	75904	33174	30601	8864	3265				
37. U.S.A.,	(s) Rh_D	Rotkin 1965	P	353	157	129	57	10	1·0008	0·0000	1·4345	2·3900
San Francisco Bay area			C	353	162	133	41	17				
38. U.S.A., Iowa		Buckwalter *et al.* 1964	P	976	438	436	83	19	1·0542	0·5965	0·9038	0·7016
			C	49979	22392	21144	4695	1748				
39. U.S.A.,		Garriga & Ghossein 1963	P	123	57	42	22	2	0·8179	0·9536	1·2313	0·6655
New York		Osborne & De George 1963	C	4738	2029	1828	636	245				
40. Peru, Lima	Adeno-carcinoma	Velarde & Carpio 1969	P	94(c)	51	34	9	0	2·1066	11·1875	1·4713	1·1290
			C	10000(c)	6895	2182	827	96				
41. Peru, Lima	Primary and exclusively epidermoid	Velarde & Carpio 1969	P	2825(c)	2036	544	223	22	0·8443	9·7662	0·9132	1·3032
			C	10000(c)	6895	2182	827	96				
				23255					1·0914	28·6839	1·0187	0·6845
				χ_{40}^2 for homogeneity of areas						123·8022		45·5931

MALIGNANT NEOPLASMS OF CORPUS UTERI

Place	Additional details	Authors		Number	O	A	B	AB	A/O Relative incidence	A/O χ_1^2 for difference from unity	B/O Relative incidence	B/O χ_1^2 for difference from unity
1. Czechoslovakia		Matoušek 1935	P	12	5	3	3	1	0·4715	1·0556	1·0685	0·0082
		Leischner 1936 M1	C	2429	796	1013	447	173				
2. Czechoslovakia		Milunič̌ová *et al.* 1969[a]	P	142	43	61	23	15	0·9842	0·0057	1·0025	0·0001
		Kout 1959 M2	C	1142	358	516	191	77				
3. France, Haut-		Larrouy 1960	P	45	4	20	8	13	5·1116	8·8432	15·2652	19·5862
Languedoc			C	4367	2015	1971	264	117				
4. Germany,		Hoffbauer 1961	P	97	43	35	12	7	0·7383	1·7660	0·7227	0·9838
Berlin			C	15824	5959	6570	2301	994				
5. Germany,		Mosler 1961	P	79	32	32	11	4	0·8018	0·7709	0·8933	0·1029
Berlin			C	6128	2188	2729	842	369				
6. Germany,		Mosler & Wehle 1961	P	288	105	130	37	16	1·0891	0·4059	0·8638	0·5658
Berlin			C	6885	2537	2884	1035	429				
7. Germany,		Prokop *et al.* 1961	P	115	42	59	11	3	1·3813	2·1981	0·9090	0·0702
Bonn			C	706	295	300	85	26				
8. Germany,		Schuberth 1961	P	19	6	10	1	2	1·3918	0·4097	0·4600	0·5169
Erfurt			C	45105	16630	19914	6026	2535				

TABLE 1 **THE ABO BLOOD GROUP SYSTEM** *(cont.)*

Place	Additional details	Authors		Number	O	A	B	AB	A/O Relative incidence	A/O χ^2_1 for difference from unity	B/O Relative incidence	B/O χ^2_1 for difference from unity
9. Germany, Frankfurt am Main		Schwenzer 1961	P	27	14	11	1	1	0·7071	0·7289	0·2571	1·7123
			C	2000	792	880	220	108				
10. Germany, Freiburg		Preisler *et al.* 1959	P	202	78	97	16	11	1·2064	1·4488	0·8394	0·3911
			C	4017	1686	1738	412	181				
11. Germany, Halle an der Saale		Mazur & Alex 1961	P	137	49	58	14	16	0·9545	0·0563	0·7183	1·1682
			C	5321	1878	2329	747	367				
12. Germany, Heidelberg		Helmbold *et al.* 1958	P	94	42	45	5	2	1·0109	0·0025	0·4475	2·8652
			C	6117	2507	2657	667	286				
13. Germany, Heidelberg		Krah *et al.* 1961	P	335	130	176	22	7	1·1963	2·3769	0·6303	3·9816
			C	34513	13748	15559	3691	1515				
14. Germany, Karl-Marx Stadt		Scheffler 1961	P	222	81	93	32	16	1·1197	0·5489	1·1318	0·3486
			C	25080	9967	10220	3479	1414				
15. Germany, Leipzig		Zuber & Andreas 1961	P	385	143	174	53	15	1·0280	0·0529	0·9416	0·1247
			C	3021	1100	1302	433	186				
16. Italy, Brindisi		Perretti & Putignano 1967	P	232	72	96	40	24	1·4775	5·5366	1·1833	0·6486
			C	1812	656	592	308	256				
17. Italy, Milano		Dambrosio 1965	P	138	48	67	21	2	1·3482	2·4775	1·7087	4·1511
		Garibaldi & Gianotti 1964 M2	C	16952	7081	7331	1813	727				
18. Italy, Torino		Cagliero 1961	P	97	38	43	11	5	1·1386	0·3200	1·1597	0·1756
			C	1500	645	641	161	53				
19. Italy, Varese	(s) Rh_D	Carrera 1963	P	61	21	34	6	0	1·7648	3·9431	1·0046	0·0001
			C	1002	436	400	124	42				
20. Norway		Bergsjö & Kolstad 1962[a]	P	493	169	267	41	16	1·1941	3·0769	1·1234	0·4219
		Heistø 1956 M1	C	8292	3135	4148	677	332				
21. Poland, Warszawa		Mogielnicki & Tarłowska 1964	P	268	84	106	59	19	1·1469	0·8163	1·0910	0·2439
			C	3409	1137	1251	732	289				
22. United Kingdom, Belfast		Macafee 1962	P	53	27	18	7	1	1·1106	0·1187	1·5079	0·9354
			C	28566	15715	9433	2702	716				
23. U.S.A., Connecticut		Janus *et al.* 1967	P	946	457	349	114	26	0·8279	6·9727	0·9336	0·4253
			C	75904	33174	30601	8864	3265				
24. U.S.A., Iowa		Buckwalter *et al.* 1964	P	54(c)	27	21	4	2	0·8237	0·4439	0·7066	0·4199
			C	49979	22392	21144	4695	1748				
				4541					1·0573	2·7257	0·9840	0·1000
				χ^2_{23} for homogeneity of areas						41·6504		39·7476

ENDOMETRIAL ADENOCARCINOMA

Place	Additional details	Authors		Number	O	A	B	AB	A/O Relative incidence	A/O χ^2_1	B/O Relative incidence	B/O χ^2_1
1. Italy, Milano		Samuel *et al.* 1968	P	115	42	58	12	3	1·3191	1·6624	1·0863	0·0572
			C	935	384	402	101	48				

MALIGNANT MELANOMA OF UTERUS

Place	Additional details	Authors		Number	O	A	B	AB	A/O Relative incidence	A/O χ^2_1	B/O Relative incidence	B/O χ^2_1
1. Peru, Lima		Velarde & Carpio 1969	P	192(c)	134	39	18	1	0·9197	0·2080	1·1199	0·1993
			C	10000	6895	2182	827	96				

CHORIOCARCINOMA

Place	Additional details	Authors		Number	O	A	B	AB	A/O Relative incidence	A/O χ^2_1	B/O Relative incidence	B/O χ^2_1
1. United Kingdom, London		Bagshawe 1976	P	314	127	141	36	10	1·2403	1·5578	1·2667	0·7568
			C*	314	143	128	32	11				

* These control figures are based on those used for a smaller and partly overlapping set of data (Bagshawe *et al.* 1971), which were themselves a weighted set based on the geographical origin of the patients (Bagshawe, personal communication, 1976).

TABLE 1 **THE ABO BLOOD GROUP SYSTEM** (*cont.*)

NEOPLASMS (*cont.*)
MALIGNANT NEOPLASMS (*cont.*)

MALIGNANT NEOPLASMS OF UTERUS (precise site unspecified)

Place	Additional details	Authors		Number	O	A	B	AB	A/O Relative incidence	A/O χ_1^2 for difference from unity	B/O Relative incidence	B/O χ_1^2 for difference from unity
1. Austria, Wien	(s) Rh_D	Speiser 1958[b]	P	1561	548	676	226	111	1·0528	0·3174	1·1643	1·3878
			C	1000	367	430	130	73				
2. Denmark, København		Johannsen 1927	P	177	61	96	13	7	1·6447	6·9485	0·7848	0·5174
			C	533	232	222	63	16				
3. Denmark, København		Thomsen 1931–2	P	239(c)	106	99	19	15	0·9760	0·0208	0·6601	2·0980
		Johannsen 1927	C	533	232	222	63	16				
4. France, Paris		Huguenin & Delage 1933	P	86(c)	39	38	7	2	0·8378	0·5049	0·8468	0·1385
		Dujarric de la Rivière *et al.* 1927 M1	C	465	184	214	39	28				
5. Germany, Berlin		Hirschfeld & Hittmair 1926	P	14	5	6	3	0	1·1473	0·0505	1·3805	0·1908
			C	750	283	296	123	48				
6. Germany, Berlin		Schröder 1955	P	658	225	288	113	32	1·1121	1·3534	1·2896	4·5871
		Pettenkofer *et al.* 1957 M1	C	12000	4437	5107	1728	728				
7. Iceland		Bjarnason *et al.* 1973	P	136	70	48	13	5	1·2022	0·9605	0·9606	0·0176
			C	26716	14783	8432	2858	643				
8. Italy, Firenze		Cutrera & Leoni 1959	P	200	76	96	20	8	1·4274	5·2941	1·2228	0·6315
			C	13633	6259	5539	1347	488				
9. Italy, Genova		Chisale 1963	P	100	36	52	6	6	1·5713	3·4051	0·8131	0·1853
			C	350	161	148	33	8				
10. Italy, Lazio		Liotta *et al.* 1957	P	203	110	64	23	6	0·6532	7·1972	0·8096	0·8317
			C	10008	4472	3983	1155	398				
11. Italy, Milano		Dossena & Lanzara 1925	P	53	25	21	6	1	1·0769	0·0497	0·9231	0·0251
		Dossena 1924 M1	C	214	100	78	26	10				
12. Italy, Napoli		Martella 1938	P	282	118	117	35	12	1·2171	1·8283	0·9979	0·0001
		Sanguigno & Aghina 1954 M1	C	1200	545	444	162	49				
13. Italy, Perugia		Benda & Gambelunghe 1962	P	422	170	190	38	24	1·1305	1·2773	0·9030	0·3083
		Benda & Menghini 1957	C	7356	3163	3127	783	283				
14. Italy, Torino		Cavalli *et al.* 1964	P	576	233	272	67	4	1·2696	5·7283	1·2867	2·6038
			C	2360	1056	971	236	97				
15. Jugoslavia, Beograd		Milošević *et al.* 1961	P	323	105	131	57	30	0·9807	0·0217	1·1219	0·4809
			C	20000	5754	8592	3268	1386				
16. Poland, Białystok		Korfel 1966	P	500(c)	136	224	96	44	1·5984	15·4765	1·2866	2·9942
			C	2277(c)	822	847	451	157				
17. Poland, Lower Silesia		Sagan *et al.* 1957	P	263	70	103	55	35	1·2740	2·2304	1·3562	2·5920
			C	2397(c)	813	939	471	174				
18. United Kingdom, London, Leytonstone	(s) A_1A_2	Walther *et al.* 1956	P	45	19	23	2	1	1·2661	0·5681	0·7084	0·2123
			C	2325	1070	1023	159	73				
19. Argentina, Buenos Aires		Muller 1955	P	83	38	37	6	2	1·1921	0·5772	0·7354	0·4884
			C	29250	13889	11344	2982	1035				
20. Peru, Lima		Muñoz-Baratta 1962	P	145(c)	78	35	24	8	1·1395	0·4114	1·6094	4·1491
			C	107938(c)	66058	26013	12629	3238				
				6066					1·1596	19·9261	1·1343	7·0094
				χ_{19}^2 for homogeneity of areas						34·2954		17·4304

MALIGNANT NEOPLASMS OF OVARY

Place	Additional details	Authors		Number	O	A	B	AB	A/O Relative incidence	A/O χ_1^2 for difference from unity	B/O Relative incidence	B/O χ_1^2 for difference from unity
1. Austria, Wien	(s) Rh_D	Speiser 1958[b]	P	318	121	135	39	23	0·9522	0·1156	0·9099	0·2011
			C	1000	367	430	130	73				
2. Czechoslovakia		Matoušek 1935	P	15	2	8	3	2	3·1431	2·0909	2·6711	1·1535
		Leischner 1936 M1	C	2429	796	1013	447	173				

TABLE 1 THE ABO BLOOD GROUP SYSTEM (*cont.*)

Place	Additional details	Authors		Number	O	A	B	AB	A/O		B/O	
									Relative incidence	χ_1^2 for difference from unity	Relative incidence	χ_1^2 for difference from unity
3. Czechoslovakia		Miluničová *et al.* 1969[a]	P	50	11	28	7	4	1·7660	2·4625	1·1928	0·1285
		Kout 1959 M2	C	1142	358	516	191	77				
4. France, Haut-		Larrouy 1960	P	25	10	11	3	1	1·1246	0·0718	2·2898	1·5683
Languedoc			C	4367	2015	1971	264	117				
5. Germany,		Schröder 1955	P	70	20	38	9	3	1·6507	3·2738	1·1555	0·1290
Berlin		Pettenkofer *et al.* 1957 M1	C	12000	4437	5107	1728	728				
6. Germany,		Hoffbauer 1961	P	91	34	40	11	6	1·0671	0·0770	0·8379	0·2588
Berlin			C	15824	5959	6570	2301	994				
7. Germany,		Mosler 1961	P	67	19	36	9	3	1·5191	2·1523	1·2309	0·2610
Berlin			C	6128	2188	2729	842	369				
8. Germany,		Mosler & Wehle 1961	P	217	75	108	28	6	1·2667	2·3960	0·9151	0·1561
Berlin			C	6885	2537	2884	1035	429				
9. Germany,		Prokop *et al.* 1961	P	49	22	23	2	2	1·0280	0·0080	0·3155	2·3737
Bonn			C	706	295	300	85	26				
10. Germany,		Schwenzer 1961	P	13	2	8	2	1	3·6000	2·6152	3·6000	1·6313
Frankfurt am Main			C	2000	792	880	220	108				
11. Germany,		Preisler *et al.* 1959	P	65	21	33	5	6	1·5244	2·2475	0·9743	0·0027
Freiburg			C	4017	1686	1738	412	181				
12. Germany, Halle		Mazur & Alex 1961	P	101	34	49	13	5	1·1621	0·4444	0·9613	0·0144
an der Saale			C	5321	1878	2329	747	367				
13. Germany,		Krah *et al.* 1961	P	150	57	72	13	8	1·1161	0·3824	0·8495	0·2806
Heidelberg			C	34513	13748	15559	3691	1515				
14. Germany,		Scheffler 1961	P	69	20	31	12	6	1·5116	2·0705	1·7189	2·1945
Karl-Marx Stadt			C	25080	9967	10220	3479	1414				
15. Germany,		Zuber & Andreas 1961	P	173	59	83	23	8	1·1885	0·9724	0·9903	0·0015
Leipzig			C	3021	1100	1302	433	186				
16. Italy, Firenze		Cutrera & Leoni 1959	P	200	78	104	18	0	1·5066	7·3765	1·0723	0·0703
			C	13633	6259	5539	1347	488				
17. Italy, Milano		Dossena & Lanzara 1925	P	23	11	9	2	1	1·0490	0·0102	0·6993	0·2001
		Dossena 1924 M1	C	214	100	78	26	10				
18. Italy, Milano		Dambrosio 1965	P	89	25	53	10	1	2·0477	8·6851	1·5623	1·4147
		Garibaldi & Gianotti 1964 M2	C	16952	7081	7331	1813	727				
19. Italy, Napoli		Martella 1938	P	11	3	3	5	0	1·2275	0·0626	5·6070	5·4905
		Sanguigno & Aghina 1954 M1	C	1200	545	444	162	49				
20. Norway		Bergsjö & Kolstad 1962[a]	P	397	139	212	31	15	1·1527	1·6195	1·0328	0·0252
		Heistø 1956 M1	C	8292	3135	4148	677	332				
21. United	(s) A_1A_2	Walther *et al.* 1956	P	33	14	15	3	1	1·1207	0·0927	1·4420	0·3253
Kingdom, London, Leytonstone			C	2325	1070	1023	159	73				
22. S. India,		Ghooi *et al.* 1970	P	51	10	11	27	3	2·5143	3·2775	5·1840	13·6853
Bhopal			C	100	48	21	25	6				
23. U.S.A., Iowa		Buckwalter *et al.* 1964	P	445(c)	183	193	51	18	1·1169	1·1382	1·3292	3·1964
			C	49979	22392	21144	4695	1748				
24. U.S.A.,		Osborne & De George	P	453	187	200	47	19	1·1871	2·5837	0·8018	1·7003
New York		1963	C	4738	2029	1828	636	249				
				3175					1·2257	25·2147	1·0908	1·8988
				χ_{23}^2 for homogeneity of areas						21·0116		34·5643

TABLE 1 **THE ABO BLOOD GROUP SYSTEM** (*cont.*)

NEOPLASMS (*cont.*)

MALIGNANT NEOPLASMS (*cont.*)

MALIGNANT NEOPLASMS OF VAGINA

Place	Additional details	Authors		Number	O	A	B	AB	A/O		B/O	
									Relative incidence	χ_1^2 for difference from unity	Relative incidence	χ_1^2 for difference from unity
1. Austria, Wien	(s) Rh_D	Speiser 1958[b]	P	77	36	28	10	3	0·6638	2·4494	0·7842	0·4277
			C	1000	367	430	130	73				
2. Germany, Berlin		Hoffbauer 1961	P	44	18	20	4	2	1·0078	0·0006	0·5755	0·9971
			C	15824	5959	6570	2301	994				
3. Germany, Berlin		Mosler 1961	P	85	35	30	16	4	0·6872	2·2430	1·1879	0·3198
			C	6128	2188	2729	842	369				
4. Germany, Berlin		Mosler & Wehle 1961	P	114	32	53	19	10	1·4570	2·7851	1·4554	1·6522
			C	6885	2537	2884	1035	429				
5. Germany, Bonn		Prokop *et al.* 1961	P	55	19	26	8	2	1·3456	0·9009	1·4613	0·7464
			C	706	295	300	85	26				
6. Germany, Erfurt		Schuberth 1961	P	10	5	4	1	0	0·6681	0·3615	0·5519	0·2943
			C	45105	16630	19914	6026	2535				
7. Germany, Freiburg		Preisler & Matthes 1961	P	47	19	23	3	2	1·1743	0·2654	0·6461	0·4903
			C	4017	1686	1738	412	181				
8. Germany, Halle an der Saale		Mazur & Alex 1961	P	55	23	29	3	0	1·0167	0·0035	0·3279	3·2829
			C	5321	1878	2329	747	367				
9. Germany, Heidelberg		Krah *et al.* 1961	P	108	42	55	8	3	1·1571	0·5054	0·7095	0·7898
			C	34513	13748	15559	3691	1515				
10. Germany, Karl-Marx Stadt		Scheffler 1961	P	19	7	6	6	0	0·8359	0·1037	2·4556	2·6043
			C	25080	9967	10220	3479	1414				
11. Germany, Leipzig		Zuber & Andreas 1961	P	175	69	75	16	15	0·9183	0·2461	0·5891	3·4913
			C	3021	1100	1302	433	186				
				789					0·9969	0·0015	0·9153	0·5220
				χ_{10}^2 for homogeneity of areas						9·8629		14·5742

MALIGNANT NEOPLASMS OF VULVA

Place	Additional details	Authors		Number	O	A	B	AB	A/O Relative incidence	A/O χ_1^2	B/O Relative incidence	B/O χ_1^2
1. Austria, Wien	(s) Rh_D	Speiser 1958[b]	P	74	23	41	10	0	1·5214	2·4151	1·2274	0·2729
			C	1000	367	430	130	73				
2. Germany, Berlin		Schröder 1955	P	31	9	13	5	4	1·2549	0·2736	1·4265	0·4046
		Pettenkofer *et al.* 1957 M1	C	12000	4437	5107	1728	728				
3. Germany, Freiburg		Preisler *et al.* 1959	P	19	5	13	1	0	2·5222	3·0777	0·8184	0·0334
			C	4017	1686	1738	412	181				
4. United Kingdom, Belfast		Macafee 1973	P	75	40	28	6	1	1·1662	0·3881	0·8724	0·0970
			C	28566	15715	9433	2702	716				
				199					1·3884	4·2043	1·1065	0·1613
				χ_3^2 for homogeneity of areas						1·9503		0·6465

MALIGNANT NEOPLASMS OF UTERUS, OVARY

Place	Additional details	Authors		Number	O	A	B	AB	A/O Relative incidence	A/O χ_1^2	B/O Relative incidence	B/O χ_1^2
1. Bulgaria	294 cervix uteri, 28 corpus uteri, 66 ovary	Zographov 1962	P	388	127	168	65	28	0·9606	0·1142	1·0201	0·0166
			C	15422	4953	6821	2485	1163				
2. Italy, Milano		Visconti *et al.* 1961[a]	P	188	69	95	18	6	1·3235	3·0795	1·0046	0·0003
			C	9607	3974	4134	1032	467				
3. Italy, Napoli		Spena & Grippo 1964	P	191	63	95	24	9	1·7402	10·7398	1·7772	5·2263
			C	2147	989	857	212	89				
				767					1·2095	5·2380	1·1494	1·3903
				χ_2^2 for homogeneity of areas						8·6956		3·8529

TABLE 1 **THE ABO BLOOD GROUP SYSTEM** (*cont.*)

Place	Additional details	Authors		Number	O	A	B	AB	A/O Relative incidence	A/O χ_1^2 for difference from unity	B/O Relative incidence	B/O χ_1^2 for difference from unity
MALIGNANT NEOPLASMS OF CORPUS UTERI, OVARY, VAGINA, VULVA												
1. N. India, Calcutta		Mitra *et al.* 1962	P C	58 2273	13 740	19 594	20 777	6 162	1·8208	2·7085	1·4652	1·1262
MALIGNANT NEOPLASMS OF FALLOPIAN TUBE, VAGINA, VULVA												
1. Italy, Milano		Dambrosio 1965 Garibaldi & Gianotti 1964 M2	P C	26 16952	12 7081	10 7331	3 1813	1 727	0·8049	0·2565	0·9764	0·0014
MALIGNANT NEOPLASMS OF UNSPECIFIED FEMALE GENITAL ORGANS												
1. Finland, Helsinki		Krokfors & Kinnunen 1954	P C	300 310	113 89	110 139	57 48	20 25	0·6863	4·0094	1·0299	0·0151
2. Germany, Berlin		Pettenkofer & Tomascheck 1961	P C	406 9000	147 3328	168 3830	70 1296	21 546	0·9931	0·0036	1·2228	1·8259
3. Germany, Heidelberg		Helmbold *et al.* 1958	P C	46 6117	19 2507	22 2657	3 667	2 286	1·0925	0·0792	0·5935	0·7019
4. Germany, Köln		Guthof 1961	P C	116 5000	40 1947	62 2305	10 516	4 232	1·3093	1·7257	0·9433	0·0267
5. Italy, Trieste		Tagliaferro 1937[a] Goldstein 1927, 1929 M1	P C	103 1766	40 681	42 672	17 284	4 129	1·0641	0·0745	1·0191	0·0040
6. N. India, Calcutta	Organs other than cervix uteri	Mitra *et al.* 1962	P C	58 2273	13 740	19 594	20 777	6 162	1·8208	2·7085	1·4652	1·1262
7. Argentina	Whites	Estevez 1963	P C	223(c) 21715(c)	104 11165	80 8123	30 1836	9 591	1·0573	0·1391	1·7542	7·2470
8. New Zealand, Auckland		Cotter *et al.* 1961	P C	434(c) 13493(c)	194 6367	194 5467	27 1218	19 441	1·1646	2·1809	0·7275	2·3440
				1686					1·0635	1·1486	1·1267	1·9659
				χ_7^2 for homogeneity of areas						9·7723		11·3249
MALIGNANT NEOPLASMS OF PROSTATE												
1. Germany, Tübingen		Brockmüller 1962	P C	256 39031	111 16283	113 16745	26 4298	6 1705	0·9899	0·0057	0·8874	0·2988
2. Italy, Milano		Visconti *et al.* 1961[a]	P C	111 9607	49 3974	46 4134	12 1032	4 467	0·9024	0·2471	0·9430	0·0328
3. Italy, Napoli		Spena & Grippo 1964	P C	93 2147	44 989	34 857	9 212	6 89	0·8917	0·2417	0·9542	0·0157
4. Italy, Torino		Cavalli *et al.* 1964	P C	152 2360	56 1056	81 971	15 236	0 97	1·5730	6·3774	1·1985	0·3656
5. Italy, Veneto		Mobilio & Torchiana 1960	P C	149 1093	56 536	81 382	8 126	4 49	2·0295	14·4436	0·6077	1·6249
6. United Kingdom, London		Bourke & Griffin 1962	P C	224(c) 10000	82 4578	113 4219	20 890	9 313	1·4953	7·5289	1·2546	0·8096
7. United Kingdom, London, Leytonstone	(s) A_1A_2	Walther *et al.* 1956	P C	45 2325	23 1070	19 1023	2 159	1 73	0·8640	0·2179	0·5852	0·5214
8. U.S.A., Iowa		Buckwalter *et al.* 1958	P C	376(c) 6313	167 2892	153 2626	37 568	19 227	1·0090	0·0060	1·1281	0·4135
9. Peru, Lima		Muñoz-Baratta 1962	P C	61(c) 107938	36 66058	16 26013	7 12629	2 3238	1·1286	0·1621	1·0171	0·0017
				1467					1·1756	7·8693	1·0140	0·0139
				χ_8^2 for homogeneity of areas						21·3610		4·0701

TABLE 1 THE ABO BLOOD GROUP SYSTEM (*cont.*)

Place	Additional details	Authors		Number	O	A	B	AB	A/O Relative incidence	A/O χ_1^2 for difference from unity	B/O Relative incidence	B/O χ_1^2 for difference from unity
NEOPLASMS (*cont.*)												
MALIGNANT NEOPLASMS (*cont.*)												
MALIGNANT NEOPLASMS OF SEMINAL VESICLE												
1. S. India, Bhopal		Ghooi *et al.* 1970	P	57	26	9	22	0	0·7912	0·2516	1·6246	1·6269
			C	100	48	21	25	6				
MALIGNANT NEOPLASMS OF PENIS												
1. N. India, Kanpur		Tyagi *et al.* 1965	P	29	8	12	8	1	2·1893	2·9299	0·8714	0·0755
			C	6000	1985	1360	2278	377				
2. S. India, Bhopal		Ghooi *et al.* 1970	P	54	16	4	24	10	0·5714	0·8221	2·8800	6·7813
			C	100	48	21	25	6				
				83					1·4591	0·6963	1·7930	3·4230
					χ_1^2 for homogeneity of areas					3·0557		3·4338
MALIGNANT NEOPLASMS OF KIDNEY												
1. France, Haut-Languedoc		Larrouy 1960	P	23	7	10	3	3	1·4605	0·5883	3·2711	2·9232
			C	4367	2015	1971	264	117				
2. Germany, Tübingen		Brockmüller 1962	P	143	61	63	13	6	1·0043	0·0006	0·8074	0·4890
			C	39031	16283	16745	4298	1705				
3. Iceland		Bjarnason *et al.* 1973	P	65	40	17	7	1	0·7451	1·0304	0·9052	0·0590
			C	26716	14783	8432	2858	643				
4. Italy, Milano		Visconti *et al.* 1961[a]	P	71	32	31	7	1	0·9313	0·0793	0·8424	0·1679
			C	9607	3974	4134	1032	467				
5. Italy, Veneto		Mobilio & Torchiana 1960	P	79	28	32	12	7	1·6036	3·1214	1·8231	2·7991
			C	1093	536	382	126	49				
6. United Kingdom, London	Nephro-blastoma in children	Atwell 1962	P	78	25	45	6	2	1·9532	7·1503	1·2345	0·2134
			C	10000	4578	4219	890	313				
7. United Kingdom, London, Leytonstone	(s) A_1A_2	Walther *et al.* 1956	P	17	8	9	0	0	1·1767	0·1112		
			C	2325	1070	1023	159	73				
8. U.S.S.R., Moscow	Nephro-blastoma in children	Bubnov & Kirdan 1972	P	167	59	61	33	14	0·9888	0·0033	0·9167	0·1402
			C	1148	395	413	241	99				
9. S. India, Bhopal		Ghooi *et al.* 1970	P	74	31	14	27	2	1·0323	0·0059	1·6723	2·0317
			C	100	48	21	25	6				
				717					1·1232	1·7349	1·1105	0·6941
					χ_8^2 for homogeneity of areas					10·3556		
				(700)	χ_7^2 for homogeneity of areas							8·1293
MALIGNANT NEOPLASMS OF BLADDER												
1. Austria, Wien	(s) S, Rh_D	Speiser 1958[a]	P	131	36	66	18	11	1·5647	4·1777	1·4115	1·2672
			C	1000	367	430	130	73				
2. Germany, Tübingen	(s) A_1A_2	Dick *et al.* 1962	P	145	45	72	21	7	1·5559	5·3926	1·7680	4·6297
			C	39031	16283	16745	4298	1705				
3. Italy, Milano		Visconti *et al.* 1961[a]	P	112	48	51	10	3	1·0214	0·0109	0·8022	0·3978
			C	9607	3974	4134	1032	467				
4. Italy, Veneto		Mobilio & Torchiana 1960	P	275	99	115	39	22	1·6299	10·2516	1·6758	5·8528
			C	1093	536	382	126	49				
5. United Kingdom, London, Leytonstone	(s) A_1A_2	Walther *et al.* 1956	P	25	16	7	1	1	0·4576	2·9486	0·4206	0·7012
			C	2325	1070	1023	159	73				

TABLE 1 **THE ABO BLOOD GROUP SYSTEM** *(cont.)*

Place	Additional details	Authors		Number	O	A	B	AB	A/O Relative incidence	A/O χ^2_1 for difference from unity	B/O Relative incidence	B/O χ^2_1 for difference from unity
6. N. India, Kanpur		Tyagi *et al.* 1965	P	18	3	5	8	2	2·4326	1·4783	2·3237	1·5479
			C	6000	1985	1360	2278	377				
7. S. India, Bhopal		Ghooi *et al.* 1970	P	22	12	3	7	0	0·5714	0·6456	1·1200	0·0447
			C	100	48	21	25	6				
8. Egypt, Alexandria		Sadek *et al.* 1965[a]	P	19	6	4	5	4	0·5763	0·7260	0·9801	0·0011
			C	3720	1142	1321	971	286				
9. Peru, Lima		Muñoz-Baratta 1962	P	40	26	11	1	2	1·0744	0·0398	0·2012	2·4759
			C	107938	66058	26013	12629	3238				
				787					1·3359	11·2958	1·3823	6·8479
				χ^2_8 for homogeneity of areas						14·3752		10·0705
MALIGNANT NEOPLASMS OF BLADDER, PROSTATE												
1. Italy, Trieste		Tagliaferro 1937[a]	P	12	2	8	2	0	4·0536	3·1194	2·3979	0·7611
		Goldstein 1927, 1929 M1	C	1766	681	672	284	129				
NEOPLASMS OF NERVOUS SYSTEM												
RETINOBLASTOMAS												
1. United Kingdom, Manchester	Children	Gaisford & Campbell 1958	P	13	3	7	2	1	2·8012	2·2259	3·8342	2·1636
			C	9370	4532	3775	788	275				
GLIOMAS												
1. United Kingdom, Manchester	Children	Gaisford & Campbell 1958	P	70	23	40	6	1	2·0879	7·8579	1·5003	0·7777
			C	9370	4532	3775	788	275				
2. U.S.A., Boston		Mayr *et al.* 1956	P	25	12	10	2	1	0·9614	0·0085	0·7068	0·2064
			C	120281	55089	47752	12990	4450				
3. U.S.A., Iowa		Buckwalter *et al.* 1959	P	62	26	31	4	1	1·2627	0·7682	0·7337	0·3320
			C	49979	22392	21144	4695	1748				
				157					1·4972	5·5510	1·0256	0·0063
				χ^2_2 for homogeneity of areas						3·0836		1·3097
ASTROCYTOMAS												
1. Italy, Padova		Iraci & Carteri 1964	P	565	255	242	52	16	1·0709	0·3688	1·0021	0·0001
			C	1000	457	405	93	45				
2. Sweden	(s) S	Strang *et al.* 1966	P	900	325	459	81	35	1·1364	2·8621	0·9523	0·1433
			C	10457	3974	4939	1040	504				
3. United Kingdom, Manchester	(s) C	Pearce & Yates 1965	P	548	238	237	51	22	1·1955	3·5795	1·2324	1·7262
			C	9370	4532	3775	788	275				
4. U.S.A., Boston		Mayr *et al.* 1956	P	159	73	64	19	3	1·0114	0·0044	1·1038	0·1468
			C	120281	55089	47752	12990	4450				
5. U.S.A., Boston		Selverstone & Cooper 1961	P	139	46	72	10	11	1·8057	9·7913	0·9219	0·0542
			C	120281	55089	47752	12990	4450				
6. U.S.A., Iowa		Buckwalter *et al.* 1959	P	215	93	101	18	3	1·1501	0·9430	0·9231	0·0962
			C	49979	22392	21144	4695	1748				
7. U.S.A., New York		Garcia *et al.* 1963	P	132	62	45	20	5	1·1634	0·3682	1·0342	0·0108
			C	219	109	68	34	8				
				2658					1·1620	11·1056	1·0308	0·1616
				χ^2_6 for homogeneity of areas						6·8117		2·0160

TABLE 1 **THE ABO BLOOD GROUP SYSTEM** *(cont.)*

Place	Additional details	Authors		Number	O	A	B	AB	A/O Relative incidence	A/O χ^2_1 for difference from unity	B/O Relative incidence	B/O χ^2_1 for difference from unity
NEOPLASMS *(cont.)*												
MALIGNANT NEOPLASMS (cont.)												
NEOPLASMS OF NERVOUS SYSTEM *(cont.)*												
GLIOBLASTOMAS												
1. United Kingdom, Manchester	(s) C	Pearce & Yates 1965	P	373	168	169	31	5	1·2077	2·8820	1·0612	0·0890
			C	9370	4532	3775	788	275				
2. United Kingdom, Oxford		Carter *et al.* 1964	P	160	74	74	11	1	1·0269	0·0256	0·8160	0·3913
		Kopeć 1970	C	11662	5237	5100	954	371				
3. U.S.A., Boston		Mayr *et al.* 1956	P	183	78	72	26	7	1·0649	0·1478	1·4136	2·3323
			C	120281	55089	47752	12990	4450				
4. U.S.A., Iowa		Buckwalter *et al.* 1959	P	128	62	57	7	2	0·9736	0·0212	0·5385	2·4063
			C	49979	22392	21144	4695	1748				
				844					1·1013	1·7179	1·0409	0·0972
				χ^2_3 for homogeneity of areas						1·3587		5·1216
EPENDYMOMAS												
1. Italy, Padova		Iraci & Carteri 1964	P	56	27	25	4	0	1·0448	0·0235	0·7280	0·3360
			C	1000	457	405	93	45				
2. United Kingdom, Manchester	(s) C	Pearce & Yates 1965	P	104	47	45	9	3	1·1494	0·4410	1·1013	0·0696
			C	9370	4532	3775	788	275				
3. U.S.A., Boston		Mayr *et al.* 1956	P	18	9	8	1	0	1·0255	0·0027	0·4712	0·5095
			C	120281	55089	47752	12990	4450				
				178					1·1020	0·3701	0·9170	0·0880
				χ^2_2 for homogeneity of areas						0·0971		0·8271
OLIGODENDROGLIOMAS												
1. Italy, Padova		Iraci & Carteri 1964	P	63	24	26	9	4	1·2224	0·4757	1·8427	2·2546
			C	1000	457	405	93	45				
2. United Kingdom, Manchester	(s) C	Pearce & Yates 1965	P	59	30	25	2	2	1·0004	0·0000	0·3834	1·7183
			C	9370	4532	3775	788	275				
				122					1·0982	0·2225	1·2711	0·4548
				χ^2_1 for homogeneity of areas						0·2532		3·5180
MEDULLOBLASTOMAS												
1. Italy, Padova		Iraci & Carteri 1964	P	46	13	27	6	0	2·3436	6·1152	2·2680	2·6141
			C	1000	457	405	93	45				
2. United Kingdom, London	Children	Atwell 1962	P	48	22	19	4	3	0·9371	0·0428	0·9352	0·0151
			C	10000	4578	4219	890	313				
3. United Kingdom, Manchester	(s) C	Pearce & Yates 1965	P	102	46	49	4	3	1·2788	1·4188	0·5001	1·7573
			C	9370	4532	3775	788	275				
4. U.S.A., Iowa		Buckwalter *et al.* 1959	P	19	8	8	3	0	1·0590	0·0132	1·7885	0·7370
			C	49979	22392	21144	4695	1748				
				215					1·3125	3·4047	1·1383	0·2200
				χ^2_3 for homogeneity of areas						4·1852		4·9035

TABLE 1 **THE ABO BLOOD GROUP SYSTEM** *(cont.)*

Place	Additional details	Authors		Number	O	A	B	AB	A/O Relative incidence	A/O χ_1^2 for difference from unity	B/O Relative incidence	B/O χ_1^2 for difference from unity
Meningiomas												
1. Italy, Padova		Iraci & Toffolo 1964[b]	P	470	184	196	70	20	1·2020	2·2276	1·8694	11·9845
			C	1000	457	405	93	45				
2. United Kingdom, Manchester		MacLeod 1937	P	18	9	7	1	1	0·9221	0·0256	0·7050	0·1092
			C	1927	939	792	148	48				
3. United Kingdom, Manchester		Yates & Pearce 1960	P	322	155	131	27	9	1·0146	0·0145	1·0018	0·0001
			C	9370	4532	3775	788	275				
4. United Kingdom, Manchester	(s) C	Pearce & Yates 1965	P	406	193	166	36	11	1·0326	0·0879	1·0728	0·1433
			C	9370	4532	3775	788	275				
5. U.S.A., Boston		Mayr *et al.* 1956	P	164	71	63	24	6	1·0237	0·0182	1·4335	2·3225
			C	120281	55089	47752	12990	4450				
				1380					1·0655	1·0344	1·3124	7·4417
				χ_4^2 for homogeneity of areas						1·3395		7·1179
Neuromas												
1. Italy, Padova	Acoustic	Iraci & Carteri 1964	P	114	35	66	7	6	2·1273	11·7854	0·9828	0·0016
			C	1000	457	405	93	45				
2. United Kingdom, London	Neuro-blastomas in children	Atwell 1962	P	83	37	35	6	5	1·0264	0·0121	0·8341	0·1686
			C	10000	4578	4219	890	313				
3. United Kingdom, Manchester	Acoustic and other	MacLeod 1937	P	23	11	9	2	1	0·9700	0·0045	1·1536	0·0341
			C	1927	939	792	148	48				
4. United Kingdom, Manchester	Neurilemoma; (s) C	Pearce & Yates 1965	P	204	101	84	15	4	0·9985	0·0001	0·8541	0·3184
			C	9370	4532	3775	788	275				
5. U.S.A., Boston	Acoustic	Mayr *et al.* 1956	P	59	26	24	7	2	1·0649	0·0493	1·1418	0·0969
			C	120281	55089	47752	12990	4450				
				483					1·1796	2·7485	0·9343	0·1409
				χ_4^2 for homogeneity of areas						9·1030		0·4788
Malignant Neurogenous Neoplasms												
1. U.S.S.R., Moscow	Children	Bubnov & Kirdan 1972	P	81	27	29	17	8	1·0273	0·0095	1·0320	0·0097
			C	1148	395	413	241	99				
Malignant Neoplasms of Brain												
1. Italy, Napoli		Spena & Grippo 1964	P	61	28	23	7	3	0·9479	0·0351	1·1663	0·1284
			C	2147	989	857	212	89				
2. United Kingdom, London, Leytonstone	(s) A_1A_2	Walther *et al.* 1956	P	13	7	4	2	0	0·5977	0·6711	1·9227	0·6574
			C	2325	1070	1023	159	73				
				74					0·8761	0·2594	1·3024	0·4863
				χ_1^2 for homogeneity of areas						0·4468		0·2995
Metastatic Neoplasms of Brain												
1. U.S.A., Iowa		Buckwalter *et al.* 1959	P	65	28	31	4	2	1·1725	0·3720	0·6813	0·5148
			C	49979	22392	21144	4695	1748				
Benign Neoplasms of Brain												
1. U.S.A., Iowa		Buckwalter *et al.* 1959	P	77	29	40	7	1	1·4607	2·4102	1·1512	0·1117
			C	49979	22392	21144	4695	1748				
2. Peru, Lima		Muñoz-Baratta 1962	P	66(c)	28	29	4	5	2·6301	13·3115	0·7472	0·2970
			C	107938(c)	66058	26013	12629	3238				
				143					1·9132	13·0577	0·9755	0·0056
				χ_1^2 for homogeneity of areas						2·6640		0·4031

TABLE 1 THE ABO BLOOD GROUP SYSTEM (*cont.*)

NEOPLASMS (*cont.*)
MALIGNANT NEOPLASMS (*cont.*)
NEOPLASMS OF NERVOUS SYSTEM (*cont.*)

UNSPECIFIED NEOPLASMS OF BRAIN

Place	Additional details	Authors		Number	O	A	B	AB	A/O Relative incidence	A/O χ_1^2 for difference from unity	B/O Relative incidence	B/O χ_1^2 for difference from unity
1. Austria, Wien	(s) S, Rh_D	Speiser 1958[a]	P	1264	444	564	171	85	1·0842	0·7195	1·0873	0·3780
			C	1000	367	430	130	73				
2. Japan, Sendai		Moniwa 1960	P	97	34	35	22	6	0·8950	0·2114	0·9074	0·1256
			C	21199	6769	7786	4827	1817				
3. U.S.A., Boston		Mayr *et al.* 1956	P	29	13	11	2	3	0·9762	0·0035	0·6524	0·3160
			C	120281	55089	47752	12990	4450				
4. U.S.A., New York	Other than astrocytomas	Garcia *et al.* 1963	P	279	133	89	45	12	1·0726	0·1153	1·0847	0·0967
			C	219	109	68	34	8				
				1669					1·0557	0·4609	1·0449	0·1615
				χ_3^2 for homogeneity of areas						0·5888		0·7549

NEOPLASMS OF SYMPATHETIC SYSTEM

Place	Additional details	Authors		Number	O	A	B	AB	A/O Relative incidence	A/O χ_1^2 for difference from unity	B/O Relative incidence	B/O χ_1^2 for difference from unity
1. United Kingdom, Manchester	Children	Gaisford & Campbell 1958	P	30	11	15	2	2	1·6371	1·5372	1·0457	0·0034
			C	9370	4532	3775	788	275				

VASCULAR NEOPLASMS OF CENTRAL NERVOUS SYSTEM

Place	Additional details	Authors		Number	O	A	B	AB	A/O Relative incidence	A/O χ_1^2 for difference from unity	B/O Relative incidence	B/O χ_1^2 for difference from unity
1. United Kingdom, Manchester	Non-glial; (s) C	Pearce & Yates 1965	P	107	53	44	8	2	0·9967	0·0003	0·8681	0·1376
			C	9370	4532	3775	788	275				

NEOPLASMS OF LYMPHATIC AND HAEMATOPOIETIC TISSUE

HODGKIN'S DISEASE, LYMPHOGRANULOMA

Place	Additional details	Authors		Number	O	A	B	AB	A/O Relative incidence	A/O χ_1^2 for difference from unity	B/O Relative incidence	B/O χ_1^2 for difference from unity
1. Czechoslovakia, Praha	Lympho-granuloma	Májský 1964	P	85	29	39	12	5	0·9356	0·0682	0·7778	0·5020
		Kout 1959 M2	C	1142	359	516	191	76				
2. Italy, Cagliari	Lympho-granuloma	Adamo 1961[a, c]	P	10	3	6	1	0	3·5346	3·1797	2·6192	0·6931
		Boero & Coraddu 1965	C	3516	2043	1156	260	57				
3. Italy, Lombardia	Lympho-granuloma	Ninni & Bedarida 1959	P	37	14	16	6	1	1·1225	0·0947	2·1122	2·1540
			C	640	276	281	56	27				
4. Italy, Milano	Lympho-granuloma	Visconti *et al.* 1961[a]	P	117	44	54	16	3	1·1798	0·6548	1·4003	1·3112
			C	9607	3974	4134	1032	467				
5. Italy, Perugia	Lympho-granuloma	Benda & Menghini 1957	P	96	51	31	11	3	0·6148	4·5061	0·8713	0·1693
			C	7356	3163	3127	783	283				
6. Netherlands, Leiden	Hodgkin's Disease; (s) A_1A_2	Does *et al.* 1972	P	46	25	19	2	0	1·0133	0·0008	0·2667	2·3084
			C	42	20	15	6	1				
7. Poland, Kraków	Lympho-granuloma; (s) children and adults	Cichecka 1965	P	160	54	58	32	16	0·8677	0·5605	0·9337	0·0941
			C	39006	12457	15419	7906	3224				
8. Poland, Warszawa	Hodgkin's Disease	Królikowska & Żupańska 1964	P	234	88	86	34	26	0·8988	0·4865	0·6558	4·3036
		Charzewski *et al.* 1965 M2	C	13744	4719	5131	2780	1114				
9. United Kingdom, London	Hodgkin's Disease	Kay & Shorter 1956	P	80	35	39	6	0	1·2122	0·6774	0·8398	0·1551
		Discombe 1954 M1	C	10000	4556	4188	930	326				
10. United Kingdom, London, Leytonstone	Hodgkin's Disease	Walther *et al.* 1956	P	11	3	8	0	0	2·7892	2·2861		
			C	2325	1070	1023	159	73				

TABLE 1 **THE ABO BLOOD GROUP SYSTEM** (*cont.*)

Place	Additional details	Authors		Number	O	A	B	AB	A/O Relative incidence	A/O χ^2_1 for difference from unity	B/O Relative incidence	B/O χ^2_1 for difference from unity
11. United Kingdom, Manchester	Hodgkin's Disease	Harris *et al.* 1972	P	46	25	17	3	1	0·7695	0·4627	0·7371	0·1724
			C	90	43	38	7	2				
12. U.S.S.R., Moscow	Lympho-granuloma in children	Bubnov & Kirdan 1972	P	229	90	73	51	15	0·7758	2·1662	0·9288	0·1460
			C	1148	395	413	241	99				
13. U.S.A., New York	Hodgkin's Disease	Levitan *et al.* 1959	P	500	224	174	73	29	0·8488	2·5393	1·0622	0·1922
			C	12917(c)	5531	5062	1697	627				
				1651					0·8998	3·3228	0·9452	0·5235
					χ^2_{12} for homogeneity of areas					14·3602		
				(1640)	χ^2_{11} for homogeneity of areas							11·6779

LYMPHOSARCOMAS

Place	Additional details	Authors		Number	O	A	B	AB	A/O Relative incidence	A/O χ^2_1 for difference from unity	B/O Relative incidence	B/O χ^2_1 for difference from unity
1. Italy, Cagliari		Adamo 1961[a, c]	P	17	3	13	0	1	7·6583	10·0688		
		Boero & Coraddu 1965	C	3516	2043	1156	260	57				
2. Peru, Lima		Muñoz-Baratta 1962	P	84(c)	40	26	17	1	1·6506	3·9543	2·2230	7·6050
			C	107938(c)	66058	26013	12629	3238				
				101					2·0265	9·0663		
					χ^2_1 for homogeneity of areas					4·9568		

RETICULOSARCOMAS

Place	Additional details	Authors		Number	O	A	B	AB	A/O Relative incidence	A/O χ^2_1 for difference from unity	B/O Relative incidence	B/O χ^2_1 for difference from unity
1. U.S.S.R., Moscow	Children	Bubnov & Kirdan 1972	P	166	46	77	33	10	1·6010	5·5814	1·1758	0·4467
			C	1148	395	413	241	99				

LYMPHOSARCOMAS, RETICULOSARCOMAS

Place	Additional details	Authors		Number	O	A	B	AB	A/O Relative incidence	A/O χ^2_1 for difference from unity	B/O Relative incidence	B/O χ^2_1 for difference from unity
1. Japan, Sendai		Moniwa 1960	P	50	12	17	18	3	1·2316	0·3047	2·1035	3·9710
			C	21199	6769	7786	4827	1817				

RETICULO-ENDOTHELIAL NEOPLASMS

Place	Additional details	Authors		Number	O	A	B	AB	A/O Relative incidence	A/O χ^2_1 for difference from unity	B/O Relative incidence	B/O χ^2_1 for difference from unity
1. United Kingdom,	Other than leukaemia	Gaisford & Campbell 1958	P	37	19	14	4	0	0·8846	0·1207	1·2108	0·1203
			C	9370	4532	3775	788	275				

RETICULOSES

Place	Additional details	Authors		Number	O	A	B	AB	A/O Relative incidence	A/O χ^2_1 for difference from unity	B/O Relative incidence	B/O χ^2_1 for difference from unity
1. Czechoslovakia, Praha		Májský 1964	P	43	9	24	8	2	1·8553	2·4252	1·6707	1·0791
		Kout 1959 M2	C	1142	359	516	191	76				
2. Poland, Kraków	(s) Children and adults	Cichecka 1965	P	102	30	48	21	3	1·2926	1·2131	1·1029	0·1183
			C	39006	12457	15419	7906	3224				
				145					1·4181	3·0219	1·2234	0·6672
					χ^2_1 for homogeneity of areas					0·6165		0·5302

LYMPHOMAS

Place	Additional details	Authors		Number	O	A	B	AB	A/O Relative incidence	A/O χ^2_1 for difference from unity	B/O Relative incidence	B/O χ^2_1 for difference from unity
1. N. India, Kanpur		Tyagi *et al.* 1965	P	30	8	5	14	3	0·9122	0·0259	1·5249	0·9020
			C	6000	1985	1360	2278	377				
2. Nigeria	Burkitt's lymphoma in Yoruba children	Williams 1966	P	100	53	23	21	3	1·1222	0·1816	0·8572	0·3122
			C	636(c)	331	128	153	24				
				130					1·0804	0·1001	1·0061	0·0007
					χ^2_1 for homogeneity of areas					0·1074		1·2135

TABLE 1 **THE ABO BLOOD GROUP SYSTEM** (*cont.*)

Place	Additional details	Authors		Number	O	A	B	AB	A/O Relative incidence	A/O χ_1^2 for difference from unity	B/O Relative incidence	B/O χ_1^2 for difference from unity
NEOPLASMS (*cont.*)												
MALIGNANT NEOPLASMS (*cont.*)												
NEOPLASMS OF LYMPHATIC AND HAEMATOPOIETIC TISSUE (*cont.*)												
OTHER AND UNSPECIFIED NEOPLASMS OF LYMPHATIC AND HAEMATOPOIETIC TISSUE												
1. Iceland		Bjarnason *et al.* 1973	P	165	77	45	30	13	1·0246	0·0167	2·0153	10·5064
			C	26716	14783	8432	2858	643				
2. Argentina	Leukaemias, lymphomas; Whites	Estevez 1963	P	68	28	34	6	0	1·6690	4·0158	1·3031	0·3453
			C	21715	11165	8123	1836	591				
				233					1·2163	1·6693	1·8570	10·0873
					χ_1^2 for homogeneity of areas					2·3632		0·7644
MYELOID LEUKAEMIA, ACUTE												
1. Poland, Kraków	(s) children and adults	Cichecka 1965	P	301	102	105	74	20	0·8317	1·7449	1·1431	0·7605
			C	39006	12457	15419	7906	3224				
2. Poland, Warszawa		Królikowska & Żupańska 1964	P	215	71	76	47	21	0·9845	0·0089	1·1237	0·3785
		Charzewski *et al.* 1965 M2	C	13744	4719	5131	2780	1114				
3. United Kingdom, England and Wales		Hewitt & Spiers 1964	P	309	158	113	30	8	0·7763	4·2141	1·0727	0·1237
			C	134641	62216	57317	11013	4095				
4. U.S.A., San Francisco	97% Whites	Lucia *et al.* 1958	P	25	13	11	1	0	0·9544	0·0129	0·3048	1·3082
			C	5175	2318	2055	585	217				
				850					0·8442	4·5636	1·1046	0·9547
					χ_3^2 for homogeneity of areas					1·4172		1·6161
MYELOID LEUKAEMIA, CHRONIC												
1. Belgium, Gent		Goeminne 1962	P	26	11	11	2	2	1·2012	0·1836	1·3715	0·1676
			C	3704	1833	1526	243	102				
2. Czechoslovakia, Praha		Májský 1964	P	75	27	34	8	6	0·8761	0·2458	0·5569	2·0148
		Kout 1959 M2	C	1142	359	516	191	76				
3. Italy, Lombardia		Ninni & Bedarida 1959	P	48	15	26	6	1	1·7025	2·5209	1·9714	1·8080
			C	640	276	281	56	27				
4. Italy, Cagliari		Adamo 1961[a, c]	P	10	3	6	0	1	3·5346	3·1797		
		Boero & Coraddu 1965	C	3516	2043	1156	260	57				
5. Poland, Kraków		Cichecka 1965	P	175	40	73	45	17	1·4744	3·8809	1·7726	6·9091
			C	39006	12457	15419	7906	3224				
6. Poland, Kraków		Gurda & Turowska 1970	P	45	11	24	8	2	1·7627	2·4209	1·1459	0·0858
			C	39006	12457	15419	7906	3224				
7. Poland, Warszawa		Królikowska & Żupańska 1964	P	262	73	113	53	23	1·4237	5·4353	1·2324	1·3179
		Charzewski *et al.* 1965 M2	C	13744	4719	5131	2780	1114				
8. U.S.A., Rochester		Tinney & Watkins 1941	P	90(c)	46	32	8	4	0·7280	1·7514	0·9783	0·0030
			C	1000(c)	450	430	80	40				
9. U.S.A., San Francisco		Lucia *et al.* 1958	P	80	31	38	7	4	1·3827	1·7648	0·8947	0·0698
			C	5175	2318	2055	585	217				
				811					1·2897	9·1541	1·2551	4·0879
					χ_8^2 for homogeneity of areas					12·2292		
				(801)	χ_7^2 for homogeneity of areas							8·2881
MYELOID LEUKAEMIAS, UNSPECIFIED												
1. Italy, Milano		Visconti *et al.* 1961[a]	P	78	27	39	8	4	1·3885	1·7057	1·1410	0·1065
			C	9607	3974	4134	1032	467				
2. United Kingdom, London		Kay & Shorter 1956	P	45	17	19	6	3	1·2159	0·3413	1·7290	1·3221
		Discombe 1954 M1	C	10000	4556	4188	930	326				
				123					1·3236	1·9463	1·3578	0·9856
					χ_1^2 for homogeneity of areas					0·1007		0·4430

TABLE 1 **THE ABO BLOOD GROUP SYSTEM** (*cont.*)

Place	Additional details	Authors		Number	O	A	B	AB	A/O Relative incidence	A/O χ^2_1 for difference from unity	B/O Relative incidence	B/O χ^2_1 for difference from unity
LYMPHATIC LEUKAEMIA, ACUTE												
1. U.S.A., San Francisco	97% Whites	Lucia *et al.* 1958	P	103	41	46	14	2	1·2655	1·1788	1·3530	0·9331
			C	5175	2318	2055	585	217				
LYMPHATIC LEUKAEMIA, CHRONIC												
1. Belgium, Gent		Goeminne 1962	P	11	8	2	0	1	0·3003	2·3111		
			C	3704	1833	1526	243	102				
2. Czechoslovakia, Praha		Májský 1964	P	73	25	27	14	7	0·7514	0·9992	1·0526	0·0220
		Kout 1959 M2	C	1142	359	516	191	76				
3. Italy, Lombardia		Ninni & Bedarida 1959	P	49	16	24	5	4	1·4733	1·3486	1·5402	0·6569
			C	640	276	281	56	27				
4. Poland, Kraków		Gurda & Turowska 1970	P	78	22	35	15	6	1·2853	0·8493	1·0743	0·0457
			C	39006	12457	15419	7906	3224				
5. Poland, Warszawa		Królikowska & Żupańska 1964	P	262	106	89	47	20	0·7722	3·1706	0·7527	2·5810
		Charzewski *et al.* 1965 M2	C	13744	4719	5131	2780	1114				
6. U.S.A., Rochester		Tinney & Watkins 1941	P	53(c)	21	21	9	2	1·0465	0·0207	2·4107	4·4638
			C	1000(c)	450	430	80	40				
7. U.S.A., San Francisco		Lucia *et al.* 1958	P	91	35	43	8	5	1·3858	2·0184	0·9057	0·0630
			C	5175	2318	2055	585	217				
				617					0·9636	0·1547	0·9688	0·0653
					χ^2_6 for homogeneity of areas					10·5632		
				(606)	χ^2_5 for homogeneity of areas							7·7671
LYMPHATIC LEUKAEMIAS, UNSPECIFIED												
1. Italy, Milano		Visconti *et al.* 1961[a]	P	56	29	18	6	3	0·5967	2·9455	0·7967	0·2552
			C	9607	3974	4134	1032	467				
2. Poland, Kraków		Cichecka 1965	P	148	48	55	27	18	0·9257	0·1521	0·8863	0·2509
			C	39006	12457	15419	7906	3224				
3. United Kingdom, London		Kay & Shorter 1956	P	36	16	19	1	0	1·2918	0·5673	0·3062	1·3168
		Discombe 1954 M1	C	10000	4556	4188	930	326				
				240					0·8863	0·6590	0·8297	0·8056
					χ^2_2 for homogeneity of areas					3·0060		1·0173
MONOCYTIC LEUKAEMIA, CHRONIC												
1. U.S.A., Rochester		Tinney & Watkins 1941	P	15(c)	6	6	1	2	1·0465	0·0061	0·9375	0·0035
			C	1000(c)	450	430	80	40				
MONOCYTIC LEUKAEMIAS, UNSPECIFIED												
1. U.S.A., San Francisco		Lucia *et al.* 1958	P	44	27	15	2	0	0·6267	2·0877	0·2935	2·7870
			C	5175	2318	2055	585	217				
LEUKAEMIAS, ACUTE												
1. Belgium, Gent		Goeminne 1962	P	28	13	12	2	1	1·1088	0·0660	1·1605	0·0381
			C	3704	1833	1526	243	102				
2. Czechoslovakia, Praha		Májský 1964	P	122	42	52	15	13	0·8614	0·4661	0·6713	1·6128
		Kout 1959 M2	C	1142	359	516	191	76				
3. Germany, Göttingen		Jörgensen 1967	P	88	34	44	8	2	1·1360	0·2755	0·9047	0·0582
			C	694	273	311	71	39				
4. Italy, Lombardia		Ninni & Bedarida 1959	P	78	35	39	2	2	1·0945	0·1327	0·2816	2·9191
			C	640	276	281	56	27				
5. Italy, Milano	Children	Bonvini 1961	P	99	28	57	10	4	1·9995	7·9434	1·7602	2·0339
			C	640	276	281	56	27				
6. Italy, Napoli	Children	Miraglia & Rolando 1962	P	158	68	64	19	7	1·1553	0·6053	0·9400	0·0508
			C	1200	545	444	162	49				

TABLE 1 **THE ABO BLOOD GROUP SYSTEM** (*cont.*)

Place	Additional details	Authors		Number	O	A	B	AB	A/O Relative incidence	A/O χ_1^2 for difference from unity	B/O Relative incidence	B/O χ_1^2 for difference from unity
NEOPLASMS (*cont.*)												
MALIGNANT NEOPLASMS (*cont.*)												
NEOPLASMS OF LYMPHATIC AND HAEMATOPOIETIC TISSUE (*cont.*)												
LEUKAEMIAS, ACUTE (*cont.*)												
7. Poland,		Gurda & Turowska 1970	P	52	17	23	9	3	1·0930	0·0773	0·8342	0·1933
Kraków			C	39006	12457	15419	7906	3224				
8. U.S.S.R.,	Children	Bubnov & Kirdan 1972	P	505	178	179	109	39	0·9618	0·0939	1·0037	0·0006
Moscow			C	1148	395	413	241	99				
9. U.S.A.,	Gentiles;	De George 1970	P	237	99	101	29	8	1·5580	6·7811	1·3276	1·2496
New York City	(s) A, Rh_D	MacMahon & Folusiak 1958	C	548	281	184	62	21				
10. U.S.A.,	(s) acute and	Tinney & Watkins 1941	P	100(c)	43	41	13	3	0·9978	0·0001	1·7006	2·4537
Rochester	subacute		C	1000(c)	450	430	80	40				
11. U.S.A.,		Kaplan 1961	P	177	84	68	21	4	1·0028	0·0003	1·1134	0·1921
San Francisco			C	20070	9473	7647	2127	823				
				1644					1·1208	3·4913	1·0465	0·2738
				χ_{10}^2 for homogeneity of areas						12·9505		10·5284
LEUKAEMIAS, CHRONIC												
1. Germany,		Jörgensen 1967	P	118	46	58	11	3	1·1068	0·2246	0·9195	0·0541
Göttingen			C	694	273	311	71	39				
2. U.S.A.,		Buckwalter *et al.* 1958	P	456(c)	226	179	40	11	0·8723	1·7393	0·9012	0·3435
Iowa			C	6313(c)	2892	2626	568	227				
3. U.S.A.,	Gentiles;	De George 1970	P	137	54	62	17	4	1·7534	7·2262	1·4268	1·3021
New York City	(s) A, Rh_D	MacMahon & Folusiak 1958	C	548	281	184	62	21				
				711					1·0172	0·0402	0·9944	0·0016
				χ_2^2 for homogeneity of areas						9·1499		1·6981
LEUKAEMIAS OTHER THAN ACUTE MYELOID												
1. United Kingdom, England and Wales		Hewitt & Spiers 1964	P	785	349	347	73	16	1·0793	1·0062	1·1817	1·6714
			C	134641	62216	57317	11013	4095				
LEUKAEMIAS, UNSPECIFIED												
1. France,		Lobstein 1958	P	60	26	32	2	0	1·0763	0·0768	0·3895	1·6444
Mulhouse			C	6423	2648	3028	523	224				
2. Italy, Genova	Children	Cordone & Tavella 1963	P	102	60	26	13	3	0·4714	8·3057	1·0571	0·0237
			C	350	161	148	33	8				
3. Italy, Milano		Visconti *et al.* 1961[a]	P	37	19	13	2	3	0·6577	1·3497	0·4053	1·4723
			C	9607	3974	4134	1032	467				
4. Italy, Perugia		Benda & Menghini 1957	P	255	98	130	20	7	1·3418	4·6645	0·8244	0·6033
			C	7356	3163	3127	783	283				
5. United Kingdom, London, Leytonstone	(s) A_1A_2	Walther *et al.* 1956	P	46	22	19	4	1	0·9033	0·1034	1·2236	0·1345
			C	2325	1070	1023	159	73				
6. United Kingdom, Manchester		MacLeod 1937	P	24	12	8	3	1	0·7904	0·2626	1·5861	0·5013
			C	1927	939	792	148	48				
7. United Kingdom, Manchester	Children	Gaisford & Campbell 1958	P	102	53	41	7	1	0·9287	0·1250	0·7596	0·4632
			C	9370	4532	3775	788	275				
8. N. India,		Tyagi *et al.* 1965	P	32	10	8	12	2	1·1676	0·1062	1·0457	0·0108
Kanpur			C	6000	1985	1360	2278	377				
9. S. India,		Ghooi *et al.* 1970	P	94	34	18	30	12	1·2101	0·2370	1·6941	2·2488
Bhopal			C	100	48	21	25	6				
10. U.S.A., Boston		Steinberg 1960	P	450(c)	203	181	49	17	1·1135	0·6267	0·8925	0·3078
		Dublin *et al.* 1964	C	605	281	225	76	23				

TABLE 1 **THE ABO BLOOD GROUP SYSTEM** (*cont.*)

Place	Additional details	Authors		Number	O	A	B	AB	A/O Relative incidence	A/O χ_1^2 for difference from unity	B/O Relative incidence	B/O χ_1^2 for difference from unity
11. U.S.A., Chicago	133 Whites, 4 Negroes	Best *et al.* 1949	P	137(c)	53	56	18	10	1·2076	0·9415	1·1357	0·2114
			C	4500(c)	1983	1735	593	189				
12. U.S.A., Michigan	Whites (s) A_1A_2	Gershowitz & Neel 1965	P	170	67	74	22	7	1·2236	1·2931	1·5688	2·9485
			C	1508	688	621	144	55				
13. U.S.A., New York	Gentiles	MacMahon & Folusiak 1958	P	639	291	235	90	23	1·2333	2·6350	1·4017	3·3312
			C	548	281	184	62	21				
14. U.S.A., New York	Jews	MacMahon & Folusiak 1958	P	665	226	261	120	58	0·9939	0·0018	1·6391	5·8782
			C	375	142	165	46	22				
15. U.S.A., Rochester	Whites	Buchanan & Higley 1921	P	115	58	39	17	1	0·7037	2·6039	1·6487	2·7533
		Tinney & Watkins 1941	C	1000(c)	450	430	80	40				
16. Brazil, Rio Grande do Sul	Whites; (s) A_1A_2	Ayres *et al.* 1966	P	51	16	23	9	3	1·6121	1·9082	3·1540	6·1173
			C	333	157	140	28	8				
17. Peru, Lima		Muñoz-Baratta 1962	P	113	70	28	13	2	1·0343	0·0228	0·9980	0·0000
			C	107938	66706	25797	12413	3022				
				3092					1·0698	1·8569	1·2198	7·2679
				χ_{16}^2 for homogeneity of areas						23·4070		21·3821
POLYCYTHAEMIA VERA												
1. Czechoslovakia, Praha		Májský 1964	P	16	3	9	4	0	2·0872	1·2054	2·5061	1·4273
		Kout 1959 M2	C	1142	359	516	191	76				
2. Poland, Kraków		Cichecka 1965	P	18	5	10	3	0	1·6158	0·7671	0·9454	0·0059
			C	39006	12457	15419	7906	3224				
3. Poland, Warszawa		Królikowska & Żupańska 1964	P	94	31	37	23	3	1·0977	0·1456	1·2594	0·6972
		Charzewski *et al.* 1965 M2	C	13744	4719	5131	2780	1114				
4. U.S.A., Madison and St. Louis		Sievers & Calabresi 1959	P	332	162	128	29	13	0·8660	1·4654	0·8222	0·9341
			C	32945	14918	13611	3248	1168				
5. U.S.A., Rochester		Tinney & Watkins 1941	P	100(c)	42	40	14	4	0·9967	0·0002	1·8750	3·5936
			C	1000(c)	450	430	80	40				
				560					0·9525	0·2655	1·1141	0·5852
				χ_4^2 for homogeneity of areas						3·3182		6·0730
MYELOFIBROSIS												
1. Poland, Kraków		Cichecka 1965	P	11	3	4	3	1	1·0772	0·0095	1·5756	0·3100
			C	39006	12457	15419	7906	3224				
2. Poland, Warszawa		Królikowska & Żupańska 1964	P	31	8	15	6	2	1·7244	1·5459	1·2731	0·1995
		Charzewski *et al.* 1965 M2	C	13744	4719	5131	2780	1114				
				42					1·5348	1·1270	1·3587	0·4623
				χ_1^2 for homogeneity of areas						0·4284		0·0472
MYELOMAS												
1. Czechoslovakia, Praha		Májský 1964	P	49	16	20	9	4	0·8697	0·1663	1·0573	0·0171
		Kout 1959 M2	C	1142	359	516	191	76				
2. Poland, Warszawa	Plasmocytoma	Królikowska & Żupańska 1964	P	33	12	13	6	2	0·9963	0·0001	0·8487	0·1073
		Charzewski *et al.* 1965 M2	C	13744	4719	5131	2780	1114				
3. United Kingdom, NE. Scotland		Allan 1970	P	120(a)	51	53	13	3	1·4949	4·1427	1·2287	0·4335
			C	8811	4478	3113	929	291				
				202					1·2525	2·0461	1·0932	0·1566
				χ_2^2 for homogeneity of areas						2·2630		0·4013

TABLE 1 **THE ABO BLOOD GROUP SYSTEM** (*cont.*)

NEOPLASMS (*cont.*)
MALIGNANT NEOPLASMS (*cont.*)
NEOPLASMS OF LYMPHATIC AND HAEMATOPOIETIC TISSUE (*cont.*)

ERYTHROLEUKAEMIA

Place	Additional details	Authors		Number	O	A	B	AB	A/O Relative incidence	A/O χ^2_1 for difference from unity	B/O Relative incidence	B/O χ^2_1 for difference from unity
1. Poland, Kraków		Cichecka 1965	P	15	5	3	7	0	0·4847	0·9830	2·2059	1·8244
			C	39006	12457	15419	7906	3224				

SARCOMAS

Place	Additional details	Authors		Number	O	A	B	AB	A/O Relative incidence	A/O χ^2_1 for difference from unity	B/O Relative incidence	B/O χ^2_1 for difference from unity
1. Germany, Berlin		Schröder 1955	P	52	19	24	6	3	1·0974	0·0913	0·8109	0·1997
		Pettenkofer *et al.* 1957 M1	C	12000	4437	5107	1728	728				
2. Switzerland, Zürich		Botsztejn 1942	P	113	47	51	15	0	0·9088	0·2012	1·3945	1·0922
			C	1000	402	480	92	26				
3. United Kingdom, London, Leytonstone		Walther *et al.* 1956	P	21	9	9	3	0	1·0459	0·0090	2·2432	1·4451
			C	2325	1070	1023	159	73				
4. United Kingdom, Manchester		MacLeod 1937	P	15	9	6	0	0	0·7904	0·1975		
			C	1927	939	792	148	48				
5. N. India, Kanpur		Tyagi *et al.* 1965	P	18	2	5	7	4	3·6489	2·3894	3·0498	1·9314
			C	6000	1985	1360	2278	377				
				219					1·0020	0·0002	1·3800	1·8846
					χ^2_4 for homogeneity of areas					2·8882		
				(204)	χ^2_3 for homogeneity of areas							2·7838

MALIGNANT NEOPLASMS DEFINED AS CANCERS OF MIXED OR UNSPECIFIED SITES

Place	Additional details	Authors		Number	O	A	B	AB	A/O Relative incidence	A/O χ^2_1 for difference from unity	B/O Relative incidence	B/O χ^2_1 for difference from unity
1. Austria, Wien		Flamm & Friedrich 1929	P	170(c)	48	91	21	10	1·4849	4·8368	1·0214	0·0065
		Corvin M1	C	10392	3635	4641	1557	559				
2. Belgium, Liège		Moureau & Firket 1934	P	200(c)	79	93	21	7	1·3121	2·9869	1·4926	2·4940
			C	3500(c)	1634	1466	291	109				
3. Belgium, Liège		Otto-Servais *et al.* 1959	P	715	339	302	54	20	0·9535	0·3238	0·9352	0·1876
			C	6000	2771	2589	472	168				
4. Finland		Mustakallio 1937	P	57	27	20	6	4	0·6126	2·6974	0·5032	2·2754
			C	2592	908	1098	401	188				
5. Finland		Streng & Ryti 1927[a]	P	51	15	25	9	2	1·3057	0·6438	1·1974	0·1762
			C	1383(c)	463	591	232	97				
6. France		Dujarric de la Rivière & Kossovitch 1929	P	60	25	25	10	0	0·9951	0·0003	1·5140	1·1332
		Kossovitch 1929 M1	C	962	405	407	107	43				
7. Italy, Milano		Mor & Sforza 1960	P	292	115	136	29	12	1·0712	0·1858	0·9433	0·0511
			C	500	202	223	54	21				
8. Italy, Napoli	Larynx, oesophagus, pancreas, thyroid, liver, kidney, bladder	Spena & Grippo 1964	P	55	27	19	6	3	0·8121	0·4717	1·0367	0·0062
			C	2147	989	857	212	89				
9. Italy, Siena	Colon, lung, breast, prostate (s) S	Prior & Vegni 1957	P	102	42	50	9	1	1·3690	2·0351	0·7582	0·5290
			C	1025	460	400	130	35				
10. Italy, Trieste		Goldstein 1929	P	218	70	90	44	14	1·3498	3·1290	1·6002	5·1626
			C	1548	611	582	240	115				
11. Netherlands		Bendien 1926	P	110	26	47	18	19	1·7255	3·5853	3·2308	8·5168
		Snyder 1926 M1	C	200	84	88	18	10				
12. Poland, Katowice	(s) into 21 sites	Kukowka 1935	P	200	64	88	36	12	1·1892	0·9299	1·3469	1·6722
		Meyer 1928 M1	C	956	352	407	147	50				
13. Switzerland, Zürich		Botsztejn 1942	P	887	383	405	77	22	0·8856	1·5292	0·8785	0·5798
			C	1000	402	480	92	26				

TABLE 1 **THE ABO BLOOD GROUP SYSTEM** (*cont.*)

Place	Additional details	Authors		Number	O	A	B	AB	A/O		B/O	
									Relative incidence	χ_1^2 for difference from unity	Relative incidence	χ_1^2 for difference from unity
14. United Kingdom, Manchester		MacLeod 1937	P C	92 1927	49 939	30 792	9 148	4 48	0·7259	1·8305	1·1653	0·1680
15. U.S.S.R., Lwów	(s) S	Szmyt 1938 Halber & Mydlarski 1925 M1	P C	50(c) 285	13 101	12 107	12 49	13 28	0·8713	0·1057	1·9027	2·1713
16. Japan, Tokyo		Terada 1929	P C	109 3097(c)	23 969	47 1190	25 651	14 287	1·6640	3·8917	1·6179	2·6903
17. U.S.A., New York	Single cancers	Tsukada *et al.* 1964	P C	620 1954	273 811	257 764	66 272	24 107	0·9993	0·0000	0·7208	4·5169
18. U.S.A., New York	Multiple cancers	Tsukada *et al.* 1964	P C	310 1954	115 811	142 764	38 272	15 107	1·3107	3·9984	0·9852	0·0055
19. U.S.A., Rochester	Whites	Buchanan & Higley 1921 Tinney & Watkins 1941	P C	292 1000(c)	140 450	119 430	22 80	11 40	0·8895	0·6819	0·8839	0·2261
20. Australia, Sydney	(s) S	Parker & Walsh 1958	P C	5117 30000	2472 14672	1963 11514	495 2912	187 902	1·0119	0·1308	1·0089	0·0278
				9707					1·0310	1·5577	1·0279	0·4981
				χ_{19}^2 for homogeneity of areas						32·4363		32·0984

MALIGNANT NEOPLASMS OF UNSPECIFIED SITES

Place	Additional details	Authors		Number	O	A	B	AB	A/O Relative incidence	A/O χ_1^2 for difference from unity	B/O Relative incidence	B/O χ_1^2 for difference from unity
1. Austria, Wien	Carcinomas, sarcomas, gliomas	Hoche & Moritsch 1926	P C	176 296	62 103	62 103	20 65	32 25	1·0000	0·0000	0·5112	4·9365
2. Bulgaria	Cancers, sarcomas, haemocyto-blastomas	Zographov 1962	P C	314 15422	95 4953	142 6821	56 2485	21 1163	1·0854	0·3747	1·1749	0·8964
3. Finland	Cancers, sarcomas	Sievers 1929	P C	138(c) 1711	40 584	65 740	23 272	10 115	1·2824	1·4242	1·2346	0·6011
4. Finland		Mustakallio 1937	P C	40 2595	13 908	22 1098	3 401	2 188	1·3995	0·9081	0·5225	1·0179
5. Germany, München	Cancers, sarcomas	Lützeler & Dormanns 1929 Kruse M1	P C	233 1300	97 552	108 559	20 125	8 64	1·0995	0·3880	0·9105	0·1253
6. Germany, Zwickau		Lickint & Tröltzsch 1929 Christiansen *et al.* 1935 M1	P C	40 5335(c)	13 2150	17 2321	8 597	2 267	1·2113	0·2690	2·2162	3·1034
7. Greece	(s) S	Hatzesoterios 1959	P C	2043 19265	857 7964	815 7578	275 2785	96 938	0·9994	0·0001	0·9176	1·3981
8. United Kingdom, St. Andrews	Carcinomas, sarcomas, rodent ulcer, leukaemias	Alexander 1921	P C	50(c) 50(c)	14 23	14 19	16 6	6 2	1·2105	0·1527	4·3810	6·3426
9. Egypt, Cairo	Includes leukaemias and Hodgkin's Disease; excludes cancers of alimentary tract	Awny & Kamel 1959	P C	307 1588	96 583	120 515	71 351	20 139	1·4150	5·3788	1·2284	1·4562
10. U.S.A., New York	(s) into 44 sites	Goldfeder & Fershing 1937 Brody *et al.* 1936 M1	P C	300 1000	131 478	105 353	47 122	17 47	1·0854	0·3038	1·4057	2·9584
11. U.S.A., Philadelphia	76% females	Pfahler & Widmann 1924 Ottenberg 1921 M1	P C	314 286	146 126	118 120	35 34	15 6	0·8486	0·8527	0·8884	0·1924
				3955					1·0514	1·6599	1·0123	0·0515
				χ_{10}^2 for homogeneity of areas						8·3922		22·9768

TABLE 1 **THE ABO BLOOD GROUP SYSTEM** (*cont.*)

NEOPLASMS (*cont.*)

MALIGNANT NEOPLASMS (*cont.*)

MALIGNANT NEOPLASMS; SITES SPECIFIED BY EXCLUSION

Place	Additional details	Authors		Number	O	A	B	AB	A/O Relative incidence	A/O χ_1^2 for difference from unity	B/O Relative incidence	B/O χ_1^2 for difference from unity
1. Austria, Wien	Other than gastric; (s) $A_1 A_2$	Weiser 1957	P	735(c)	267	331	99	38	1·0179	0·0435	1·0025	0·0004
			C	10000	3631	4422	1343	604				
2. Czechoslovakia, Praha	Other than breast and lung	Jakoubková & Májský 1965	P	79	20	30	19	10	1·0407	0·0181	1·7806	3·0082
			C	1142	358	516	191	77				
3. Germany, Tübingen	Other than breast and gastric	Völter *et al.* 1970	P	2018	790	917	201	110	1·1287	5·9191	0·9639	0·2067
		Dick *et al.* 1962	C	39031	16283	16745	4298	1705				
4. Poland, Warszawa	Other than oesophagus, gastric, intestines, bile ducts	Kosiński *et al.* 1959	P	119	39	48	16	16	1·1868	0·6140	0·7833	0·6625
			C	4270	1537	1594	805	334				
5. United Kingdom, England and Wales	Childhood cancer other than leukaemia	Hewitt & Spiers 1964	P	780	352	330	68	30	1·0176	0·0517	1·0913	0·4328
			C	134641	62216	57317	11013	4095				
6. United Kingdom, Sheffield	Other than breast	Green & Dunsford 1954	P	207	92	85	23	7	0·9828	0·0128	1·3950	1·9240
		Kopeć 1970	C	4435	2020	1899	362	154				
7. Philippines, Santo Tomas	Other than gastric	Tan 1962	P	100	51	20	26	3	0·7306	1·2020	0·9129	0·1184
			C	500	231	124	129	16				
				4038					1·0674	3·6249	1·0199	0·0197
				χ_6^2 for homogeneity of areas						4·2363		6·3333

BENIGN NEOPLASMS

BENIGN NEOPLASMS OF SALIVARY GLANDS

Place	Additional details	Authors		Number	O	A	B	AB	A/O Relative incidence	A/O χ_1^2 for difference from unity	B/O Relative incidence	B/O χ_1^2 for difference from unity
1. United Kingdom, Manchester	Adeno-lymphomas	Garrett *et al.* 1971	P	32(a)	12	16	2	2	1·5542	1·3072	0·9564	0·0034
			C	1554(a)	746	640	130	38				
2. United Kingdom, Manchester	Mixed salivary adenoma	Garrett *et al.* 1971	P	290(a)	147	117	21	5	0·9277	0·3082	0·8198	0·6223
			C	1554(a)	746	640	130	38				
3. United Kingdom, Glasgow	Pleomorphic adenoma	Cameron 1958	P	294	92	170	23	9	3·0800	71·9383	1·2469	0·8656
			C	5898	3177	1906	637	178				
4. U.S.A., New York	Parotid glands	Osborne & De George 1962	P	251	96	106	33	16	1·2256	1·9806	1·0966	0·1989
			C	4738	2029	1828	636	245				
5. U.S.A., New York	Submaxillary glands	Osborne & De George 1962	P	24	7	12	3	2	1·9028	1·8213	1·3673	0·2046
			C	4738	2029	1828	636	245				
				891					1·5554	33·2950	1·0598	0·2050
				χ_4^2 for homogeneity of areas						44·0606		1·6899

BENIGN NASOPHARYNGEAL NEOPLASMS

Place	Additional details	Authors		Number	O	A	B	AB	A/O Relative incidence	A/O χ_1^2 for difference from unity	B/O Relative incidence	B/O χ_1^2 for difference from unity
1. Peru, Lima		Muñoz-Baratta 1962	P	38(c)	23	10	5	0	1·1041	0·0683	1·1371	0·0678
			C	107938(c)	66058	26013	12629	3238				

BENIGN NEOPLASMS OF DIGESTIVE SYSTEM

Place	Additional details	Authors		Number	O	A	B	AB	A/O Relative incidence	A/O χ_1^2 for difference from unity	B/O Relative incidence	B/O χ_1^2 for difference from unity
1. Japan, Sendai		Moniwa 1960	P	67	22	25	16	4	0·9879	0·0017	1·0199	0·0036
			C	21199	6769	7786	4827	1817				

BENIGN ABDOMINAL NEOPLASMS

Place	Additional details	Authors		Number	O	A	B	AB	A/O Relative incidence	A/O χ_1^2 for difference from unity	B/O Relative incidence	B/O χ_1^2 for difference from unity
1. Peru, Lima		Muñoz-Baratta 1962	P	88(c)	38	28	14	8	1·8712	6·3233	1·9271	4·3985
			C	107938(c)	66058	26013	12629	3238				

TABLE 1 **THE ABO BLOOD GROUP SYSTEM** *(cont.)*

Place	Additional details	Authors		Number	O	A	B	AB	A/O Relative incidence	A/O χ_1^2 for difference from unity	B/O Relative incidence	B/O χ_1^2 for difference from unity
POLYPS OF COLON												
1. U.S.A., New York	Adenomatous; Whites	Fleming *et al.* 1967	P	326	139	128	43	16	1·1134	0·6794	1·0090	0·0023
			C	2525	1122	928	344	131				
2. U.S.A., New York	Papillary adenomas; Whites	Fleming *et al.* 1967	P	47	32	9	5	1	0·3400	8·0617	0·5096	1·9331
			C	2525	1122	928	344	131				
3. U.S.A., New York	Polyposis; Whites	Fleming *et al.* 1967	P	18	11	6	1	0	0·6595	0·6677	0·2965	1·3500
			C	2525	1122	928	344	131				
				391					0·9613	0·1086	0·8975	0·4020
				χ_2^2 for homogeneity of areas						9·3002		2·8834
BENIGN NEOPLASMS OF FEMUR												
1. Peru, Lima		Muñoz-Baratta 1962	P	27(c)	15	5	6	1	0·8465	0·1042	2·0923	2·3348
			C	107938(c)	66058	26013	12629	3238				
BENIGN NEOPLASMS OF BREAST												
1. Germany, Berlin		Wehle 1957	P	80	28	32	16	4	0·9677	0·0160	1·4778	1·5459
			C	21104	7725	9123	2987	1269				
BENIGN NEOPLASMS OF UTERUS												
1. Germany, Berlin	Myomas	Wehle 1957	P	1446	502	628	223	93	1·0593	0·8678	1·1489	2·7743
			C	21104	7725	9123	2987	1269				
2. Italy, Brindisi	Fibromyomas	Perretti & Putignano 1967	P	1380	412	664	212	92	1·7859	47·0560	1·0960	0·7046
			C	1812	656	592	308	256				
3. Italy, Milano	Fibromas	Dossena & Lanzara 1925	P	64	27	29	7	1	1·3770	1·0849	0·9972	0·0000
		Dossena 1924 M1	C	214	100	78	26	10				
4. Italy, Milano	Fibromyomas	Dambrosio 1965	P	285	127	118	31	9	0·8974	0·7041	0·9534	0·0559
		Garibaldi & Gianotti 1964 M2	C	16952	7081	7331	1813	727				
5. Italy, Torino	Fibromyomas	Cagliero 1961	P	755	345	304	87	19	0·8867	1·5563	1·0103	0·0047
			C	1500	645	641	161	53				
6. Italy, Varese	Fibromas; (s) Rh_D	Carrera 1963	P	229	97	106	16	10	1·1911	1·2468	0·5800	3·5683
			C	1002	436	400	124	42				
7. Portugal	Fibromyomas	Lessa & Alarcão 1947	P	317	132	163	17	5	1·1091	0·6576	0·6502	2·4827
			C	1748	732	815	145	56				
8. N. India, Lucknow	Fibromas	Nath *et al.* 1963	P	109	30	20	53	6	0·9163	0·0892	1·4477	2·5372
			C	3330(c)	1035	753	1263	279				
9. Japan, Sendai	Fibromyomas	Moniwa 1960	P	424	129	162	94	39	1·0918	0·5430	1·0218	0·0249
			C	21199	6769	7786	4827	1817				
10. Japan, Sendai	Other than fibromyomas	Moniwa 1960	P	51	13	20	10	8	1·3375	0·6649	1·0787	0·0324
			C	21199	6769	7786	4827	1817				
11. Egypt, Cairo	Fibromas	Awny & Kamel 1959	P	125(c)	36	50	32	7	1·5723	3·9813	1·4764	2·3871
			C	1588(c)	583	515	351	139				
12. U.S.A., Rochester	Fibromas; Whites	Buchanan & Higley 1921	P	137	54	64	13	6	1·2403	1·1986	1·3542	0·8345
		Tinney & Watkins 1941	C	1000(c)	450	430	80	40				
13. Peru, Lima		Muñoz-Baratta 1962	P	150	78	50	14	8	1·6278	7·2219	0·9388	0·0472
			C	107938	66058	26013	12629	3238				
				5472					1·1662	20·0232	1·0732	2·2060
				χ_{12}^2 for homogeneity of areas						46·8492		13·2478

TABLE 1 **THE ABO BLOOD GROUP SYSTEM** (*cont.*)

Place	Additional details	Authors		Number	O	A	B	AB	A/O Relative incidence	A/O χ_1^2 for difference from unity	B/O Relative incidence	B/O χ_1^2 for difference from unity
NEOPLASMS (*cont.*)												
BENIGN NEOPLASMS (*cont.*)												
BENIGN NEOPLASMS OF OVARY												
1. Germany, Berlin	Cysts	Wehle 1957	P	360	101	165	72	22	1·3833	6·4993	1·8436	15·4293
			C	21104	7725	9123	2987	1269				
2. Italy, Milano	Cysts	Dossena & Lanzara 1925	P	23	9	9	4	1	1·2821	0·2519	1·7094	0·7018
		Dossena 1924 M1	C	214	100	78	26	10				
3. Japan, Sendai		Moniwa 1960	P	428	137	170	97	24	1·0788	0·4274	0·9929	0·0028
			C	21199	6769	7786	4827	1817				
4. U.S.A., New York		Osborne & De George 1963	P	260	98	114	35	13	1·2912	3·2627	1·1394	0·4169
			C	4738	2029	1828	636	245				
				1071					1·2360	8·1867	1·2673	8·1867
				χ_3^2 for homogeneity of areas						2·2549		8·3638
BENIGN NEOPLASMS OF TESTIS												
1. Peru, Lima		Muñoz-Baratta 1962	P	34	15	8	5	6	1·3544	0·4799	1·7436	1·1585
			C	107938	66058	26013	12629	3238				
BENIGN NEOPLASMS OF BLADDER												
1. Peru, Lima		Muñoz-Baratta 1962	P	41	24	8	4	5	0·8465	0·1666	0·8718	0·0645
			C	107938	66058	26013	12629	3238				
UNSPECIFIED NEOPLASMS												
CHROMOPHOBE ADENOMA OF PITUITARY												
1. Italy, Padova		Iraci & Toffolo 1964[a]	P	117	46	54	13	4	1·3246	1·7598	1·3887	0·9663
			C	1000	457	405	93	45				
2. United Kingdom, Birmingham		Aird *et al.* 1960	P	25	15	9	1	0	0·6774	0·8510	0·4047	0·7660
			C	9590	4559	4038	751	242				
3. United Kingdom, Bristol		Aird *et al.* 1960	P	24	10	11	3	0	1·0465	0·0107	1·5750	0·4683
			C	1989	861	905	164	59				
4. United Kingdom, Cardiff		Aird *et al.* 1960	P	25	11	10	3	1	1·0262	0·0034	1·2780	0·1373
			C	874	403	357	86	28				
5. United Kingdom, Liverpool		Aird *et al.* 1960	P	37	15	19	3	0	1·6684	2·1859	1·1207	0·0323
			C	8202	4124	3131	736	211				
6. United Kingdom, London		Aird *et al.* 1960	P	171	80	67	18	6	0·9088	0·3283	1·1574	0·3078
			C	10000	4578	4219	890	313				
7. United Kingdom, Manchester		Aird *et al.* 1960	P	44	26	12	6	0	0·5341	3·2082	1·2104	0·1756
			C	5431	2570	2221	490	150				
8. United Kingdom, Manchester		Pearce & Yates 1965	P	160	79	62	17	2	0·9422	0·1211	1·2376	0·6228
			C	9370	4532	3775	788	275				
9. United Kingdom, Oxford		Aird *et al.* 1960	P	82	36	40	4	2	1·1303	0·2805	0·5761	1·0865
			C	6492	2888	2839	557	208				
10. Sweden	(s) S	Strang 1968	P	400	154	186	39	21	0·9718	0·0664	0·9677	0·0323
			C	10457	3974	4939	1040	504				
11. U.S.A., New York	Whites	Damon 1957	P	150	71	50	21	8	0·7520	2·2147	1·1137	0·1713
			C	1848	802	751	213	82				
12. U.S.A., New York	Negroes	Damon 1957	P	34	20	8	6	0	0·7406	0·4740	0·8373	0·1331
			C	370	187	101	67	15				
				1269					0·9572	0·4923	1·0792	0·5946
				χ_{11}^2 for homogeneity of areas						11·0117		4·3050

TABLE 1 **THE ABO BLOOD GROUP SYSTEM** (*cont.*)

Place	Additional details	Authors		Number	O	A	B	AB	A/O Relative incidence	A/O χ_1^2 for difference from unity	B/O Relative incidence	B/O χ_1^2 for difference from unity
ADENOMAS OF PITUITARY, OTHER THAN CHROMOPHOBE												
1. Italy, Padova		Iraci & Toffolo 1964[a]	P	33	19	8	5	1	0·4751	3·0382	1·2932	0·2489
			C	1000	457	405	93	45				
NEOPLASMS OF PITUITARY												
1. United Kingdom, Manchester	May include malignant	MacLeod 1937	P	61	29	26	3	3	1·0630	0·0495	0·6563	0·4720
			C	1927	939	792	148	48				
2. United Kingdom, Manchester	Non-glial (s) C	Pearce & Yates 1965	P	276	129	119	24	4	1·1075	0·6261	1·0700	0·0899
			C	9370	4532	3775	788	275				
				337					1·0993	0·6573	1·0094	0·0019
				χ_1^2 for homogeneity of areas						0·0183		0·5600
NEOPLASMS OF SALIVARY GLANDS												
1. Italy, Cagliari		Boero & Coraddu 1965	P	73	24	45	3	1	3·3137	22·0000	0·9822	0·0008
			C	3516	2043	1156	260	57				
NEOPLASMS OF ALIMENTARY TRACT												
1. Spain, Málaga		Franquelo Ramos & Eloy-Garcia 1966	P	83	23	33	15	12	1·6013	2·8621	5·0174	20·7767
			C	1195	577	517	75	26				
NEOPLASMS OF SPLEEN												
1. Germany, München	Post-mortem	Lützeler & Dormanns 1929	P	148	69	64	13	2	0·9159	0·2288	0·8320	0·3342
		Kruse M1	C	1300	552	559	125	64				
NEOPLASMS OF FEMALE GENITAL ORGANS, BENIGN OR MALIGNANT												
1. Poland	(s) A	Kozaczenko 1966	P	567	174	233	109	51	1·3247	7·8111	1·2403	3·0824
			C	67356	24695	24964	12473	5224				
NEOPLASMS OF NEPHROGENITAL RIDGE												
1. United Kingdom, Manchester	Include Wilms' tumour	Gaisford & Campbell 1958	P	26	17	7	1	1	0·4943	2·4553	0·3383	1·1078
			C	9370	4532	3775	788	275				
EPITHELIAL NEOPLASMS												
1. United Kingdom, Manchester		Gaisford & Campbell 1958	P	18	4	13	1	0	3·9017	5·6610	1·4378	0·1054
			C	9370	4532	3775	788	275				
2. Peru, Lima		Muñoz-Baratta 1962	P	40(c)	31	2	6	1	0·1638	6·1470	1·0124	0·0008
			C	107938	66058	26013	12629	3238				
				58					1·1666	0·1171	1·0623	0·0213
				χ_1^2 for homogeneity of areas						11·6909		0·0848
NEOPLASMS OTHER THAN CANCERS, BENIGN OR MALIGNANT												
1. U.S.A., Rochester	Whites	Buchanan & Higley 1921	P	65	33	21	10	1	0·6660	2·0039	1·7045	1·9604
		Tinney & Watkins 1941	C	1000 (c)	450	430	80	40				

TABLE 1 THE ABO BLOOD GROUP SYSTEM (*cont.*)

Place	Additional details	Authors		Number	O	A	B	AB	A/O Relative incidence	A/O χ_1^2 for difference from unity	B/O Relative incidence	B/O χ_1^2 for difference from unity
ENDOCRINE AND METABOLIC DISEASES												
NON-TOXIC GOITRE												
1. United Kingdom, Liverpool	Single adenoma; (s) ABH secretion	Kitchin *et al.* 1959	P	34	12	21	0	1	2·4455	5·2285		
			C	208	109	78	15	6				
2. United Kingdom, Liverpool	Multiple adenoma; (s) ABH secretion	Kitchin *et al.* 1959	P	179	96	61	18	4	0·8880	0·2894	1·3625	0·6747
			C	208	109	78	15	6				
3. Japan, Sendai		Moniwa 1960	P	102	31	38	23	10	1·0657	0·0688	1·0404	0·0206
			C	21199	6769	7786	4827	1817				
				315					1·1075	0·4586	1·1432	0·3616
					χ_2^2 for homogeneity of areas					5·1281		
				(281)·	χ_1^2 for homogeneity of areas							0·3338
THYROTOXICOSIS												
1. Austria, Wien	Exophthalmic	Flamm & Friedrich 1929 Corvin M1	P	23(c)	10	6	3	4	0·4699	2·1345	0·7004	0·2921
			C	10392	3635	4641	1557	559				
2. Finland		Streng & Ryti 1927[b]	P	22	11	8	2	1	0·6014	1·1863	0·4117	1·3248
			C	2595	908	1098	401	188				
3. Finland		Mustakallio 1937	P	59	28	26	5	0	0·7679	0·9155	0·4043	3·4261
			C	2595	908	1098	401	188				
4. Germany, München		Hermanns & Kronberg 1927	P	25	24	1	0	0	0·0409	9·6395		
			C	265	110	112	27	16				
5. United Kingdom, Liverpool	Primary thyrotoxicosis, diffuse goitre; (s) ABH secretion	Kitchin *et al.* 1959	P	104	47	39	13	5	1·1596	0·3181	2·0099	2·8002
			C	208	109	78	15	6				
6. United Kingdom, Liverpool	Secondary thyrotoxicosis, multiple adenoma; (s) ABH secretion	Kitchin *et al.* 1959	P	24	12	10	2	0	1·1645	0·1130	1·2111	0·0557
			C	208	109	78	15	6				
7. United Kingdom, Glasgow		Jackson *et al.* 1965	P	851	462	286	87	16	1·0319	0·1513	0·9392	0·2532
			C	5898	3177	1906	637	178				
8. United Kingdom, Northern Ireland I[1]		Dawson *et al.* 1966	P	88	59	18	9	2	0·4712	7·7843	0·8798	0·1274
			C	20722	11068	7166	1919	569				
9. United Kingdom Northern Ireland II[2]		Dawson *et al.* 1966	P	185	114	52	17	2	0·7752	2·3065	0·8474	0·4040
			C	43570	24054	14154	4233	1129				
10. United Kingdom, Northern Ireland III[3]		Dawson *et al.* 1966	P	34	22	6	5	1	0·5348	1·8356	1·1884	0·1201
			C	4020	2306	1176	441	97				
11. United Kingdom, Belfast		Macafee 1967[a]	P	212	127	61	20	4	0·8002	2·0334	0·9159	0·1323
			C	28566	15715	9433	2702	716				
12. Japan, Niigata		Hirose & Honma 1962	P	109	35	41	28	5	0·9388	0·0746	1·0165	0·0042
			C	12253	3624	4522	2852	1255				
13. Japan, Sendai		Moniwa 1960	P	214	70	75	53	16	0·9315	0·1806	1·0618	0·1072
			C	21199	6769	7786	4827	1817				
				1950					0·8929	4·4328	0·9535	0·3828
					χ_{12}^2 for homogeneity of areas					24·2405		
				(1925)	χ_{11}^2 for homogeneity of areas							8·6644

[1] Armagh, Banbridge, Ballymena, Enniskillen, Lurgan, Newtownards.
[2] Ballymoney, Belfast, Coleraine, Dungannon, Limavady, Lisburn, Londonderry, Magherafelt, Omagh, Whiteabbey.
[3] Downpatrick, Newcastle, Newry.

TABLE 1 THE ABO BLOOD GROUP SYSTEM (*cont.*)

Place	Additional details	Authors		Number	O	A	B	AB	A/O Relative incidence	A/O χ_1^2 for difference from unity	B/O Relative incidence	B/O χ_1^2 for difference from unity
GOITRE												
1. Austria, Wien		Flamm & Friedrich 1929	P	47(c)	19	18	6	4	0·7420	0·8193	0·7372	0·4220
		Corvin M1	C	10392	3635	4641	1557	559				
2. Finland		Lindgren 1934	P	163	68	61	26	8	0·7358	2·8802	0·8107	0·7877
		Mustakallio 1943 M1	C	3313	1145	1396	540	232				
3. Finland		Mustakallio 1937	P	195	74	73	36	12	0·8158	1·4185	1·1016	0·2085
			C	2595	908	1098	401	188				
4. Germany, München		Lützeler & Dormanns 1929	P	206	95	79	25	7	0·8212	1·4494	1·1621	0·3741
		Kruse M1	C	1300	552	559	125	64				
5. Germany, Oberbayern		Hermanns & Kronberg 1927	P	74	14	51	4	5	3·5778	14·9005	1·1640	0·0628
			C	265	110	112	27	16				
6. Germany, Oberbayern		Brockmüller 1962	P	597	258	264	52	23	0·9950	0·0032	0·7636	3·1094
			C	39031	16283	16745	4298	1705				
7. Italy, Cuneo		Beffa *et al.* 1960	P	111	49	49	10	3	1·1138	0·2532	0·9546	0·0161
			C	912	421	378	90	23				
8. Italy, Milano		Mor & Sforza 1960	P	308	122	152	24	10	1·1286	0·6043	0·7359	1·2826
			C	500	202	223	54	21				
9. Italy, Napoli	(s) S	Cocchia *et al.* 1963	P	300	140	127	22	11	1·1105	0·3579	0·7969	0·5403
			C	300	142	116	28	14				
10. Italy, Potenza	(s) S	Pietrandolfi & Pesce 1961	P	40	17	17	5	1	1·4766	1·1395	0·8298	0·1229
			C	334	158	107	56	13				
11. Italy, Torino		Beffa *et al.* 1960	P	255	104	127	19	5	1·1900	1·5328	0·8101	0·6479
			C	2072	878	901	198	95				
12. Portugal		Lessa & Ruffié 1960	P	24(c)	10	14	0	0	1·2788	0·3500		
			C	3353(c)	1424	1559	250	120				
13. U.S.S.R., Caucasus, Karachay-Cherkesskaya A.Obl.	Females	Lauer 1929	P	397(c)	175	131	67	24	0·8010	1·5065	0·8360	0·6364
			C	269(c)	107	100	49	13				
14. U.S.S.R., Caucasus, Karachay-Cherkesskaya A.Obl.	(s) S	Grikurov 1936	P	214	91	75	40	8	1·0200	0·0127	1·0580	0·0694
			C	811	349	282	145	35				
15. U.S.S.R., Tadzhikistan, Kurgan-Tyube District	Uzbeks; (s) S	Sakharov 1933	P	175	68	43	55	9	0·7831	1·1970	0·8220	0·8797
			C	566	187	151	184	44				
16. U.S.S.R., Uzbekistan, Ak-Darinskiy District	Uzbeks; (s) S	Sakharov 1933	P	499	145	177	138	39	0·9591	0·0768	0·7614	3·0498
			C	697	176	224	220	77				
17. U.S.S.R., Uzbekistan, Ak-Darinskiy District	Mixed population	Sakharov 1933	P	64	25	14	21	4	0·9600	0·0089	1·4400	0·8157
			C	82	36	21	21	4				
18. U.S.S.R., Uzbekistan, Samarkand District	Tadzhiks; (s) S	Sakharov 1933	P	167	48	53	51	15	0·9452	0·0565	1·0350	0·0205
			C	393	113	132	116	32				
19. U.S.S.R., Uzbekistan, Samarkand District	Uzbeks; (s) S	Sakharov 1933	P	87	23	27	33	4	1·1868	0·2865	1·4043	1·2096
			C	307	92	91	94	30				
				3923					0·9931	0·0270	0·8919	3·8723
					χ_{18}^2 for homogeneity of areas					28·8267		
				(3899)	χ_{17}^2 for homogeneity of areas							10·3831

TABLE 1 **THE ABO BLOOD GROUP SYSTEM** (*cont.*)

Place	Additional details	Authors		Number	O	A	B	AB	A/O Relative incidence	A/O χ_1^2 for difference from unity	B/O Relative incidence	B/O χ_1^2 for difference from unity
ENDOCRINE AND METABOLIC DISEASES (*cont.*)												
CRETINISM												
1. Italy, Cuneo		Beffa *et al.* 1960	P	77	35	40	2	0	1·2729	0·9935	0·2673	3·2114
			C	912	421	378	90	23				
DIABETES MELLITUS												
1. Austria, Wien	(s) S, Rh_D	Speiser 1958[a]	P	239	79	103	43	14	1·1128	0·4165	1·5366	3·9830
			C	1000	367	430	130	73				
2. Austria, Wien	(s) S	Mähr 1959	P	1300	443	576	202	79	1·1097	1·1986	1·2873	3·6181
		Speiser 1958	C	1000	367	430	130	73				
3. Belgium, Bruxelles	(s) S	Cornil & Pirart 1961	P	564	218	272	52	22	1·2891	6·7003	1·2744	2·0961
			C	3337(c)	1496	1448	280	113				
4. Belgium, Liège	(s) S	Otto-Servais *et al.* 1959	P	1392	624	592	151	25	1·0154	0·0579	1·4206	11·5166
			C	6000	2771	2589	472	168				
5. Czechoslovakia, Praha		Miluničová & Dominec 1966	P	121	45	43	26	7	0·7963	1·0037	1·0146	0·0030
		Miluničová & Sottner 1965 M2	C	878	295	354	168	61				
6. Czechoslovakia, Praha	(s) S	Miluničová *et al.* 1969[a]	P	400	141	165	62	32	0·9752	0·0326	0·7721	2·0539
		Miluničová & Sottner 1965 M2	C	878	295	354	168	61				
7. Denmark	Mothers; (s) Rh_D	Klebe & Nielsen 1972	P	652	281	281	70	20	0·9428	0·4620	1·0096	0·0049
			C	12123	5046	5352	1245	480				
8. Denmark, Köbenhavn	(s) S, A	Andersen & Lauritzen 1960	P	1009	471	408	96	34	0·8280	7·6256	0·7984	3·9644
			C	49137(a)	20351	21290	5195	2301				
9. Finland		Sievers 1929	P	117(c)	38	53	16	10	1·1007	0·1908	0·9040	0·1081
			C	1711	584	740	272	115				
10. Finland		Mustakallio 1937	P	101	30	45	18	8	1·2404	0·8064	1·3586	1·0155
			C	2595	908	1098	401	188				
11. Finland		Streng & Ryti 1927[a]	P	72	18	34	11	9	1·4798	1·7292	1·2196	0·2577
			C	1383	463	591	232	97				
12. Germany, Berlin		Wende 1965	P	1100	380	516	160	44	1·1498	4·0527	1·0889	0·7766
			C	21104	7725	9123	2987	1269				
13. Germany, Erlangen, Nürnberg		Berg *et al.* 1967	P	49	14	28	6	1	1·2941	0·5032	1·2298	0·1442
			C	193	66	102	23	2				
14. Germany, Hamburg-Eppendorf	(s) S, A, A_1A_2	Sauer *et al.* 1963	P	1709	641	768	210	90	1·1794	6·1420	1·0601	0·3522
			C	3086	1262	1282	390	152				
15. Germany, Oberbayern		Hermanns & Kronberg 1927	P	16	3	7	6	0	2·2917	1·3915	8·1481	8·0580
			C	265	110	112	27	16				
16. Germany, Zwickau		Lickint & Tröltzsch 1929	P	100	40	44	12	4	1·0190	0·0073	1·0804	0·0541
		Christiansen *et al.* 1935 M1	C	5335(c)	2150	2321	597	267				
17. Hungary, Budapest	(s) S	Révai & König 1968	P	308	77	133	56	42	1·3579	4·5039	1·3695	3·1668
			C	23000	7570	9632	4020	1778				
18. Italy		Lang 1959	P	2751	1288	1052	284	127	1·0412	0·8872	0·9375	0·9137
			C	42735	20426	16023	4804	1482				
19. Italy, Milano	(s) S, A	Serra *et al.* 1963	P	900	351	434	89	26	1·3423	8·7968	1·1851	1·0733
			C	1000	444	409	95	52				
20. Italy, Modena	(s) S, A	Tedeschi & Cavazzuti 1959	P	436	169	193	55	19	1·2790	4·4361	1·6391	7·7848
			C	1799	831	742	165	61				
21. Norway, Oslo	(s) A_1A_2	Berg *et al.* 1967	P	176	69	91	13	3	1·0396	0·0560	0·8722	0·1946
			C	3089	1199	1521	259	110				
22. Poland, Kołobrzeg		Grabowska 1969	P	2037	642	845	407	143	1·1188	1·5394	1·2317	3·4273
			C	1000	340	400	175	85				
23. Poland, Wrocław	Children	Wartenberg & Wąsikowa 1971	P	145	55	52	27	11	0·6437	3·5331	0·7481	1·0338
			C	325	96	141	63	25				

TABLE 1 **THE ABO BLOOD GROUP SYSTEM** *(cont.)*

Place	Additional details	Authors		Number	O	A	B	AB	A/O Relative incidence	A/O χ^2_1 for difference from unity	B/O Relative incidence	B/O χ^2_1 for difference from unity
24. Portugal		Lessa & Ruffié 1960	P C	26(c) 3353(c)	13 1424	9 1559	3 250	1 120	0·6324	1·1091	1·3145	0·1802
25. San Marino	(s) S	Dominici 1965	P C	92 3350	41 1533	36 1392	12 305	3 120	0·9670	0·0210	1·4711	1·3345
26. Switzerland, Genève		Zeytinoglu 1957	P C	393 23796	162 9686	170 11303	46 1951	15 856	0·8993	0·9207	1·4097	4·1333
27. United Kingdom, Liverpool	(s) A	Woodrow 1974 Kopeć 1970	P C	143 12084	68 6066	58 4591	12 1094	5 333	1·1270	0·4420	0·9785	0·0048
28. United Kingdom, London	(s) S, ABH secretion	Doll *et al.* 1961	P C	102 610	39 272	45 262	12 60	6 16	1·1979	0·5889	1·3949	0·8565
29. United Kingdom, Oxford	(s) S, A	McConnell *et al.* 1956	P C	500 6492	213 2888	233 2839	31 557	23 208	1·1128	1·1790	1·7546	2·0277
30. United Kingdom, SW. Lancashire	(s) S, A	McConnell *et al.* 1956	P C	634 6510	280 3146	265 2648	61 546	28 170	1·1244	1·7103	1·2553	2·3374
31. United Kingdom, W. Cheshire	(s) S, A	McConnell *et al.* 1956	P C	199 1247	86 546	98 521	11 135	4 45	1·1942	1·2314	0·5173	3·8866
32. United Kingdom, Glasgow	(s) S, A	Craig & Wang 1955	P C	817 7418	411 3853	296 2485	80 817	30 263	1·1167	1·8809	0·9180	0·4463
33. United Kingdom, Belfast		Macafee 1964[b]	P C	865 28566	446 15715	307 9433	91 2702	21 716	1·1467	3·3030	1·1867	2·1489
34. N. India, Chandigarh	(s) S	Jolly *et al.* 1969	P C	818 6204	298 1912	174 1373	295 2382	51 537	0·8131	4·1338	0·7946	6·8751
35. N. India, Delhi	(s) S, A	Lamba *et al.* 1974	P C	416 6338(c)	138 1864	71 1383	178 2481	29 610	0·6934	5·9331	0·9691	0·0715
36. N. India, Lucknow		Nath *et al.* 1963	P C	57 3330(c)	14 1035	21 753	18 1263	4 279	2·0618	4·3145	1·0536	0·0212
37. Egypt, Cairo	(s) S	Bibawi & Khatwa 1961	P C	951 10045	279 3279	408 3570	132 2448	132 748	1·3432	13·1477	0·6337	17·5236
38. Republic of South Africa	Bantu	Buckwalter *et al.* 1961	P C	23 7105	10 3197	8 2022	5 1527	0 359	1·2649	0·2445	1·0468	0·0070
39. Republic of South Africa	Asiatic Indians	Buckwalter *et al.* 1961	P C	60 7462	18 2788	15 1721	24 2490	3 463	1·3500	0·7312	1·4929	1·6389
40. Canada, Toronto	Juveniles	Simpson *et al.* 1962	P C	101 36990	49 17029	41 14636	9 3930	2 1395	0·9735	0·0160	0·7959	0·3954
41. U.S.A., Iowa	(s) S	Buckwalter 1964	P C	1489 49979	656 22392	634 21144	164 4695	35 1748	1·0235	0·1691	1·1923	3·9272
42. Trinidad	Chinese, Europeans, Negroes; (s) S	Henry & Poon-King 1961 Arneaud & Young 1955 M1	P C	156 4866	75 2294	46 1173	30 1076	5 323	1·1995	0·9098	0·8528	0·5280
43. Trinidad	Asiatic Indians; (s) S	Henry & Poon-King 1961	P C	199 1000	57 396	47 248	80 280	15 76	1·3166	1·6675	1·9850	13·0061
				23735					1·0727	18·8268	1·0487	4·1313
				χ^2_{42} for homogeneity of areas						80·9002		112·8194

TABLE 1 **THE ABO BLOOD GROUP SYSTEM** (*cont.*)

ENDOCRINE AND METABOLIC DISEASES (*cont.*)

DIABETES MELLITUS: PATIENTS UNDER 20 YEARS

These data are included in the totals shown in the main Diabetes Mellitus Table.

Place	Additional details	Authors		Number	O	A	B	AB	A/O Relative incidence	A/O χ_1^2 for difference from unity	B/O Relative incidence	B/O χ_1^2 for difference from unity
1. Denmark, København	Under 20 years; (s) S	Andersen & Lauritzen 1960	P C	316 49137(a)	164 20351	119 21290	28 5195	5 2301	0·6936	9·1743	0·6688	3·8473
2. Italy, Milano	Under 20 years; (s) S	Serra *et al.* 1964	P C	64 1000	27 444	30 409	6 95	1 52	1·2062	0·4682	1·0386	0·0066
3. Poland, Wrocław	Children	Wartenberg & Wąsikowa 1971	P C	145 325	55 96	52 141	27 63	11 25	0·6437	3·5331	0·7481	1·0338
4. United Kingdom, Liverpool	Juveniles	Woodrow 1974 Kopeć 1970	P C	91 12084	44 6066	37 4591	6 1094	4 333	1·1111	0·2212	0·7561	0·4104
5. United Kingdom, Oxford	Under 20 years	McConnell *et al.* 1956	P C	40 6492	16 2888	17 2839	1 557	6 208	1·0808	0·0495	0·3241	1·1927
6. United Kingdom, SW. Lancashire	Under 20 years	McConnell *et al.* 1956	P C	39 6510	14 3146	21 2648	4 546	0 170	1·7821	2·7882	1·6464	0·7682
7. United Kingdom, W. Cheshire	Under 20 years	McConnell *et al.* 1956	P C	30 1247	10 546	15 521	5 135	0 45	1·5720	1·2008	2·0222	1·6035
8. Canada, Toronto	Juveniles	Simpson *et al.* 1962	P C	101 36990	49 17029	41 14636	9 3930	2 1395	0·9735	0·0160	0·7959	0·3954
				826					0·8804	2·6722	0·8022	2·9512
					χ_7^2 for homogeneity of areas					14·7791		6·3067

DIABETES MELLITUS: PATIENTS OVER 20 YEARS

These data are included in the totals shown in the main Diabetes Mellitus Table.

Place	Additional details	Authors		Number	O	A	B	AB	A/O Relative incidence	A/O χ_1^2 for difference from unity	B/O Relative incidence	B/O χ_1^2 for difference from unity
1. Austria, Wien	Men and women; (s) S, Rh_D	Speiser 1958[a]	P C	239 1000	79 367	103 430	43 130	14 73	1·1128	0·4165	1·5366	3·9830
2. Austria, Wien	Men and women; (s) S	Mähr 1959	P C	1300 1000	443 367	576 430	202 130	79 73	1·1097	1·1986	1·2873	3·6181
3. Belgium, Bruxelles	Men and women; (s) S	Cornil & Pirart 1961	P C	564 3337(c)	218 1496	272 1448	52 280	22 113	1·2891	6·7003	1·2744	2·0961
4. Belgium, Liège	Men and women	Otto-Servais *et al.* 1959	P C	1392 6000	624 2771	592 2589	151 472	25 168	1·0154	0·0579	1·4206	11·5166
5. Czechoslovakia, Praha	Over 40 years	Miluničová & Dominec 1966 Miluničová & Sottner 1965 M2	P C	56 878	20 295	19 354	15 168	2 61	0·7917	0·5015	1·3170	0·6011
6. Czechoslovakia, Praha	Men and women; (s) S	Miluničová *et al.* 1969[a] Miluničová & Sottner 1965 M2	P C	400 878	141 295	165 354	62 168	32 61	0·9752	0·0326	0·7721	2·0539
7. Denmark	Mothers; (s) Rh_D	Klebe & Nielsen 1972	P C	652 12123	281 5046	281 5352	70 1245	20 480	0·9428	0·4620	1·0096	0·0049
8. Denmark, København	Over 20 years; (s) S	Andersen & Lauritzen 1960	P C	693 49137(a)	307 20351	289 21290	68 5195	29 2301	0·8999	1·6353	0·8677	1·4186
9. Germany, Hamburg-Eppendorf	Over 40 years; (s) S	Sauer *et al.* 1963	P C	1325 3086	468 1262	616 1282	173 390	68 152	1·2957	12·6050	1·1962	2·8538

TABLE 1 THE ABO BLOOD GROUP SYSTEM (*cont.*)

Place	Additional details	Authors		Number	O	A	B	AB	A/O Relative incidence	A/O χ_1^2 for difference from unity	B/O Relative incidence	B/O χ_1^2 for difference from unity
10. Hungary, Budapest	Men and women; (s) S	Révai & König 1968	P	308	77	133	56	42	1·3575	4·5039	1·3695	3·1668
			C	23000	7570	9632	4020	1778				
11. Italy, Milano	Over 20 years	Serra *et al.* 1964	P	836	324	404	83	25	1·3536	8·9341	1·1973	1·1647
			C	1000	444	409	95	52				
12. Italy, Modena	Over 30 years; (s) S	Tedeschi & Cavazzuti 1959	P	369	143	160	49	17	1·2531	3·2238	1·7257	8·5879
			C	1799	831	742	165	61				
13. United Kingdom, Liverpool	Mature	Woodrow 1974	P	52	24	21	6	1	1·1561	0·2347	1·3862	0·5096
		Kopeć 1970	C	12084	6066	4591	1094	333				
14. United Kingdom, Oxford	Over 20 years	McConnell *et al.* 1956	P	460	197	216	30	17	1·1154	1·1435	0·7896	1·3764
			C	6492	2888	2839	557	208				
15. United Kingdom, SW. Lancashire	Over 20 years	McConnell *et al.* 1956	P	595	266	244	57	28	1·0898	0·8650	1·2347	1·8944
			C	6510	3146	2648	546	170				
16. United Kingdom, W. Cheshire	Over 20 years	McConnell *et al.* 1956	P	169	76	83	6	4	1·1445	0·6290	0·3193	6·8936
			C	1247	546	521	135	45				
17. United Kingdom, Glasgow	Over 30 years	Craig & Wang 1955	P	689	338	255	71	25	1·1698	3·2666	0·9906	0·0048
			C	7418	3853	2485	817	263				
18. United Kingdom, Belfast	Men and women	Macafee 1964[b]	P	865	446	307	91	21	0·9067	1·6195	0·9168	0·5311
			C	11327	5522	4192	1229	384				
19. N. India, Delhi	Over 20 years	Lamba *et al.* 1974	P	408	137	71	175	28	0·7141	4·9722	0·9812	0·0256
			C	6338	1864	1383	2481	610				
				11372					1·0804	11·0011	1·1170	9·9464
				χ_{18}^2 for homogeneity of areas						42·0009		42·3546

DIABETES MELLITUS: YOUNGER PATIENTS/OLDER PATIENTS

Place	Additional details	Authors		Number	O	A	B	AB	A/O Relative incidence	A/O χ_1^2 for difference from unity	B/O Relative incidence	B/O χ_1^2 for difference from unity
1. Denmark, Köbenhavn		Andersen & Lauritzen 1960	Under 20	*316*	*164*	*119*	*28*	*5*	*0·7708*	*3·1940*	*0·7708*	*1·1340*
			Over 20	*693*	*307*	*289*	*68*	*29*				
2. Italy, Milano		Serra *et al.* 1964	Under 20	*64*	*27*	*30*	*6*	*1*	*0·8911*	*0·1751*	*0·8675*	*0·0924*
			Over 20	*836*	*324*	*404*	*83*	*25*				
3. United Kingdom, Oxford		McConnell *et al.* 1956	Under 20	*40*	*16*	*17*	*1*	*6*	*0·9690*	*0·0076*	*0·4104*	*0·7205*
			Over 20	*460*	*197*	*216*	*30*	*17*				
4. United Kingdom, Liverpool		Woodrow 1974	Juvenile	*91*	*44*	*37*	*6*	*4*	*0·9610*	*0·0114*	*0·5455*	*0·9238*
			Mature	*52*	*24*	*21*	*6*	*1*				
5. United Kingdom, SW. Lancashire		McConnell 1956	Under 20	*39*	*14*	*21*	*4*	*0*	*1·6352*	*1·9054*	*1·3333*	*0·2414*
			Over 20	*595*	*266*	*244*	*57*	*28*				
6. United Kingdom, W. Cheshire		McConnell 1956	Under 20	*30*	*10*	*15*	*5*	*0*	*1·3735*	*0·5251*	*6·3333*	*7·1006*
			Over 20	*169*	*76*	*83*	*6*	*4*				
				580/2805					*0·9052*	*0·8748*	*0·9146*	*0·2367*
				χ_5^2 for homogeneity of areas						*4·9438*		*9·9760*
7. Italy, Modena	(s) S	Tedeschi & Cavazzutti 1959	Under 30	*27*	*9*	*14*	*3*	*1*	*1·3903*	*0·5546*	*0·9728*	*0·0016*
			Over 30	*369*	*143*	*160*	*49*	*17*				
8. United Kingdom, Glasgow		Craig & Wang 1955	Under 30	*128*	*73*	*41*	*9*	*5*	*0·7445*	*1·9368*	*0·5869*	*2·0018*
			Over 30	*689*	*338*	*255*	*71*	*25*				
				155/1058					*0·8366*	*0·8705*	*0·6597*	*1·5872*
				χ_1^2 for homogeneity of areas						*1·6209*		*0·4162*

TABLE 1 **THE ABO BLOOD GROUP SYSTEM** *(cont.)*

Place	Additional details	Authors		Number	O	A	B	AB	A/O Relative incidence	A/O χ_1^2 for difference from unity	B/O Relative incidence	B/O χ_1^2 for difference from unity
ENDOCRINE AND METABOLIC DISEASES *(cont.)*												
DIABETES MELLITUS: YOUNGER PATIENTS/OLDER PATIENTS *(cont.)*												
9. Czechoslovakia, Praha		Miluničová & Dominec 1966	Under 40 Over 40	*65* *56*	*25* *20*	*24* *19*	*11* *15*	*5* *2*	*1·0105*	*0·0006*	*0·5867*	*1·1488*
10. Germany, Hamburg-Eppendorf	(s) S	Sauer *et al.* 1963	Under 40 Over 40	*384* *1325*	*173* *468*	*152* *616*	*37* *173*	*22* *68*	*0·6675*	*10·1351*	*0·5786*	*7·3533*
				449/1381					*0·6902*	*9·2780*	*0·5797*	*8·5006*
				χ_1^2 for homogeneity of areas						*0·8577*		*0·0015*
			Younger/ Older	*1184/5244*					*0·8095*	*8·1755*	*0·7212*	*7·2103*
				χ_9^2 for homogeneity of areas						*10·2702*		*13·5079*
DIABETES MELLITUS: MALES/FEMALES												
1. Austria, Wien		Speiser 1958	M F	*126* *113*	*46* *33*	*61* *42*	*16* *27*	*3* *11*	*1·0419*	*0·0183*	*0·4251*	*4·8270*
2. Austria, Wien		Mähr 1959	M F	*500* *800*	*175* *268*	*224* *352*	*76* *126*	*25* *54*	*0·9745*	*0·0397*	*0·9237*	*0·2062*
3. Belgium, Bruxelles		Cornil & Pirart 1961	M F	*209* *355*	*77* *141*	*105* *167*	*24* *28*	*3* *19*	*1·1513*	*0·5580*	*1·5696*	*2·0852*
4. Belgium, Liège		Otto-Servais *et al.* 1959	M F	*367* *633*	*159* *284*	*168* *270*	*34* *69*	*6* *10*	*1·1114*	*0·5730*	*0·8801*	*0·3035*
5. Czechoslovakia, Praha		Miluničová *et al.* 1969[a]	M F	*187* *213*	*75* *66*	*65* *100*	*32* *30*	*15* *17*	*0·5720*	*5·7927*	*0·9387*	*0·0430*
6. Denmark, Köbenhavn		Andersen & Lauritzen 1960	M F	*522* *487*	*249* *222*	*211* *197*	*46* *50*	*16* *18*	*0·9549*	*0·0116*	*0·8202*	*0·7814*
7. Germany, Hamburg-Eppendorf		Sauer *et al.* 1963	M F	*808* *901*	*304* *337*	*370* *398*	*91* *119*	*43* *47*	*1·0306*	*0·0790*	*0·8477*	*1·0641*
8. Hungary, Budapest		Révai & König 1968	M F	*153* *155*	*36* *41*	*72* *61*	*27* *29*	*18* *24*	*1·3443*	*1·0615*	*1·0603*	*0·0278*
9. Italy, Milano		Serra *et al.* 1963	M F	*372* *528*	*129* *222*	*190* *244*	*41* *48*	*12* *14*	*1·3401*	*3·9636*	*1·4700*	*2·5819*
10. Italy, Modena		Tedeschi & Cavazzuti 1959	M F	*201* *235*	*79* *90*	*87* *106*	*23* *32*	*12* *7*	*0·9350*	*0·1009*	*0·8188*	*0·4056*
11. San Marino		Dominici 1965	M F	*59* *33*	*24* *17*	*22* *14*	*11* *1*	*2* *1*	*1·1131*	*0·0528*	*7·7917*	*3·5379*
12. United Kingdom, London		Doll *et al.* 1961	M F	*40* *62*	*14* *25*	*21* *24*	*3* *9*	*2* *4*	*1·5625*	*0·9923*	*0·5952*	*0·4842*
13. United Kingdom, Oxford		McConnell *et al.* 1956	M F	*181* *319*	*74* *139*	*91* *142*	*10* *21*	*6* *17*	*1·2037*	*0·8877*	*0·8945*	*0·0739*
14. United Kingdom, SW. Lancashire		McConnell *et al.* 1956	M F	*221* *413*	*91* *189*	*101* *164*	*19* *42*	*10* *18*	*1·2791*	*1·8770*	*0·9396*	*0·0419*
15. United Kingdom, W. Cheshire		McConnell *et al.* 1956	M F	*82* *117*	*30* *56*	*46* *52*	*5* *6*	*1* *3*	*1·6513*	*2·7295*	*1·5556*	*0·4672*
16. United Kingdom, Glasgow		Craig & Wang 1955	M F	*276* *541*	*151* *260*	*93* *202*	*23* *57*	*9* *21*	*0·7888*	*2·1519*	*0·6948*	*1·8549*
17. N. India, Chandigarh		Jolly *et al.* 1969	M F	*535* *283*	*197* *101*	*115* *59*	*191* *104*	*32* *19*	*0·9993*	*0·0000*	*0·9416*	*0·1215*
18. N. India, Delhi		Lamba *et al.* 1974	M F	*249* *167*	*82* *56*	*46* *25*	*102* *76*	*19* *10*	*1·2566*	*0·9322*	*0·9166*	*0·1432*
19. Egypt, Cairo		Bibawi & Khatwa 1961	M F	*323* *628*	*81* *198*	*160* *248*	*40* *92*	*42* *90*	*1·5771*	*7·5009*	*1·0628*	*0·0697*

TABLE 1 **THE ABO BLOOD GROUP SYSTEM** *(cont.)*

Place	Additional details	Authors		Number	O	A	B	AB	A/O Relative incidence	A/O χ^2_1 for difference from unity	B/O Relative incidence	B/O χ^2_1 for difference from unity
20. U.S.A., Iowa		Buckwalter 1964	M	*612*	*265*	*261*	*72*	*14*	*1·0324*	*0·0793*	*1·1547*	*0·6656*
			F	*877*	*391*	*373*	*92*	*21*				
21. Trinidad	Chinese, Europeans, Negroes	Henry & Poon-King 1961	M	*33*	*12*	*12*	*8*	*1*	*1·8529*	*1·7948*	*1·9091*	*1·5506*
			F	*123*	*63*	*34*	*22*	*4*				
22. Trinidad	Asiatic Indians	Henry & Poon-King 1961	M	*80*	*20*	*19*	*35*	*6*	*1·2554*	*0·3127*	*1·4389*	*1·0358*
			F	*119*	*37*	*28*	*45*	*9*				
				6136/8102					*1·0803*	*3·9863*	*0·9722*	*0·2576*
				χ^2_{21} for homogeneity of areas						*27·5233*		*22·1146*
DIABETES, KIMMELSTIEL-WILSON SYNDROME												
1. Switzerland, Genève		Zeytinoglu 1957	P	39	5	31	2	1	5·3130	12·0002	1·9859	0·6718
			C	23796	9686	11303	1951	856				
TOXAEMIA OF PREGNANCY												
1. Germany, Leipzig		Kyank & Kulisch 1958	P	846(c)	307	349	140	50	0·8682	2·2361	1·0913	0·4831
			C	1831(c)	627	821	262	121				
2. United Kingdom, London		Pearson & Pinker 1956	P	675	296	298	58	23	1·1666	3·3066	0·8725	0·8551
			C	10411	4809	4150	1080	372				
3. United Kingdom, London		Dickins *et al.* 1956	P	448	237	170	30	11	0·7663	6·1536	0·6964	3·1178
			C	3203	1469	1375	267	92				
4. United Kingdom, London		Dickins *et al.* 1956	P	262	106	116	29	11	1·1352	0·7660	1·6534	4·6779
			C	1523	695	670	115	43				
5. United Kingdom, Newport (Mon.)		Andrews 1959	P	149	65	67	12	5	1·0431	0·0508	1·0251	0·0054
			C	938	422	417	76	23				
6. U.S.S.R., Leningrad	(s) Rh_D	Golovachev & Bokarius 1972	P	2234	784	866	462	122	1·0036	0·0038	0·9626	0·3068
			C	5889	2037	2242	1247	363				
7. Israel, Jerusalem	(s) Rh_D	Harlap & Davies 1974	P	176	50	65	46	15	1·2110	1·0213	1·4944	3·8020
			C	11004	3744	4019	2305	936				
8. Japan, Sendai		Moniwa 1960	P	79	30	27	16	6	0·7824	0·8520	0·7479	0·8772
			C	21199	6769	7786	4827	1817				
				4869					0·9903	0·0710	0·9954	0·0052
				χ^2_7 for homogeneity of areas						14·3192		14·1201
PELLAGRA												
1. Egypt		el-Hefnawi *et al.* 1963	P	20	7	7	5	1	0·9383	0·0141	0·9460	0·0090
			C	5200	1674	1784	1264	478				
RICKETS												
1. Austria, Vöcklabruck	Infants; (s) S	Kircher 1968	P	557	243	211	75	28	0·9470	0·2883	1·1471	0·9110
			C	3405	1468	1346	395	196				
COELIAC DISEASE												
1. United Kingdom, Birmingham		Langman *et al.* 1969	P	116(c)	44	60	10	2	1·5100	4·2859	1·2918	0·5310
			C	19789	9225	8331	1623	610				
2. United Kingdom, London Inner Area		Langman *et al.* 1969	P	70	38	25	6	1	0·7138	1·7108	0·8091	0·2322
			C	33026	15121	13937	2951	1017				
3. United Kingdom, London Outer Area		Langman *et al.* 1969	P	23	15	8	0	0	0·5351	2·0356		
			C	10289	4586	4571	843	289				
				209					1·0466	0·0943	1·0765	0·0721
				χ^2_2 for homogeneity of areas						7·9380		
				(186) χ^2_1 for homogeneity of areas								0·6911

TABLE 1 THE ABO BLOOD GROUP SYSTEM (*cont.*)

Place	Additional details	Authors		Number	O	A	B	AB	A/O Relative incidence	A/O χ_1^2 for difference from unity	B/O Relative incidence	B/O χ_1^2 for difference from unity
ENDOCRINE AND METABOLIC DISEASES (*cont.*)												
NON-TROPICAL SPRUE												
1. U.S.A., Boston		Joske & Benson 1958	P	28	20	7	1	0	0·4550	3·1803	0·2016	2·4315
			C	2330(c)	1109	853	275	93				
HAEMOCHROMATOSIS												
1. Belgium, Bruxelles	Idiopathic	Cornil & Pirart 1961	P	24	14	9	1	0	0·6642	0·9106	0·3816	0·8627
			C	3337	1496	1448	280	113				
2. Australia, Sydney	(s) A_1A_2	Bradley & Walsh 1965	P	56	26	24	4	2	1·1763	0·3282	0·7751	0·2246
		Walsh 1947 M1	C	30000	14672	11514	2912	902				
				80					0·9887	0·0023	0·6672	0·7193
				χ_1^2 for homogeneity of areas						1·2366		0·3680
SPASMOPHILIA												
1. Austria, Vöcklabruck	Infants	Kircher 1968	P	100	45	41	10	4	0·9937	0·0008	0·8259	0·2918
			C	3405	1468	1346	395	196				
HYPOGAMMAGLOBULINAEMIA												
1. United Kingdom	Non-lymphopenic	Mollison & Hill 1969	P	145	64	66	8	7	1·1190	0·4035	0·6430	1·3739
		Discombe & Meyer 1952 M1	C	10000	4578	4219	890	313				
2. U.S.A., Minnesota	Non-lymphopenic	Meuwissen *et al.* 1969	P	49(c)	32	9	6	2	0·2464	12·4233	0·6429	0·8313
			C	300(c)	120	137	35	8				
				194					0·8717	0·7240	0·6429	2·2052
				χ_1^2 for homogeneity of areas						12·1028		0·0000
DISEASES OF THE BLOOD												
HYPOCHROMIC ANAEMIA												
1. Austria, Vöcklabruck	Infants; (s) S	Kircher 1968	P	393	157	169	46	21	1·1740	1·8769	1·0889	0·2316
			C	3405	1468	1346	395	196				
2. Italy, Lombardia		Ninni & Bedarida 1959	P	61	27	25	7	2	0·9095	0·1070	1·2778	0·2984
			C	640	276	281	56	27				
3. N. India, Lucknow	Microcytic, due to ancylostomiasis	Nath *et al.* 1963	P	182	68	42	60	12	0·8490	0·6570	0·7231	3·1735
			C	3330(c)	1035	753	1263	279				
4. N. India, Lucknow	Normocytic	Nath *et al.* 1963	P	221	68	48	80	25	0·9702	0·0241	0·9641	0·0462
			C	3330(c)	1035	753	1263	279				
5. Peru, Lima		Muñoz-Baratta 1962	P	41(c)	13	17	6	5	3·3208	10·6074	2·4142	3·1876
			C	107938(c)	66058	26013	12629	3238				
				898					1·1074	1·4895	0·9675	0·1157
				χ_4^2 for homogeneity of areas						11·7829		6·8216
PERNICIOUS ANAEMIA												
1. Austria, Wien	(s) S, Rh_D	Speiser 1958[a]	P	202	68	90	27	17	1·1296	0·4812	1·1209	0·2096
			C	1000	367	430	130	73				
2. Denmark, København		Køster *et al.* 1955	P	111	44	47	14	6	0·9842	0·0057	1·1861	0·3067
			C	14304	5804	6299	1557	644				
3. Finland		Mustakallio 1937	P	16	1	9	4	2	7·4426	3·6195	9·0574	3·8735
			C	2595	908	1098	401	188				

TABLE 1 **THE ABO BLOOD GROUP SYSTEM** (*cont.*)

Place	Additional details	Authors		Number	O	A	B	AB	A/O		B/O	
									Relative incidence	χ_1^2 for difference from unity	Relative incidence	χ_1^2 for difference from unity
4. Finland	Cryptogenic	Kaipainen & Vuorinen	P	138(c)	40	60	23	15	1·1722	0·5313	1·2055	0·4432
		1960	C	891	304	389	145	53				
		Mäkelä *et al.* 1959 M2										
5. France, Mulhouse	Biermer's	Lobstein 1958	P	51	23	23	1	4	0·8745	0·2051	0·2201	2·1905
			C	6423	2648	3028	523	224				
6. Italy, Lombardia		Ninni & Bedarida 1959	P	81	31	38	9	3	1·2040	0·5241	1·4309	0·7787
			C	640	276	281	56	27				
7. Poland, Katowice		Machalski *et al.* 1968	P	94	23	45	19	7	1·6295	3·5477	1·5745	2·0919
			C	3606	1216	1460	638	292				
8. Poland, Kraków		Cichecka 1965	P	57	12	32	8	5	2·1544	5·1345	1·0504	0·0116
			C	39006	12457	15419	7906	3224				
9. Poland, Warszawa		Królikowska & Żupańska	P	209	54	91	39	25	1·5499	6·4181	1·2260	0·9278
		1964	C	13744	4719	5131	2780	1114				
		Charzewski *et al.* 1965 M2										
10. United Kingdom, Cambridge		Aird *et al.* 1956	P	110	51	49	8	2	1·0056	0·0008	0·9664	0·0078
			C	3438	1571	1501	255	111				
11. United Kingdom, London		Aird *et al.* 1956	P	244	90	135	12	7	1·6276	12·5063	0·6858	1·4847
			C	10000	4578	4219	890	313				
12. United Kingdom, Manchester		MacLeod 1937	P	193	80	75	25	13	1·1115	0·3969	1·9827	7·7663
			C	1927	939	792	148	48				
13. United Kingdom, Newcastle upon Tyne		Aird *et al.* 1956	P	109	55	45	7	2	1·0261	0·0163	0·6357	1·2674
			C	13572	6598	5261	1321	392				
14. United Kingdom, Oxford		Aird *et al.* 1956	P	258	112	120	18	8	1·0899	0·4128	0·8333	0·4992
			C	6395	2888	2839	557	111				
15. United Kingdom, Sheffield		Aird *et al.* 1956	P	123	47	58	10	8	1·3586	2·3495	1·2399	0·3669
			C	3111	1451	1318	249	93				
16. United Kingdom, Glasgow		Aird *et al.* 1956	P	270	135	96	31	8	1·1853	1·5485	1·1453	0·4428
			C	5898	3177	1906	637	178				
17. U.S.A., Boston		Hoskins *et al.* 1965	P	158(c)	68	63	21	6	1·3460	2·8009	1·2575	0·8169
			C	5236(c)	2602	1791	639	204				
18. U.S.A., California		Creger & Sortor 1956	P	115(c)	43	59	12	1	1·6997	6·9582	1·2429	0·4412
			C	20070(c)	9473	7647	2127	823				
19. U.S.A., Chicago	Whites; (s) A_1A_2	Ladenson *et al.* 1949	P	119	34	62	17	6	1·8316	6·7406	1·7538	2·9224
		Wiener *et al.* 1944 M1	C	562	228	227	65	42				
20. U.S.A., Chicago	Negroes; (s) A_1A_2	Ladenson *et al.* 1949	P	41	20	16	4	1	1·3375	0·6152	0·4553	1·8722
		Wiener *et al.* 1944 M1	C	231	107	64	47	13				
21. U.S.A., Iowa		Buckwalter & Knowler	P	158	59	76	14	9	1·3642	3·1934	1·1317	0·1727
		1958	C	49979	22392	21144	4695	1748				
22. U.S.A., Rochester	Whites	Buchanan & Higley 1921	P	457	189	202	46	20	1·1185	0·8444	1·3690	2·3639
		Tinney & Watkins 1941	C	1000(c)	450	430	80	40				
23. U.S.A., Rochester		Tinney & Watkins 1941	P	105(c)	42	42	12	9	1·0465	0·0396	1·6071	1·8472
			C	1000(c)	450	430	80	40				
24. Peru, Lima		Muñoz-Baratta 1962	P	27(c)	18	5	2	2	0·7054	0·4765	0·5812	0·5300
			C	107938(c)	66058	26013	12629	3238				
				3446					1·2524	32·3099	1·1929	7·8940
				χ_{23}^2 for homogeneity of areas						27·0572		25·7411

TABLE 1 **THE ABO BLOOD GROUP SYSTEM** (*cont.*)

Place	Additional details	Authors		Number	O	A	B	AB	A/O Relative incidence	A/O χ_1^2 for difference from unity	B/O Relative incidence	B/O χ_1^2 for difference from unity
DISEASES OF THE BLOOD (*cont.*)												
MACROCYTIC ANAEMIA												
1. United Kingdom, Manchester		MacLeod 1937	P C	17 1927	9 938	7 792	0 148	1 48	0·9221	0·0256		
2. Peru, Lima		Muñoz-Baratta 1962	P C	30 107938	18 66058	5 26013	5 12629	2 3238	0·7054	0·4765	1·4530	0·5460
				47					0·8064	0·3619		
					χ_1^2 for homogeneity of areas					0·1402		
HAEMOLYTIC ANAEMIA												
CONGENITAL												
1. Poland, Kraków		Cichecka 1965	P C	33 39006	12 12457	13 15419	7 7906	1 3224	0·8752	0·1107	0·9191	0·0314
2. Poland, Warszawa		Królikowska & Żupańska 1964 Charzewski *et al.* 1965 M2	P C	26 13744	7 4719	13 5131	5 2780	1 1114	1·7080	1·3015	1·2125	0·1081
3. U.S.A., San Francisco	Whites	Hunt & Lucia 1953 Reed 1968 M2	P C	31 8962	15 4067	11 3639	5 958	0 298	0·8196	0·2504	1·4151	0·4499
				90					1·0202	0·0068	1·1436	0·1992
					χ_2^2 for homogeneity of areas					1·6558		0·3902
ACQUIRED												
1. Austria, Wien		Lal & Speiser 1957	P C	97 10000	39 3631	38 4422	11 1343	9 604	0·8001	0·9485	0·7626	0·6250
2. Poland, Kraków		Cichecka 1965	P C	79 39006	21 12457	35 15419	17 7906	6 3224	1·3465	1·1595	1·2755	0·5553
3. Poland, Warszawa		Królikowska & Żupańska 1964 Charzewski *et al.* 1965 M2	P C	83 13744	33 4719	26 5131	16 2780	8 1114	0·7246	1·5000	0·8230	0·4063
4. United Kingdom, Sheffield		Dunsford & Owen 1960	P C	127 6000(c)	60 2723	51 2597	7 515	9 165	0·8912	0·3581	0·6169	1·4422
5. U.S.A., San Francisco		Hunt & Lucia 1953 Reed 1968 M2	P C	27 8962	21 4067	2 3639	4 958	0 298	0·1064	9·1553	0·8086	0·1509
6. Australia, Sydney		Clemens & Walsh 1955	P C	66 30000	42 14672	23 11514	1 2912	0 902	0·6978	1·9195	0·1200	4·3905
				479					0·8234	3·4099	0·8176	1·5863
					χ_5^2 for homogeneity of areas					11·6311		5·9826
HAEMOLYTIC ANAEMIA												
1. United Kingdom, Manchester	Congenital or acquired	MacLeod 1937	P C	65 1927	30 939	26 792	6 148	3 48	1·0275	0·0099	1·2689	0·2729
2. Peru, Lima	Unspecified	Muñoz-Baratta 1962	P C	23(c) 107938(c)	15 66058	4 26013	2 12629	2 3238	0·6772	0·4798	0·6974	0·2291
				88					0·9494	0·0449	1·0807	0·0396
					χ_1^2 for homogeneity of areas					0·4448		0·4625
HAEMOLYTIC JAUNDICE												
1. U.S.A., Rochester		Tinney & Watkins 1941	P C	58 1000(c)	30 450	22 430	3 80	3 40	0·7674	0·8407	0·5625	0·8680

TABLE 1 THE ABO BLOOD GROUP SYSTEM (*cont.*)

Place	Additional details	Authors		Number	O	A	B	AB	A/O Relative incidence	A/O χ_1^2 for difference from unity	B/O Relative incidence	B/O χ_1^2 for difference from unity
APLASTIC ANAEMIA												
1. Poland, Kraków		Cichecka 1965	P C	63 39006	21 12457	28 15419	12 7906	2 3224	1·0772	0·0662	0·9004	0·0840
2. United Kingdom, Manchester		MacLeod 1937	P C	18 1927	11 939	5 792	1 148	1 48	0·5389	1·3033	0·5768	0·2756
3. Peru, Lima		Muñoz-Baratta 1962	P C	27 107938	17 66058	5 26013	3 12629	2 3238	0·7469	0·3290	0·9231	0·0163
				108					0·8853	0·2856	0·8730	0·2045
				χ_2^2 for homogeneity of areas						1·4129		0·1715
SECONDARY ANAEMIA												
1. Finland		Mustakallio 1937	P C	78 2595	32 908	26 1098	15 401	5 188	0·6719	2·2045	1·0614	0·0350
2. Peru, Lima		Muñoz-Baratta 1962	P C	307(c) 107938(c)	191 66058	62 26013	33 12629	21 3238	0·8243	1·7428	0·9037	0·2876
				385					0·7865	3·4987	0·9423	0·1340
				χ_1^2 for homogeneity of areas						0·4486		0·1886
VARIOUS ANAEMIAS												
1. Peru, Lima	Chronic	Muñoz-Baratta 1962	P C	41(c) 107938(c)	23 66058	5 26013	8 12629	5 3238	0·5520	1·4494	1·8194	2·1248
2. Peru, Lima	Nutritional	Muñoz-Baratta 1962	P C	44(c) 107938(c)	22 66058	10 26013	7 12629	5 3238	1·1543	0·1415	1·6643	1·3773
3. Peru, Lima	Postinfective	Muñoz-Baratta 1962	P C	50(c) 107938(c)	24 66058	8 26013	10 12629	8 3238	0·8465	0·1666	2·1794	4·2815
4. Peru, Lima	Due to renal insufficiency	Muñoz-Baratta 1962	P C	23(c) 107938(c)	7 66058	8 26013	5 12629	3 3238	2·9022	4·2373	3·7362	5·0657
HAEMOPHILIA												
1. Czechoslovakia, Praha		Májský 1964 Kout 1959 M2	P C	30 1142	11 359	13 516	5 191	1 76	0·8222	0·2220	0·8544	0·0829
2. Poland, Kraków		Cichecka 1965	P C	51 39006	17 12457	13 15419	11 7906	10 3224	0·6178	1·7067	1·0195	0·0025
3. Poland, Warszawa		Królikowska & Żupańska 1964 Charzewski *et al.* 1965 M2	P C	112 13744	41 4719	45 5131	17 2780	9 1114	1·0094	0·0019	0·7038	1·4722
4. U.S.A., Rochester		Tinney & Watkins 1941	P C	38(c) 1000(c)	13 450	21 430	3 80	1 40	1·6905	2·1354	1·2981	0·1602
				231					0·9071	0·0040	0·8491	0·6504
				χ_3^2 for homogeneity of areas						4·0620		1·0674
IDIOPATHIC THROMBOCYTOPENIC PURPURA												
1. Poland, Kraków	Schönlein-Henoch syndrome; children	Cichecka 1965	P C	112 39006	29 12457	59 15419	18 7906	6 3224	1·6437	4·7877	0·9780	0·0055
2. Poland, Kraków	Werlhof's disease	Cichecka 1965	P C	61 39006	10 12457	24 15419	23 7906	4 3224	1·9390	3·0917	3·6240	11·5380
3. Poland, Warszawa	Thrombo-penia	Królikowska & Żupańska 1964 Charzewski *et al.* 1965 M2	P C	47 13744	19 4719	20 5131	7 2780	1 1114	0·9681	0·0102	0·6254	1·1237
4. U.S.A., Rochester		Tinney & Watkins 1941	P C	53(c) 1000(c)	19 450	27 430	6 80	1 40	1·4871	1·6717	1·7763	1·4106
5. Peru, Lima	Purpura haemor-rhagica	Muñoz-Baratta 1962	P C	61 107938	41 66058	9 26013	6 12629	5 3238	0·5574	2·5195	0·7655	0·3737
				334					1·2925	3·5637	1·2535	1·6668
				χ_4^2 for homogeneity of areas						8·5171		12·7846

TABLE 1 **THE ABO BLOOD GROUP SYSTEM** (*cont.*)

Place	Additional details	Authors		Number	O	A	B	AB	A/O Relative incidence	A/O χ_1^2 for difference from unity	B/O Relative incidence	B/O χ_1^2 for difference from unity
DISEASES OF THE BLOOD (*cont.*)												
HAEMOPHILIA AND PURPURA												
1. U.S.A.,		Buchanan & Higley 1921	P	40	19	16	4	1	0·8813	0·1335	1·1842	0·0902
Rochester		Tinney & Watkins 1941	C	1000(c)	450	430	80	40				
TROPICAL EOSINOPHILIA												
1. N. India,		Anand 1961	P	224	46	81	72	25	2·4177	16·3042	2·1491	11·8610
Dehra Dun			C	470	173	126	126	45				
2. N. India,		Anand 1961	P	188	39	60	76	13	2·8205	13·5922	2·1747	9·1059
Delhi			C	196	77	42	69	8				
3. N. India,		Anand 1961	P	318	87	105	108	18	1·9310	11·6195	1·6415	6·9646
Delhi			C	410	160	100	121	29				
4. N. India,		Nath *et al.* 1963	P	50	13	18	11	8	1·9032	3·0727	0·6934	0·7905
Lucknow			C	3330(c)	1035	753	1263	279				
				780					2·2174	43·0102	1·7541	21·9835
				χ_3^2 for homogeneity of areas						1·5784		6·7384
MENTAL DISORDERS												
PSYCHOSES												
SENILE DEMENTIA												
1. Austria, Wien		Pilcz 1927	P	54(c)	23	14	11	6	0·5050	3·8766	0·7876	0·4005
		Hoche & Moritsch 1926 M1	C	1000	331	399	201	69				
2. Czechoslovakia,		Leischner 1936	P	20	5	10	4	1	1·5716	0·6762	1·4246	0·2762
Praha			C	2429	796	1013	447	173				
3. Germany,		Saleck 1932	P	198	78	97	14	9	1·0171	0·0096	0·6342	2·0462
Tübingen			C	700	265	324	75	36				
4. Greece,		Zervopoulos *et al.* 1967	P	39	9	20	8	2	2·1467	3·5989	3·5033	6·5834
Makedhonia and Thraki			C	4480	1876	1942	476	186				
5. Hungary,		Somogyi & Angyal 1931	P	43	16	19	7	1	0·9227	0·0537	0·8045	0·2212
Budapest			C	1000	331	426	180	63				
6. Italy, Arezzo		Marzi & Turchini 1952	P	21	6	12	3	0	2·3934	2·9291	2·1471	1·1138
			C	473	219	183	51	20				
7. Italy, Milano		Bravetta 1930	P	37	14	16	6	1	1·2857	0·4609	1·8437	1·5223
		Cuboni M1	C	1500	684	608	159	49				
8. Italy, Padova		Bianchini 1937	P	96	43	39	11	3	1·0237	0·0094	1·1903	0·2184
		Pennati & Bianchini 1930 M1	C	500	228	202	49	21				
9. Italy, Siena		D'Ormea & Centini 1942	P	43(c)	18	17	6	2	0·9761	0·0051	1·3172	0·3392
		Lecchini 1930 M1	C	8720	3758	3636	951	375				
10. Italy, Vercelli		Giuli 1959	P	57	28	22	7	0	0·8816	0·1844	0·8308	0·1823
			C	1000	432	385	130	53				
11. Poland,		Meyer 1928	P	45(c)	12	21	10	2	1·6241	1·6939	3·0934	6·2956
Lower Silesia		Kruse M1	C	600	245	264	66	25				
12. United Kingdom,		Thomas & Hewitt 1939	P	94	44	38	7	5	0·8316	0·5514	0·6531	0·9152
England			C	374	156	162	38	18				
				747					1·0376	0·1791	1·1352	0·9787
				χ_{11}^2 for homogeneity of areas						13·8702		19·1356

TABLE 1 **THE ABO BLOOD GROUP SYSTEM** *(cont.)*

Place	Additional details	Authors		Number	O	A	B	AB	A/O		B/O	
									Relative incidence	χ_1^2 for difference from unity	Relative incidence	χ_1^2 for difference from unity
Postencephalitic Psychoses												
1. Italy, Vercelli		Giuli 1959	P C	12 1000	4 432	6 385	2 130	0 53	1·6831	0·6430	1·6615	0·3392
Schizophrenia												
1. Austria, Wien		Pilcz 1927 Hoche & Moritsch 1926 M1	P C	96 1000	35 331	41 399	12 201	8 69	0·9718	0·0140	0·5646	2·7252
2. Czechoslovakia, Bohemia	Paranoid	Prokop *et al.* 1938	P C	587(c) 725(c)	149 225	294 310	108 140	36 50	1·4321	7·2539	1·1649	0·8455
3. Czechoslovakia, Bohemia	Other than paranoid	Prokop *et al.* 1938	P C	1180(c) 725(c)	421 225	470 310	224 140	65 50	0·8103	3·6356	0·8551	1·3296
4. Czechoslovakia, Nitra		Miššík 1962	P C	257 1000	90 345	97 402	44 188	26 65	0·9250	0·2270	0·8972	0·2800
5. Czechoslovakia, Praha		Leischner 1936	P C	312 2429	107 796	120 1013	68 447	17 173	0·8813	0·8021	1·1317	0·5557
6. France, Seine		Kossovitch & Sérane 1941 Khérumian *et al.* 1958 M2	P C	178 30621	71 13755	86 13312	17 2505	4 1049	1·2516	1·9416	1·3147	1·0195
7. Germany, Schleswig-Holstein		Gundel & Tornquist 1929	P C	774 19461	202 7664	344 8461	193 2412	35 924	1·5426	23·1764	3·0359	115·5025
8. Germany, Tübingen		Saleck 1932	P C	2380 700	1028 265	994 324	245 75	113 36	0·7909	6·2293	0·8421	1·3329
9. Greece, Makedhonia and Thraki	Catatonic	Zervopoulos *et al.* 1967	P C	38 4480	15 1876	16 1942	5 476	2 186	1·0304	0·0069	1·3137	0·2765
10. Greece, Makedhonia and Thraki	Hebephrenic	Zervopoulos *et al.* 1967	P C	215 4480	86 1876	85 1942	28 476	16 186	0·9548	0·0876	1·2832	1·2440
11. Greece, Makedhonia and Thraki	Paranoid	Zervopoulos *et al.* 1967	P C	192 4480	73 1876	86 1942	24 476	9 186	1·1380	0·6340	1·2957	1·1572
12. Greece, Makedhonia and Thraki	Simple	Zervopoulos *et al.* 1967	P C	97 4480	36 1876	42 1942	10 476	9 186	1·1270	0·2716	1·0948	0·0629
13. Hungary, Budapest		Somogyi & Angyal 1931	P C	411 1000	134 331	175 426	74 180	28 63	1·0147	0·0115	1·0155	0·0080
14. Italy		Laurà 1938	P C	78(c) 200(c)	30 86	32 73	12 31	4 10	1·2566	0·5803	1·1097	0·0675
15. Italy		Andreani 1954	P C	67(c) 970(c)	30 472	27 389	5 81	5 28	1·0920	0·1033	0·9712	0·0034
16. Italy, Ancona		Fattovich 1928	P C	134 1500(c)	72 684	36 607	18 159	8 50	0·5634	7·3511	1·0755	0·0686
17. Italy, Arezzo	Hebephrenic	Marzi & Turchini 1952	P C	43 473	16 219	19 183	6 51	2 20	1·4211	0·9868	1·6103	0·8959
18. Italy, Arezzo	Paranoid	Marzi & Turchini 1952	P C	91 473	44 219	36 183	8 51	3 20	0·9791	0·0073	0·7807	0·3564
19. Italy, Catania		di Mauro 1936 del Carpio 1929 M1	P C	89 500	49 235	32 171	8 73	0 21	0·8975	0·1894	0·5256	2·5329
20. Italy, Milano		Bravetta 1930 Cuboni M1	P C	192 1500	92 684	76 608	20 159	4 49	0·9293	0·1979	0·9352	0·0654
21. Italy, Padova		Bianchini 1937 Pennati & Bianchini 1930 M1	P C	154(c) 500	70 228	66 202	14 49	4 21	1·0642	0·0999	0·9306	0·0468
22. Italy, Perugia		Pennacchi 1928 Pennacchi 1931 M1	P C	162(c) 1000	47 367	58 462	54 137	3 34	0·9803	0·0091	3·0778	25·3690

TABLE 1 **THE ABO BLOOD GROUP SYSTEM** (*cont.*)

MENTAL DISORDERS (*cont.*)
PSYCHOSES (*cont.*)
SCHIZOPHRENIA (*cont.*)

Place	Additional details	Authors		Number	O	A	B	AB	A/O Relative incidence	A/O χ_1^2 for difference from unity	B/O Relative incidence	B/O χ_1^2 for difference from unity
23. Italy, Siena		d'Ormea & Centini 1942	P	102(c)	45	48	6	3	1·1025	0·2182	0·5269	2·1587
		Lecchini 1930 M1	C	8720	3758	3636	951	375				
24. Italy, Vercelli		Giuli 1959	P	291	123	116	34	18	1·0582	0·1478	0·9186	0·1517
			C	1000	432	385	130	53				
25. Poland		Wilczkowski 1927	P	227	69	94	46	18	1·2654	2·0340	1·2564	1·3223
			C	2613	914	984	485	230				
26. Poland, Kielce		Gala & Gala 1966	P	158(c)	48	66	32	12	1·2626	1·3843	1·2765	1·0442
			C	1644	534	636	305	119				
27. Poland, Kraków		Turowska *et al.* 1968	P	197(c)	51	74	46	16	0·9341	0·1500	1·1831	0·7122
		Socha 1966 M2	C	5201	1627	2113	1037	424				
28. Poland, Lower Silesia		Meyer 1928	P	526(c)	204	222	76	24	1·0099	0·0056	1·3829	2·8187
		Kruse M1	C	600	245	264	66	25				
29. Poland, Warszawa	(s) S	Rosiński 1960	P	617	208	246	137	26	1·0248	0·0667	1·1265	1·1523
			C	40000	13347	15403	7804	3446				
30. Switzerland, Basel	Catatonic	Würz 1928	P	151	63	73	8	7	0·9859	0·0065	0·7115	0·7931
			C	3017	1255	1475	224	63				
31. Switzerland, Basel	Hebephrenic	Würz 1928	P	49	18	26	3	2	1·2290	0·4453	0·9338	0·0119
			C	3017	1255	1475	224	63				
32. Switzerland, Basel	Paranoid	Würz 1928	P	69	29	36	3	1	1·0562	0·0469	0·5796	0·7974
			C	3017	1255	1475	224	63				
33. Switzerland, Basel	Mixed forms	Würz 1928	P	65	27	35	1	2	1·1030	0·1431	0·2075	2·3727
			C	3017	1255	1475	224	63				
34. United Kingdom, England		Thomas & Hewitt 1939	P	67	27	28	8	4	0·9986	0·0000	1·2164	0·1970
			C	374	156	162	38	18				
35. United Kingdom, England	Delusional insanity	Thomas & Hewitt 1939	P	65	24	31	8	2	1·2438	0·5503	1·3684	0·4934
			C	374	156	162	38	18				
36. United Kingdom, Chorley, Leyland, Preston	(s) $A_1 A_2$	Masters 1967	P	87	41	41	5	0	1·3745	1·8103	0·7023	0·5106
			C	652	334	243	58	17				
37. U.S.S.R., Kiev	(s) S	Chominskij & Schustova 1928	P	276	79	122	48	27	1·2980	3·0468	1·0119	0·0039
			C	3840	1254	1492	753	341				
38. U.S.A., Brooklyn	Catatonic	Herman & Derby 1937	P	209	92	78	25	14	0·9320	0·1828	0·7806	1·0719
			C	1444	609	554	212	69				
39. U.S.A., Brooklyn	Paranoid	Herman & Derby 1937	P	218	93	84	34	7	0·9929	0·0019	1·0502	0·0516
			C	1444	609	554	212	69				
40. U.S.A., Brooklyn	Simple, hebephrenic	Herman & Derby 1937	P	81	36	31	11	3	0·9466	0·0474	0·8778	0·1360
			C	1444	609	554	212	69				
41. U.S.A., Iowa	(s) S	Buckwalter *et al.* 1959	P	1209	575	481	109	44	0·8859	3·7540	0·9041	0·9098
			C	49979	22392	21144	4695	1748				
42. U.S.A., Mississippi	(s) ABH secretion	Lafferty *et al.* 1960	P	110	56	43	10	1	0·7515	0·9699	1·6429	0·7257
			C	100	46	47	5	2				
43. Argentina, Buenos Aires		Espejo Solá 1931	P	107	62	38	5	2	0·8427	0·3732	0·5914	0·8058
			C	127	66	48	9	4				
				12608					1·0172	0·4983	1·1663	20·7444
		χ_{42}^2 for homogeneity of areas								68·7037		153·2420

TABLE 1 **THE ABO BLOOD GROUP SYSTEM** (*cont.*)

Place	Additional details	Authors		Number	O	A	B	AB	A/O Relative incidence	A/O χ_1^2 for difference from unity	B/O Relative incidence	B/O χ_1^2 for difference from unity
MANIC-DEPRESSIVE PSYCHOSES												
1. Austria, Wien		Pilcz 1927	P	61(c)	23	20	10	8	0·7214	1·0774	0·7160	0·7369
		Hoche & Moritsch 1926 M1	C	1000	331	399	201	69				
2. Austria, Wien	Psychotic depressions	Pilcz 1927	P	62(c)	24	27	10	1	0·9333	0·0566	0·6862	0·9479
		Hoche & Moritsch 1926 M1	C	1000	331	399	201	69				
3. Czechoslovakia, Nitra		Miššík 1962	P	35	8	17	7	3	1·8237	1·9081	1·6057	0·8124
			C	1000	345	402	188	65				
4. Czechoslovakia, Praha		Leischner 1936	P	98	34	36	22	6	0·8320	0·5691	1·1523	0·2563
			C	2429	796	1013	447	173				
5. Germany, Tübingen		Saleck 1932	P	140	58	60	16	6	0·8461	0·6850	0·9747	0·0068
			C	700	265	324	75	36				
6. Germany, Tübingen	Melancholia	Saleck 1932	P	114	55	37	15	7	0·5502	6·8548	0·9636	0·0135
			C	700	265	324	75	36				
7. Greece, Makedhonia and Thraki		Zervopoulos *et al.* 1967	P	40	16	19	4	1	1·1471	0·1622	0·9853	0·0007
			C	4480	1876	1942	476	186				
8. Hungary, Budapest		Somogyi & Angyal 1931	P	35	13	14	7	1	0·8368	0·2066	0·9902	0·0004
			C	1000	331	426	180	63				
9. Italy		Laurà 1938	P	22(c)	11	6	5	0	0·6426	0·6913	1·2610	0·1606
			C	200(c)	86	73	31	10				
10. Italy		Andreani 1954	P	44(c)	19	19	4	2	1·2134	0·3402	1·2268	0·1317
			C	970(c)	472	389	81	28				
11. Italy, Ancona		Fattovich 1928	P	47	34	9	3	1	0·2983	10·1884	0·3796	2·5327
			C	1500(c)	684	607	159	50				
12. Italy, Milano		Bravetta 1930	P	25(c)	15	7	3	0	0·5250	1·9527	0·8604	0·0555
		Cuboni M1	C	1500	684	608	159	49				
13. Italy, Padova		Bianchini 1937	P	113(c)	51	47	14	1	1·0402	0·0309	1·2773	0·5172
		Pennati & Bianchini 1930 M1	C	500	228	202	49	21				
14. Italy, Siena		D'Ormea & Centini 1942	P	69(c)	26	31	8	4	1·2323	0·6123	1·2159	0·2319
		Lecchini 1930 M1	C	8720	3758	3636	951	375				
15. Italy, Vercelli		Giuli 1959	P	172	68	74	21	9	1·2211	1·2042	1·0262	0·0093
			C	1000	432	385	130	53				
16. Poland, Lower Silesia		Meyer 1928	P	32	9	10	11	2	1·0311	0·0043	4·5370	10·3364
		Kruse M1	C	600	245	264	66	25				
17. United Kingdom, England		Thomas & Hewitt 1939	P	257	107	117	26	7	1·0530	0·0874	0·9975	0·0001
			C	374	156	162	38	18				
18. United Kingdom, Chorley, Leyland, Preston	(s) A_1A_2	Masters 1967	P	35	25	7	3	0	0·3849	4·7998	0·6910	0·3470
			C	652	334	243	58	17				
19. U.S.S.R., Kiev		Chominskij & Schustova 1928	P	27	9	9	5	4	0·8405	0·1350	0·9252	0·0193
			C	3840	1254	1492	753	341				
20. U.S.A., Brooklyn		Herman & Derby 1937	P	188	79	71	28	10	0·9880	0·0049	1·0182	0·0059
			C	1444	609	554	212	69				
21. U.S.A., Iowa	(s) S	Buckwalter *et al.* 1959	P	154	71	60	20	3	0·8949	0·3994	1·3435	1·3549
			C	49979	22392	21144	4695	1748				
22. U.S.A., North Carolina		Parker *et al.* 1961	P	86	51	26	4	5	0·5866	4·8264	0·4160	2·8259
		Hervey *et al.* 1951 M1	C	5080	2392	2079	451	158				
				1856					0·8880	4·5266	1·0483	0·3488
				χ_{21}^2 for homogeneity of areas						32·2696		20·9544

TABLE 1 **THE ABO BLOOD GROUP SYSTEM** (*cont.*)

Place	Additional details	Authors		Number	O	A	B	AB	A/O		B/O	
									Relative incidence	χ_1^2 for difference from unity	Relative incidence	χ_1^2 for difference from unity
MENTAL DISORDERS (*cont.*)												
PSYCHOSES (*cont.*)												
PARANOIA												
1. Austria, Wien		Pilcz 1927	P	59	23	24	10	2	0·8656	0·2296	0·7160	0·7369
		Hoche & Moritsch 1926 M1	C	1000	331	399	201	69				
2. Germany, Tübingen		Saleck 1932	P	77	38	32	5	2	0·6888	2·1579	0·4649	2·4099
			C	700	265	324	75	36				
3. Hungary, Budapest		Somogyi & Angyal 1931	P	17	11	0	4	2			0·6687	0·4634
			C	1000	331	426	180	63				
4. Italy, Catanzaro		Asaro 1955	P	65	29	20	15	1	1·0138	0·0019	1·6529	1·9473
		Formaggio & Ferutta 1955 M1	C	303	147	100	46	10				
				218					0·8197	1·4405	0·8916	0·2810
				(201)	χ_2^2 for homogeneity of areas					0·9489		
					χ_3^2 for homogeneity of areas							5·1366
ARTERIOSCLEROTIC PSYCHOSES												
1. U.S.A., Iowa	(s) S	Buckwalter *et al.* 1959	P	271	139	99	31	2	0·7543	4·5739	1·0637	0·0959
			C	49979	22392	21144	4695	1748				
CONFUSIONAL PSYCHOSES												
1. Italy, Arezzo		Marzi & Turchini 1952	P	40	18	17	5	0	1·1302	0·1205	1·1928	0·1111
			C	473	219	183	51	20				
2. Italy, Milano		Bravetta 1930	P	82(c)	39	35	6	2	1·0096	0·0016	0·6618	0·8516
		Cuboni M1	C	1500	684	608	159	49				
3. Italy, Padova		Bianchini 1937	P	62(c)	23	24	11	4	1·1778	0·2834	2·2254	4·0198
		Pennati & Bianchini 1930 M1	C	500	228	202	49	21				
				184					1·0832	0·2304	1·2737	0·8690
					χ_2^2 for homogeneity of areas					0·1751		4·1135
DYSTHYMIA												
1. Italy, Arezzo		Marzi & Turchini 1952	P	120	52	50	15	3	1·1507	0·4000	1·2387	0·4163
			C	473	219	183	51	20				
INVOLUTIONAL PSYCHOSES												
1. Czechoslovakia, Nitra		Miššík 1962	P	71	24	28	13	6	1·0012	0·0000	0·9940	0·0003
			C	1000	345	402	188	65				
2. U.S.A., Brooklyn		Herman & Derby 1937	P	160	68	57	31	4	0·9215	0·1875	1·3096	1·3642
			C	1444	609	554	212	69				
3. U.S.A., Iowa	(s) S	Buckwalter *et al.* 1959	P	107	48	42	14	3	0·9266	0·1297	1·3911	1·1775
			C	49979	22392	21144	4695	1748				
				338					0·9383	0·2536	1·2574	1·9649
					χ_2^2 for homogeneity of areas					0·0636		0·5771
SYMPTOMATIC PSYCHOSES												
1. Czechoslovakia, Praha		Leischner 1936	P	21	10	6	5	0	0·4715	2·1024	0·8904	0·0444
			C	2429	796	1013	447	173				
UNSPECIFIED PSYCHOSES												
1. Czechoslovakia, Nitra		Miššík 1962	P	42	13	17	8	4	1·1223	0·0943	1·1293	0·0704
			C	1000	345	402	188	65				

TABLE 1 **THE ABO BLOOD GROUP SYSTEM** (*cont.*)

Place	Additional details	Authors		Number	O	A	B	AB	A/O Relative incidence	A/O χ_1^2 for difference from unity	B/O Relative incidence	B/O χ_1^2 for difference from unity
2. Finland		Mustakallio 1937	P	80	27	32	12	9	0·9801	0·0057	1·0064	0·0003
			C	2595	908	1098	401	188				
3. Italy, Catanzaro		Asaro 1955	P	231	100	86	38	7	1·2642	1·4302	1·2143	0·5815
		Formaggio & Ferutta 1955 M1	C	303	147	100	46	10				
NEUROSES												
Psychopathy												
1. Austria, Wien		Pilcz 1927	P	99	24	29	32	14	1·0024	0·0001	2·1957	7·6449
		Hoche & Moritsch 1926 M1	C	1000	331	399	201	69				
2. Czechoslovakia, Nitra		Miššík 1962	P	26	9	12	4	1	1·1443	0·0909	0·8156	0·1125
			C	1000	345	402	188	65				
3. Czechoslovakia, Praha		Leischner 1936	P	78	28	31	11	8	0·8700	0·2763	0·6996	0·9810
			C	2429	796	1013	447	173				
4. Finland		Mustakallio 1937	P	215	69	99	28	19	1·1865	1·0992	0·9189	0·1331
			C	2595	908	1098	401	188				
5. Germany, Schleswig-Holstein		Gundel & Tornquist 1929	P	217	59	106	30	22	1·6274	8·9043	1·6157	4·5280
			C	19461	7664	8461	2412	924				
6. Hungary, Budapest		Somogyi & Angyal 1931	P	129	39	60	21	9	1·1954	0·6694	0·9902	0·0012
			C	1000	331	426	180	63				
7. U.S.S.R., Kiev		Chominskij & Schustova 1928	P	17	11	4	2	0	0·3056	4·1040	0·3028	2·4069
			C	3840	1254	1492	753	341				
				781					1·1993	4·3101	1·1761	1·9710
				χ_6^2 for homogeneity of areas						10·8341		13·8366
Anxiety Neuroses												
1. Denmark, Helsingør		Kjaersgaard 1959	P	51	17	22	7	5	1·2381	0·3998	1·9986	2·0747
		Goldschmidt 1961 M2	C	474	199	208	41	26				
Depressive Neuroses												
1. Denmark, Helsingør		Kjaersgaard 1959	P	162	69	68	19	6	0·9429	0·0887	1·3365	0·8715
		Goldschmidt 1961 M2	C	474	199	208	41	26				
2. U.S.A., North Carolina	Whites	Parker *et al.* 1961	P	67	27	34	5	1	1·4488	2·0412	0·9822	0·0013
		Hervey *et al.* 1951 M1	C	5080	2392	2079	451	158				
				229					1·1040	0·3949	1·2234	0·5907
				χ_1^2 for homogeneity of areas						1·7350		0·2821
Hysteria												
1. Austria, Wien		Pilcz 1927	P	76	26	39	7	4	1·2444	0·6864	0·4434	3·4946
		Hoche & Moritsch 1926 M1	C	1000	331	399	201	69				
2. Czechoslovakia, Praha		Leischner 1936	P	23	13	5	4	1	0·3022	5·1289	0·5479	1·0954
			C	2429	796	1013	447	173				
3. Denmark, Helsingør		Kjaersgaard 1959	P	52	15	28	6	3	1·7859	2·9970	1·9415	1·6752
		Goldschmidt 1961 M2	C	474	199	208	41	26				
				151					1·1616	0·6024	0·7435	1·0647
				χ_2^2 for homogeneity of areas						8·2099		5·2005
Neurasthenia												
1. Denmark, Helsingør		Kjaersgaard 1959	P	33	15	14	3	1	0·8929	0·0867	0·9707	0·0021
		Goldschmidt 1961 M2	C	474	199	208	41	26				
2. Germany, Oberbayern		Hermanns & Kronberg 1927	P	78	41	22	9	6	0·5270	4·6697	0·8943	0·0687
			C	265	110	112	27	16				
				111					0·6068	3·5773	0·9164	0·0597
				χ_1^2 for homogeneity of areas						1·1791		0·0111

TABLE 1 THE ABO BLOOD GROUP SYSTEM (*cont.*)

MENTAL DISORDERS (*cont.*)
NEUROSES (*cont.*)

UNSPECIFIED NEUROSES

Place	Additional details	Authors		Number	O	A	B	AB	A/O Relative incidence	A/O χ_1^2 for difference from unity	B/O Relative incidence	B/O χ_1^2 for difference from unity
1. Czechoslovakia, Nitra		Miššík 1962	P	46	10	17	13	6	1·4590	0·8688	2·3856	4·0832
			C	1000	345	402	188	65				

ALCOHOLISM

Place	Additional details	Authors		Number	O	A	B	AB	A/O Relative incidence	A/O χ_1^2 for difference from unity	B/O Relative incidence	B/O χ_1^2 for difference from unity
1. Austria, Wien		Pilcz 1927	P	95	29	49	15	2	1·4017	1·8873	0·8518	0·2358
		Hoche & Moritsch 1926 M1	C	1000	331	399	201	69				
2. Czechoslovakia, Nitra		Miššík 1962	P	77	33	27	11	6	0·7022	1·7190	0·6117	1·8665
			C	1000	345	402	188	65				
3. Czechoslovakia, Praha		Leischner 1936	P	93	21	47	17	8	1·7587	4·4802	1·4416	1·2167
			C	2429	796	1013	447	173				
4. Germany, Tübingen		Saleck 1932	P	43	15	19	6	3	1·0360	0·0099	1·4133	0·4779
			C	700	265	324	75	36				
5. Italy, Ancona	Alcoholic psychoses	Fattovich 1928	P	38	21	16	1	0	0·8586	0·2054	0·2049	2·3818
			C	1500(c)	684	607	159	50				
6. Italy, Vercelli		Giuli 1959	P	65	28	27	9	1	1·0820	0·0800	1·0681	0·0277
			C	1000	432	385	130	53				
7. United Kingdom	English; (s) ABH secretion	Camps *et al.* 1969	P	403(a)	185	167	40	11	1·0251	0·0225	1·0347	0·0159
			C	284	134	118	28	4				
8. United Kingdom	Scottish; (s) ABH secretion	Camps *et al.* 1969	P	263(a)	137	94	27	5	0·9430	0·1269	1·0777	0·0805
			C	507	257	187	47	16				
9. United Kingdom	Irish; (s) ABH secretion	Camps *et al.* 1969	P	175(a)	92	61	19	3	1·2314	1·3277	0·9328	0·0654
			C	973	533	287	118	35				
10. U.S.A., Brooklyn	Alcoholic psychoses	Herman & Derby 1937	P	78	33	33	9	3	1·0993	0·1399	0·7834	0·4031
			C	1444	609	554	212	69				
11. U.S.A., Iowa	Alcoholic psychoses; (s) S	Buckwalter *et al.* 1959	P	62	37	17	8	0	0·4866	6·0379	1·0312	0·0062
			C	49979	22392	21144	4695	1748				
				1392					1·0339	0·2275	0·9733	0·6750
				χ_{10}^2 for homogeneity of areas						15·8093		6·1025

MENTAL RETARDATION

Place	Additional details	Authors		Number	O	A	B	AB	A/O Relative incidence	A/O χ_1^2 for difference from unity	B/O Relative incidence	B/O χ_1^2 for difference from unity
1. Austria, Wien	Amentia	Pilcz 1927	P	29	9	18	2	0	1·6591	1·4887	0·3659	1·6323
		Hoche & Moritsch 1926 M1	C	1000	331	399	201	69				
2. Czechoslovakia, Nitra	Oligophrenia	Miššík 1962	P	29	9	11	5	4	1·0489	0·0110	1·0195	0·0012
			C	1000	345	402	188	65				
3. Germany, Schleswig-Holstein	Imbecility	Gundel & Tornquist 1929	P	209	65	86	51	7	1·1984	1·2021	2·4931	23·4825
			C	19461	7664	8461	2412	924				
4. Germany, Tübingen	Imbecility	Saleck 1932	P	330	134	140	38	18	0·8545	1·1514	1·0020	0·0001
			C	700	265	324	75	36				
5. Greece, Makedhonia and Thraki	Mental deficiency	Zervopoulos *et al.* 1967	P	125	55	50	11	9	0·8782	0·4300	0·7882	0·5068
			C	4480	1876	1942	476	186				
6. Hungary, Budapest	Oligophrenia	Somogyi & Angyal 1931	P	69	25	28	9	7	0·8702	0·2383	0·6620	1·0655
			C	1000	331	426	180	63				
7. Italy	Phrenasthenia	Andreani 1954	P	120(c)	57	52	8	3	1·1069	0·2489	0·8178	0·2575
			C	970(c)	472	389	81	28				
8. Italy	Phrenasthenia	Laurà 1938	P	46(c)	26	16	4	0	0·7250	0·8191	0·4268	2·1813
			C	200(c)	86	73	31	10				

TABLE 1 **THE ABO BLOOD GROUP SYSTEM** (*cont.*)

Place	Additional details	Authors		Number	O	A	B	AB	A/O Relative incidence	A/O χ_1^2 for difference from unity	B/O Relative incidence	B/O χ_1^2 for difference from unity
9. Italy, Ancona	Phrenasthenia	Fattovich 1928	P	35	13	17	5	0	1·4736	1·0825	1·6546	0·8907
			C	1500(c)	684	607	159	50				
10. Italy, Arezzo	Phrenasthenia	Marzi & Turchini 1952	P	106	54	43	7	2	0·9529	0·0448	0·5566	1·8496
			C	473	219	183	51	20				
11. Italy, Catania	Phrenasthenia	di Mauro 1936	P	30(c)	14	6	10	0	0·5890	1·1291	2·2994	3·6609
		del Carpio 1929 M1	C	500	235	171	73	21				
12. Italy, Catanzara	Phrenasthenia	Asaro 1955	P	112	62	35	12	3	0·8298	0·5657	0·6185	1·8032
		Formaggio & Ferutta 1955 M1	C	303	147	100	46	10				
13. Italy, Ferrara	Phrenasthenia in children	Caselli 1955	P	105	53	44	6	2	1·0415	0·0286	0·6009	1·1220
		Ceppelini 1953 M1	C	279	138	110	26	5				
14. Italy, Milano	Phrenasthenia	Bravetta 1930	P	204(c)	96	77	20	11	0·9023	0·3983	0·8962	0·1761
		Cuboni M1	C	1500	684	608	159	49				
15. Italy, Padova	Phrenasthenia	Bianchini 1937	P	103(c)	49	42	8	4	0·9675	0·0204	0·7597	0·4439
		Pennati & Bianchini 1930 M1	C	500	228	202	49	21				
16. Italy, Siena	Phrenasthenia	D'Ormea & Centini 1942	P	64(c)	23	23	13	5	1·0336	0·0124	2·2335	5·3052
		Lecchini 1930 M1	C	8720	3758	3636	951	375				
17. Italy, Vercelli	Oligophrenia, phrenasthenia	Giuli 1959	P	130	61	43	19	7	0·7910	1·2339	1·0351	0·0150
			C	1000	432	385	130	53				
18. Poland, Lower Silesia	Idiocy	Meyer 1928	P	34(c)	10	18	4	2	1·6705	1·6109	1·4848	0·4232
		Kruse M1	C	600	245	264	66	25				
19. Poland, Lower Silesia	Imbecility	Meyer 1928	P	105(c)	42	50	13	0	1·1048	0·1922	1·1490	0·1608
		Kruse M1	C	600	245	264	66	25				
20. U.S.S.R., Kiev	Oligophrenia	Chominskij & Schustova 1928	P	29	13	10	4	2	0·6465	1·0663	0·5124	1·3586
			C	3840	1254	1492	753	341				
21. Egypt	Primary amentia (69) Mongolism (4)	Khalil 1960	P	73	23	29	17	4	1·1581	0·2743	0·9900	0·0010
			C	10045(c)	3279	3570	2448	748				
22. U.S.A., Iowa	Mental deficiency; (s) S	Buckwalter *et al.* 1959	P	194	94	82	16	2	0·9238	0·2738	0·8118	0·5923
			C	49979	22392	21144	4695	1748				
				2281					0·9671	0·4547	1·0784	1·0376
				χ_{21}^2 for homogeneity of areas						13·0681		45·8923

DISEASES OF THE NERVOUS SYSTEM AND SENSE ORGANS

MUSCULAR DYSTROPHY

Place	Additional details	Authors		Number	O	A	B	AB	A/O Relative incidence	A/O χ_1^2	B/O Relative incidence	B/O χ_1^2
1. U.S.A., Oklahoma	(s) type of dystrophy	Brandt & Welsh 1962	P	49	25	19	3	2	0·9326	0·0525	0·5636	0·8797
			C	25067	11995	9775	2554	743				

HUNTINGTON'S CHOREA

Place	Additional details	Authors		Number	O	A	B	AB	A/O Relative incidence	A/O χ_1^2	B/O Relative incidence	B/O χ_1^2
1. U.S.A., Kansas City		Schimke & Ziegler 1970	P	70	21	38	9	2	1·9928	6·3685	2·1821	3·7855
			C	6313	2892	2626	568	227				

MULTIPLE SCLEROSIS

Place	Additional details	Authors		Number	O	A	B	AB	A/O Relative incidence	A/O χ_1^2	B/O Relative incidence	B/O χ_1^2
1. Germany, Essen	(s) $A_1 A_2$	Bertrams & Kuwert 1976	P	802	319	348	103	32	1·0750	0·4809	1·1371	0·6865
			C	1000	405	411	115	69				
2. Germany, Tübingen		Saleck 1932	P	31	12	16	2	1	1·0905	0·0492	0·5889	0·4670
			C	700	265	324	75	36				
3. United Kingdom, S. Scotland, N. Northumberland		Simpson *et al.* 1965	P	87	47	26	11	3	0·7920	0·9093	1·1229	0·1195
			C	54477	27702	19350	5774	1651				
4. United Kingdom, Tyneside, NE. Durham		Simpson *et al.* 1965	P	67	34	28	4	1	0·9987	0·0000	0·5637	1·1701
			C	8225	3900	3216	814	295				

TABLE 1 **THE ABO BLOOD GROUP SYSTEM** (*cont.*)

Place	Additional details	Authors		Number	O	A	B	AB	A/O		B/O	
									Relative incidence	χ_1^2 for difference from unity	Relative incidence	χ_1^2 for difference from unity
DISEASES OF THE NERVOUS SYSTEM AND SENSE ORGANS (*cont.*)												
MULTIPLE SCLEROSIS (*cont.*)												
5. United Kingdom, N. England (exc. parts mentioned in 3 and 4)		Simpson *et al.* 1965	P	353	180	136	29	8	0·9302	0·4015	0·9347	0·1126
			C	31717	15502	12592	2672	951				
6. United Kingdom, Bath		McAlpine *et al.* 1965	P	15	6	9	0	0	1·4878	0·5577		
			C	833	367	370	73	23				
7. United Kingdom, Birmingham		McAlpine *et al.* 1965	P	22	15	5	2	0	0·3691	3·7221	0·7579	0·1354
			C	19789	9225	8331	1623	610				
8. United Kingdom, Exeter		McAlpine *et al.* 1965	P	50	20	23	5	2	1·3129	0·7296	1·4457	0·4931
			C	563	266	233	46	18				
9. United Kingdom, London		Pratt 1963	P	329	178	118	27	6	0·7192	7·6352	0·7772	1·4755
			C	33026	15121	13937	2951	1017				
10. United Kingdom, Manchester		McAlpine *et al.* 1965	P	51	32	14	3	2	0·5163	4·2408	0·5149	1·2049
			C	12233	5849	4956	1065	363				
11. United Kingdom, Newcastle upon Tyne		MacDonald *et al.* 1976	P	136(a)	77	50	7	2	0·8425	0·8675	0·4786	3·4315
			C	5371	2643	2037	502	189				
12. United Kingdom, Newcastle upon Tyne		Roberts 1976	P	188	109	59	15	5	0·7023	4·6271	0·7245	1·3277
			C	5371	2643	2037	502	189				
13. U.S.A., Boston		Alexander *et al.* 1950	P	111	56	44	9	2	0·9064	0·2375	0·6816	1·1387
		Mayr *et al.* 1956 M1	C	120281	55089	47752	12990	4450				
				2242					0·8903	5·0069	0·8860	2·0302
					χ_{12}^2 for homogeneity of areas					16·1521		
				(2227)	χ_{11}^2 for homogeneity of areas							9·7323
PARKINSON'S DISEASE												
1. Germany, Tübingen		Saleck 1932	P	49	19	24	4	2	1·0331	0·0105	0·7439	0·2738
			C	700	265	324	75	36				
2. Sweden		Strang 1965	P	245	113	100	22	10	0·7120	5·9747	0·7439	1·5760
			C	10457	3974	4939	1040	504				
3. United Kingdom, Northern Ireland		Kak & Gordon 1970	P	187	100	48	30	9	0·7831	1·9278	1·6200	5·3182
			C	27650	14931	9152	2765	802				
				481					0·7651	6·7363	1·1145	0·5173
					χ_2^2 for homogeneity of areas					1·1767		6·6507
EPILEPSY												
1. Austria, Wien		Pilcz 1927	P	46(c)	15	19	10	2	1·0508	0·0197	1·0978	0·0499
		Hoche & Moritsch 1926 M1	C	1000	331	399	201	69				
2. Czechoslovakia, Praha		Leischner 1936	P	76	20	42	9	5	1·6501	3·2986	0·8013	0·2980
			C	2429	796	1013	447	173				
3. Germany, Schleswig-Holstein		Gundel & Tornquist 1929	P	259	98	120	17	24	1·1091	0·5712	0·5512	5·1001
			C	19461	7664	8461	2412	924				
4. Germany, Tübingen		Saleck 1932	P	181	74	80	20	7	0·8842	0·4606	0·9550	0·0264
			C	700	265	324	75	36				

TABLE 1 THE ABO BLOOD GROUP SYSTEM (*cont.*)

Place	Additional details	Authors		Number	O	A	B	AB	A/O		B/O	
									Relative incidence	χ_1^2 for difference from unity	Relative incidence	χ_1^2 for difference from unity
5. Greece, Makedhonia and Thraki		Zervopoulos *et al.* 1967	P	79	28	33	10	8	1·1385	0·2509	1·4076	0·8447
			C	4480	1876	1942	476	186				
6. Hungary, Budapest		Somogyi & Angyal 1931	P	46	17	21	7	1	0·9598	0·0150	0·7572	0·3680
			C	1000	331	426	180	63				
7. Italy		Andreani 1954	P	73(c)	30	30	12	1	1·2134	0·5242	2·3309	5·4611
			C	970(c)	472	389	81	28				
8. Italy		Laurà 1938	P	33(c)	10	15	6	2	1·7671	1·6884	1·6645	0·8360
			C	200(c)	86	73	31	10				
9. Italy, Ancona		Fattovich 1928	P	23	16	7	0	0	0·4930	2·3994		
			C	1500(c)	684	607	159	50				
10. Italy, Arezzo		Marzi & Turchini 1952	P	27	15	9	3	0	0·7180	0·5842	0·8588	0·0546
			C	473	219	183	51	20				
11. Italy, Cagliari	(s) S	Benassi & Atzeni 1934	P	58	30	18	10	0	1·0229	0·0052	2·1439	3·6444
			C	499	283	166	44	6				
12. Italy, Catanzara		Asaro 1955	P	44	19	17	7	1	1·3153	0·5855	1·1773	0·1190
		Formaggio & Ferutta 1955 M1	C	303	147	100	46	10				
13. Italy, Milano		Bravetta 1930	P	183(c)	78	82	12	11	1·1827	1·0011	0·6618	1·6396
		Cuboni M1	C	1500	684	608	159	49				
14. Italy, Padova		Bianchini 1937	P	46(c)	20	18	7	1	1·0158	0·0022	1·6286	1·0928
		Pennati & Bianchini 1937 M1	C	500	228	202	49	21				
15. Italy, Pisa		Favilli 1959	P	134	67	50	15	2	0·7166	2·3871	1·0510	0·0215
			C	386	169	176	36	5				
16. Italy, Siena		D'Ormea & Centini 1942	P	87(c)	38	22	19	8	0·5984	3·6471	1·9758	5·7776
		Lecchini 1930 M1	C	8720	3758	3636	951	375				
17. Italy, Vercelli		Giuli 1959	P	38	14	15	7	2	1·2022	0·2372	1·6615	1·1494
			C	1000	432	385	130	53				
18. Italy, Volterra		Favilli 1959	P	117	57	44	14	2	0·7412	1·7287	1·1530	0·1653
			C	386(c)	169	176	36	5				
19. Norway, Oslo	(s) A	Brendemoen 1960	P	511	178	266	48	19	1·1726	2·6634	1·2823	2·2994
			C	33580(c)	12982	16545	2730	1323				
20. Poland, Kielce		Gala & Gala 1966	P	72(c)	19	14	36	3	0·6766	1·1986	3·6280	19·4457
			C	1644	584	636	305	119				
21. Poland, Lower Silesia		Meyer 1928	P	127(c)	44	48	23	12	1·0124	0·0030	1·9404	5·1434
		Kruse M1	C	600	245	264	66	25				
22. United Kingdom, Berkshire and Oxfordshire	Women	Fedrick 1972	P	164	57	82	14	11	1·5202	5·8289	1·1992	0·3667
			C	12902	5815	5503	1191	393				
23. U.S.S.R., Kiev		Chominskij & Schustova 1928	P	52	18	21	8	5	0·9806	0·0037	0·7402	0·4956
			C	3840	1254	1492	753	341				
24. U.S.S.R., Perm		Karnaukhova 1930	P	355	103	103	110	39	0·8679	0·9657	1·0856	0·3326
			C	4600	1353	1559	1331	357				
25. Japan, Sendai		Moniwa 1960	P	86	22	33	23	8	1·3041	0·9270	1·4661	1·6393
			C	21199	6769	7786	4827	1817				
26. U.S.A., Brooklyn	With psychosis	Herman & Derby 1937	P	35	10	17	4	4	1·8688	2·4094	1·1491	0·0542
			C	1444	609	554	212	69				
27. U.S.A., Iowa	(s) S	Buckwalter *et al.* 1959	P	78	47	22	5	4	0·4957	7·3697	0·5074	2·0781
			C	49979	22392	21144	4695	1748				
28. Argentina, Buenos Aires		Dimitri *et al.* 1939	P	20	12	4	4	0	0·3763	2·8633	1·4229	0·3724
			C	15045	6702	5937	1570	836				
29. Australia	Whites; (s) A_1A_2	Simmons *et al.* 1944	P	22	14	6	1	1	0·5104	1·8999	0·3487	1·0360
		Bryce *et al.* 1950–1 M1	C	176943	84034	70565	17215	5129				
				3072					1·0231	0·2844	1·2168	10·4511
					χ_{28}^2 for homogeneity of areas					45·2545		
				(3049)	χ_{27}^2 for homogeneity of areas							49·4607

TABLE 1 **THE ABO BLOOD GROUP SYSTEM** *(cont.)*

Place	Additional details	Authors		Number	O	A	B	AB	A/O Relative incidence	A/O χ_1^2 for difference from unity	B/O Relative incidence	B/O χ_1^2 for difference from unity
DISEASES OF THE NERVOUS SYSTEM AND SENSE ORGANS *(cont.)*												
KURU												
1. New Guinea, Eastern Highlands	Fore; all A are A_1	Simmons *et al.* 1961	P	192	79	69	40	4	0·7151	2·7401	1·3266	1·2232
			C	356	131	160	50	15				
2. New Guinea, Eastern Highlands	North Fore; all A are A_1	Simmons *et al.* 1972	P	94	42	30	19	3	0·9573	0·0274	1·1194	0·1346
			C	428	193	144	78	13				
3. New Guinea, Eastern Highlands	South Fore; all A are A_1	Simmons *et al.* 1972	P	158	58	68	26	6	1·2305	1·1768	1·2468	0·7577
			C	1086	445	424	160	57				
4. New Guinea, Eastern Highlands	Other than Fore; all A are A_1	Simmons *et al.* 1972	P	48	23	15	10	0	1·0165	0·0023	1·3972	0·7415
			C	1168	572	367	178	51				
				492					0·9609	0·1189	1·2615	2·5956
				χ_3^2 for homogeneity of areas						3·8278		0·2614
MOTOR NEURONE DISEASE												
1. United Kingdom, Newcastle upon Tyne		Vejjajiva *et al.* 1965	P	40	18	12	10	0	0·8480	0·1944	3·0241	7·7306
			C	4619	2259	1776	415	169				
2. U.S.A., Maryland	Amyotrophic lateral sclerosis	Myrianthopoulos & Leyshon 1967	P	346	130	147	52	17	1·2115	1·3009	1·4286	2·2164
			C	346	150	140	42	14				
				386					1·1409	0·7384	1·7439	7·3409
				χ_1^2 for homogeneity of areas						0·7569		2·6061
BLEPHARITIS												
1. Italy, Perugia		Giannantoni 1928	P	28	9	12	4	3	1·5758	0·5708	1·1556	0·0328
			C	32	13	11	5	3				
UVEITIS												
1. Japan, Tokyo	(s) ABH secretion	Oda 1971	P	239	72	82	51	34	0·8761	0·2058	0·8854	0·1365
			C	100	30	39	24	7				
REFRACTIVE ERRORS OF EYE												
HYPEROPIA												
1. Italy, Perugia		Giannantoni 1928	P	25	6	12	4	3	2·3636	1·7709	1·7333	0·4362
			C	32	13	11	5	3				
2. Poland, Białystok	(s) S	Wilk *et al.* 1969	P	287	84	121	54	28	1·5013	3·4569	1·3592	1·2989
			C	191	74	71	35	11				
				312					1·5732	4·7871	1·3909	1·6582
				χ_1^2 for homogeneity of areas						0·4407		0·0769
MYOPIA												
1. Italy, Firenze	Over 10 diopters	Scialdone & Pantalone 1963	P	409(c)	90	234	61	24	2·9379	75·2647	3·1495	47·6389
			C	100000(c)	45910	40630	9880	3580				
2. Italy, Perugia		Giannantoni 1928	P	26	14	5	4	3	0·4221	1·6938	0·7429	0·1477
			C	32	13	11	5	3				
3. Poland, Białystok	(s) S	Wilk *et al.* 1969	P	84	24	36	15	9	1·5634	2·0576	1·3214	0·5164
			C	191	74	71	35	11				
				519					2·5515	67·8905	2·6200	41·3025
				χ_2^2 for homogeneity of areas						11·1256		7·0005

TABLE 1 **THE ABO BLOOD GROUP SYSTEM** (*cont.*)

Place	Additional details	Authors		Number	O	A	B	AB	A/O Relative incidence	A/O χ_1^2 for difference from unity	B/O Relative incidence	B/O χ_1^2 for difference from unity
ASTIGMATISM												
1. Poland, Białystok	(s) S	Wilk *et al.* 1969	P	98	26	39	19	14	1·5634	2·1775	1·5451	1·4212
			C	191	74	71	35	11				
REFRACTION DIFFERENT IN EACH EYE												
1. Poland, Białystok	(s) S	Wilk *et al.* 1969	P	159	56	62	24	17	1·1539	0·3328	0·9061	0·0956
			C	191	74	71	35	11				
CATARACT												
1. Italy, Perugia		Giannantoni 1928	P	30	6	19	2	3	3·7424	4·4990	0·8667	0·0217
			C	32	13	11	5	3				
2. Canada, Winnipeg		Reed 1960	P	152	81	54	12	5	0·7830	1·9268	0·5929	2·8412
			C	23005	10510	8949	2626	920				
				182					0·8795	0·5736	0·6141	2·7243
				χ_1^2 for homogeneity of areas						5·8522		0·1386
GLAUCOMA												
1. Germany, Jena	Primary	Lobeck 1932	P	70	26	38	4	2	1·0385	0·0148	0·6391	0·5223
			C	149	54	76	13	6				
2. Italy, Firenze	Simple, chronic	Miani 1958	P	100	48	45	6	1	1·0594	0·0766	0·5808	1·5667
			C	13633	6259	5539	1347	488				
3. Italy, Perugia		Giannantoni 1928	P	24	7	10	4	3	1·6883	0·6679	1·4857	0·2340
			C	32	13	11	5	3				
4. N. India, Sitapur	56 open-angle, 39 narrow-angle, 5 unclassifiable; (s) ABH secretion	Garg & Pahwa 1965 Tyagi 1968 M2	P	100	19	45	30	6	3·1633	17·5837	1·3286	0·9344
			C	13105	4103	3072	4876	1054				
5. Japan, Nagoya		Mikuchi 1931	P	42	11	18	10	3	1·1511	0·1306	1·1771	0·1343
			C	1161	325	462	251	123				
				336					1·4114	6·6127	1·0254	0·0164
				χ_4^2 for homogeneity of areas						11·8608		3·3753
DISEASES OF THE CIRCULATORY SYSTEM												
RHEUMATIC FEVER												
1. Finland		Sievers 1929	P	243(c)	79	104	44	16	1·0389	0·0576	1·1958	0·7844
			C	1711	584	740	272	115				
2. Finland		Mustakallio 1937	P	271	88	118	47	18	1·1089	0·4888	1·2094	0·9972
			C	2595	908	1098	401	188				
3. Poland, Katowice		Machalski *et al.* 1968	P	239	77	101	46	15	1·0925	0·3207	1·1386	0·4541
			C	3606	1216	1460	638	292				
4. United Kingdom, Buckinghamshire		Glynn *et al.* 1956	P	525	213	223	57	32	1·0987	0·9341	1·3829	4·5406
			C	15046	6775	6456	1311	504				
5. Republic of South Africa	Bantu	Buckwalter *et al.* 1961	P	70	34	24	10	2	1·1161	0·1678	0·6158	1·8032
			C	7105	3197	2022	1527	359				
6. Republic of South Africa	Indians	Buckwalter *et al.* 1961	P	73	22	22	25	4	1·6200	2·5338	1·2724	0·6730
			C	7462	2788	1721	2490	463				
7. U.S.A., Boston		Dublin *et al.* 1964	P	608	276	246	55	31	1·1131	0·7322	0·7368	2·4220
			C	605	281	225	76	23				
8. U.S.A., Iowa	(s) S, A_1A_2	Buckwalter *et al.* 1962	P	752	301	344	73	34	1·2103	5·7639	1·1567	1·2262
			C	49979	22392	21144	4695	1748				
9. U.S.A., Michigan	Whites; (s) A_1A_2	Gershowitz & Neel 1965	P	104	49	40	12	3	0·9044	0·2083	1·1701	0·2200
			C	1508	688	621	144	55				
10. Australia, Sydney	(s) A_1A_2	Walsh & Kooptzoff 1956	P	259	110	114	24	11	1·2107	1·6468	0·7905	0·9209
			C	1123	500	428	138	57				
				3144					1·1376	9·0415	1·1012	2·3314
				χ_9^2 for homogeneity of areas						3·8124		11·7101

TABLE 1 **THE ABO BLOOD GROUP SYSTEM** (*cont.*)

Place	Additional details	Authors		Number	O	A	B	AB	A/O		B/O	
									Relative incidence	χ_1^2 for difference from unity	Relative incidence	χ_1^2 for difference from unity
DISEASES OF THE CIRCULATORY SYSTEM (*cont.*)												
RHEUMATIC HEART DISEASE												
1. France, Paris	Endocarditis in children	Pham-Huu-Trung *et al.* 1961	P C	434 257	189 113	187 112	47 27	11 5	0·9983	0·0001	1·0408	0·0221
2. Hungary, Budapest	Carditis in under 22-year-olds	Zih & Thoma 1967	P C	770 2966	206 975	371 1247	123 527	70 217	1·4081	12·4925	1·1047	0·6229
3. Italy, Bergamo		Gualandri & Ballabio 1965	P C	67 401	27 194	29 161	6 36	5 10	1·2942	0·8025	1·1975	0·1373
4. Italy, Bologna		Gualandri & Ballabio 1965	P C	49 186	20 81	22 92	6 9	1 4	0·9685	0·0086	2·7000	2·9006
5. Italy, Brescia		Gualandri & Ballabio 1965	P C	108 571	30 281	65 226	9 49	4 15	2·6940	17·3205	1·7204	1·7479
6. Italy, Como		Gualandri & Ballabio 1965	P C	96 293	35 141	48 112	9 31	4 9	1·7265	4·5585	1·1696	0·1371
7. Italy, Foggia		Gualandri & Ballabio 1965	P C	51 122	18 55	20 48	10 12	3 7	1·2731	0·4034	2·5463	3·3981
8. Italy, Mantova		Gualandri & Ballabio 1965	P C	67 193	25 86	33 81	7 15	2 11	1·4015	1·2084	1·6053	0·8579
9. Italy, Milano		Gualandri & Ballabio 1965	P C	376 935	142 384	168 402	47 101	19 48	1·1301	0·8274	1·2584	1·2940
10. Italy, Sicilia		Gualandri & Ballabio 1965	P C	43 51	12 18	29 20	2 10	0 3	2·1750	2·7030	0·3000	1·9618
11. Italy, Varese		Gualandri & Ballabio 1965	P C	48 561	10 262	28 226	7 52	3 21	3·2460	9·6303	3·5269	5·9746
12. Italy, Venezia		Gualandri & Ballabio 1965	P C	77 973	28 463	35 359	8 114	6 37	1·6121	3·2941	1·1604	0·1289
13. Poland		Sowińska *et al.* 1968	P C	242 836	75 259	93 319	50 180	24 78	1·0068	0·0015	0·9593	0·0405
14. United Kingdom, Bristol and West of England		Maxted 1940	P C	200 4388	94 2137	89 1818	12 304	5 129	1·1129	0·5002	0·8974	0·1199
15. United Kingdom, Bristol	(s) isolated mitral, isolated aortic, and multi-valvular	David 1970 Kopeć 1970	P C	165 3284	60 1430	82 1485	13 275	10 94	1·3160	2·4922	1·1267	0·1450
16. United Kingdom, Liverpool	Carditis; (s) S	Clarke *et al.* 1960	P C	263 16057	105 7842	116 6294	36 1519	6 402	1·3765	5·5395	1·7700	8·5395
17. United Kingdom, Taplow		Glynn 1959	P C	609 15046	255 6775	256 6456	64 1311	34 504	1·0535	0·3344	1·2970	3·3062
18. United Kingdom, Glasgow	Mitral	Addis 1959	P C	538 5898	280 3177	175 1906	65 637	18 178	1·0418	0·1654	1·1578	1·0301
19. United Kingdom, Cardiff	Carditis, mitral stenosis	Hooper 1960 Kopeć 1970	P C	213 1053	90 485	86 430	25 103	12 35	1·0778	0·2069	1·3080	1·1447
20. United Kingdom, Belfast	Mitral stenosis	Macafee 1965[b]	P C	431 28566	203 15715	156 9433	57 2702	15 716	1·2802	5·3046	1·6331	10·5031
21. Egypt		Khattab & Ismail 1960	P C	120 10000	32 3598	51 3360	29 2393	8 649	1·7066	5·5551	1·3626	1·4410
22. Canada, Edmonton		Sartor & Fraser 1964	P C	136 2171	56 998	55 842	19 239	6 92	1·1641	0·6040	1·4168	1·6038
				5103					1·2306	36·5332	1·2845	24·6475
				χ_{21}^2 for homogeneity of areas						37·4200		22·4303

TABLE 1 **THE ABO BLOOD GROUP SYSTEM** (*cont.*)

Place	Additional details	Authors		Number	O	A	B	AB	A/O Relative incidence	A/O χ_1^2 for difference from unity	B/O Relative incidence	B/O χ_1^2 for difference from unity
MALIGNANT HYPERTENSION												
1. U.S.A., New York	Whites; (s) S	Perera & Adler 1960	P	90	50	30	8	2	0·6738	2·8697	0·5562	2·3405
		Miller *et al.* 1951 M2	C	5000(c)	2190	1950	630	230				
2. U.S.A., New York	Negroes; (s) S	Perera & Adler 1960	P	90	56	11	17	6	0·4464	4·5967	0·6459	1·7699
		Miller *et al.* 1951 M1	C	200	100	44	47	9				
				180					0·6011	6·6006	0·6063	4·0227
				χ_1^2 for homogeneity of areas						0·8658		0·0877
HYPERTENSION												
1. Austria, Wien	(s) S, Rh_D	Speiser 1958[a]	P	250	95	107	31	17	0·9613	0·0625	0·9212	0·1266
			C	1000	367	430	130	73				
2. Czechoslovakia	(s) S	Mikolášek & Miluničová 1967	P	383	126	155	72	30	1·0028	0·0005	1·1002	0·4167
			C	176000	58520	71790	30395	15295				
3. Finland		Mustakallio 1937	P	45	12	18	12	3	1·2404	0·3295	2·2643	3·9231
			C	2595	908	1098	401	188				
4. Germany, Köln	(s) S	Wiechmann & Paal 1927	P	500(c)	188	185	77	50	0·9009	0·7295	1·5530	6·7187
			C	1100(c)	455	497	120	28				
5. Germany, Oberbayern		Hermanns & Kronberg 1927	P	36	10	19	5	2	1·8661	2·2805	2·0370	1·4625
			C	265	110	112	27	16				
6. Poland, Wrocław		Zuber 1966	P	322	116	136	51	19	0·9231	0·3871	0·7098	4·0405
			C	9722(c)	3095	3931	1917	779				
7. Romania, Bucureşti	(s) S, A	Săhleanu *et al.* 1960	P	467	184	174	73	36	0·9776	0·0369	0·9355	0·1888
			C	1970	764	739	324	143				
8. United Kingdom, Scotland	(s) S	Maxwell & Maxwell 1955	P	2147	1138	722	237	50	0·9837	0·0922	0·9822	0·0492
			C	7418	3853	2485	817	263				
9. N. India, Lucknow		Nath *et al.* 1963	P	52	15	9	24	4	0·8247	0·2063	1·3112	0·6667
			C	3330(c)	1035	753	1263	279				
10. U.S.A.		Pell *et al.* 1957	P	303	130	135	31	7	1·1587	1·3654	1·1272	0·3406
			C	5876	2699	2419	571	187				
11. U.S.A.		Pell *et al.* 1957	P	89	27	41	13	8	1·5888	3·3310	1·2737	0·4910
			C	1713	701	670	265	77				
12. U.S.A.		Pell *et al.* 1957	P	69	34	27	6	2	0·8653	0·3048	0·7612	0·3691
			C	2073	936	859	217	61				
13. U.S.A.		Pell *et al.* 1957	P	47	19	21	3	4	1·1684	0·2377	0·6390	0·5140
			C	2734	1202	1137	297	98				
				4710					0·9994	0·0003	1·0327	0·4002
				χ_{12}^2 for homogeneity of areas						9·3636		18·9073
HYPOTENSION												
1. Germany, Oberbayern		Hermanns & Kronberg 1927	P	65	21	29	8	7	1·3563	0·9276	1·5520	0·8833
			C	265	110	112	27	16				
ANGINA PECTORIS AND CORONARY OCCLUSION WITHOUT INFARCTION (OR WITHOUT SPECIFIED INFARCTION)												
1. Denmark, København	Coronary occlusion; (s) S	Gjørup 1963	P	846	345	372	93	36	0·9935	0·0071	1·0049	0·0016
			C	14304	5804	6299	1557	644				
2. Irish Republic, Dublin	Angina pectoris	Maurer *et al.* 1969	P	84	42	32	9	1	1·3902	1·9700	1·0998	0·0671
			C	117287	65548	35923	12771	3045				
3. Irish Republic, Dublin	Acute coronary insufficiency	Maurer *et al.* 1969	P	93	53	31	7	2	1·0673	0·0828	0·6779	0·9341
			C	117287	65548	35923	12771	3045				
4. Poland, Kraków	Coronary occlusion without infarction	Jaegermann 1964	P	90	34	31	19	6	0·7366	1·5117	0·8805	0·1969
		Socha 1966	C	39006	12457	15419	7906	3224				

TABLE 1 **THE ABO BLOOD GROUP SYSTEM** *(cont.)*

Place	Additional details	Authors		Number	O	A	B	AB	A/O		B/O	
									Relative incidence	χ_1^2 for difference from unity	Relative incidence	χ_1^2 for difference from unity
DISEASES OF THE CIRCULATORY SYSTEM *(cont.)*												
ANGINA PECTORIS AND CORONARY OCCLUSION WITHOUT INFARCTION (OR WITHOUT SPECIFIED INFARCTION) *(cont.)*												
5. United Kingdom, Aberdeen	Ischaemic heart disease without infarction; men	Allan & Dawson 1968	P	151	71	56	20	4	1·1180	0·3816	1·3025	1·0637
			C	7092	3565	2515	771	241				
6. United Kingdom, Edinburgh	Effort angina; men	Oliver & Cumming 1962	P	96	52	37	6	1	0·9967	0·0002	0·5029	2·5130
			C	5000	2506	1789	575	130				
7. N. India, Patna	Myocardial ischaemia or angina pectoris	Srivastava *et al.* 1966	P	111	23	43	37	8	2·7261	14·8826	1·3179	1·0710
			C	9257	2909	1995	3551	802				
8. Republic of South Africa, Cape Peninsula	Angina pectoris; Afrikaans speaking Whites	Bronte-Stewart *et al.* 1962	P	44	23	14	3	4	0·7468	0·7257	0·5314	1·0445
			C	1902	876	714	215	97				
9. Republic of South Africa, Cape Peninsula	Angina pectoris; English speaking Whites	Bronte-Stewart *et al.* 1962	P	47	17	21	6	3	1·3160	0·6937	1·5272	0·7750
			C	2080	913	857	211	99				
10. Republic of South Africa, Cape Peninsula	Angina pectoris; Whites exc. Afrikaans and English speaking	Bronte-Stewart *et al.* 1962	P	17	7	8	1	1	1·3531	0·3307	0·5273	0·3526
			C	567	251	212	68	36				
11. Republic of South Africa, Cape Peninsula	Angina pectoris; Jewish	Bronte-Stewart *et al.* 1962	P	29	13	9	6	1	0·6341	1·0765	1·0054	0·0001
			C	1115	403	440	185	87				
12. Republic of South Africa, Cape Peninsula	Angina pectoris; Coloured	Bronte-Stewart *et al.* 1962	P	23	9	5	6	3	0·6970	0·4082	1·2349	0·1545
			C	702	276	220	149	57				
				1631					1·0548	0·9098	1·0120	0·0204
				χ_{11}^2 for homogeneity of areas						21·1611		8·1536
MYOCARDIAL INFARCTION												
1. Belgium	35–54 years old	Houte & Kesteloot 1972	P	643	286	290	39	28	1·1042	1·3787	0·7688	2·3249
			C	24511	11344	10417	2012	738				
2. Finland, Turku		Kalliomäki & Saarimaa 1962	P	359	118	156	59	26	1·0576	0·1935	0·8799	0·5960
			C	4129	1348	1685	766	330				
3. Greece, Athínai		Sakellaropoulos & Costeas 1970	P	354(c)	146	155	36	17	1·0381	0·1012	0·7399	2·5399
		Valaoras 1970 M2	C	9066	3664	3747	1221	434				
4. Greece, Athínai		Koïdakis *et al.* 1970	P	182	56	91	25	10	1·6555	8·7610	1·3436	1·5066
			C	304317	124716	122413	41439	15749				
5. Irish Republic, Dublin		Maurer *et al.* 1969	P	286	151	102	28	5	1·2326	2·6547	0·9517	0·0577
			C	117287	65548	35923	12771	3045				
6. Poland	Under 45 years	Ciswicka-Sznajderman *et al.* 1973	P	55	12	23	13	7	2·0680	2·9738	2·1151	2·4159
			C	104	41	38	21	4				
7. Poland, Kraków	Post-mortem	Jaegermann 1964	P	115(c)	38	44	23	10	0·9355	0·0905	0·9537	0·0321
		Socha 1966	C	39006	12457	15419	7906	3224				
8. Poland, Łódź	Fatal	Geraga *et al.* 1972	P	32	6	13	7	6	2·2560	2·7101	2·3650	2·3865
		Sabliński 1959 M2	C	8311	3132	3008	1545	626				
9. Poland, Łódź	Survivors	Geraga *et al.* 1972	P	137	55	41	27	14	0·7762	1·4851	0·9952	0·0004
		Sabliński 1959 M2	C	8311	3132	3008	1545	626				
10. Poland, Lublin	(s) Rh_D	Szczepański & Jach 1973	P	1279	372	557	249	101	1·4759	16·3068	1·5273	12·2427
			C	1100	413	419	181	87				

TABLE 1 **THE ABO BLOOD GROUP SYSTEM** (*cont.*)

Place	Additional details	Authors		Number	O	A	B	AB	A/O		B/O	
									Relative incidence	χ_1^2 for difference from unity	Relative incidence	χ_1^2 for difference from unity
11. United Kingdom, Aberdeen	Men	Allan & Dawson 1968	P C	202 7092	82 3565	92 2515	24 771	4 241	1·5904	9·0663	1·3533	1·6513
12. United Kingdom, Edinburgh	Men	Oliver & Cumming 1962	P C	204 5000	101 2506	75 1789	21 575	7 130	1·0402	0·0642	0·9062	0·1627
13. Israel	Jewish men over 40, born in Austria, Hungary, Romania; (s) G	Medalie *et al.* 1971	P C	76(a) 1654	22 580	30 733	16 222	8 119	1·0790	0·0706	1·9001	3·6085
14. Israel	Jewish men over 40, born in Germany; (s) A_1A_2	Medalie *et al.* 1971	P C	25(a) 489	9 175	7 193	8 88	1 33	0·7052	0·4604	1·7677	1·2817
15. Israel	Jewish men over 40, born in Poland; (s) A_1A_2	Medalie *et al.* 1971	P C	65(a) 1242	17 420	31 512	13 213	4 97	1·4959	1·6996	1·5079	1·1810
16. Israel	Jewish men over 40, born in Bulgaria and Jugoslavia; (s) G	Medalie *et al.* 1971	P C	17(a) 375	3 98	8 170	4 74	2 33	1·5373	0·3897	1·7658	0·5326
17. Israel	Jewish men over 40, born in U.S.S.R.; (s) A_1A_2	Medalie *et al.* 1971	P C	36(a) 551	13 197	15 216	6 94	2 44	1·0524	0·0170	0·9673	0·0043
18. Israel	Jewish men over 40, born in Turkey, Israel, Syria; (s) G	Medalie *et al.* 1971	P C	85(a) 1810	23 601	34 667	17 390	11 152	1·3320	1·0806	1·1390	0·1590
19. Israel	Jewish men over 40, born in Iraq; (s) A_1A_2	Medalie *et al.* 1971	P C	38(a) 1125	11 253	15 438	7 296	5 138	0·7877	0·3478	0·5439	1·5381
20. Israel	Jewish men over 40, born in Egypt; (s) A_1A_2	Medalie *et al.* 1971	P C	18(a) 525	4 176	8 182	4 120	2 47	1·9341	1·1267	1·4667	0·2854
21. Israel	Jewish men over 40, born in Morocco; (s) A_1A_2	Medalie *et al.* 1971	P C	12(a) 421	4 159	5 107	0 125	3 30	1·8575	0·8235		
22. N. India, Patna		Srivastava *et al.* 1966	P C	87 9257	17 2909	35 1995	29 3551	6 802	3·0021	13·6952	1·3975	1·1923
23. S. India, Bombay		Godbole 1960	P C	110 3600	34 1228	31 953	35 1096	10 323	1·1749	0·4088	1·1534	0·3411
24. Malaya, Singapore	Chinese	Saha *et al.* 1973	P C	213 15262	91 6644	54 3967	50 3814	18 837	0·9938	0·0013	0·9571	0·0611
25. Malaya, Singapore	Indians	Saha *et al.* 1973	P C	199 5000	68 1951	52 1051	57 1680	22 318	1·4195	3·4670	0·9735	0·0217
26. Malaya, Singapore	Malays	Saha *et al.* 1973	P C	51 5461	20 2098	13 1369	13 1596	5 398	0·9961	0·0001	0·8544	0·1933
27. Republic of South Africa, Cape Peninsula	Afrikaans-speaking Whites	Bronte-Stewart *et al.* 1962	P C	132 1902	63 876	52 714	12 215	5 97	1·0127	0·0042	0·7761	0·6120
28. Republic of South Africa, Cape Peninsula	English-speaking Whites	Bronte-Stewart *et al.* 1962	P C	240 2080	77 913	119 857	34 211	10 99	1·6464	10·5113	1·9105	8·6904

TABLE 1 **THE ABO BLOOD GROUP SYSTEM** (*cont.*)

Place	Additional details	Authors		Number	O	A	B	AB	A/O Relative incidence	A/O χ_1^2 for difference from unity	B/O Relative incidence	B/O χ_1^2 for difference from unity
DISEASES OF THE CIRCULATORY SYSTEM (*cont.*)												
MYOCARDIAL INFARCTION (*cont.*)												
29. Republic of South Africa, Cape Peninsula	Whites exc. Afrikaans and English speaking	Bronte-Stewart *et al.* 1962	P	61	19	28	12	2	1·7448	3·1927	2·3313	4·6323
			C	567	251	212	68	36				
30. Republic of South Africa, Cape Peninsula	Jewish	Bronte-Stewart *et al.* 1962	P	124	38	54	24	8	1·3016	1·4008	1·3758	1·3417
			C	1115	403	440	185	87				
31. Republic of South Africa, Cape Peninsula	Coloured	Bronte-Stewart *et al.* 1962	P	75	18	37	16	4	2·5788	9·8887	1·6465	1·9369
			C	702	276	220	149	57				
32. U.S.A.	Men under 40; (s) Rh_D	Gertler & White 1954	P	81	26	37	14	4	1·9253	4·3093	1·7692	1·8925
			C	145	69	51	21	4				
33. U.S.A.		Pell & D'Alonzo 1961	P	226	101	98	21	6	1·2284	1·0806	0·9897	0·0010
			C	245	119	94	25	7				
34. U.S.A.	Men	Nefzger *et al.* 1969	P	816(c)	295	395	90	36	1·4742	22·7099	1·2504	3·0771
			C	6611(c)	2955	2684	721	251				
35. Argentina, Buenos Aires	Jewish	Neuman *et al.* 1961	P	221	66	86	52	17	1·3529	3·3340	1·9821	13·2020
			C	8259	3283	3162	1305	509				
36. Argentina, Buenos Aires	Non-Jewish	Neuman *et al.* 1961	P	63	24	23	9	7	1·2465	0·5622	1·8002	2·2185
			C	3953	1925	1480	401	147				
37. Australia, Melbourne	Mostly British	Denborough 1962	P	205(c)	74	103	22	6	1·6575	10·9849	1·4512	2·3492
			C	176943	84034	70565	17215	5129				
				7124					1·2927	76·2639	1·1882	18·0048
					χ_{36}^2 for homogeneity of areas					61·0888		
				(7112)	χ_{35}^2 for homogeneity of areas							58·2656
MYOCARDIAL INFARCTION, CORONARY INSUFFICIENCY, ANGINA PECTORIS, PRESENT/ABSENT												
1. U.S.A., Framingham	(s) S	Havlik *et al.* 1969	Present	*273*	*138*	*97*	*31*	*7*	*0·8339*	*1·7573*	*0·9601*	*0·0391*
			Absent	*3852*	*1795*	*1513*	*420*	*124*				
MYOCARDISM												
1. Finland		Mustakallio 1937	P	143	39	76	16	12	1·6115	5·5792	0·9290	0·0592
			C	2595	908	1098	401	188				
INTRACEREBRAL ARTERIOVENOUS ANEURISM												
1. Sweden	(s) S	Strang 1967	P	150	67	52	21	10	0·6245	6·4053	1·1977	0·5103
			C	10457	3974	4939	1040	504				
CEREBRAL STROKE												
1. Romania, Bucureşti	Fatal; type not diagnosed post-mortem	Ionescu *et al.* 1976	P	649	221	281	103	44	0·9815	0·0418	0·9257	0·4064
			C	20705	6811	8823	3429	1642				
ARTERIOSCLEROSIS												
1. Czechoslovakia, Praha	Athero-sclerosis	Leischner 1936	P	63	20	28	12	3	1·1001	0·1035	1·0685	0·0320
			C	2429	796	1013	447	173				
2. Finland		Sievers 1929	P	223(c)	76	89	43	15	0·9242	0·2264	1·2148	0·9056
			C	1711	584	740	272	115				
3. Finland		Mustakallio 1937	P	128	38	62	18	10	1·3492	2·0183	1·0726	0·0574
			C	2595	908	1098	401	188				
4. Finland,		Streng & Ryti 1927[a]	P	113	34	51	19	9	1·1751	0·4926	1·1152	0·1344
			C	1383(c)	463	591	232	97				
5. Germany, München	(s) A	Lützeler & Dormanns 1929 Kruse M1	P	310	142	131	28	9	0·9110	0·4756	0·8708	0·3643
			C	1300	552	559	125	64				

TABLE 1 **THE ABO BLOOD GROUP SYSTEM** *(cont.)*

Place	Additional details	Authors		Number	O	A	B	AB	A/O Relative incidence	A/O χ^2_1 for difference from unity	B/O Relative incidence	B/O χ^2_1 for difference from unity
6. Poland, Katowice	Athero-matosis	Machalski *et al.* 1968	P	251	87	94	46	24	0·8999	0·4707	1·0077	0·0017
			C	3606	1216	1460	638	292				
7. Poland, Kielce	Cerebral atheromatosis	Gala & Gala 1966	P	31(c)	9	9	12	1	0·9182	0·0323	2·5530	4·4048
			C	1644	584	636	305	119				
8. Poland, Kraków	Presence of atheromatous lesions in the coronary arteries; (s) S	Jaegermann 1964	P	505	160	220	93	32	1·1680	2·1766	0·9645	0·0751
			C	19634	6478	7626	3904	1626				
9. United Kingdom, Leeds, York	Occlusive peripheral arterio-sclerosis; men	Hall *et al.* 1971	P	554	216	268	52	18	1·3737	11·9887	1·2843	2·6086
			C	98064	45399	41006	8510	3149				
10. United Kingdom, Glasgow	Peripheral vascular disease or arterio-sclerosis	MacAndrew 1969	P	378	165	153	50	10	1·5099	11·2159	1·4307	4·0610
			C	1936	1034	635	219	48				
11. U.S.A., Boston	Arterio-sclerosis obliterans; (s) S	Weiss 1972	P	502	192	233	60	17	1·5679	17·8001	1·2686	2·1775
			C	2583	1230	952	303	98				
12. U.S.A., Brooklyn	Cerebral arteriosclerosis (with psychosis)	Herman & Derby 1937	P	224	101	79	31	13	0·8598	0·8770	0·8817	0·3267
			C	1444	609	554	212	69				
				3282					1·2058	20·7369	1·1282	4·3078
				χ^2_{11} for homogeneity of areas						27·1408		10·8413

ATHEROSCLEROSIS, WITH OCCLUSION/WITHOUT OCCLUSION

Place	Additional details	Authors		Number	O	A	B	AB	A/O Relative incidence	A/O χ^2_1	B/O Relative incidence	B/O χ^2_1
1. United Kingdom, London		Kingsbury 1971	With	*506*	*174*	*261*	*53*	*18*	*1·8061*	*7·4449*	*1·0372*	*0·0132*
			Without	*129*	*59*	*49*	*17*	*4*				

BUERGER'S DISEASE

Place	Additional details	Authors		Number	O	A	B	AB	A/O Relative incidence	A/O χ^2_1	B/O Relative incidence	B/O χ^2_1
1. Japan, Niigata		Hirose & Honma 1962	P	66	13	37	6	10	2·2810	6·5100	0·5865	1·1660
			C	12253	3624	4522	2852	1255				

ARTERIOSCLEROTIC HEART DISEASE

Place	Additional details	Authors		Number	O	A	B	AB	A/O Relative incidence	A/O χ^2_1	B/O Relative incidence	B/O χ^2_1
1. Denmark, København		Viskum 1973	P	253	111	112	19	11	0·9297	0·2907	0·6381	3·2323
		Andersen 1955 M1	C	14304	5804	6299	1557	644				

ACROCYANOSIS

Place	Additional details	Authors		Number	O	A	B	AB	A/O Relative incidence	A/O χ^2_1	B/O Relative incidence	B/O χ^2_1
1. Italy, Trentino		Nardelli 1928	P	43	17	19	6	1	1·3671	0·7659	2·0147	1·7878
		Formentano 1951 M1	C	279	137	112	24	6				

THROMBOSIS AND EMBOLISM

Place	Additional details	Authors		Number	O	A	B	AB	A/O Relative incidence	A/O χ^2_1	B/O Relative incidence	B/O χ^2_1
1. Germany, München	Post-mortem	Lützeler & Dormanns 1929	P	162	67	66	22	7	0·9727	0·0227	1·4500	1·9671
		Kruse M1	C	1300	552	559	125	64				
2. Germany, Tübingen	Thrombo-embolism; (s) S	Völter *et al.* 1970	P	975	360	484	91	40	1·3074	14·4663	0·9577	0·1332
		Dick *et al.* 1962	C	39031	16283	16745	4298	1705				
3. Romania, Bucureşti	Cerebral thrombosis; diagnosed post-mortem	Ionescu *et al.* 1976	P	329	104	151	46	28	1·1208	0·7881	0·8785	0·5279
			C	20705	6811	8823	3429	1642				
4. United Kingdom	Thrombo-embolism; non-pregnant women not on oral contraceptives	Jick *et al.* 1969	P	28	9	15	3	1	1·8652	2·1853	1·8178	0·8035
			C	190177	88782	79334	16280	5781				

TABLE 1 **THE ABO BLOOD GROUP SYSTEM** *(cont.)*

Place	Additional details	Authors		Number	O	A	B	AB	A/O Relative incidence	A/O χ_1^2 for difference from unity	B/O Relative incidence	B/O χ_1^2 for difference from unity
DISEASES OF THE CIRCULATORY SYSTEM *(cont.)*												
THROMBOSIS AND EMBOLISM *(cont.)*												
5. United Kingdom, Nottingham	Venous thrombo-embolism; medical patients	Talbot *et al.* 1970	P	153	68	68	15	2	1·0853	0·2270	1·2646	0·6755
			C	60606	28006	25806	4885	1909				
6. United Kingdom, Nottingham	Venous thrombo-embolism; surgical patients	Talbot *et al.* 1970	P	147	59	67	18	3	1·2324	1·3668	1·7491	4·2968
			C	60606	28006	25806	4885	1909				
7. United Kingdom, Nottingham	Pulmonary embolism; fatal	Talbot *et al.* 1970	P	163	67	78	10	8	1·2634	1·9653	0·8557	0·2109
			C	60606	28006	25806	4885	1909				
8. United Kingdom, Nottingham	Venous thrombo-embolism	Talbot *et al.* 1972	P	478	176	229	63	10	1·2674	3·7864	1·8251	9·9660
			C	950	413	424	81	32				
9. U.S.A.	Thrombo-embolism; medical patients and non-pregnant women not on oral contraceptives	Jick *et al.* 1969	P	83	29	43	8	3	1·9157	7·0911	1·1198	0·0783
			C	2583	1230	952	303	98				
10. U.S.A., Rochester	Pulmonary embolism	Mayo & Fergeson 1953	P	173	81	74	13	5	0·9561	0·0664	0·9028	0·1006
		Tinney & Watkins 1941	C	1000(c)	450	430	80	40				
				2691					1·2299	22·0826	1·1351	3·1639
				χ_9^2 for homogeneity of areas						9·8827		15·5959
THROMBOEMBOLISM IN PREGNANT OR PUERPERAL WOMEN												
1. Sweden		Jick *et al.* 1969	P	82	16	48	15	3	2·2221	7·6269	3·1606	10·2020
			C	18944	6827	9217	2025	875				
2. United Kingdom		Jick *et al.* 1969	P	40	15	20	3	2	1·4921	1·3725	1·0907	0·0188
			C	190177	88782	79334	16280	5781				
3. United Kingdom, England and Wales	Pulmonary embolism during pregnancy or puerperium	U.K. Department of Health 1972	P	58(c)	19	32	4	3	1·8275	4·3108	1·0829	0·0209
			C	10000	4578	4219	890	313				
4. United Kingdom, Nottingham		Talbot *et al.* 1970	P	100	34	49	9	8	1·5640	4·0095	1·5176	1·2360
			C	60606	28006	25806	4885	1909				
5. United Kingdom, Aberdeen	Superficial puerperal thrombo-phlebitis; (s) Rh_D	Allan & Stewart 1971	P	607	262	253	69	23	1·3824	13·1979	1·2654	2·9581
			C	27093	13742	9599	2860	892				
6. U.S.A.		Jick *et al.* 1969	P	44	13	25	3	3	2·4846	6·9733	0·9368	0·0103
			C	2583	1230	952	303	98				
				931					1·5147	32·1817	1·3820	7·9972
				χ_5^2 for homogeneity of areas						5·3093		6·4489
THROMBOEMBOLISM IN WOMEN ON ORAL CONTRACEPTIVES												
1. Sweden		Jick *et al.* 1969	P	59	10	36	8	5	2·6665	7·5130	2·6971	4·3627
			C	18944	6827	9217	2025	875				
2. Sweden		Westerholm *et al.* 1971	P	50	10	29	7	4	2·4675	6·0524	2·4068	3·1669
			C	15802	6048	7108	1759	887				
3. United Kingdom		Jick *et al.* 1969	P	72	17	42	11	2	2·7648	12·5124	3·5287	10·6134
			C	190177	88782	79334	16280	5781				
4. U.S.A.		Jick *et al.* 1969	P	55	9	32	8	6	4·5938	16·1190	3·6084	6·8550
			C	2583	1230	952	303	98				
				236					2·9649	40·4703	3·0746	24·4424
				χ_3^2 for homogeneity of areas						1·7265		0·5556

TABLE 1 THE ABO BLOOD GROUP SYSTEM (*cont.*)

Place	Additional details	Authors		Number	O	A	B	AB	A/O Relative incidence	A/O χ_1^2 for difference from unity	B/O Relative incidence	B/O χ_1^2 for difference from unity
ARTERITIS												
1. Italy, Milano		Mor & Sforza 1960	P	128	44	59	20	5	1·2146	0·7699	1·7003	2·9292
			C	500	202	223	54	21				
VARICOSE VEINS OF LOWER EXTREMITIES												
1. Italy, Chieri, Torino		Capitolo *et al.* 1965	P	307	120	131	45	11	1·0874	0·3528	1·4216	3·0953
			C	1218	508	510	134	66				
HAEMORRHAGES												
1. Romania, Bucureşti	Cerebral; diagnosed post-mortem	Ionescu *et al.* 1976	P	482	176	199	81	26	0·8728	1·6891	0·9141	0·4369
			C	20705	6811	8823	3429	1641				
2. Peru, Lima	Cerebral	Muñoz-Baratta 1962	P	22(c)	8	7	5	2	2·2220	2·3793	3·2692	4·3160
			C	107938(c)	66058	26013	12629	3238				
3. Peru, Lima	Gastro-intestinal	Muñoz-Baratta 1962	P	834(c)	615	144	65	10	0·5946	31·3388	0·5528	20·5374
			C	107938(c)	66058	26013	12629	3238				
4. Peru, Lima	Gastro-intestinal	Muñoz-Baratta 1962	P	701(c)	471	136	62	32	0·7333	10·1016	0·6885	7·5910
			C	107938(c)	66058	26013	12629	3238				
5. Peru, Lima	Nasal	Muñoz-Baratta 1962	P	46(c)	33	7	4	2	0·5387	2·2096	0·6340	0·7405
			C	107938(c)	66058	26013	12629	3238				
6. Japan, Sendai	Pregnancy or childbirth	Moniwa 1960	P	85	24	31	17	13	1·1230	0·1812	0·9933	0·0004
			C	21199	6769	7786	4827	1817				
7. Peru, Lima	Postpartum	Muñoz-Baratta 1962	P	32(c)	20	6	6	0	0·7618	0·3415	1·5692	0·9366
			C	107938(c)	66058	26013	12629	3238				
8. Peru, Lima	Postoperative	Muñoz-Baratta 1962	P	81(c)	59	13	6	3	0·5595	3·5896	0·5319	2·1690
			C	107938(c)	66058	26013	12629	3238				
9. Peru, Lima	Haemoptysis	Muñoz-Baratta 1962	P	150(c)	82	27	24	17	0·8362	0·6497	1·5309	3·3614
			C	107938(c)	66058	26013	12629	3238				
10. Peru, Lima	Haematuria	Muñoz-Baratta 1962	P	45(c)	20	15	7	3	1·9046	3·5561	1·8307	1·8952
			C	107938(c)	66058	26013	12629	3238				
				2478					0·7486	31·8088	0·8011	10·6987
				χ_9^2 for homogeneity of areas						24·2277		31·2857
DISEASES OF THE RESPIRATORY SYSTEM												
RESPIRATORY INFECTIONS												
1. Austria, Vöcklabruck	Infants; (s) S	Kircher 1968	P	673	266	289	81	37	1·1849	3·3314	1·1317	0·7924
			C	3405	1468	1346	395	196				
2. Finland		Mustakallio 1937	P	125	42	53	25	5	1·0435	0·0406	1·3478	1·3218
			C	2595	908	1098	401	188				
				798					1·1608	3·0692	1·1766	1·7618
				χ_1^2 for homogeneity of areas						0·3028		0·3524
BRONCHOPNEUMONIA												
1. Denmark, Köbenhavn	Danes	Viskum 1973	P	177	71	73	22	11	0·9474	0·1040	1·1551	0·3443
		Andersen 1955 M1	C	14304	5804	6299	1557	644				
2. United Kingdom, London	Autopsies on children under 13	Carter & Heslop 1957	P	171	69	77	18	7	1·2109	1·3109	1·3419	1·2113
			C	10000	4578	4219	890	313				
3. United Kingdom, Glasgow	Autopsies on children under 13	Struthers 1951	P	148	47	68	21	12	2·0953	14·8757	2·0926	7·7067
			C	6011	3063	2115	654	179				
				496					1·2893	6·3612	1·4608	6·4216
				χ_2^2 for homogeneity of areas						9·9294		2·8407

TABLE 1 THE ABO BLOOD GROUP SYSTEM (*cont.*)

Place	Additional details	Authors		Number	O	A	B	AB	A/O Relative incidence	A/O χ_1^2 for difference from unity	B/O Relative incidence	B/O χ_1^2 for difference from unity
DISEASES OF THE RESPIRATORY SYSTEM (*cont.*)												
PNEUMONIA												
1. Finland		Sievers 1929	P	421(c)	146	169	71	35	0·9135	0·5169	1·0441	0·0708
			C	1711	584	740	272	115				
2. Finland		Mustakallio 1937	P	40	15	16	7	2	0·8821	0·1200	1·0567	0·0143
			C	2595	908	1098	401	188				
3. Germany, München		Lützeler & Dormanns 1929	P	201	94	82	19	6	0·8614	0·8419	0·8926	0·1767
		Kruse M1	C	1300	552	559	125	64				
4. Greece, Athínai		Diamantopoulos 1928	P	33	10	12	10	1	1·3397	0·4567	3·6284	7·9617
			C	1216	537	481	148	50				
				695					0·9099	1·0145	1·1125	0·6955
				χ_3^2 for homogeneity of areas						0·9210		7·5280
BRONCHITIS												
1. Denmark, Köbenhavn	Chronic; Danes	Viskum 1973	P	347	148	149	38	12	0·9276	0·4088	0·9571	0·0567
		Andersen 1955 M1	C	14304	5804	6299	1557	644				
2. Finland		Sievers 1929	P	204	71	89	32	12	0·9893	0·0041	0·9677	0·0213
			C	1711	584	740	272	115				
3. Finland		Streng & Ryti 1927[a]	P	144	56	61	19	8	0·8534	0·6599	0·6771	1·9756
			C	1383(c)	463	591	232	97				
4. Germany, Erlangen, Nürnberg	Chronic or recurrent	Berg, G. *et al.* 1967	P	48	19	20	5	4	0·6811	1·1552	0·7551	0·2535
			C	193	66	102	23	2				
5. United Kingdom, London	Bronchitis and/or emphysema	Lewis & Woods 1961	P	258	130	97	26	5	0·8096	2·4158	1·0288	0·0169
			C	10000	4578	4219	890	313				
				1001					0·8828	3·0467	0·9189	0·6185
				χ_4^2 for homogeneity of areas						1·5971		1·7055
EMPHYSEMA												
1. Germany, München		Lützeler & Dormanns 1929	P	91	38	38	13	2	0·9875	0·0028	1·5107	1·5058
		Kruse M1	C	1300	552	559	125	64				
2. Poland, Wrocław		Zuber 1966	P	151	46	73	27	5	1·2495	1·3772	0·9476	0·0485
			C	9722(c)	3095	3931	1917	779				
				242					1·1398	0·7798	1·1132	0·2947
				χ_1^2 for homogeneity of areas						0·6002		1·2596
ATROPHIC OZENOUS RHINITIS												
1. Italy, Barletta		Rizzi 1963	P	20	13	3	2	2	0·3087	3·3624	0·4752	0·9577
		Liaci & Scarano 1959 M2	C	8347	3858	2884	1249	356				
PLEURISY												
1. Finland		Sievers 1929	P	189(c)	56	81	36	16	1·1415	0·5265	1·3803	2·0354
			C	1711	584	740	272	115				
2. Finland		Mustakallio 1937	P	46	16	23	6	1	1·1883	0·2768	0·8491	0·1149
			C	2595	908	1098	401	188				
3. Poland, Wrocław		Zuber 1966	P	97	24	51	14	8	1·6731	4·2825	0·9418	0·0316
			C	9722	3095	3931	1917	779				
				332					1·2847	3·4822	1·1685	0·7921
				χ_2^2 for homogeneity of areas						1·6036		1·3898

TABLE 1 **THE ABO BLOOD GROUP SYSTEM** *(cont.)*

Place	Additional details	Authors		Number	O	A	B	AB	A/O Relative incidence	A/O χ_1^2 for difference from unity	B/O Relative incidence	B/O χ_1^2 for difference from unity
SPONTANEOUS PNEUMOTHORAX												
1. Denmark, København	Danes	Viskum 1973	P	85	32	36	13	4	1·0366	0·0218	1·5144	1·5802
		Andersen 1955 M1	C	14304	5804	6299	1557	644				
BRONCHIECTASIS												
1. United Kingdom, London		Lewis & Woods 1961	P	78	35	35	5	3	1·0851	0·1158	0·7348	0·4129
			C	10000	4578	4219	890	313				
DISEASES OF THE DIGESTIVE SYSTEM												
DENTAL CARIES												
1. Germany, Göttingen		Jörgensen 1967	P	251	86	124	30	11	1·2657	2·0893	1·3413	1·3750
			C	694	273	311	71	39				
DENTAL CARIES, EXTENSIVE/NONE AT ALL												
1. U.S.A., New York		Thompson 1931	Extens.	*36*	*18*	*12*	*3*	*3*	*0·8148*	*0·1230*	*0·6111*	*0·2983*
			None	*24*	*11*	*9*	*3*	*1*				
PERIODONTOSIS												
1. France, Bordeau	(s) S, Rh_D	Toussaint & Mériaux 1970	P	1784	794	792	150	48	1·0044	0·0050	1·1894	2·3195
			C	3216	1448	1438	230	100				
GASTRITIS												
1. Finland		Sievers 1929	P	98(c)	21	50	24	3	1·8790	5·6286	2·4538	8·5106
			C	1711	584	740	272	115				
2. United Kingdom, Bristol	Erosive; (s) S	Thompson *et al.* 1968	P	40	15	23	2	0	1·5295	1·6378	0·7146	0·1991
		Roberts 1948	C	40740	17939	17984	3347	1470				
3. Egypt, Alexandria		Sadek *et al.* 1965[a]	P	205	65	81	35	24	1·0773	0·1888	0·6333	4·5505
			C	3720	1142	1321	971	286				
				343					1·3064	4·0939	0·9690	0·0337
				χ_2^2 for homogeneity of areas						3·3612		13·2265
APPENDICITIS												
1. Austria, Wien		Flamm & Friedrich 1929	P	82(c)	24	36	15	7	1·1749	0·3713	1·4591	1·3068
		Corvin M1	C	10392	3635	4641	1557	559				
2. Finland		Sievers 1929	P	122(c)	31	56	27	8	1·4256	2·3647	1·8700	5·2463
			C	1711	584	740	272	115				
3. Germany, Tübingen		Völter *et al.* 1970	P	443	171	217	42	13	1·2340	4·1794	0·9305	0·1732
		Dick *et al.* 1962	C	39031	16283	16745	4298	1705				
4. Japan, Niigata		Hirose & Honma 1962	P	1910	590	684	430	206	0·9291	1·4801	0·9261	1·2686
			C	12253	3624	4522	2852	1255				
5. Japan, Sendai	Acute	Moniwa 1960	P	887	303	314	191	79	0·9009	1·6094	0·8840	1·7108
			C	21199	6769	7786	4827	1817				
6. U.S.A., New Haven	Acute; Whites	Pearson 1964	P	581	243	232	82	24	0·9751	0·0485	1·3222	2·8137
		Niederman *et al.* 1962 M2	C	1000	431	422	110	37				
				4025					0·9863	0·1190	0·9744	0·2823
				χ_5^2 for homogeneity of areas						9·9344		12·2370
HERNIA OF ABDOMINAL CAVITY												
1. Japan, Sendai	Without mention of obstruction	Moniwa 1960	P	169	54	62	38	15	0·9982	0·0001	0·9868	0·0039
			C	21199	6769	7786	4827	1817				

TABLE 1 THE ABO BLOOD GROUP SYSTEM (*cont.*)

Place	Additional details	Authors		Number	O	A	B	AB	A/O Relative incidence	A/O χ^2_1 for difference from unity	B/O Relative incidence	B/O χ^2_1 for difference from unity
DISEASES OF THE DIGESTIVE SYSTEM (*cont.*)												
HERNIA OF UNSPECIFIED SITE												
1. Austria, Wien		Flamm & Friedrich 1929	P	80(c)	24	38	14	4	1·2401	0·6764	1·3619	0·8367
		Corvin M1	C	10392	3635	4641	1557	559				
INTESTINAL OBSTRUCTION												
1. Japan, Sendai	Without mention of hernia	Moniwa 1960	P	262	67	104	68	23	1·3495	3·6199	1·4233	4·1542
			C	21199	6769	7786	4827	1817				
ULCERATIVE COLITIS												
1. Czechoslovakia, Praha		Veselý 1969[a]	P	57	23	21	7	6	0·6352	2·1487	0·5720	1·6051
			C	1142(c)	359	516	191	76				
2. United Kingdom, Oxford		Smith & Truelove 1961	P	317	147	124	33	13	0·9420	0·2349	1·3137	1·9467
			C	12820	6010	5382	1027	401				
3. United Kingdom, West Midlands		Winstone *et al.* 1960	P	277	132	117	21	7	0·9533	0·1407	0·9036	0·1848
			C	39084	17983	16720	3166	1215				
4. U.S.A., Connecticut	25% Jewish	Thayer & Bove 1965	P	170	66	74	20	10	1·2489	1·7207	1·1204	0·1981
			C	94167	41433	37196	11206	4332				
5. U.S.A., Iowa		Buckwalter *et al.* 1958	P	184(c)	80	82	15	7	1·1288	0·5776	0·9547	0·0265
			C	6313(c)	2892	2626	568	227				
6. U.S.A., Rochester	Chronic	Mayo & Fergeson 1953	P	87(c)	35	33	15	4	0·9867	0·0028	2·4107	7·0413
		Tinney & Watkins 1941	C	1000(c)	450	430	80	40				
				1092					1·0030	0·0021	1·1445	1·5674
				χ^2_5 for homogeneity of areas						4·8234		9·4350
ANAL FISSURE OR FISTULA												
1. Japan, Sendai		Moniwa 1960	P	107	30	46	16	15	1·3331	1·4931	0·7479	0·8772
			C	21199	6769	7786	4827	1817				
PERITONITIS												
1. Japan, Sendai		Moniwa 1960	P	61	22	21	13	5	0·8299	0·3726	0·8286	0·2879
			C	21199	6769	7786	4827	1817				
DISEASES OF INTESTINES OR PERITONEUM												
1. Japan, Sendai	Other than peritonitis	Moniwa 1960	P	121	45	52	12	12	1·0046	0·0005	0·3740	9·1353
			C	21199	6769	7786	4827	1817				
CIRRHOSIS OF LIVER												
1. Austria, Wien	(s) S, Rh_D	Speiser 1958[a]	P	355	110	172	48	25	1·3345	4·1736	1·2319	1·0781
			C	1000	367	430	130	73				
2. Austria, Wien	Alcoholic or posthepatitic; (s) S	Wewalka 1960	P	250	59	144	34	13	2·0041	19·8110	1·5580	4·1499
			C	10000	3631	4422	1343	604				
3. Czechoslovakia, Bohemia		Kordač 1965	P	304	95	130	55	24	1·1050	0·5448	1·1422	0·6136
			C	80518	27051	33501	13711	6255				
4. Czechoslovakia, Praha		Veselý 1969[a]	P	142	45	61	23	13	0·9431	0·0792	0·9607	0·0218
			C	1142(c)	359	516	191	76				
5. France, Mulhouse	Alcoholic	Lobstein 1958	P	179	67	88	16	8	1·1486	0·7110	1·2091	0·4523
			C	6423	2648	3028	523	224				
6. Germany, München		Lützeler & Dormanns 1929	P	15	7	4	3	1	0·5643	0·8259	1·8926	0·8374
		Kruse M1	C	1300	552	559	125	64				
7. Poland, Katowice		Machalski & Wantoła 1967	P	218	54	90	53	21	1·3863	3·3905	1·8690	9·7027
			C	2950(c)	994	1195	522	239				
8. Portugal		Lessa & Ruffié 1960	P	362(c)	138	190	28	6	1·2576	3·7919	1·1557	0·4394
			C	3353(c)	1424	1559	250	120				

TABLE 1 **THE ABO BLOOD GROUP SYSTEM** (*cont.*)

Place	Additional details	Authors		Number	O	A	B	AB	A/O Relative incidence	A/O χ_1^2 for difference from unity	B/O Relative incidence	B/O χ_1^2 for difference from unity
9. United Kingdom, Region I		Zuckerman 1966	P		15	14			1·0120	0·0010		
			C		27934	25763						
10. United Kingdom, Region II		Zuckerman 1966	P		8	12			1·6326	1·1520		
			C		7743	7114						
11. United Kingdom, Region III		Zuckerman 1966	P		34	43			1·4695	2·8005		
			C		9379	8072						
12. United Kingdom, Region IV		Zuckerman 1966	P		25	31			1·2177	0·5368		
			C		21360	21751						
13. N. India, Lucknow		Nath *et al.* 1963	P	137	33	48	43	13	1·9993	8·9827	1·0678	0·0778
			P	3330(c)	1035	753	1263	279				
14. Japan, Niigata	Banti's disease	Hirose & Honma 1962	P	74	15	41	11	7	2·1905	6·7161	0·9318	0·0315
			C	12253	3624	4522	2852	1255				
15. U.S.A., Iowa	Portal	Buckwalter *et al.* 1964	P	273(c)	126	110	29	8	0·9245	0·3595	1·0977	0·2036
			C	49979	22392	21144	4695	1748				
16. U.S.A., Iowa	Other than portal	Buckwalter *et al.* 1964	P	62(c)	28	28	3	3	1·0590	0·0460	0·5110	1·2206
			C	49979	22392	21144	4695	1748				
17. Mexico		Lisker *et al.* 1964	P	322(c)	182	107	27	6	1·1382	1·0759	0·9860	0·0045
			C	6843(c)	4021	2077	605	140				
18. Peru, Lima		Muñoz-Baratta 1962	P	144(c)	89	36	15	4	1·0272	0·0184	0·8816	0·2037
			C	107938(c)	66058	26013	12629	3238				
				2837+?					1·2372	24·8769	1·1811	6·6605
					χ_{17}^2 for homogeneity of areas					30·1399		
				(2837)	χ_{13}^2 for homogeneity of areas							12·3764

CHOLELITHIASIS

Place	Additional details	Authors		Number	O	A	B	AB	A/O Relative incidence	A/O χ_1^2 for difference from unity	B/O Relative incidence	B/O χ_1^2 for difference from unity
1. Austria, Wien		Flamm & Friedrich 1929	P	71(c)	20	40	10	1	1·5665	2·6685	1·1673	0·1586
		Corvin M1	C	10392	3635	4641	1557	559				
2. Czechoslovakia, Praha		Veselý 1969[b]	P	680	194	311	115	60	1·1122	0·8635	1·1111	0·5071
			C	1142	358	516	191	77				
3. Denmark, København		Jordal 1956	P	413	174	174	47	18	0·9214	0·5664	1·0069	0·0017
			C	14304	5804	6299	1557	644				
4. Denmark, København	(s) S, A	Kjølbye & Lykkegaard Nielsen 1959	P	1369	511	643	142	73	1·1817	7·5162	1·0957	0·8788
			C	23842	9814	10450	2489	1089				
5. France, Colmar		Lobstein & Voegtlin 1959	P	236	83	126	16	11	1·2644	2·6429	0·8190	0·5182
			C	5570	2188	2627	515	240				
6. France, Mulhouse		Lobstein & Voegtlin 1959	P	602	213	306	55	28	1·2563	6·0056	1·3074	2·8544
			C	6423	2648	3028	523	224				
7. Germany, Berlin		Schmauss *et al.* 1968	P	3082	1070	1396	398	218	1·1660	11·8732	0·9340	1·1470
			C	15154	5642	6313	2247	952				
8. Germany, München		Lützeler & Dormanns 1929	P	110	42	50	11	7	1·1756	0·5519	1·1566	0·1699
		Kruse M1	C	1300	552	559	125	64				
9. Italy, Milano		Rotelli & Corippo 1959	P	414	166	198	38	12	0·9855	0·0184	0·8481	0·8011
			C	8000	3090	3740	834	336				
10. Italy, Milano		Mor & Sforza 1960	P	553	232	248	55	18	0·9683	0·0584	0·8868	0·3139
			C	500	202	223	54	21				
11. Italy, Napoli	(s) S	Cocchia *et al.* 1963	P	300	126	158	9	7	1·5350	6·1364	0·3622	6·3726
			C	300	142	116	28	14				
12. Italy, Potenza		Pesce & Pontrandolfi 1961	P	48	18	19	9	2	1·3293	0·7211	1·1419	0·1020
		Pontrandolfi & Pesce 1960 M2	C	1259	539	428	236	56				
13. Italy, Trieste		Guarini & Furlani 1968	P	409	126	199	69	15	2·0481	38·3938	1·9667	19·6513
			C	11679	5405	4168	1505	601				

TABLE 1 **THE ABO BLOOD GROUP SYSTEM** (*cont.*)

Place	Additional details	Authors		Number	O	A	B	AB	A/O Relative incidence	A/O χ_1^2 for difference from unity	B/O Relative incidence	B/O χ_1^2 for difference from unity
DISEASES OF THE DIGESTIVE SYSTEM (*cont.*)												
CHOLELITHIASIS (*cont.*)												
14. Poland, Katowice		Machalski *et al.* 1968	P	526	150	215	113	48	1·1938	2·4465	1·4358	7·3078
			C	3606(c)	1216	1460	638	292				
15. Poland, Poznań		Woszczyk 1966	P	1320	420	537	237	126	1·2047	7·0165	1·0214	0·0588
			C	7951	2773	2943	1532	703				
16. Poland, Warszawa		Czaplicki *et al.* 1964	P	621	182	271	105	63	1·4358	12·5042	1·1015	0·5529
			C	4270	1537	1594	805	334				
17. Sweden, Göteborg	(s) S	Bodvall & Övergaard 1966	P	979	356	491	83	49	1·1877	2·8707	0·9245	0·2098
			C	855	341	396	86	32				
18. Japan, Niigata		Hirose & Honma 1962	P	1941	596	748	419	178	1·0058	0·0095	0·8933	2·7129
			C	12253	3624	4522	2852	1255				
19. Japan, Sendai		Moniwa 1960	P	234	79	80	51	24	0·8804	0·6381	0·9053	0·3035
			C	21199	6769	7786	4827	1817				
20. U.S.A., Los Angeles		Hauch & Moore 1963	P	628	307	246	37	38	0·9204	0·8919	0·6568	5·6183
			C	11851	5548	4830	1018	455				
21. Peru, Lima		Muñoz-Baratta 1962	P	124(c)	82	22	15	5	0·6813	2·5520	0·9568	0·0247
			C	107938	66058	26013	12629	3238				
				14660					1·1468	43·8033	1·0079	0·0722
				χ_{20}^2 for homogeneity of areas						63·1423		50·1931
CHOLECYSTITIS												
1. Italy, Potenza	Acute and chronic	Pesce & Pontrandolfi 1961	P	32	5	13	10	4	3·2743	5·0045	4·5678	7·5384
		Pontrandolfi & Pesce 1960 M2	C	1259	539	428	236	56				
2. Poland, Białystok	(s) S	Korfel *et al.* 1967	P	912(c)	248	428	163	73	1·6964	37·8406	1·2274	3·6103
			C	5372	1959	1993	1049	371				
3. N. India, Lucknow	Chronic	Nath *et al.* 1963	P	79	25	18	30	6	0·9896	0·0011	0·9834	0·0037
			C	3330(c)	1035	753	1263	279				
4. Japan, Sendai	Without mention of calculi	Moniwa 1960	P	117	27	40	32	18	1·2880	1·0278	1·6620	3·7600
			C	21199	6769	7786	4827	1817				
5. Peru, Lima		Muñoz-Baratta 1962	P	442(c)	298	105	31	8	0·8948	0·9560	0·5441	10·3718
			C	107938	66058	26013	12629	3238				
				1582					1·3409	20·8809	1·0916	1·1141
				χ_4^2 for homogeneity of areas						23·9491		24·1700
CHOLELITHIASIS OR CHOLECYSTITIS												
1. Germany, Göttingen		Jörgensen 1967	P	396	142	195	44	15	1·2054	1·8328	1·1914	0·6456
			C	694	273	311	71	39				
2. Germany, Greifswald		Ludwig 1964	P	830	290	401	93	46	1·1186	1·9874	0·9049	0·6663
			C	13100	4760	5884	1687	769				
3. U.S.A., Rochester		Mayo & Fergeson 1953	P	117	52	42	18	5	0·8453	0·5939	1·9471	4·9607
		Tinney & Watkins 1941	C	1000(c)	450	430	80	40				
				1343					1·1092	2·4876	1·0462	0·2018
				χ_2^2 for homogeneity of areas						1·9265		6·0708
DISEASES OF GALL-BLADDER OR BILIARY DUCTS												
1. Italy, Verona	With or without calculi; (s) S	Bonzanini 1961	P	640	262	309	53	16	1·2351	5·6551	0·9854	0·0086
			C	5500	2460	2349	505	186				
2. Poland, Warszawa	Excluding cancer	Kosiński *et al.* 1959	P	551	171	233	124	23	1·3138	6·5256	1·3845	6·6978
			C	4270	1537	1594	805	334				

TABLE 1 THE ABO BLOOD GROUP SYSTEM (*cont.*)

Place	Additional details	Authors		Number	O	A	B	AB	A/O Relative incidence	A/O χ_1^2 for difference from unity	B/O Relative incidence	B/O χ_1^2 for difference from unity
3. Japan, Sendai	Other than cholelithiasis and cholecystitis	Moniwa 1960	P	69	21	31	12	5	1·2834	0·7766	0·8013	0·3736
			C	21199	6769	7786	4827	1817				
4. U.S.A., Rochester	Acute and chronic; Whites	Buchanan & Higley 1921	P	176	95	62	13	6	0·6830	4·6592	0·7697	0·6703
		Tinney & Watkins 1941	C	1000(c)	450	430	80	40				
				1436					1·1742	6·6769	1·1396	2·0578
				χ_3^2 for homogeneity of areas						10·9396		5·6925
JAUNDICE												
1. U.S.A., Rochester	All causes; Whites	Buchanan & Higley 1921	P	173	64	83	20	6	1·3572	2·8953	1·7578	3·9599
		Tinney & Watkins 1941	C	1000(c)	450	430	80	40				
DISEASES OF THE PANCREAS												
1. Czechoslovakia, Praha	Pancreatitis	Veselý 1969[b]	P	167	49	72	26	20	1·0195	0·0095	0·9946	0·0004
			C	1142	358	516	191	77				
2. Germany, Erlangen, Nürnberg	Pancreatitis, acute or chronic	Berg, G. *et al.* 1967	P	27	12	12	3	0	0·6471	0·9889	0·7174	0·2321
			C	193	66	102	23	2				
3. Japan, Sendai		Moniwa 1960	P	50	12	16	16	6	1·1592	0·1493	1·8698	2·6790
			C	21199	6769	7786	4827	1817				
				244					0·9799	0·0156	1·1578	0·5129
				χ_2^2 for homogeneity of areas						1·1321		2·3986
GASTRIC ULCERS												
1. Austria, Wien	(s) Rh_D, S	Speiser 1956	P	1028	393	441	129	65	0·9214	1·2608	0·8875	1·2597
			C	10000	3631	4422	1343	604				
2. Czechoslovakia		Vahala *et al.* 1970	P	127	44	54	16	13	0·8515	0·5622	0·6816	1·5758
		Kout 1959 M2	C	1142	358	516	191	77				
3. Czechoslovakia, Praha	(s) A_1A_2	Kubičková & Veselý 1966	P	406	134	181	57	34	0·9371	0·2378	0·7973	1·5533
			C	1142	358	516	191	77				
4. Denmark	Corpus; (s) S	Sørensen 1957	P	75	32	34	8	1	1·0018	0·0001	1·0133	0·0011
			C	12123	5046	5352	1245	480				
5. Denmark, Köbenhavn		Køster *et al.* 1955	P	337	156	139	28	14	0·8210	2·7913	0·6691	3·7610
			C	14304	5804	6299	1557	644				
6. Denmark, Köbenhavn		Jordal 1956	P	415	184	187	31	13	0·9364	0·3881	0·6280	5·6191
			C	14304	5804	6299	1557	644				
7. Denmark, Köbenhavn		Blegvad 1960[b]	P	102	44	39	12	7	0·8167	0·8418	1·0166	0·0025
		Andersen 1955 M1	C	14304	5804	6299	1557	644				
8. Finland		Streng & Ryti 1927[a]	P	46	16	19	9	2	0·9303	0·0439	1·1226	0·0742
			C	1383	463	591	232	97				
9. France, Colmar		Lobstein & Voegtlin 1959	P	153	60	72	16	5	0·9995	0·0000	1·1329	0·1910
			C	5570	2188	2627	515	240				
10. France, Mulhouse		Lobstein & Voegtlin 1959	P	237	108	96	25	8	0·7773	3·1125	1·1720	0·4887
			C	6423	2648	3028	523	224				
11. France, Paris		Khérumian & Moullec 1959	P	1008	437	423	115	33	0·9694	0·2063	1·3580	8·4751
			C	207588	91414	91276	17714	7184				
12. Germany, Berlin		Scholz 1963	P	400	167	150	60	23	0·9291	0·3895	1·2947	2·6218
			C	3960	1654	1599	459	248				
13. Germany, Erlangen, Nürnberg		Berg, G. *et al.* 1967	P	78	33	32	8	5	0·6275	2·5112	0·6957	0·6156
			C	193	66	102	23	2				
14. Germany, Leipzig		Gedicke & Wellhöner 1961	P	321	128	133	44	6	0·9283	0·3277	0·8933	0·3795
			C	3174	1198	1341	461	174				

TABLE 1 **THE ABO BLOOD GROUP SYSTEM** (*cont.*)

Place	Additional details	Authors		Number	O	A	B	AB	A/O Relative incidence	A/O χ_1^2 for difference from unity	B/O Relative incidence	B/O χ_1^2 for difference from unity
DISEASES OF THE DIGESTIVE SYSTEM (*cont.*)												
GASTRIC ULCERS (*cont.*)												
15. Germany, Marburg		Borschell 1961	P	200	97	83	16	4	0·7103	3·9593	0·4108	9·1470
			C	696	254	306	102	34				
16. Germany, Tübingen		Brockmüller 1962	P	397	174	160	45	18	0·8942	1·0325	0·9798	0·0148
			C	39031	16283	16745	4298	1705				
17. Hungary		István & Széll 1961	P	438	153	183	76	26	0·9392	0·3219	0·9339	0·2333
			C	23000	7567	9637	4025	1771				
18. Hungary	Pylorus	István & Széll 1961	P	165	60	67	24	14	0·8768	0·5430	0·7520	1·3836
			C	23000	7567	9637	4025	1771				
19. Italy, Aquila		Curtoni & Morgante 1964	P	210(c)	123	63	16	8	0·6430	7·9520	0·6446	2·6781
			C	8920(c)	4321	3442	872	285				
20. Italy, Campania		Pollara & Melina 1957	P	300	145	115	31	9	0·9415	0·1768	0·6638	3·4692
			C	1000	444	374	143	39				
21. Italy, Lombardia		Ninni & Bedarida 1959	P	356	158	129	59	10	0·8019	2·2915	1·8404	8·3133
			C	640	276	281	56	27				
22. Italy, Milano		Mangani 1957	P	19	4	11	3	1	2·6436	2·7681	2·8881	1·9243
		Visconti *et al.* 1961	C	9607	3974	4134	1032	467				
23. Italy, Milano		Rotelli & Corippo 1959	P	168	64	82	20	2	1·0586	0·1140	1·1578	0·3198
			C	8000	3090	3740	834	336				
24. Italy, Milano		Camerini Riviera 1960	P	165	68	81	8	8	1·2215	1·3777	0·5036	3·2457
			C	2346	1006	981	235	124				
25. Italy, Milano		Mor & Sforza 1960	P	285	115	133	25	12	1·0476	0·0843	0·8132	0·5925
			C	500	202	223	54	21				
26. Italy, Milano		Visconti *et al.* 1961[b]	P	343	152	130	42	19	0·8226	2·5840	1·0643	0·1229
			C	9607	3975	4133	1032	467				
27. Italy, Palermo		Carlo & Ridulfo 1958	P	69	31	22	9	7	0·9723	0·0095	0·8029	0·3176
			C	980	448	327	162	43				
28. Italy, Pavia		Prosser 1957	P	122	56	50	11	5	0·7377	2·4075	0·7278	0·9155
			C	8000	3090	3740	834	336				
29. Italy, Perugia		Benda & Menghini 1957	P	383	176	166	30	11	0·9540	0·1794	0·6886	3·4287
			C	7356	3163	3127	783	283				
30. Italy, Roma		Misiti *et al.* 1968	P	26	10	12	3	1	1·3409	0·4688	1·1776	0·0616
			C	20051	8973	8030	2286	762				
31. Italy, Siena	(s) S	Prior & Vegni 1957	P	73	33	28	8	4	0·9758	0·0085	0·8578	0·1424
			C	1025	460	400	130	35				
32. Italy, Verona	(s) S	Bonzanini 1961	P	85	38	39	5	3	1·0748	0·0986	0·6410	0·8650
			C	5500	2460	2349	505	186				
33. Norway, Oslo		Heistø 1956	P	412	179	189	31	13	0·7980	4·4512	0·8020	1·2286
			C	8292	3135	4148	677	332				
34. Poland		Belec *et al.* 1971	P	196	73	74	28	21	0·9323	0·1779	0·6511	3·6838
		Charzewski *et al.* 1965 M2	C	13744	4719	5131	2780	1114				
35. Poland, Katowice		Machalski *et al.* 1968	P	284	85	126	48	25	1·2346	2·0945	1·0763	0·1545
			C	3606	1216	1460	638	292				
36. Poland, Kraków		Socha 1960	P	2361	890	825	455	191	0·7578	30·9404	0·8112	12·3904
			C	37766	12151	14863	7658	3094				
37. Poland, Lower Silesia		Sagan *et al.* 1957	P	67	26	27	12	2	0·8991	0·1454	0·7967	0·4129
			C	2397	813	939	471	174				
38. Poland, Lublin		Spruch & Dacka 1968	P	336	120	122	73	21	0·9157	0·3643	1·1290	0·5040
			C	1150	399	443	215	93				
39. Poland, Opole		Gołąbek 1965	P	44	16	18	9	1	0·9946	0·0002	0·9150	0·0441
			C	1453	488	552	300	113				
40. Poland, Poznań		Wojtowicz *et al.* 1960	P	436	170	154	82	30	0·8536	1·9175	0·8731	0·9649
			C	7951	2773	2943	1532	703				
41. Poland, Poznań		Woszczyk 1966	P	498	199	169	92	38	0·8002	4·2677	0·8368	1·8773
		Wojtowicz *et al.* 1960	C	7951	2773	2943	1532	703				

TABLE 1 THE ABO BLOOD GROUP SYSTEM (*cont.*)

Place	Additional details	Authors		Number	O	A	B	AB	A/O Relative incidence	A/O χ_1^2 for difference from unity	B/O Relative incidence	B/O χ_1^2 for difference from unity
42. Poland, Warszawa		Kosiński *et al.* 1959	P C	384 4270	164 1537	133 1594	61 805	26 334	0·7820	4·0608	0·7102	4·8037
43. Poland, Warszawa		Czaplicki *et al.* 1964	P C	127 4270	51 1537	44 1594	20 805	12 334	0·8319	0·7767	0·7488	1·1709
44. Portugal		Lessa & Ruffié 1960	P C	1292(c) 3353(c)	626 1424	536 1559	95 250	35 120	0·7821	12·5683	0·8644	1·2618
45. Romania	(s) ABH secretion	Fodor & Urcan 1966	P C	94 222	21 75	49 80	18 52	6 15	2·1875	6·5279	1·2363	0·3314
46. Romania, Sibiu		Coroianu *et al.* 1958	P C	34 3850	12 1425	15 1540	4 693	3 192	1·1567	0·1399	0·6854	0·4253
47. Spain, Málaga		Franquelo Ramos & Eloy-Garcia 1966	P C	44 1195	14 577	26 517	2 75	2 26	2·0727	4·6779	1·0990	0·0152
48. Spain, Viscaya	Basques	Goti Iturriaga & Velasco Alonso 1965	P C	19 386	11 198	8 168	0 14	0 6	0·8571	0·1047		
49. Spain, Viscaya	Non-Basques	Goti Iturriaga & Velasco-Alonso 1965	P C	21 336	7 151	12 154	1 24	1 7	1·6809	1·1270	0·8988	0·0096
50. Sweden, Luleå		Hedenstedt 1961	P C	109 8163	37 3024	57 3972	8 806	7 361	1·1729	0·5630	0·8112	0·2850
51. Switzerland, Basel	(s) S	Moor-Jankowski *et al.* 1961	P C	437 2076	168 842	219 912	32 229	18 93	1·2035	2·6804	0·7004	2·9669
52. United Kingdom, Bristol	Type 1*	Johnson *et al.* 1964	P C	189 3284	95 1430	82 1485	5 275	7 94	0·8312	1·4189	0·2737	7·8145
53. United Kingdom, Liverpool		McConnell 1961 Kopeć 1956 M1	P C	232 9301	118 4633	85 3575	28 841	1 252	0·9335	0·2282	1·3072	1·5740
54. United Kingdom, Liverpool		McConnell 1966	P C	377 15377	185 7527	151 6015	31 1450	10 385	1·0214	0·0363	0·8698	0·5052
55. United Kingdom, London	(s) S	Aird *et al.* 1954	P C	599 10000	314 4578	228 4219	46 890	11 313	0·7879	7·0802	0·7536	3·0482
56. United Kingdom, London	Type 1*	Johnson 1965	P C	2188 19473	1026 9173	923 7898	181 1798	58 604	1·0448	0·8387	0·9000	1·5487
57. United Kingdom, Manchester	(s) S	Aird *et al.* 1954	P C	232 9370	122 4532	90 3775	15 788	5 275	0·8856	0·7452	0·7071	1·5729
58. United Kingdom, Middlesbrough	(s) S	Grahame 1961	P C	232 4540	113 2149	103 1873	0 386	16 132	1·0458	0·1026		
59. United Kingdom, Middlesbrough	Type 1*	Johnson *et al.* 1964	P C	217 1678	101 777	99 668	14 164	3 69	1·1401	0·7549	0·6567	1·9930
60. United Kingdom, Newcastle upon Tyne	(s) S	Aird *et al.* 1954	P C	184 13572	102 6598	58 5261	16 1321	8 392	0·7131	4·1736	0·7835	0·8132
61. United Kingdom, Oxford	With metaplasia	Glober *et al.* 1972	P C	53 11662	28 5237	20 5100	4 954	1 371	0·7335	1·1159	0·7842	0·2059
62. United Kingdom, Oxford	Without metaplasia	Glober *et al.* 1972	P C	41 11662	25 5237	14 5100	2 954	0 371	0·5750	2·7380	0·4392	1·2511
63. United Kingdom, Preston	Type 1*	Johnson *et al.* 1964	P C	101 2061	37 938	52 857	7 208	5 58	1·5382	3·8244	0·8532	0·1435

* For details of classification see text, p. 29.

TABLE 1 **THE ABO BLOOD GROUP SYSTEM** (*cont.*)

Place	Additional details	Authors		Number	O	A	B	AB	A/O		B/O	
									Relative incidence	χ_1^2 for difference from unity	Relative incidence	χ_1^2 for difference from unity
DISEASES OF THE DIGESTIVE SYSTEM (*cont.*)												
GASTRIC ULCERS (*cont.*)												
64. United Kingdom, Glamorgan I		Beasley 1960[a]	P	546	289	207.	44	6	0·8758	1·8265	0·6768	5·1728
			C	3514	1658	1356	373	127				
65. United Kingdom, Glamorgan II		Beasley 1960[a]	P	431	220	169	32	10	0·7854	5·0900	0·7100	3·0301
			C	4570	2011	1967	412	180				
66. United Kingdom, Newport		Beasley 1960[b]	P	690	372	254	49	15	0·6914	11·7235	0·7078	3·0700
			C	907	403	398	75	31				
67. United Kingdom, Belfast	Type 1*	Johnson *et al.* 1964	P	186	82	85	14	5	1·3655	3·9799	0·7671	0·8307
			C	11327	5522	4192	1229	384				
68. United Kingdom, Belfast		Macafee 1965[a]	P	325	187	109	24	5	0·9711	0·0587	0·7464	1·8022
			C	28566	15715	9433	2702	716				
69. S. India, Bombay		Joshi *et al.* 1958	P	18	6	6	4	2	1·2886	0·1918	0·7470	0·2034
			C	3600	1228	953	1096	323				
70. S. India, Bombay	Perforated	Joshi *et al.* 1958	P	10	5	1	3	1	0·2577	1·5297	0·6723	0·2947
			C	3600	1228	953	1096	323				
71. N. Vietnam		Nguyen Duong Quang *et al.* 1960	P	199	64	50	75	10	1·7824	9·1044	1·8472	12·6389
			C	6750	3080	1350	1954	366				
72. China, Shanghai		Dao *et al.* 1958	P	66	29	18	10	9	0·6394	2·2013	0·4074	5·9564
			C	7684	2461	2389	2083	751				
73. Japan, Niigata	High gastric	Hirose & Honma 1962	P	394	142	154	50	48	0·8691	1·4017	0·4474	23·3769
			C	12253	3624	4522	2852	1255				
74. Japan, Niigata	Mid gastric	Hirose & Honma 1962	P	2163	785	672	507	199	0·6861	43·5645	0·8207	10·0835
			C	12253	3624	4522	2852	1255				
75. Japan, Niigata	Prepyloric	Hirose & Honma 1962	P	382	104	125	103	50	0·9632	0·0774	1·2585	2·6491
			C	12253	3624	4522	2852	1255				
76. Japan, Niigata	Multiple form	Hirose & Honma 1962	P	563	175	150	188	46	0·6716	12·4314	1·3346	7·2230
			C	12253	3624	4522	2852	1255				
77. Japan, Sendai	Antrum, pylorus; (s) A	Kurokawa & Masuda 1958 Moniwa 1960	P	256	86	78	61	31	0·7885	2·2835	0·9947	0·0010
			C	21199	6769	7786	4827	1817				
78. Japan, Sendai	Corpus; (s) A	Kurokawa & Masuda 1958 Moniwa 1960	P	819	315	262	165	77	0·7231	14·4625	0·7345	9·9239
			C	21199	6769	7786	4827	1817				
79. Japan, Sendai	Fornix, subcardiac; (s) A	Kurokawa & Masuda 1958 Moniwa 1960	P	77	30	21	17	9	0·6086	3·0366	0·7946	0·5711
			C	21199	6769	7786	4827	1817				
80. Japan, Sendai	Multiple form; (s) A	Kurokawa & Masuda 1958 Moniwa 1960	P	60	17	20	16	7	1·0228	0·0047	1·3198	0·6329
			C	21199	6769	7786	4827	1817				
81. Japan, Sendai		Moniwa 1960	P	511	195	158	112	46	0·7044	10·4628	0·8054	3·2485
			C	21199	6769	7786	4827	1817				
82. Japan, Tokyo	(s) S	Uetake *et al.* 1958	P	682	239	244	142	57	0·8419	3·5457	0·8390	2·7215
			C	77625	24165	29305	17113	7042				
83. U.S.A., Iowa City and New York		Glass *et al.* 1962 Osborne & De George 1962	P	28	12	13	2	1	1·2025	0·2107	0·5317	0·6816
			C	4738	2029	1828	636	245				
84. U.S.A., Iowa	(s) A_1A_2, S	Newman *et al.* 1961	P	184	104	54	19	7	0·5710	9·8580	0·7143	1·5954
			C	1261	563	512	144	42				
85. U.S.A., Iowa		Buckwalter 1962	P	817(c)	437	297	58	25	0·7196	18·8326	0·6332	10·5501
			C	49979(c)	22391	21146	4693	1749				

* For details of classification see text p. 29.

TABLE 1 **THE ABO BLOOD GROUP SYSTEM** (*cont.*)

Place	Additional details	Authors		Number	O	A	B	AB	A/O Relative incidence	A/O χ_1^2 for difference from unity	B/O Relative incidence	B/O χ_1^2 for difference from unity
86. Mexico		Lisker *et al.* 1964	P	225	124	80	18	3	1·2499	2·3370	0·9650	0·0193
			C	6843	4022	2076	605	140				
87. Chile, Valparaiso		Jackson *et al.* 1959	P	142	75	38	26	3	0·9088	0·2197	2·2715	11·7976
			C	2500	1435	800	219	46				
88. Peru, Lima		Muñoz-Baratta 1962	P	240(c)	153	50	24	13	0·8299	1·3078	0·8205	0·8105
			C	107938(c)	66058	26013	12629	3238				
				30391					0·8692	107·4638	0·8726	49·6415
					χ_{87}^2 for homogeneity of areas					191·9718		
				(30140)	χ_{85}^2 for homogeneity of areas							186·0383
GASTRIC ULCERS, BLEEDING												
1. Greece, Athínai		Merikas *et al.* 1966	P	125	60	47	8	10	0·8115	1·1418	0·3674	7·0515
			C	18325	7465	7206	2709	945				
2. United Kingdom, London		Langman & Doll 1965	P	343	183	127	21	12	0·7530	5·8322	0·5903	5·1062
		Discombe & Meyer 1952 M1	C	10000	4578	4219	890	313				
3. United Kingdom, NE. Scotland		Johnston *et al.* 1973	P	77	47	20	7	3	0·6121	3·3543	0·7179	0·6639
			C	8811	4478	3113	929	291				
4. United Kingdom, Glasgow	(s) S	Peebles Brown *et al.* 1956	P	55	35	15	3	2	0·7144	1·1776	0·4275	1·9852
			C	5898	3177	1906	637	178				
				600					0·7440	10·7511	0·5401	12·9784
					χ_3^2 for homogeneity of areas					0·7548		1·8284
GASTRIC ULCERS, NOT BLEEDING												
1. Greece, Athínai		Merikas *et al.* 1966	P	216	91	93	23	9	1·0587	0·1479	0·6965	2·3802
			C	18325	7465	7206	2709	945				
2. United Kingdom, London		Langman & Doll 1965	P	429	188	185	44	12	1·0678	0·3847	1·2039	1·1714
		Discombe & Meyer 1952 M1	C	10000	4578	4219	890	313				
3. United Kingdom, Glasgow		Peebles Brown *et al.* 1956	P	245	139	75	24	7	0·8994	0·5264	0·8611	0·4404
			C	5898	3177	1906	637	178				
				890					1·0194	0·0672	0·9563	0·1435
					χ_2^2 for homogeneity of areas					0·9917		3·8485
GASTRIC ULCERS, BLEEDING/NOT BLEEDING												
1. Greece, Athínai		Merikas *et al.* 1966	Bl.	*125*	*60*	*47*	*8*	*10*	*0·7665*	*1·1849*	*0·5275*	*2·0858*
			No Bl.	*216*	*91*	*93*	*23*	*9*				
2. United Kingdom, London		Langman & Doll 1965	Bl.	*343*	*183*	*127*	*21*	*12*	*0·7052*	*5·0705*	*0·4903*	*6·2616*
			No Bl.	*429*	*188*	*185*	*44*	*12*				
3. United Kingdom, Glasgow		Peebles Brown *et al.* 1956	Bl.	*55*	*35*	*15*	*3*	*2*	*0·7943*	*0·4582*	*0·4964*	*1·1942*
			No Bl.	*245*	*139*	*75*	*24*	*7*				
				523/890					*0·7312*	*6·5626*	*0·5004*	*9·5220*
					χ_2^2 for homogeneity of areas					*0·1510*		*0·0196*
STOMAL ULCERS												
1. United Kingdom, London	Perforated	Langman *et al.* 1967	P	79	50	25	3	1	0·5425	6·1849	0·3086	3·8967
		Discombe & Meyer 1952 M1	C	10000	4578	4219	890	313				
2. United Kingdom, London	Clinical history not known	Langman *et al.* 1967	P	216	132	67	14	3	0·5508	15·4965	0·5456	4·5699
		Discombe & Meyer 1952 M1	C	10000	4578	4219	890	313				
3. United Kingdom, Glasgow		Peebles Brown *et al.* 1956	P	79	55	14	5	5	0·4243	8·1265	0·4534	2·8429
			C	5898	3177	1906	637	178				
				374					0·5271	29·1885	0·4822	10·5410
					χ_2^2 for homogeneity of areas					0·6194		0·7685

TABLE 1 THE ABO BLOOD GROUP SYSTEM (*cont.*)

Place	Additional details	Authors		Number	O	A	B	AB	A/O Relative incidence	A/O χ_1^2 for difference from unity	B/O Relative incidence	B/O χ_1^2 for difference from unity
DISEASES OF THE DIGESTIVE SYSTEM (*cont.*)												
STOMAL ULCERS (*cont.*)												
STOMAL ULCERS, BLEEDING												
1. United Kingdom, London		Langman *et al.* 1967	P	63	38	19	6	0	0·5425	4·7090	0·8122	0·2227
		Discombe & Meyer 1952 M1	C	10000	4578	4219	890	313				
STOMAL ULCERS, NOT BLEEDING												
1. United Kingdom, London,		Langman *et al.* 1967	P	152	85	57	8	2	0·7276	3·3962	0·4841	3·8103
		Discombe & Meyer 1952 M1	C	10000	4578	4219	890	313				
STOMAL ULCERS, BLEEDING/NOT BLEEDING												
1. United Kingdom, London		Langman *et al.* 1967	Bl.	*63*	*38*	*19*	*6*	*0*	*0·7456*	*0·7962*	*1·6776*	*0·8119*
			No Bl.	*152*	*85*	*57*	*8*	*2*				
DUODENAL ULCERS												
1. Austria, Wien	(s) Rh_D, S	Speiser 1956	P	1160	476	479	130	75	0·8263	7·7622	0·7384	8·5063
			C	10000	3631	4422	1343	604				
2. Austria, Wien	(s) A_1A_2	Weiser 1957	P	449	201	172	54	22	0·7027	11·0299	0·7264	4·1699
			C	10000	3631	4422	1343	604				
3. Czechoslovakia		Vahala *et al.* 1970	P	173	78	62	26	7	0·5515	10·5164	0·6248	3·7300
		Kout 1959 M2	C	1142	358	516	191	77				
4. Czechoslovakia, Praha	Without resection	Veselý & Kubíčková 1969	P	814(c)	280	327	132	75	0·8103	3·8967	0·8836	0·7983
			C	1142	358	516	191	77				
5. Czechoslovakia, Praha	With resection	Veselý & Kubíčková 1969	P	597(c)	233	205	101	58	0·6104	17·5268	0·8125	1·9405
			C	1142	358	516	191	77				
6. Czechoslovakia, Praha		Kubíčková & Veselý 1972	P	1026	376	411	154	85	0·7584	7·7862	0·7677	4·0679
			C	1142	358	516	191	77				
7. Denmark, København		Køster *et al.* 1955	P	680	342	261	60	17	0·7032	17·4980	0·6540	8·8386
			C	14304	5804	6299	1557	644				
8. Denmark, København		Jordal 1956	P	1223	588	479	110	46	0·7506	19·9772	0·6974	11·1951
			C	14304	5804	6299	1557	644				
9. France, Colmar		Lobstein & Voegtlin 1959	P	180	89	63	18	10	0·5896	9·9890	0·8593	0·3326
			C	5570	2188	2627	515	240				
10. France, Mulhouse		Lobstein & Voegtlin 1959	P	372	192	139	26	15	0·6331	15·9382	0·6856	3·0994
			C	6423	2648	3028	523	224				
11. France, Paris		Khérumian & Moullec 1959	P	1195(c)	593	450	115	37	0·7600	19·1619	1·0008	0·0001
			C	207588	91414	91276	17714	7184				
12. Germany, Erlangen, Nürnberg		Berg, G. *et al.* 1967	P	92	38	36	14	4	0·6130	3·0297	1·0572	0·0198
			C	193	66	102	23	2				
13. Germany, Leipzig		Klaus 1963	P	1236	547	461	173	55	0·7644	14·4700	0·9173	0·7733
			C	5000	1920	2117	662	301				
14. Germany, Tübingen	(s) A_1A_2	Dick *et al.* 1962	P	489	244	177	54	14	0·7054	12·3413	0·8384	1·3553
			C	39031	16283	16745	4298	1705				
15. Greece, Athinai		Papayannopoulos 1958	P	147	62	58	22	5	1·0526	0·0783	1·1813	0·4474
		Constantoulis & Paidoussis 1957 M1	C	21635	9408	8361	2826	1040				
16. Hungary		István & Széll 1961	P	467	167	186	83	31	0·8745	1·5493	0·9344	0·2502
			C	23000	7567	9637	4025	1771				
17. Italy, Aquila		Curtoni & Morgante 1964	P	473(c)	239	165	55	14	0·8667	1·9015	1·1403	0·7263
			C	8920(c)	4321	3442	872	285				

TABLE 1 **THE ABO BLOOD GROUP SYSTEM** (*cont.*)

Place	Additional details	Authors		Number	O	A	B	AB	A/O Relative incidence	A/O χ_1^2 for difference from unity	B/O Relative incidence	B/O χ_1^2 for difference from unity
18. Italy, Campania		Pollara & Melina 1957	P	300	159	108	27	6	0·8064	2·2620	0·5272	7·7934
			C	1000	444	374	143	39				
19. Italy, Lombardia		Ninni & Bedarida 1959	P	523	235	170	92	26	0·7105	6·7431	1·9295	11·8011
			C	640	276	281	56	27				
20. Italy, Milano		Mangani 1957	P	47	20	21	3	3	1·0094	0·0009	0·5776	0·7833
		Visconti *et al.* 1961	C	9607	3974	4134	1032	467				
21. Italy, Milano		Rotelli & Corippo 1959	P	532	256	202	58	16	0·6519	19·3732	0·8394	1·3515
			C	8000	3090	3740	834	336				
22. Italy, Milano		Camerini Riviera 1960	P	309	133	125	32	19	0·9638	0·0775	1·0300	0·0198
			C	2346	1006	981	235	124				
23. Italy, Milano		Mor & Sforza 1960	P	437	222	151	52	12	0·6161	11·4070	0·8762	0·3700
			C	500	202	223	54	21				
24. Italy, Milano	(s) S	Visconti *et al.* 1961[b]	P	740	383	256	72	29	0·6429	27·8457	0·7241	5·8818
			C	9607	3975	4133	1032	467				
25. Italy, Palermo		Carlo & Ridulfo 1958	P	388	190	116	52	30	0·8364	1·6636	0·7569	2·3590
			C	980(c)	448	327	162	43				
26. Italy, Pavia		Prosser 1957	P	345	181	109	38	17	0·4975	31·8697	0·7779	1·8916
			C	8000	3090	3740	834	336				
27. Italy, Perugia		Benda & Menghini 1957	P	628	336	218	58	16	0·6563	21·6340	0·6973	5·9593
			C	7356	3163	3127	783	283				
28. Italy, Roma	Includes gastric ulcers associated with duodenal ones	Misiti *et al.* 1968	P	316	156	112	32	16	0·8023	3·1167	0·8052	1·2290
			C	20051(c)	8973	8030	2286	762				
29. Italy, Siena	(s) S	Prior & Vegni 1957	P	130	57	58	10	5	1·1702	0·6259	0·6208	1·7841
			C	1025	460	400	130	35				
30. Italy, Verona	(s) S	Bonzanini 1961	P	455	225	187	34	9	0·8704	1·8139	0·7361	2·5900
			C	5500	2460	2349	505	186				
31. Jugoslavia, Beograd		Glidžić & Krajinović 1964	P	444	163	160	80	41	0·7608	5·5967	1·0568	0·1501
			C	5495	1826	2356	848	465				
32. Jugoslavia, Zagreb		Luketić *et al.* 1959	P	126	44	51	22	9	0·9429	0·0811	0·9599	0·0244
			C	15832	5381	6615	2803	1033				
33. Norway, Oslo		Heistø 1956	P	579	282	250	30	17	0·6700	19·7818	0·4926	12·9606
			C	8292	3135	4148	677	332				
34. Poland		Belec *et al.* 1971	P	804	342	248	157	57	0·6669	22·2862	0·7793	6·3061
		Charzewski *et al.* 1965 M2	C	13744	4719	5131	2780	1114				
35. Poland, Katowice		Machalski *et al.* 1968	P	553	235	187	87	44	0·6628	15·2298	0·7056	6·7030
			C	3606	1216	1460	638	292				
36. Poland, Kraków		Socha 1960	P	1880	779	594	258	149	0·6234	71·6593	0·7292	23·2503
			C	37766	12151	14863	7658	3094				
37. Poland, Lower Silesia		Sagan *et al.* 1957	P	77	33	25	13	6	0·6559	2·4497	0·6800	1·3452
			C	2397	813	939	471	174				
38. Poland, Lublin		Spruch & Dacka 1968	P	256	94	88	51	23	0·8432	1·0870	1·0069	0·0013
			C	1150	399	443	215	93				
39. Poland, Opole		Gołąbek 1965	P	91	32	42	11	6	1·1603	0·3753	0·5592	2·6495
			C	1453	488	552	300	113				
40. Poland, Poznań		Wojtowicz *et al.* 1960	P	494	200	142	104	48	0·6690	12·6815	0·9412	0·2347
			C	7951	2773	2943	1532	703				
41. Poland, Poznań		Woszczyk 1966	P	343	130	117	63	33	0·8480	1·6044	0·8772	0·6987
		Wojtowicz *et al.* 1960	C	7951	2773	2943	1532	703				
42. Poland, Warszawa		Kosiński *et al.* 1959	P	263	88	93	58	24	1·0190	0·0152	1·2584	1·7323
			C	4270	1537	1594	805	334				
43. Poland, Warszawa		Czaplicki *et al.* 1964	P	149	63	50	22	14	0·7653	1·9265	0·6667	2·5989
			C	4270	1537	1594	805	334				
44. Romania	(s) ABH secretion	Fodor & Urcan 1966	P	352	130	136	53	33	0·9808	0·0092	0·5880	4·7689
			C	222	75	80	52	15				
45. Romania, Sibiu		Coroianu *et al.* 1958	P	78	31	30	15	2	0·8955	0·1821	0·9950	0·0003
			C	3850(c)	1425	1540	693	192				

TABLE 1 **THE ABO BLOOD GROUP SYSTEM** (*cont.*)

Place	Additional details	Authors		Number	O	A	B	AB	A/O Relative incidence	A/O χ_1^2 for difference from unity	B/O Relative incidence	B/O χ_1^2 for difference from unity
DISEASES OF THE DIGESTIVE SYSTEM (*cont.*)												
DUODENAL ULCERS (*cont.*)												
46. Spain, Málaga		Franquelo Ramos & Eloy-Garcia 1966	P C	126 1195	61 577	49 517	14 75	2 26	0·8965	0·2950	1·7657	3·1416
47. Spain, Viscaya	Basques	Goti-Iturriaga & Velasco Alonso 1965	P C	95 386	38 198	53 168	4 14	0 6	1·6438	4·3964	1·4887	0·4488
48. Spain, Viscaya	Non-Basques	Goti-Iturriaga & Velasco Alonso 1965	P C	143 336	74 151	61 154	6 24	2 7	0·8083	1·0532	0·5101	1·9829
49. Sweden, Luleå		Hedenstedt 1961	P C	212 8163	98 3024	82 3972	23 806	9 361	0·6370	8·8481	0·8805	0·2929
50. Switzerland, Basel	(s) S	Moor-Jankowski *et al.* 1961	P C	582 2076	249 842	262 912	50 229	21 93	0·9714	0·0829	0·7383	3·1124
51. United Kingdom, Chorley, Leyland, Preston		Masters 1967	P C	26 652	22 334	3 243	0 58	0 17	0·1874	7·2648		
52. United Kingdom, Liverpool		McConnell 1966	P C	860 15377	505 7527	263 6015	62 1450	30 385	0·6517	30·1442	0·6373	10·7197
53. United Kingdom, Liverpool		Evans *et al.* 1968	P C	100 6510	55 3146	30 2648	13 546	2 170	0·6480	3·6044	1·3619	0·9810
54. United Kingdom, London	(s) S	Aird *et al.* 1954*	P C	812 10000	460 4578	263 4219	65 890	24 313	0·6204	35·4370	0·7268	5·3855
55. United Kingdom, Manchester	(s) S	Aird *et al.* 1954	P C	423 9370	225 4532	148 3775	37 788	13 275	0·7897	4·7708	0·9458	0·0943
56. United Kingdom, Middlesbrough	(s) Rh_D, S	Grahame 1961	P C	722 4540	426 2149	251 1873	32 386	13 132	0·6760	20·9109	0·4182	20·7349
57. United Kingdom, Newcastle upon Tyne	(s) S	Aird *et al.* 1954	P C	482 13572	288 6598	157 5261	30 1321	7 392	0·6837	14·2002	0·5203	11·3197
58. Israel	Ashkenazi Jews	Birnbaum & Menczel 1959	P C	158(c) 946(c)	73 362	54 390	23 136	8 58	0·6866	3·7652	0·8386	0·4602
59. Israel	Oriental Jews	Birnbaum & Menczel 1959	P C	58(c) 137(c)	28 50	17 46	9 27	4 14	0·6599	1·2675	0·5952	1·3202
60. Israel	Sephardi Jews	Birnbaum & Menczel 1959	P C	42(c) 252(c)	16 102	10 81	14 47	2 22	0·7870	0·3106	1·8989	2·4923
61. N. India, Rajasthan, Udaipur		Sharma *et al.* 1969	P C	186 3799	99 1300	32 879	42 1346	13 274	0·4780	12·5923	0·4097	22·4732
62. S. India, Bombay		Joshi *et al.* 1958	P C	226 3600	88 1228	47 953	74 1096	17 323	0·6882	4·0466	0·9422	0·1333
63. S. India, Bombay		Joshi *et al.* 1958	P C	154 3600	49 1228	45 953	40 1096	20 323	1·1834	0·6371	0·9146	0·1689
64. S. India, Bombay		Vachhrajani & Shenoy 1959	P C	98 1834	48 747	20 422	24 505	6 160	0·7376	1·2431	0·7396	1·3824
65. North Vietnam		Nguyen Duong Quang *et al.* 1960	P C	465 6750	219 3080	71 1350	150 1954	25 366	0·7397	4·6126	1·0796	0·4863
66. China, Shanghai		Dao *et al.* 1958	P C	141 7684	58 2461	34 2389	36 2083	13 751	0·6039	5·3584	0·7333	2·0957
67. Japan, Niigata		Hirose & Honma 1962	P C	1610 12253	535 3624	521 4522	358 2852	196 1255	0·7804	14·3388	0·8503	4·9728

* From this set the data included in Langman & Doll 1965 (see Langman *et al.* 1967) have been excluded.

TABLE 1 **THE ABO BLOOD GROUP SYSTEM** *(cont.)*

Place	Additional details	Authors		Number	O	A	B	AB	A/O		B/O	
									Relative incidence	χ_1^2 for difference from unity	Relative incidence	χ_1^2 for difference from unity
68. Japan, Sendai		Kurokawa & Masuda 1958	P	775	290	250	143	92	0·7495	10·7673	0·6915	12·6057
		Moniwa 1960	C	21199	6769	7786	4827	1817				
69. Japan, Sendai		Moniwa 1960	P	333	112	101	88	32	0·7840	3·0996	1·1018	0·4554
			C	21199	6769	7786	4827	1817				
70. Japan, Tokyo	(s) S	Uetake *et al.* 1958	P	291	112	90	58	31	0·6626	8·4198	0·7313	3·7291
			C	77625	24165	29305	17113	7042				
71. Egypt, Alexandria		Sadek *et al.* 1965[a]	P	228	102	60	48	18	0·5085	16·2720	0·5535	10·7534
			C	3720	1142	1321	971	286				
72. Nigeria	Yoruba	Ball 1962	P	390	235	75	72	8	0·7699	3·8307	0·6805	8·0591
			C	26027	13411	5559	6038	1019				
73. Nigeria, Ibadan	Yoruba	Davey & Elebute 1963	P	421	238	89	86	8	0·8865	0·9200	0·8012	3·0401
			C	19257	9876	4166	4454	761				
74. U.S.A., Iowa City, and New York		Glass *et al.* 1962	P	72	36	27	6	3	0·8325	0·5105	0·5317	2·0304
		Osborne & De George 1962	C	4738	2029	1828	636	245				
75. U.S.A., Iowa	(s) A_1A_2, S	Newman *et al.* 1961	P	479	257	163	44	15	0·6974	9·4412	0·6694	4·5598
			C	1261	563	512	144	42				
76. U.S.A., Iowa		Buckwalter 1962	P	2386(c)	1288	825	215	58	0·6782	72·4554	0·7964	9·1132
			C	49979(c)	22391	21146	4693	1749				
77. U.S.A., Los Angeles	25% Negroes	Ventzke & Grossman 1962	P	100	50	35	8	7	0·8668	0·4172	0·5771	2·0728
		Reed 1968 M2	C	11949	5529	4465	1533	422				
78. U.S.A., Rochester		Mayo & Fergeson 1953	P	165(c)	78	71	14	2	0·9526	0·0750	1·0096	0·0009
		Tinney & Watkins 1941	C	1000(c)	450	430	80	40				
79. U.S.A., St. Louis	Whites	Sievers 1959	P	23	13	7	2	1	0·5902	1·2645	0·7066	0·2089
			C	32945	14918	13611	3248	1168				
80. Mexico		Lisker *et al.* 1964	P	326	213	76	27	10	0·6913	7·3360	0·8427	0·6713
			C	6843	4022	2076	605	140				
81. Chile, Valparaiso		Jackson *et al.* 1959	P	113	72	32	8	1	0·7972	1·0907	0·7281	0·6988
			C	2500	1435	800	219	46				
82. Peru, Lima		Muñoz-Baratta 1962	P	839(c)	534	193	71	41	0·9178	1·0350	0·6955	8·2172
			C	107938(c)	66058	26013	12629	3238				
83. Venezuela, Maracay		Arias & Bermúdez 1963	P	86	46	23	12	5	0·7836	0·6633	1·1413	0·1118
			C	202	105	67	24	6				
				37160					0·7315	624·0396	0·8001	161·4559
					χ_{82}^2 for homogeneity of areas					150·5906		
				(37134)	χ_{81}^2 for homogeneity of areas							156·5601

Duodenal Ulcers, Bleeding

Place	Additional details	Authors		Number	O	A	B	AB	A/O		B/O	
									Relative incidence	χ_1^2 for difference from unity	Relative incidence	χ_1^2 for difference from unity
1. Czechoslovakia, Praha		Veselý & Kubíčková 1969	P	151(c)	60	52	28	11	0·6013	6·3686	0·8747	0·2967
			C	1142	358	516	191	77				
2. Greece, Athinai		Merikas *et al.* 1966	P	856	431	288	100	37	0·6922	22·3084	0·6394	15·6021
			C	18325	7465	7206	2709	945				
3. United Kingdom, Liverpool, and SW. Lancashire	(s) ABH secretion, S	Horwich *et al.* 1966	P	128	78	39	6	5	0·5940	6·9302	0·4432	3·6457
			C	6510	3146	2648	546	170				
4. United Kingdom, London		Langman *et al.* 1967	P	545	323	180	33	9	0·6047	27·7853	0·5255	11·9138
			C	10000	4578	4219	890	313				
5. United Kingdom, Newcastle upon Tyne		Pringle *et al.* 1964	P	75	41	25	6	3	0·7676	1·0733	0·7724	0·3451
		Kopeć 1970	C	5969	2903	2306	550	210				
6. United Kingdom, NE. Scotland		Johnston *et al.* 1973	P	434(c)	251	136	39	8	0·7794	5·2270	0·7490	2·7021
		Kopeć 1970	C	8811	4478	3113	929	291				
7. United Kingdom, Glasgow	(s) S	Peebles Brown *et al.* 1956	P	459	279	136	33	11	0·8125	3·6605	0·5899	7·7869
			C	5898	3177	1906	637	178				
				2648					0·6963	66·7506	0·6439	37·6534
					χ_6^2 for homogeneity of areas					6·6027		4·6390

TABLE 1 THE ABO BLOOD GROUP SYSTEM (*cont.*)

Place	Additional details	Authors		Number	O	A	B	AB	A/O Relative incidence	A/O χ_1^2 for difference from unity	B/O Relative incidence	B/O χ_1^2 for difference from unity
DISEASES OF THE DIGESTIVE SYSTEM (*cont.*)												
DUODENAL ULCERS (*cont.*)												
Duodenal Ulcers, Not Bleeding												
1. Czechoslovakia, Praha		Veselý & Kubíčková 1969	P	611(c)	223	251	87	50	0·7809	4·6330	0·7312	4·0809
			C	1142	358	516	191	77				
2. Greece, Athínai		Merikas *et al.* 1966	P	1000	423	378	136	63	0·9257	1·1273	0·8860	1·4343
			C	18325	7465	7206	2709	945				
3. United Kingdom, Liverpool, and SW. Lancashire	(s) ABH secretion, S	Horwich *et al.* 1966	P	674	351	244	60	19	0·8259	4·7895	0·9849	0·0107
			C	6510	3146	2648	546	170				
4. United Kingdom, London		Langman *et al.* 1967	P	780	408	292	60	20	0·7766	10·0982	0·7564	3·8081
			C	10000	4578	4219	890	313				
5. United Kingdom, Newcastle upon Tyne		Pringle *et al.* 1964	P	100	59	37	3	1	0·7895	1·2486	0·2684	4·9089
		Kopeć 1970	C	5969	2903	2306	550	210				
6. United Kingdom, Glasgow	(s) S	Peebles Brown *et al.* 1956	P	1183	668	381	112	22	0·9507	0·5154	0·8362	2·5989
			C	5898	3177	1906	637	178				
				4348					0·8639	16·6472	0·8349	10·3739
				χ_5^2 for homogeneity of areas						5·7648		6·4679
Duodenal Ulcers, Bleeding/Not Bleeding												
1. Czechoslovakia, Praha		Veselý & Kubíčková 1969	Bl.	151	60	52	28	11	0·7700	1·5400	1·1962	0·4705
			No Bl.	611	223	251	87	50				
2. Greece, Athínai		Merikas *et al.* 1966	Bl.	856	431	288	100	37	0·7478	7·8209	0·7216	4·8305
			No Bl.	1000	423	378	136	63				
3. United Kingdom, Liverpool, and SW. Lancashire	(s) ABH secretion, S	Horwich *et al.* 1966	Bl.	128	78	39	6	5	0·7193	2·3906	0·4500	3·2041
			No Bl.	674	351	244	60	19				
4. United Kingdom, London		Langman *et al.* 1967	Bl.	545	323	180	33	9	0·7787	4·3089	0·6947	2·5271
			No Bl.	780	408	292	60	20				
5. United Kingdom, Newcastle upon Tyne		Pringle *et al.* 1964	Bl.	75	41	25	6	3	0·9723	0·0073	2·8780	2·0643
			No Bl.	100	59	37	3	1				
6. United Kingdom, Glasgow	(s) S	Peebles Brown *et al.* 1956	Bl.	459	279	136	33	11	0·8546	1·6394	0·7054	2·7487
			No Bl.	1183	668	381	112	22				
				2214/4348					0·7856	16·4062	0·7650	7·7812
				χ_5^2 for homogeneity of areas						1·3009		8·0640
ULCERS TO THE RIGHT OF THE GASTRIC ANGULUS												
1. United Kingdom, Bristol	Type 3*	Johnson *et al.* 1964	P	73	35	30	6	2	0·8254	0·5819	0·8914	0·0662
			C	3284	1430	1485	275	94				
2. United Kingdom, London	Type 3*	Johnson 1965	P	743	415	258	58	12	0·7220	16·2633	0·7130	5·6315
			C	19473	9173	7898	1798	604				
3. United Kingdom, Middlesbrough	Type 3*	Johnson *et al.* 1964	P	96	61	30	4	1	0·5721	5·9407	0·3107	4·9915
			C	1678	777	668	164	69				
4. United Kingdom, Preston	Type 3*	Johnson *et al.* 1964	P	44	26	13	5	0	0·5473	3·0898	0·8672	0·0830
			C	2061	938	857	208	58				
5. United Kingdom, Belfast	Type 3*	Johnson *et al.* 1964	P	102	75	18	7	2	0·3161	19·1330	0·4194	4·8047
			C	11327	5522	4192	1229	384				
				1058					0·6675	34·5016	0·6677	11·1520
				χ_4^2 for homogeneity of areas						10·5070		4·4249

* For details of classification see text p. 29.

TABLE 1 THE ABO BLOOD GROUP SYSTEM (*cont.*)

Place	Additional details	Authors		Number	O	A	B	AB	A/O Relative incidence	A/O χ^2_1 for difference from unity	B/O Relative incidence	B/O χ^2_1 for difference from unity
BOTH GASTRIC AND DUODENAL ULCERS PRESENT												
1. Czechoslovakia,		Kubíčková & Veselý 1966	P	112	39	51	16	6	0·9073	0·1895	0·7690	0·7177
Praha		Kout 1959 M2	C	1142	358	516	191	77				
2. Denmark,	(s) S	Sørensen 1957	P	531	278	189	46	18	0·6410	21·3305	0·6706	6·0604
Köbenhavn			C	12123	5046	5352	1245	480				
3. Denmark,		Køster *et al.* 1955	P	30	13	11	4	2	0·7797	0·3684	1·1470	0·0574
Köbenhavn			C	14304	5804	6299	1557	644				
4. Italy		Lang 1959	P	748	402	226	88	32	0·7167	15·8005	0·9308	0·3650
			C	42735	20426	16023	4804	1482				
5. Italy, Forli		Maltoni & Canali 1956	P	255	137	95	20	3	0·8092	2·1106	0·7737	0·9793
			C	1350	636	545	120	49				
6. Italy, Genova		Spandonari &	P	221(c)	124	77	17	3	0·6543	8·2327	0·5512	5·1547
		Carboneschi 1957	C	5893	2569	2438	639	247				
		Calzia 1967 M2										
7. United	Type 2*	Johnson *et al.* 1964	P	71	39	25	4	3	0·6173	3·4729	0·5333	1·4114
Kingdom,			C	3284	1430	1485	275	94				
Bristol												
8. United		McConnell 1966	P	48	30	13	4	1	0·5423	3·3879	0·6921	0·4765
Kingdom,			C	15377	7527	6015	1450	385				
Liverpool												
9. United	Type 2*	Johnson 1965	P	767	407	292	45	23	0·8333	5·4389	0·5641	12·9349
Kingdom,			C	19473	9173	7898	1798	604				
London												
10. United	(s) S	Grahame 1961	P	126	90	24	12	0	0·3060	26·0809	0·7423	0·9107
Kingdom,			C	4540	2149	1873	386	132				
Middlesbrough												
11. United	Type 2*	Johnson *et al.* 1964	P	129	83	29	15	2	0·4064	16·4394	0·8562	0·2798
Kingdom,			C	1678	777	668	164	69				
Middlesbrough												
12. United	Type 2*	Johnson *et al.* 1964	P	58	42	12	4	0	0·3127	12·3546	0·4295	2·5540
Kingdom,			C	2061	938	857	208	58				
Preston												
13. United		Peebles Brown *et al.* 1956	P	38	24	9	5	0	0·6251	1·4374	1·0391	0·0060
Kingdom,			C	5898	3177	1906	637	178				
Glasgow												
14. United	Type 2*	Johnson *et al.* 1964	P	59	41	15	3	0	0·4819	5·8249	0·3288	3·4497
Kingdom,			C	11327	5522	4192	1229	384				
Belfast												
15. North Vietnam		Nguyen Duong Quang	P	78	26	11	38	3	0·9652	0·0096	2·3038	10·6145
		et al. 1960	C	6750	3080	1350	1954	366				
16. Japan, Niigata		Hirose & Honma 1962	P	537	188	155	101	93	0·6607	13·9977	0·6827	9·1971
			C	12253	3624	4522	2852	1255				
17. Japan, Sendai		Kurokawa & Masuda	P	115	40	32	29	14	0·6955	2·3326	1·0167	0·0046
		1958	C	21199	6769	7786	4827	1817				
		Moniwa 1960										
18. Japan, Tokyo	(s) S	Uetake *et al.* 1958	P	125	33	44	37	11	1·0995	0·1693	1·5832	3·6761
			C	77625	24165	29305	17113	7042				
19. U.S.A.,		Glass *et al.* 1962	P	100	48	40	8	4	0·9250	0·1298	0·5317	2·6978
Iowa City and		Osborne & De George	C	4738	2029	1828	636	245				
New York		1962										
				4148					0·7011	96·9575	0·7970	18·0034
				χ^2_{18} for homogeneity of areas						42·1506		43·5442
PEPTIC ULCERS, SITE UNSPECIFIED												
1. Austria, Wien		Flamm & Friedrich 1929	P	39	13	19	5	2	1·1447	0·1405	0·8979	0·0417
		Corvin M1	C	10392	3635	4641	1557	559				
2. Austria, Wien	(s) A_1A_2	Weiser 1957	P	251(c)	100	103	34	14	0·8458	1·3886	0·9192	0·1754
			C	10000	3631	4422	1343	604				

* For details of classification see text p. 29.

TABLE 1 **THE ABO BLOOD GROUP SYSTEM** (*cont.*)

Place	Additional details	Authors		Number	O	A	B	AB	A/O Relative incidence	A/O χ_1^2 for difference from unity	B/O Relative incidence	B/O χ_1^2 for difference from unity
DISEASES OF THE DIGESTIVE SYSTEM (*cont.*)												
PEPTIC ULCERS, SITE UNSPECIFIED (*cont.*)												
3. Finland		Sievers 1929	P	129(c)	47	57	17	8	0·9571	0·0459	0·7766	0·7478
			C	1711	584	740	272	115				
4. Finland		Mustakallio 1937	P	73	28	31	7	7	0·9156	0·1112	0·5661	1·7774
			C	2595	908	1098	401	188				
5. Germany, München		Lützeler & Dormanns 1929	P	35	20	14	1	0	0·6912	1·0907	0·2208	2·1528
		Kruse M1	C	1300	552	559	125	64				
6. Hungary, Nyiregyháza		Major 1960	P	126	59	44	14	9	0·6232	5·1816	0·4255	7·7955
			C	1603	529	633	295	146				
7. Italy		Balestra & Mattioli 1958	P	950	437	418	76	19	0·9947	0·0038	0·6259	10·2889
		Tranquilli-Leali 1934 M1	C	1830	781	751	217	81				
8. Italy, Napoli	(s) S	Cocchia *et al.* 1963	P	300	166	95	25	14	0·7006	3·9315	0·7638	0·8180
			C	300	142	116	28	14				
9. Italy, Roma		Ugelli 1936	P	244	127	81	29	7	0·7589	2·3885	0·8417	0·4411
		Siciliano & Mittiga 1953 M1	C	414	188	158	51	17				
10. Portugal		Lessa & Alarcão 1947	P	482	227	217	30	8	0·8586	2·0026	0·6672	3·5605
			C	1748	732	815	145	56				
11. United Kingdom, York	Males	Hall *et al.* 1971	P	1526	846	557	87	36	0·7289	33·0617	0·5486	28·1243
			C	98064	45399	41006	8510	3149				
12. United Kingdom, Glasgow		Wallace 1954	P	184	118	43	14	9	0·5650	10·0620	0·5595	4·1428
			C	7418	3853	2485	817	263				
13. N. India, Calcutta		Ghosh *et al.* 1957	P	287	99	59	96	33	0·8002	1·6267	0·9295	0·2282
			C	2026	670	499	699	158				
14. N. India, Lucknow		Nath *et al.* 1963	P	105	43	20	34	8	0·6393	2·6492	0·6480	3·4597
			C	3330(c)	1035	753	1263	279				
15. Egypt, Cairo		Awny & Kamel 1959	P	150	45	54	39	12	1·3584	2·1137	1·4395	2·5314
			C	1588	583	515	351	139				
16. Kenya, Nairobi	Africans	Mangat & Harries 1961	P	37	27	5	2	3	0·3648	4·2611	0·1776	5·5442
			C	3825	1913	971	798	143				
17. Republic of South Africa	Bantu	Buckwalter *et al.* 1961	P	92	48	28	14	2	0·9223	0·1140	0·6106	2·6095
			C	7105	3197	2022	1527	359				
18. Republic of South Africa	Indians	Buckwalter *et al.* 1961	P	162	54	35	56	17	1·0500	0·0495	1·1611	0·6011
			C	7462	2788	1721	2490	463				
19. Republic of South Africa	Coloured	Buckwalter *et al.* 1964	P	67(c)	30	18	16	3	0·5771	2·8931	0·8195	0·3416
			C	352(c)	126	131	82	13				
20. Republic of South Africa	Whites	Buckwalter *et al.* 1961	P	290	152	106	28	4	0·7884	3·3752	0·7125	2·6137
			C	6431	2893	2559	748	231				
21. U.S.A.		Pell *et al.* 1957	P	128	60	46	17	5	0·8465	0·7095	1·3411	1·1106
			C	6051	2769	2508	585	189				
22. U.S.A.		Pell *et al.* 1957	P	20	9	6	3	2	0·6799	0·5305	0·8715	0·0421
			C	1782	719	705	275	83				
23. U.S.A.		Pell *et al.* 1957	P	68	36	27	4	1	0·8155	0·6205	0·4739	1·9679
			C	2074	934	859	219	62				
24. U.S.A.		Pell *et al.* 1957	P	82	42	29	8	3	0·7211	1·7818	0·7691	0·4503
			C	2699	1179	1129	292	99				
25. U.S.A., Iowa	Negroes	Buckwalter *et al.* 1958	P	173	97	44	29	3	0·8407	0·8876	0·7305	2·1516
			C	6722	3301	1781	1351	289				
26. U.S.A., Rochester	Whites	Buchanan & Higley 1921	P	172	102	55	8	7	0·5643	10·0642	0·4412	4·4785
		Tinney & Watkins 1941	C	1000(c)	450	430	80	40				
27. Brazil, São Paulo		Leite & Goffi 1958	P	124	61	44	12	7	0·8906	0·3219	0·9280	0·0525
			C	1818	868	703	184	63				
				6296					0·7971	56·5238	0·7336	43·8080
				χ^2_{26} for homogeneity of areas						34·8836		44·4411

TABLE 1 **THE ABO BLOOD GROUP SYSTEM** (*cont.*)

Place	Additional details	Authors		Number	O	A	B	AB	A/O Relative incidence	A/O χ_1^2 for difference from unity	B/O Relative incidence	B/O χ_1^2 for difference from unity
DISEASES OF THE GENITO-URINARY SYSTEM												
DISEASES OF KIDNEY												
1. Austria, Wien	Nephroses; (s) S, Rh_D	Speiser 1958[a]	P	141	55	62	18	6	0·9621	0·0379	0·9239	0·0744
			C	1000	367	430	130	73				
2. Austria, Wien	Nephritis; (s) S, Rh_D	Speiser 1958[a]	P	232	79	106	36	11	1·1452	0·6771	1·2865	1·2478
			C	1000	367	430	130	73				
3. Japan, Sendai	Chronic nephritis	Moniwa 1960	P	72	26	20	22	4	0·6688	1·8242	1·1866	0·3473
			C	21199	6769	7786	4827	1817				
4. Japan, Sendai	Infections of kidney	Moniwa 1960	P	59	20	26	11	2	1·1302	0·1688	0·7713	0·4775
			C	21199	6769	7786	4827	1817				
5. U.S.A., Michigan	Nephritis–nephrosis; White children; (s) A_1A_2	Gershowitz & Neel 1965	P	70	36	27	6	1	0·8309	0·5054	0·7963	0·2558
			C	1508	688	621	144	55				
6. U.S.A., Rochester	Whites	Buchanan & Higley 1921	P	62	37	21	4	0	0·5940	3·4271	0·6081	0·8480
		Tinney & Watkins 1941	C	1000(c)	450	430	80	40				
7. Germany, München	Contracted kidney	Lützeler & Dormanns 1929	P	159	74	67	14	4	0·8941	0·3913	0·8355	0·3411
		Kruse 1928 M1	C	1300	552	559	125	64				
CALCULUS OF URINARY SYSTEM												
1. Czechoslovakia, Praha	Kidney	Veselý 1969[c]	P	383	142	154	64	23	0·7524	4·4293	0·8448	0·9270
			C	1142	358	516	191	77				
2. Italy, Ancona	Kidney; (s) chemical composition	Sciarra & Memeo 1957	P	197	91	80	16	10	0·9307	0·2066	2·6221	10·9209
		Formentano 1951 M1	C	2799(c)	1372	1296	92	39				
3. Italy, Milano	Kidney	Mor & Sforza 1960	P	164	70	66	21	7	0·8541	0·6401	1·1222	0·1557
			C	500	202	223	54	21				
4. Italy, Milano		Rotelli & Corippo 1959	P	120	62	44	12	2	0·5863	7·2250	0·7171	1·0950
			C	8000	3090	3740	834	336				
5. Italy, Milano	(s) S, chemical composition	Pisani & Acerbi 1960	P	1824	741	883	160	235	1·2220	8·9415	0·9243	0·4817
		Formentano & Morganti 1951 M1	C	2346(c)	1006	981	235	124				
6. Italy, Veneto	Kidney, ureter	Mobilio & Torchiana 1960	P	264	111	105	35	13	1·3273	3·4832	1·3413	1·8201
			C	1093	536	382	126	49				
7. Turkey, Ankara	Bladder	Kafkas & Gercel 1967	P	222(c)	69	110	22	21	1·0446	0·0724	0·6335	3·2136
			C	2000(c)	612	934	308	146				
8. Turkey, Ankara	Kidney, ureter	Kafkas & Gercel 1967	P	778(c)	230	385	120	43	1·0968	0·8851	1·0367	0·0740
			C	2000(c)	612	934	308	146				
9. N. India	Kidney	Anand 1964[a]	P	187	54	61	63	9	2·0898	7·3991	1·3282	1·2729
			C	187	74	40	65	8				
10. Japan, Sendai	Kidney, ureter	Moniwa 1960	P	131	50	49	22	10	0·8520	0·6306	0·6170	3·5427
			C	21199	6769	7786	4827	1817				
				4270					1·0667	2·4667	0·9857	0·0560
				χ_9^2 for homogeneity of areas						31·4462		23·5036
NON-GONOCOCCAL URETHRITIS												
1. United Kingdom, Newcastle upon Tyne	(s) S	Schofield 1966	P	345	157	144	33	11	1·1750	1·9414	1·1397	0·4633
			C	54579	27008	21082	4981	1508				
HYPERPLASIA OF PROSTATE												
1. Austria, Wien		Flamm & Friedrich 1929	P	31(c)	9	16	6	0	1·3924	0·6295	1·5564	0·7022
		Corvin M1	C	10392	3635	4641	1557	559				
2. Germany, Göttingen	(s) A	Jörgensen 1967	P	410	143	211	39	17	1·2952	3·5959	1·0487	0·0448
			C	694	273	311	71	39				

TABLE 1 THE ABO BLOOD GROUP SYSTEM (*cont.*)

Place	Additional details	Authors		Number	O	A	B	AB	A/O Relative incidence	A/O χ^2_1 for difference from unity	B/O Relative incidence	B/O χ^2_1 for difference from unity
DISEASES OF THE GENITO-URINARY SYSTEM (*cont.*)												
HYPERPLASIA OF PROSTATE (*cont.*)												
3. Germany, München		Lützeler & Dormanns 1929 Kruse M1	P	53	28	19	5	1	0·6701	1·7433	0·7886	0·2298
			C	1300	552	559	125	64				
4. Italy, Aquila		Curtoni & Morgante 1964	P	180(c)	80	72	21	7	1·1298	0·5538	1·3008	1·1243
			C	8920(c)	4321	3442	872	285				
5. Italy, Milano		Rotelli & Corippo 1959	P	204	70	104	26	4	1·2275	1·7155	1·3762	1·8786
			C	8000	3090	3740	834	336				
6. Italy, Milano		Mor & Sforza 1960	P	105	47	40	16	2	0·7709	1·2150	1·2734	0·5448
			C	500	202	223	54	21				
7. Italy, Pavia		Prosser 1959	P	200	76	92	20	12	1·0001	0·0000	0·9750	0·0099
			C	8000	3090	3740	834	336				
8. Italy, Veneto		Mobilio & Torchiana 1960	P	644	307	244	57	36	1·1152	1·0042	0·7898	1·8191
			C	1093	536	382	126	49				
9. United Kingdom, London	Myo-adenoma	Bourke & Griffin 1962	P	271(c)	117	113	26	15	1·0480	0·1231	1·1431	0·3698
			C	10000	4578	4219	890	313				
10. United Kingdom, Monmouth		Beasley 1964	P	445	193	204	36	12	1·0549	0·2355	0·8928	0·3311
			C	2268	986	988	206	88				
11. Turkey, Ankara		Kafkas & Gercel 1967	P	1000(c)	305	448	167	80	1·0880	0·5025	1·0995	0·3707
			C	2000(c)	612	934	308	146				
12. N. India, Lucknow		Nath *et al.* 1963	P	62	17	11	26	8	0·8894	0·0904	1·2533	0·5148
			C	3330(c)	1035	753	1263	279				
13. Peru, Lima		Muñoz-Baratta 1962	P	96(c)	61	21	13	1	0·8742	0·2820	1·1147	0·1263
			C	107938(c)	66058	26013	12629	3238				
				3701					1·0507	1·4061	1·0605	0·8878
				χ^2_{12} for homogeneity of areas						9·9603		7·3102
OTHER DISEASES OF MALE GENITAL ORGANS												
1. S. India, Gwalior	Azoospermia	Gupta & Gupta 1965	P	50	32	5	13	0	0·2019	10·9967	0·3467	10·2555
			C	4720	1460	1130	1711	419				
2. Japan, Sendai	Other than hyperplasia of prostate	Moniwa 1960	P	49	15	23	8	3	1·3331	0·7484	0·7479	0·4394
			C	21199	6769	7786	4827	1817				
DISEASES OF FEMALE GENITAL ORGANS												
1. Finland	Salpingitis	Mustakallio 1937	P	28	6	15	5	2	2·0674	2·2414	1·8869	1·0889
			C	2595	908	1098	401	188				
2. Japan, Sendai	Salpingitis, oophoritis	Moniwa 1960	P	184	57	66	48	13	1·0067	0·0013	1·1809	0·7138
			C	21199	6769	7786	4827	1817				
3. Japan, Sendai	Infective diseases of uterus, vagina, and vulva	Moniwa 1960	P	131	39	50	29	13	1·1146	0·2563	1·0428	0·0290
			C	21199	6769	7786	4827	1817				
4. Japan, Sendai	Uterovaginal prolapse	Moniwa 1960	P	72	22	30	14	6	1·1855	0·3663	0·8924	0·1106
			C	21199	6769	7786	4827	1817				
DISORDERS OF MENSTRUATION												
1. Czechoslovakia	Menopausal metrorrhagia	Miluničová *et al.* 1969[a]	P	170	58	71	26	15	0·8493	0·7399	0·8402	0·4755
			C	1142	358	516	191	77				
2. United Kingdom, Liverpool	Menorrhagia	Evans *et al.* 1968	P	466	240	164	49	13	0·8118	3·9645	1·1764	0·9875
			C	6510	3146	2648	546	170				
3. Japan, Sendai		Moniwa 1960	P	87	28	31	17	11	0·9625	0·0214	0·8514	0·2727
			C	21199	6769	7786	4827	1817				

TABLE 1 THE ABO BLOOD GROUP SYSTEM (*cont.*)

Place	Additional details	Authors	Number		O	A	B	AB	A/O Relative incidence	A/O χ_1^2 for difference from unity	B/O Relative incidence	B/O χ_1^2 for difference from unity
PERINATAL DISORDERS												
ABORTION, MOTHERS/CONTROLS												
1. Denmark	(s) normal and abnormal foetuses	Lauritsen *et al.* 1975	Mothers	288	122	122	28	16	1·0236	0·0232	1·0787	0·1271
			C	8818(c)	3854	3765	820	379				
2. Germany, Würzburg		Krieg & Kasper 1968	Mothers	61	20	34	5	2	1·4710	1·8648	0·9354	0·0177
			C	10130(c)	3970	4588	1061	511				
3. Portugal		Lessa & Alarcão 1947	Mothers	677	270	305	51	51	1·0146	0·0219	0·9536	0·0716
			C	1748	732	815	145	56				
4. Sweden, Scania		Grubb & Sjöstedt 1954–5	Mothers	183	68	90	18	7	1·3077	2·6973	1·0772	0·0767
			C	5668	2401	2430	590	247				
5. Japan, Sendai		Moniwa 1960	Mothers	61	23	17	17	4	0·6426	1·9067	1·0365	0·0125
			C	21199	6769	7786	4827	1817				
6. Canada, Vancouver		Takano & Miller 1972	Mothers	229	119	85	21	4	0·8409	1·4530	0·6716	2·7758
		Stout 1976	C	9714	4369	3711	1148	486				
7. U.S.A., California	Whites	Peritz 1971	Mothers	312	145	129	31	7	0·9943	0·0022	0·9076	0·2324
		Reed 1968 M2	C	8962	4067	3639	958	298				
8. U.S.A., New York City	Whites	Cohen & Sayre 1968	Mothers	2223	1127	787	229	80	0·7751	20·2837	0·6482	25·6795
		Osborne & De George 1926	C	4738	2029	1828	636	245				
9. U.S.A., Salt Lake City		McNeil *et al.* 1954	Mothers	85	48	26	9	2	0·6058	3·9332	0·9043	0·0716
		Matson & Schrader 1941 M1	C	985	463	414	96	12				
10. U.S.A., San Francisco	Whites	Allen 1964	Mothers	18	8	7	3	0	0·9779	0·0019	1·5920	0·4705
		Reed 1968 M2	C	8962	4067	3639	958	298				
11. Australia, Western Australia		Vos & Tovell 1967	Mothers	422(c)	209	154	45	14	0·6819	5·4707	0·8090	0·6868
			C	10457	4781	4287	1081	308				
				4559					0·8716	13·3433	0·7812	17·3482
			χ_{10}^2 for homogeneity of areas							24·3153		12·8740
ABORTION, FOETUSES/CONTROLS												
1. Denmark	(s) normal and abnormal	Lauritsen *et al.* 1975	Foetuses	72	33	29	7	3	0·8996	0·1752	0·9970	0·0001
			C	8818(c)	3854	3765	820	379				
2. Germany, Würzberg	Normal	Krieg & Kasper 1968	Foetuses	61	13	32	10	6	2·1300	5·2625	2·8783	6·2751
			C	10130(c)	3970	4588	1061	511				
				133					1·2425	1·1556	1·6852	3·0885
			χ_1^2 for homogeneity of areas							4·2821		3·1867
ABORTION, MOTHERS OF NORMAL/MOTHERS OF ABNORMAL FOETUSES												
1. Denmark		Lauritsen *et al.* 1975	Normal	*116*	*50*	*44*	*12*	*10*	*0·8123*	*0·5779*	*1·4400*	*0·6044*
			Abnormal	*139*	*60*	*65*	*10*	*4*				
ABORTION, FOETUSES NORMAL/ABNORMAL												
1. Denmark		Lauritsen *et al.* 1975	Normal	*42*	*11*	*22*	*7*	*2*	*5·0000*	*7·0067*		
			Abnormal	*21*	*15*	*6*	*0*	*0*				
ABORTIONS/LIVE BIRTHS (MOTHERS)												
1. Sweden, Scania		Grubb & Sjöstedt 1954–5	Ab.	*183*	*68*	*90*	*18*	*7*	*1·2890*	*1·4859*	*1·1859*	*0·2443*
			L.B.	*260*	*112*	*115*	*25*	*8*				
2. U.S.A., New York City		Cohen & Sayre 1968	Ab.	*2223*	*1127*	*787*	*229*	*80*	*0·9051*	*4·5370*	*0·7987*	*9·4999*
			L.B.	*153044*	*72456*	*55900*	*18434*	*6254*				
3. U.S.A., Salt Lake City		McNeil *et al.* 1954	Ab.	*85*	*48*	*26*	*9*	*2*	*0·8349*	*0·4378*	*1·1667*	*0·1360*
			L.B.	*319*	*168*	*109*	*27*	*15*				
4. Australia, Western Australia		Vos & Tovell 1967	Ab.	*422*	*209*	*154*	*45*	*14*	*0·6818*	*5·4723*	*0·8090*	*0·6869*
			L.B.	*300*	*124*	*134*	*33*	*9*				
				2913/153923					*0·8992*	*5·9937*	*0·8198*	*8·5799*
			χ_3^2 for homogeneity of areas							*5·9393*		*1·9872*

TABLE 1 **THE ABO BLOOD GROUP SYSTEM** *(cont.)*

Place	Additional details	Authors		Number	O	A	B	AB	A/O Relative incidence	A/O χ_1^2 for difference from unity	B/O Relative incidence	B/O χ_1^2 for difference from unity
PERINATAL DISORDERS *(cont.)*												
PREMATURE INFANTS/CONTROLS												
1. Austria, Vöcklabruck	(s) S	Kircher 1968	P	312	109	144	46	13	1·4408	7·6038	1·5684	5·9355
			C	3405	1468	1346	395	196				
2. Italy, Alessandria		Canestri 1963	P	390(c)	148	179	45	18	1·1377	1·1011	1·1791	0·7543
			C	1690(c)	698	742	180	70				
3. Italy, Genova		Cordone & Marchi 1964	P	332	151	139	28	14	1·0014	0·0011	0·9047	0·1273
			C	350	161	148	33	8				
4. Italy, Milano		Bonvini & Zanetti 1961	P	500	206	216	49	29	1·0299	0·0520	1·1723	0·5408
			C	640	276	281	56	27				
5. U.S.A., Cleveland	About 80% Negroes	Plotkin 1958	P	100	39	27	31	3	1·2069	0·5414	1·6551	4·1706
			C	2200(c)	1039	596	499	66				
				1634					1·1554	4·9175	1·2994	7·3783
				χ_4^2 for homogeneity of areas						4·3808		4·1502
PREMATURE/FULL-TERM INFANTS												
1. Italy, Alessandria		Canestri 1963	Prem.	*390*	*148*	*179*	*45*	*18*	*1·3265*	*1·8476*	*1·1486*	*0·1933*
			Full-term	*155*	*68*	*62*	*18*	*7*				
2. Italy, Genova		Cordone & Marchi 1963	Prem.	*332*	*151*	*139*	*28*	*14*	*0·9991*	*0·0000*	*0·6601*	*1·8435*
			Full-term	*202*	*89*	*82*	*25*	*6*				
3. U.S.A., Cleveland	About 80% Negroes	Plotkin 1958	Prem.	*100*	*39*	*27*	*31*	*3*	*1·2805*	*0·8929*	*1·6857*	*4·2456*
			Full-term	*1033*	*492*	*266*	*232*	*43*				
				822/1390					*1·1697*	*1·1528*	*1·1503*	*0·7121*
				χ_2^2 for homogeneity of areas						*1·5877*		*5·5703*
POST-TERM INFANTS												
1. Italy, Alessandria		Canestri 1963	P	52	28	13	11	0	0·4368	5·9456	1·5234	1·3262
			C	1690	698	742	180	70				
ECTOPIC PREGNANCY												
1. Japan, Sendai		Moniwa 1960	P	113	24	41	35	13	1·4852	2·3586	2·0451	7·2504
			C	21199	6769	7786	4827	1817				
DISEASES OF THE SKIN												
ANGIODERMATITIS												
1. Italy, Foggia		Altobella 1967–8	P	50	20	25	5	0	1·5821	2·2129	0·6592	0·6724
			C	1000	443	350	168	39				
SEBORRHOEIC DERMATITIS												
1. Italy, Trentino		Nardelli 1928	P	22	10	9	3	0	1·1009	0·0406	1·7125	0·6000
		Formentano 1951 M1	C	279	137	112	24	6				
2. United Kingdom, Glasgow		MacSween & Syme 1965	P	45	19	14	10	2	1·2282	0·3383	2·6250	6·0276
			C	5898	3177	1906	637	178				
				67					1·1814	0·3448	2·3678	6·3449
				χ_1^2 for homogeneity of areas						0·0341		0·2827
SOLAR DERMATITIS												
1. Egypt	(s) S	el-Hefnawi *et al.* 1963	P	20	10	5	5	0	0·4692	1·9018	0·6622	0·5638
			C	5200	1674	1784	1264	478				
DERMATITIS MEDICAMENTOSA												
1. Japan, Okayama		Ohmichi 1928	P	15	4	6	4	1	1·0660	0·0098	1·1976	0·0649
		After Furuhata 1933 M1	C	6936	1921	2703	1604	708				

TABLE 1 **THE ABO BLOOD GROUP SYSTEM** (*cont.*)

Place	Additional details	Authors		Number	O	A	B	AB	A/O Relative incidence	A/O χ^2_1 for difference from unity	B/O Relative incidence	B/O χ^2_1 for difference from unity
DERMATITIS, UNSPECIFIED												
1. Finland		Mustakallio 1937	P	25	8	6	7	4	0·6202	0·7770	1·9813	1·7223
			C	2595	908	1098	401	188				
ROSACEA												
1. United Kingdom Glasgow		MacSween & Syme 1965	P	78	37	25	16		1·1262	0·2083		
			C	5898	3177	1906	637	178				
LUPUS ERYTHEMATOSUS												
1. Italy, Trentino		Nardelli 1928	P	10	4	4	2	0	1·2232	0·0786	2·8542	1·3767
		Formentano 1951 M1	C	279	137	112	24	6				
2. United Kingdom, Glasgow		MacSween & Syme 1965	P	33	24	5	4		0·3473	4·6131		
			C	5898	3177	1906	637	178				
3. Egypt	(s) S	el-Hefnawi *et al.* 1963	P	110	45	34	26	5	0·7090	2·2408	0·7652	1·1539
			C	5200	1674	1784	1264	478				
				153					0·8574	4·3985	0·8414	0·5181
					χ^2_2 for homogeneity of areas					2·5340		
				(120)	χ^2_1 for homogeneity of areas							2·0125
PSORIASIS												
1. Germany, Giessen, Kassel, Marburg		Wendt 1968	P	418	171	179	42	26	0·8390	1·8039	0·7758	1·5102
			C	857	319	398	101	39				
2. Germany, Göttingen		Jörgensen 1967	P	206	84	87	23	12	0·9092	0·2995	1·0528	0·0362
			C	694	273	311	71	39				
3. Germany, München		Poehlmann 1929	P	268	154	75	31	8	0·5672	11·8561	0·7867	1·0417
		Fürst 1927 M1	C	660	297	255	76	32				
4. Italy, Foggia		Altobella 1967–8	P	240	130	70	30	10	0·6815	5·4258	0·6085	5·0115
			C	1000	443	350	168	39				
5. Italy, Napoli		Villano & Santoianni 1972	P	40	18	10	8	4	0·9596	0·0057	1·2063	0·0934
			C	40	19	11	7	3				
6. Italy, Piemonte		Ferrari 1930	P	88(c)	32	43	10	3	1·2911	0·8758	1·1343	0·0889
		Mino 1923 M1	C	234	98	102	27	7				
7. Italy, Trentino		Nardelli 1928	P	42	23	17	2	0	0·9041	0·0857	0·4964	0·8281
		Formentano 1951 M1	C	279	137	112	24	6				
8. Poland, Warszawa		Straszyński 1925[a]	P	32	9	14	6	3	1·4449	0·7336	1·2564	0·1854
			C	2613	914	984	485	230				
9. Sweden, Northern		Beckman *et al.* 1974	P	122	39	61	12	10	1·4177	2·8908	1·1315	0·1398
			C	59862	24003	26481	6527	2851				
10. United Kingdom, Leeds		Hargreaves & Hellier 1958	P	200	98	81	18	3	0·9547	0·0867	1·1214	0·1800
			C	2056	983	851	161	61				
11. United Kingdom, Glasgow		MacSween & Syme 1965	P	231	119	74	38		1·0365	0·0565		
			C	5898	3177	1906	637	178				
12. S. India, Gwalior		Gupta, S. R. & Gupta 1966	P	105	44	24	33	4	0·7059	1·8396	0·6404	3·6574
			C	4720	1461	1129	1711	419				
13. Egypt	(s) S	el-Hefnawi *et al.* 1963	P	110	13	45	30	22	3·2481	13·8366	3·0562	11·1792
			C	5200	1674	1784	1264	478				
				2102					0·9140	2·6607	0·9022	1·4766
					χ^2_{12} for homogeneity of areas					37·1356		
				(1871)	χ^2_{11} for homogeneity of areas							22·4752

TABLE 1 **THE ABO BLOOD GROUP SYSTEM** *(cont.)*

Place	Additional details	Authors		Number	O	A	B	AB	A/O Relative incidence	A/O χ_1^2 for difference from unity	B/O Relative incidence	B/O χ_1^2 for difference from unity
DISEASES OF THE SKIN *(cont.)*												
PITYRIASIS ROSEA												
1. United Kingdom, Glasgow		MacSween & Syme 1965	P	24	14	7	3		0·8334	0·1543		
			C	5898	3177	1906	637	178				
LICHEN PLANUS												
1. United Kingdom, Glasgow		MacSween & Syme 1965	P	17	7	10	0	0	2·3812	3·0888		
			C	5898	3177	1906	637	178				
2. Egypt	(s) S	el-Hefnawi *et al.* 1963	P	51	17	16	13	5	0·8831	0·1261	1·0128	0·0012
			C	5200	1674	1784	1264	478				
				68					1·2308	0·5285		
				χ_1^2 for homogeneity of areas						3·7432		
PRURIGO												
1. Poland, Warszawa	Hebra's	Straszyński 1925[a]	P	39	19	4	15	1	0·1955	8·7393	1·4878	1·2890
			C	2613	914	984	485	230				
2. Egypt	(s) S	el-Hefnawi *et al.* 1963	P	96	36	36	22	2	0·9383	0·0714	0·8093	0·5997
			C	5200	1674	1784	1264	478				
				135					0·7336	2·0065	1·0193	0·0078
				χ_1^2 for homogeneity of areas						6·8042		1·8809
LICHEN SIMPLEX CHRONICUS												
1. United Kingdom, Glasgow		MacSween & Syme 1965	P	58	30	16	12		0·8890	0·1432		
			C	5898	3177	1906	637	178				
PRURITUS												
1. United Kingdom, Glasgow	All types	MacSween & Syme 1965	P	22	12	9	1		1·2501	0·2552		
			C	5898	3177	1906	637	178				
ALOPECIA												
1. United Kingdom, Glasgow	All types	MacSween & Syme 1965	P	79	35	32	12		1·5240	2·9263		
			C	5898	3177	1906	637	178				
2. Japan, Okayama	Aerata	Ohmichi 1928	P	40	12	15	8	5	0·8884	0·0929	0·7984	0·2419
		After Furahata 1933 M1	C	6936	1921	2703	1604	708				
				119					1·3054	1·6418		
				χ_1^2 for homogeneity of areas						1·3774		
ACNE VULGARIS												
1. United Kingdom, Glasgow		MacSween & Syme 1965	P	204	106	73	25		1·1479	0·7917		
			C	5898	3177	1906	637	178				
2. S. India, Gwalior		Gupta *et al.* 1967	P	300	74	109	84	33	1·7086	6·0397	0·8663	0·4510
			C	300	87	75	114	24				
				504					1·3118	4·6190		
				χ_1^2 for homogeneity of areas						2·2124		
JUVENILE ACNE												
1. Italy, Trentino		Nardelli 1928	P	26	11	9	6	0	1·0008	0·0000	3·1136	4·2083
		Formentano 1951 M1	C	279	137	112	24	6				

TABLE 1 **THE ABO BLOOD GROUP SYSTEM** *(cont.)*

Place	Additional details	Authors		Number	O	A	B	AB	A/O Relative incidence	A/O χ_1^2 for difference from unity	B/O Relative incidence	B/O χ_1^2 for difference from unity
ACNE VULGARIS AND SEBORRHOEA												
1. Egypt	(s) S	el-Hefnawi *et al.* 1963	P	100	32	32	26	10	0·9383	0·0636	1·0760	0·0756
			C	5200	1674	1784	1264	478				
ULCER OF SKIN												
1. United Kingdom, Glasgow		MacSween & Syme 1965	P	57	27	21	9		1·2964	0·7884		
			C	5898	3177	1906	637	178				
VITILIGO												
1. N. India, Calcutta		Dutta *et al.* 1969	P	250	83	41	104	22	0·5873	7·6217	1·0131	0·0076
			C	10032	3045	2561	3766	660				
2. N. India, Uttar Pradesh	Hindus and Sikhs	Srivastava & Shukla 1965	P	424	115	87	175	47	1·1145	0·5706	1·2040	2·3422
			C	19255	5971	4053	7547	1684				
3. N. India, Uttar Pradesh	Moslems	Srivastava & Shukla 1965	P	101	33	18	39	11	0·6452	2·2014	1·0427	0·0305
			C	5191	1566	1324	1775	526				
4. N. India, Varanasi		Singh & Shanker 1966	P	100	30	20	27	23	0·9108	0·1015	0·9147	0·1095
			C	2583	873	639	859	212				
5. N. India, Varanasi		Sehgal & Dube 1968	P	173	29	45	84	15	2·4906	11·8374	2·2674	12·0268
			C	615	191	119	244	61				
6. S. India, Gwalior		Gupta, S. R. & Gupta 1966	P	102	40	16	28	18	0·5176	4·8683	0·5977	4·2729
			C	4720	1461	1129	1711	419				
7. Japan, Okayama		Ohmichi 1928	P	17	4	8	5	0	1·4214	0·3289	1·4970	0·3609
		After Furuhata 1933 M1	C	6936	1921	2703	1604	708				
8. Egypt	(s) S	el-Hefnawi *et al.* 1963	P	80	24	28	20	8	1·0947	0·1043	1·1036	0·1045
			C	5200	1674	1784	1264	478				
				1247					0·9476	0·4037	1·1164	2·3175
					χ_7^2 for homogeneity of areas					27·2305		16·9374
FRECKLES												
1. Egypt	(s) S	el-Hefnawi *et al.* 1963	P	70	40	14	12	4	0·3284	12·7047	0·3973	7·7651
			C	5200	1674	1784	1264	478				
DISEASES OF THE MUSCULOSKELETAL SYSTEM AND CONNECTIVE TISSUE												
RHEUMATOID ARTHRITIS												
1. Finland	Polyarthritis	Streng & Ryti 1927	P	83	25	34	14	10	1·0654	0·0549	1·1176	0·1048
			C	1383(c)	463	591	232	97				
2. Italy, Pietra Ligure		Cerrato & Ghibaudi 1968	P	167	99	51	14	3	0·4810	17·0124	0·5450	4·2827
			C	2631	1083	1160	281	107				
3. Poland, Kraków		Kruszewski 1966	P	403	123	163	89	28	1·0725	0·3405	1·1464	0·9553
			C	44245	14155	17490	8934	3666				
4. Romania, Bucureşti		Stoia *et al.* 1969	P	701	211	296	144	50	1·1793	3·2683	1·3504	7·5090
			C	26229(c)	8922	10613	4509	2185				
5. United Kingdom, Buckinghamshire		Glynn *et al.* 1956	P	209	95	86	22	6	0·9500	0·1172	1·1968	0·5671
			C	15046	6775	6456	1311	504				
6. U.S.S.R., Slavyansk	Polyarthritis	Penzik 1930	P	600	256	215	88	41	0·7416	9·9564	0·5396	24·0220
			C	13482	4515	5113	2876	978				
7. U.S.S.R., Slavyansk	Polyarthritis	Kaminsky 1928	P	797	442	163	147	45	0·3256	142·8050	0·5221	43·8363
			C	13482	4515	5113	2876	978				
				2960					0·7274	51·1159	0·7959	17·6577
					χ_6^2 for homogeneity of areas					122·4388		63·6195
ANKYLOSING SPONDYLITIS												
1. Poland, Kraków		Kruszewski 1966	P	169	47	71	35	16	1·2226	1·1381	1·1799	0·5468
			C	44245	14155	17490	8934	3666				
2. Romania, Bucureşti		Stoia *et al.* 1969	P	183	62	71	37	13	0·9627	0·0475	1·1808	0·6354
			C	26229(c)	8922	10613	4509	2185				
				352					1·0750	0·3190	1·1804	1·1822
					χ_1^2 for homogeneity of areas					0·8666		0·0000

TABLE 1 **THE ABO BLOOD GROUP SYSTEM** *(cont.)*

Place	Additional details	Authors		Number	O	A	B	AB	A/O Relative incidence	A/O χ_1^2 for difference from unity	B/O Relative incidence	B/O χ_1^2 for difference from unity
DISEASES OF THE MUSCULOSKELETAL SYSTEM AND CONNECTIVE TISSUE *(cont.)*												
DEGENERATIVE OSTEO-ARTHRITIS												
1. Poland, Kraków		Kruszewski 1966	P	120	40	42	26	12	0·8498	0·5414	1·0299	0·0136
			C	44245	14155	17490	8934	3666				
ARTHRITIS, UNSPECIFIED												
1. Finland		Mustakallio 1937	P	49	16	24	6	3	1·2404	0·4372	0·8491	0·1149
			C	2595	908	1098	401	188				
URIC ACID DIATHESIS												
1. Italy, Milano	Arthritis, articular rheumatism, gout	Dossena & Lanzara 1925	P	30	14	10	5	1	0·9158	0·0399	1·3736	0·3150
		Dossena 1924 M1	C	214	100	78	26	10				
OSTEOMYELITIS, PERIOSTITIS												
1. Japan, Sendai		Moniwa 1960	P	123	37	50	26	10	1·1748	0·5489	0·9854	0·0033
			C	21199	6769	7786	4827	1817				
PERTHES' DISEASE												
1. United Kingdom, Glasgow		Cameron & Izatt 1962	P	142	73	50	15	4	1·1417	0·5083	1·0248	0·0073
			C	5898	3177	1906	637	178				
DUPUYTREN'S DISEASE												
1. Norway, Bergen		Mikkelsen 1967	P	80	34	36	7	3	0·9677	0·0185	1·1370	0·0940
			C	4859	2071	2266	375	147				
BONE FRACTURES												
1. Denmark, København	Classical fracture of femoral neck	Thorsøe 1960	P	334	109	171	35	19	1·4455	8·8432	1·1970	0·8383
		Andersen 1955 M1	C	14304	5804	6299	1557	644				
2. Denmark, København	Lateral fracture of femoral neck	Thorsøe 1960	P	192	92	72	25	3	0·7211	4·2610	1·0130	0·0032
		Andersen 1955 M1	C	14304	5804	6299	1557	644				
3. United Kingdom, Belfast	Fracture of femoral neck; (s) S	Macafee 1973	P	248	138	79	27	4	0·9537	0·1119	1·1379	0·3733
			C	28566	15715	9433	2702	716				
4. U.S.A., Iowa	Fracture of hip	Buckwalter *et al.* 1957	P	981	410	441	95	35	1·1850	5·3037	1·1756	1·7374
			C	6313	2892	2625	570	226				
5. U.S.A., Iowa	Fractures other than hip	Buckwalter *et al.* 1957	P	252	112	103	26	11	1·0132	0·0089	1·1778	0·5412
			C	6313	2892	2625	570	226				
6. Germany, Tübingen		Völter *et al.* 1970	P	642	255	297	69	21	1·1326	2·0916	1·0251	0·0329
		Dick *et al.* 1962	C	39031	16283	16745	4298	1705				
				2649					1·1153	6·2543	1·1180	2·5857
				χ_5^2 for homogeneity of areas						14·3659		0·9406
CONGENITAL ANOMALIES												
SPINA BIFIDA CYSTICA												
1. N. India, Chandigarh		Sidana *et al.* 1970	P	72	25	18	24	5	1·0027	0·0001	0·7706	0·8222
			C	6204	1912	1373	2382	537				
HYDROCEPHALUS												
1. U.S.A., Michigan	Whites; (s) A_1A_2	Gershowitz & Neel 1965	P	145	60	69	11	5	1·2741	1·7143	0·8759	0·1513
			C	1508	688	621	144	55				

TABLE 1 THE ABO BLOOD GROUP SYSTEM (*cont.*)

Place	Additional details	Authors		Number	O	A	B	AB	A/O Relative incidence	A/O χ^2_1 for difference from unity	B/O Relative incidence	B/O χ^2_1 for difference from unity
DEAF-MUTISM												
1. Italy, Cuneo		Beffa *et al.* 1960	P	155	59	77	13	6	1·4535	4·0015	1·0307	0·0085
			C	912	421	378	90	23				
2. Italy, Foggia		Beffa *et al.* 1960	P	130	65	43	19	3	0·7741	1·4152	0·7562	0·9668
			C	661	282	241	109	29				
3. Italy, Torino		Beffa *et al.* 1960	P	140	75	48	14	3	0·6237	6·1216	0·8277	0·3930
			C	2072	878	901	198	95				
				425					0·9045	0·7821	0·8515	0·8454
				χ^2_2 for homogeneity of areas						10·7562		0·5229
CONGENITAL HEART DEFECTS												
Tetralogy of Fallot												
1. Germany, Göttingen	(s) whether operated or not	Jörgensen *et al.* 1968	P	316	120	135	43	18	0·9875	0·0070	1·3778	2·0835
			C	694	273	311	71	39				
2. United Kingdom, Bristol		David 1970	P	84	37	33	12	2	0·8589	0·3944	1·7757	2·8751
		Kopeć 1970	C	3284	1430	1485	275	94				
				400					0·9499	0·1616	1·4872	4·5665
				χ^2_1 for homogeneity of areas						0·2398		0·3921
Ventricular Septal Defects												
1. Germany, Göttingen	(s) whether operated or not	Jörgensen *et al.* 1968	P	612	254	258	64	36	0·8916	0·8957	0·9688	0·0269
			C	694	273	311	71	39				
2. Norway, Oslo		Brendemoen 1969	P	110	36	67	4	3	1·4066	2·6905	0·5145	1·5795
		Heistø 1956 M1	C	8292	3135	4148	677	332				
3. United Kingdom, Bristol		David 1970	P	112	52	45	13	2	0·8333	0·7765	1·3000	0·6850
		Kopeć 1970	C	3284	1430	1485	275	94				
				834					0·9642	0·1526	0·9849	0·0094
				χ^2_2 for homogeneity of areas						4·2101		2·2820
Atrial Septal Defects												
1. Germany, Göttingen	(s) whether operated or not	Jörgensen *et al.* 1968	P	296	130	123	31	12	0·8306	1·5186	0·9169	0·1304
			C	694	273	311	71	39				
2. Norway, Oslo		Brendemoen 1969	P	186	82	94	7	3	0·8664	0·8793	0·3953	5·4917
		Heistø 1956 M1	C	8292	3135	4148	677	332				
3. United Kingdom, Bristol		David 1970	P	114	49	53	8	4	1·0416	0·0408	0·8490	0·1790
		Kopeć 1970	C	3284	1430	1485	275	94				
				596					0·8874	1·5898	0·7713	2·0493
				χ^2_2 for homogeneity of areas						1·8103		3·7518
Aortic Stenosis												
1. Germany, Göttingen	(s) whether operated or not	Jörgensen *et al.* 1968	P	242	105	104	26	7	0·8695	0·7522	0·9521	0·0366
			C	694	273	311	71	39				
2. Germany, Göttingen	Stenosis of aortic isthmus; (s) whether operated or not	Jörgensen *et al.* 1968	P	127	51	58	11	7	0·9983	0·0001	0·8293	0·2731
			C	694	273	311	71	39				
3. United Kingdom, Bristol		David 1970	P	19	10	8	1	0	0·7704	0·3007	0·5200	0·3079
		Kopeć 1970	C	3284	1430	1485	275	94				
				388					0·9049	0·6563	0·8941	0·2995
				χ^2_2 for homogeneity of areas						0·3967		0·3181

TABLE 1 **THE ABO BLOOD GROUP SYSTEM** (*cont.*)

Place	Additional details	Authors		Number	O	A	B	AB	A/O Relative incidence	A/O χ_1^2 for difference from unity	B/O Relative incidence	B/O χ_1^2 for difference from unity
CONGENITAL ANOMALIES (*cont.*)												
CONGENITAL HEART DEFECTS (*cont.*)												
PULMONARY STENOSIS												
1. Germany, Göttingen	(s) whether operated or not	Jörgensen *et al.* 1968	P	211	72	111	23	5	1·3533	3·0746	1·2283	0·5622
			C	694	273	311	71	39				
2. United Kingdom, Bristol		David 1970	P	52	20	29	3	0	1·3963	1·2992	0·7800	0·1593
		Kopeć 1970	C	3284	1430	1485	275	94				
				263					1·3643	4·3652	1·1409	0·2762
				χ_1^2 for homogeneity of areas						0·0086		0·4453
HEART DEFECTS, NOT FURTHER SPECIFIED												
1. Germany, Göttingen	(s) whether operated or not	Jörgensen *et al.* 1968	P	623	256	279	63	25	0·9567	0·1365	0·9463	0·0814
			C	694	273	311	71	39				
2. N. India, Chandigarh		Sidana *et al.* 1970	P	105	35	26	38	6	1·0345	0·0168	0·8715	0·3389
			C	6204	1912	1373	2382	537				
3. Canada, Edmonton		Sartor & Fraser 1964	P	268	108	120	26	14	1·3170	3·8322	1·0053	0·0005
			C	2171	998	842	239	92				
4. U.S.A., Cook County	Negro children; (s) A_1A_2	Lev *et al.* 1967	P	138	65	39	27	7	1·1294	0·1721	1·2084	0·3157
			C	130	64	34	22	10				
5. U.S.A., Denver		Lubs *et al.* 1972	P	37	16	19	1	1	1·3842	0·9082	0·3312	1·1452
		Charney 1969	C	3648	1717	1473	324	134				
6. U.S.A., Iowa		Buckwalter *et al.* 1964	P	467(c)	216	202	35	14	0·9904	0·0096	0·7728	1·9855
			C	49979	22392	21144	4695	1748				
7. U.S.A., Michigan	Whites; (s) A_1A_2	Gershowitz & Neel 1965	P	122	55	45	17	5	0·9065	0·2219	1·4768	1·7796
			C	1508	688	621	144	55				
8. U.S.A., New Haven	Whites	Lubs *et al.* 1972	P	21	8	11	0	2	1·5480	0·8788		
			C	3467(c)	1557	1383	385	142				
				1781					1·0512	0·7143	0·9463	0·3505
				χ_7^2 for homogeneity of areas						5·4618		
				(1760) χ_6^2 for homogeneity of areas								5·2963
CLEFT PALATE OR CLEFT LIP												
1. Germany, Göttingen		Jörgensen 1967	P	565	229	243	67	26	0·9315	0·3280	1·1250	0·3744
			C	694	273	311	71	39				
2. Poland, Wrocław		Handzel & Nowakowski 1961	P	90	23	39	20	8	1·4290	1·8359	1·5123	1·8217
		Kelus 1953 M1	C	19063	6313	7491	3630	1629				
3. N. India, Chandigarh		Sidana *et al.* 1970	P	35	13	5	17	0	0·5356	1·4014	1·0497	0·0172
			C	6204	1912	1373	2382	537				
				690					0·9795	0·0357	1·1931	1·4015
				χ_2^2 for homogeneity of areas						3·5296		0·8117
PYLORIC STENOSIS												
1. Germany, Göttingen	Pylorospasm	Jörgensen 1967	P	208	81	96	20	11	1·0404	0·0528	0·9494	0·0337
			C	694	273	311	71	39				
2. United Kingdom, Oxford	Infantile hypertrophic	Hobbs 1968	P	62	24	28	5	5	1·2463	0·6209	0·9800	0·0017
			C	6452	2926	2739	622	165				
3. United Kingdom, Belfast	Infantile hypertrophic	Dodge 1971	P	486	271	130	71	14	0·6019	17·7476	1·1998	1·2997
			C	1495	719	573	157	46				
				756					0·7658	8·2226	1·1217	0·7355
				χ_2^2 for homogeneity of areas						10·1987		0·5996

TABLE 1 **THE ABO BLOOD GROUP SYSTEM** (*cont.*)

Place	Additional details	Authors		Number	O	A	B	AB	A/O Relative incidence	A/O χ^2_1 for difference from unity	B/O Relative incidence	B/O χ^2_1 for difference from unity
MALFORMATIONS												
1. Japan, Sendai	Of digestive system	Moniwa 1960	P	249	93	93	40	23	0·8694	0·8995	0·6031	7·0795
			C	21199	6769	7786	4827	1817				
2. N. India, Chandigarh	Ano-rectal	Sidana *et al.* 1970	P	26	9	8	7	2	1·2378	0·1918	0·6243	0·8707
			C	6204	1912	1373	2382	537				
3. Japan, Sendai	Malposition of uterus	Moniwa 1960	P	210	59	77	50	24	1·1346	0·5279	1·1884	0·7987
			C	21199	6769	7786	4827	1817				
4. N. India, Chandigarh	Hypospadias	Sidana *et al.* 1970	P	23	5	5	11	2	1·3926	0·2733	1·7659	1·1080
			C	6204	1912	1373	2382	537				
5. Italy, Milano	Of urinary tract; (s) S	Pisani & Acerbi 1960	P	470	211	209	40	10	1·0158	0·0208	0·8115	1·2465
		Formentano & Morganti 1951 M1	C	2346	1006	981	235	124				
6. Japan, Sendai	Of genito-urinary system	Moniwa 1960	P	71	23	20	18	10	0·7560	0·8346	1·0975	0·0870
			C	21199	6769	7786	4827	1817				
7. Italy, Milano	Dislocation of hip	Tranquilli-Leali 1938	P	140	52	47	32	9	0·9660	0·0294	2·0157	9·6194
			C	16773(c)	7108	6651	2170	844				
8. Romania, Iassi	Osteo-articular	Niculescu *et al.* 1969	P	83(c)	24	44	9	6	1·4488	2·1300	0·7198	0·7068
			C	41674	13804	17468	7192	3210				
9. Sweden	Osteogenesis imperfecta; (s) A_1A_2	Smårs *et al.* 1961	P	152	63	62	21	6	0·7732	1·2646	1·6296	1·8287
			C	225	88	112	18	7				
10. Japan, Sendai	Of bone and joint	Moniwa 1960	P	117	28	51	26	12	1·5835	3·8000	1·3022	0·9353
			C	21199	6769	7786	4827	1817				
11. United Kingdom, Glasgow	Naevi (all types)	MacSween & Syme 1965	P	37	20	12	5		1·0001	0·0000		
			C	5898	3177	1906	637	178				
12. Egypt	Xeroderma pigmentosum; (s) S	el-Hefnawi *et al.* 1963	P	24	18	3	3	0	0·1564	8·8259	0·2207	5·8486
			C	5200	1674	1784	1264	478				
13. Romania, Iassi	Other than osteo-articular	Niculescu *et al.* 1969	P	45	17	14	9	5	0·6508	1·4153	1·0161	0·0015
			C	41674	13804	17468	7192	3210				
14. Austria, Wien	Unspecified	Flamm & Friedrich 1929	P	23(c)	6	11	4	2	1·4359	0·5073	1·5564	0·4687
		Corvin M1	C	10392	3635	4641	1557	559				
DOWN'S SYNDROME (MONGOLISM)												
1. Austria, Wien		Orel 1927	P	44	15	21	7	1	1·1614	0·1869	0·7685	0·3188
			C	1000	331	399	201	69				
2. Germany, Hamburg		Manitz 1932	P	26	11	14	1	0	1·1497	0·1195	0·2743	1·5325
		Haselhorst 1930 M1	C	8680	3403	3767	1128	382				
3. United Kingdom, England		Penrose 1932	P	158	65	78	12	3	1·0766	0·1137	1·1815	0·1583
			C	226	96	107	15	8				
4. United Kingdom, Liverpool	(s) S, ABH secretion	Evans *et al.* 1966	P	82	37	37	5	3	1·2514	0·9251	0·7015	0·5517
		McConnell 1966	C	15377	7527	6015	1450	385				
5. United Kingdom, London	(s) A_1A_2	Lang-Brown *et al.* 1952–3	P	148	81	53	9	5	0·6361	6·2914	0·5623	2·6000
			C	3459	1503	1546	297	113				
6. U.S.S.R., Moscow		Nazarov & Chovdyrova 1972	P	860(c)	280	342	179	59	1·0819	0·9292	1·0415	0·1757
			C	31896	10679	12056	6555	2606				
7. Canada, Manitoba		Chown & Lewis 1963	P	119	58	43	11	7	0·7804	1·4633	0·6911	1·2230
			C	3100	1341	1274	368	117				
8. U.S.A.		Benda & Bixby 1939	P	125	60	48	12	5	0·9182	0·1918	0·7831	0·5916
			C	10536	4730	4121	1208	477				
9. U.S.A., Colony		Goodman & Thomas 1966	P	225	108	91	18	8	1·1757	0·6517	1·5385	1·2366
			C	225	120	86	13	6				
10. U.S.A., Greenville		Goodman & Thomas 1966	P	42	20	21	0	1	1·3781	0·4952		
			C	42	21	16	3	2				

TABLE 1 **THE ABO BLOOD GROUP SYSTEM** (*cont.*)

Place	Additional details	Authors		Number	O	A	B	AB	A/O Relative incidence	A/O χ_1^2 for difference from unity	B/O Relative incidence	B/O χ_1^2 for difference from unity
CONGENITAL ANOMALIES (*cont.*)												
DOWN'S SYNDROME (MONGOLISM) (*cont.*)												
11. U.S.A., Kingston		Goodman & Thomas 1966	P	149	74	55	13	7	0·9649	0·0203	1·1818	0·1432
			C	149	74	57	11	7				
12. U.S.A., Michigan and Ohio		Shaw & Gershowitz 1962	P	793	325	349	94	25	1·1897	3·3503	1·3819	4·7310
			C	1508	688	621	144	55				
13. U.S.A., Michigan	(s) A_1A_2	Shaw & Gershowitz 1963	P	207	80	94	22	11	1·3018	2·6544	1·3139	1·1232
			C	1508	688	621	144	55				
14. U.S.A., Morganton		Goodman & Thomas 1966	P	40	16	22	1	1	1·9643	1·9871	0·2500	1·4642
			C	40	20	14	5	1				
15. U.S.A., Oxford		Goodman & Thomas 1966	P	125	56	57	7	5	0·8821	0·2206	0·7222	0·3638
			C	125	52	60	9	4				
16. U.S.A., Polk	Whites; (s) Rh_D	Kaplan, S. *et al.* 1964	P	290	123	118	34	15	0·9274	0·2865	0·6734	3·6216
			C	1578	609	630	250	89				
17. Australia	Whites; (s) A_1A_2	Simmons *et al.* 1944	P	24	10	9	2	3	1·0718	0·0228	0·9763	0·0010
		Bryce *et al.* 1950–1 M1	C	176943	84034	70565	17215	5129				
				3457					1·0550	1·5826	1·0087	0·0189
					χ_{16}^2 for homogeneity of areas					18·3273		
				(3415)	χ_{15}^2 for homogeneity of areas							19·8171
ALLERGIES												
ECZEMA												
1. Germany, Berlin	(s) A_1A_2	Dorn 1959	P	192	71	83	29	9	0·9722	0·0165	0·8797	0·1906
			C	250	84	101	39	26				
2. Italy, Perugia	Acute	Narducci 1928	P	30	8	17	3	2	1·6880	1·4526	1·0046	0·0000
		Pennachi 1931 M1	C	1000	367	462	137	34				
3. Italy, Perugia	Chronic	Narducci 1928	P	56	28	16	8	4	0·4539	6·0504	0·7654	0·4187
		Pennachi 1931 M1	C	1000	367	462	137	34				
4. Italy, Trentino		Nardelli 1928	P	87	36	45	5	1	1·5290	2·7225	0·7928	0·1947
		Formentano 1951 M1	C	279	137	112	24	6				
5. United Kingdom, Glasgow	Atopic incl. infantile	MacSween & Syme 1965	P	52	28	17	7		1·0120	0·0015		
			C	5898	3177	1906	637	178				
6. S. India, Gwalior	Chronic	Gupta & Gupta 1966	P	250	62	63	103	22	1·3149	2·2328	1·4186	4·5098
			C	4720	1461	1129	1711	419				
7. Egypt	Infantile; (s) S	el-Hefnawi *et al.* 1963	P	216	80	74	38	24	0·8680	0·7380	0·6291	5·3436
			C	5200	1674	1784	1264	478				
				883					1·0318	0·1254	0·9709	0·0743
					χ_6^2 for homogeneity of areas					13·0889		
				(831)	χ_5^2 for homogeneity of areas							10·5831
URTICARIA												
1. United Kingdom, SW. England	Donors	Farr 1960	P	32	12	15	4	1	1·2640	0·3659	1·7692	0·9763
		Roberts 1948	C	120874	53744	53150	10126	3854				
2. United Kingdom, Glasgow	Papular and non-papular	MacSween & Syme 1965	P	39	16	13	5	5	1·3543	0·6558	1·5586	0·7449
			C	5898	3177	1906	637	178				
3. Egypt	In adults; (s) S	el-Hefnawi *et al.* 1963	P	33	11	10	9	3	0·8530	0·1315	1·0836	0·0317
			C	5200	1674	1784	1264	478				
4. Egypt	Papular; (s) S	el-Hefnawi *et al.* 1963	P	155	47	51	39	18	1·0182	0·0077	1·0989	0·1843
			C	5200	1674	1784	1264	478				
				259					1·0047	0·0010	1·1937	1·0159
					χ_3^2 for homogeneity of areas					1·1599		0·9213

TABLE 1 **THE ABO BLOOD GROUP SYSTEM** *(cont.)*

Place	Additional details	Authors		Number	O	A	B	AB	A/O Relative incidence	A/O χ_1^2 for difference from unity	B/O Relative incidence	B/O χ_1^2 for difference from unity
DERMATITIS												
1. United Kingdom, Glasgow	Venenata	MacSween & Syme 1965	P	88	49	27	12		0·9185	0·1241		
			C	5898	3177	1906	637	178				
2. Egypt	Contact; (s) S	el-Hefnawi *et al.* 1963	P	82	26	26	24	6	0·9383	0·0519	1·2225	0·4951
			C	5200	1674	1784	1264	478				
				170					0·9269	0·1726		
				χ_1^2 for homogeneity of areas						0·0034		
DERMATOSES												
1. Italy, Foggia		Altobella 1967–8	P	260	60	160	40	0	3·3752	52·7909	1·7579	6·3809
			C	1000	443	350	168	39				
ASTHMA												
1. Denmark København	Bronchial	Viskum 1973	P	39	17	16	2	4	0·8672	0·1668	0·4386	1·2141
		Andersen 1955 M1	C	14304	5804	6299	1557	644				
2. Italy, Cagliari	Bronchial	Adamo 1961[b]	P	50	40	6	2	2	0·2651	9·1321	0·3929	1·6489
		Boero & Coraddu 1965	C	3516	2043	1156	260	57				
3. United Kingdom, SW. England		Farr 1960	P	46	19	23	3	1	1·2241	0·4250	0·8380	0·0809
		Roberts 1948	C	120874	53744	53150	10126	3854				
4. United Kingdom, London	Bronchial; Whites	Lewis & Woods 1961	P	669	294	287	64	24	1·0593	0·4514	1·1197	0·6280
			C	10000	4578	4219	890	313				
5. N. India, Delhi		Anand 1964[b]	P	545	139	110	243	53	1·2354	1·5915	1·9454	21·0430
			C	617	217	139	195	66				
6. Japan, Sendai		Moniwa 1960	P	78	22	26	24	6	1·0275	0·0087	1·5298	2·0662
			C	21199	6769	7786	4827	1817				
7. Egypt	Bronchial; children	Khalil 1960	P	51	12	12	20	7	0·9185	0·0432	2·2324	4·8114
			C	10045(c)	3279	3570	2448	748				
8. U.S.A., Colorado	(s) Rh_D	Charney 1969	P	206	72	105	23	6	1·6999	11·4090	1·6929	4·5402
			C	3648	1717	1473	324	134				
				1684					1·1286	3·7198	1·4671	20·2960
				χ_7^2 for homogeneity of areas						19·5079		15·7367
HAY FEVER												
1. United Kingdom, SW. England		Farr 1960	P	109	43	51	13	2	1·1993	0·7725	1·6046	2·2287
		Roberts 1948	C	120874	53744	53150	10126	3854				
2. U.S.A., Colorado	(s) Rh_D	Charney 1969	P	211	106	75	22	8	0·8248	1·5450	1·0999	0·1548
			C	3648	1717	1473	324	134				
				320					0·9435	0·2195	1·2641	1·4858
				χ_1^2 for homogeneity of areas						2·0980		0·8977
ASTHMA AND/OR HAY FEVER												
1. Australia, Melbourne	(s) S	Denborough & Downing 1968	P	435	212	166	48	9	0·8877	0·6541	1·3379	1·3897
			C	411	195	172	33	11				
ASTHMA AND/OR HAY FEVER, PRESENT/ABSENT												
1. U.S.A., Seattle	Whites; (s) S, A_1A_2	Vanarsdel & Motulsky 1959	Present	*926*	*383*	*416*	*95*	*32*	*1·0723*	*0·8128*	*0·9922*	*0·0040*
			Absent	*4731*	*2016*	*2042*	*504*	*169*				

TABLE 1 **THE ABO BLOOD GROUP SYSTEM** (*cont.*)

Place	Additional details	Authors		Number	O	A	B	AB	A/O Relative incidence	A/O χ_1^2 for difference from unity	B/O Relative incidence	B/O χ_1^2 for difference from unity
ALLERGIES (*cont.*)												
UNSPECIFIED OR MIXED ALLERGIES												
1. Germany, Berlin	Other than eczema; (s) A_1A_2	Dorn 1959	P	176	60	72	36	8	0·9980	0·0001	1·2923	0·8020
			C	250	84	101	39	26				
2. Egypt, Cairo	Asthma, eczema migraine, rhinitis, urticaria	el-Mehairy & el-Tarabishi 1966	P	500	154	157	118	71	0·9364	0·3213	1·0263	0·0431
			C	10045	3279	3570	2448	748				
3. Mexico, Distrito Federal	Mestizos	Salázar-Mallén *et al.* 1969	P	100	61	29	9	1	1·1885	0·2848	1·1988	0·1227
			C	100	65	26	8	1				
				776					0·9687	0·1042	1·0709	0·3744
				χ_2^2 for homogeneity of areas						0·5020		0·5934

TABLE 1.1
THE ABO BLOOD GROUP SYSTEM
COMPARISON BETWEEN A_1 AND A_2

	Place	Additional details	Authors		Number	A_1	A_2	A_1/A_2 Relative incidence	A_1/A_2 χ_1^2 for difference from unity
LEPROSY									
Lepromatous	1. Brazil, Curitiba	Whites	Salzano *et al.* 1967	P	224(c)	69	17	0·9020	0·0471
				C	120(c)	36	8		
	2. Brazil, Florianópolis	Whites	Salzano *et al.* 1967	P	168(c)	56	14	0·7347	0·4297
				C	119(c)	48	9		
	3. Brazil, Pôrto Alegre	Whites	Salzano *et al.* 1967	P	329(c)	110	29	0·7457	0·9012
				C	333(c)	117	23		
					721			0·7760	1·2477
					χ_2^2 homogeneity for areas				0·1303
Tuberculoid	1. Brazil, Curitiba	Whites	Salzano *et al.* 1967	P	32(c)	11	0		
				C	120(c)	36	8		
	2. Brazil, Florianópolis	Whites	Salzano *et al.* 1967	P	20(c)	10	1	1·8750	0·3208
				C	119(c)	48	9		
	3. Brazil, Pôrto Alegre	Whites	Salzano *et al.* 1967	P	65(c)	22	7	0·6178	0·9648
				C	333(c)	117	23		
					85			0·7406	0·4484
					χ_1^2 for homogeneity of areas				0·8372

TABLE 1.1 **THE ABO BLOOD GROUP SYSTEM:** COMPARISON BETWEEN A_1 AND A_2 (*cont.*)

	Place	Additional details	Authors		Number	A_1	A_2	A_1/A_2 Relative incidence	χ_1^2 for difference from unity
DIABETES MELLITUS	1. Germany, Hamburg-Eppendorf		Sauer *et al.* 1963	P	1709	611	157	1·2359	3·6536
				C	3086	973	309		
	2. Norway, Oslo		Berg, K. *et al.* 1967	P	176	74	17	0·8358	0·4168
				C	3089	1276	245		
					1885			1·1713	2·3607
				χ_1^2 for homogeneity of areas					1·7097
RHEUMATIC FEVER	1. U.S.A., Iowa		Buckwalter *et al.* 1962*	P	540	202	47	0·8030	1·2123
				C	1355	471	88		
	2. U.S.A., Michigan	Whites	Gershowitz & Neel 1965	P	104	34	6	1·7574	1·5509
				C	1508	474	147		
	3. Australia, Sydney		Walsh & Kooptzoff 1956	P	259	92	22	1·1930	0·4463
				C	1123	333	95		
					903			0·9944	0·0014
				χ_2^2 for homogeneity of areas					3·2081
GASTRIC ULCERS	1. Czechoslovakia, Praha		Kubičková & Veselý 1966	P	406	158	23	1·2049	0·5330
				C	1142	439	77		
	2. U.S.A., Iowa		Newman *et al.* 1961	P	184	43	11	0·8113	0·3419
				C	1261	424	88		
	3. U.S.A., Iowa		Buckwalter 1962*	P	349	101	15	1·2580	0·5898
				C	1355	471	88		
					939			1·1168	0·4193
				χ_2^2 for homogeneity of areas					1·0454
DUODENAL ULCERS	1. Austria, Wien		Weiser 1957	P	449	139	33	0·7708	1·7288
				C	10000	3738	684		
	2. Czechoslovakia, Praha		Kubičková & Veselý 1972*	P	934	298	58	0·9012	0·3018
				C	1142	439	77		
	3. Germany, Tübingen		Dick *et al.* 1962	P	489	155	22	1·4794	2·9333
				C	39031	13839	2906		
	4. U.S.A., Iowa		Newman *et al.* 1961	P	479	140	23	1·2633	0·8492
				C	1261	424	88		
					2351			1·0181	0·0284
				χ_3^2 for homogeneity of areas					5·7847
DOWN'S SYNDROME	1. United Kingdom, London		Lang-Brown *et al.* 1952–3	P	148	47	6	2·2251	3·3369
				C	3459	1204	342		
	2. U.S.A., Michigan and Ohio		Shaw & Gershowitz 1962*	P	370	131	39	1·0417	0·0395
				C	1508	474	147		
	3. U.S.A., Michigan		Shaw & Gershowitz 1963	P	207	75	19	1·2242	0·5461
				C	1508	474	147		
					725			1·2038	1·4541
				χ_2^2 for homogeneity of areas					2·4684

* A's tested for A_1 and A_2 represent only a part of those quoted in Table 1.

TABLE 2
THE MN BLOOD GROUP SYSTEM

	Place	Additional details	Authors		Number	MM	MN	NN	MM/MN+NN Relative incidence	χ_1^2 for difference from unity
INFECTIVE AND PARASITIC DISEASES										
BACTERIAL INFECTIONS										
TUBERCULOSIS										
Pulmonary	1. Czechoslovakia, Praha	Males; (s) A	Miluničová & Dominec 1966 Kout 1959 M2	P C	106 1142	38 383	51 563	17 196	1·1074	0·2317
	2. Australia, Sydney	(s) MNS	Kooptzoff & Walsh 1957	P C	470 140	124 39	249 67	97 34	0·9281	0·1197
					576				1·0153	0·0101
				χ_1^2 for homogeneity of areas						0·3412
Sites Unspecified	Belgium, Liège		Moureau & Firket 1934	P C	250(c) 3100(c)	74 895	127 1561	49 644	1·0359	0·0598
LEPROSY										
Lepromatous	1. Philippines, Cebu		Lechat *et al.* 1968	P C	249 429	82 128	124 237	43 64	1·1547	0·7054
	2. Brazil, Curitiba	Whites	Salzano *et al.* 1967	P C	171(c) 120(c)	58 39	82 61	31 20	1·0660	0·0638
	3. Brazil, Florianópolis	Whites	Salzano *et al.* 1967	P C	168(c) 119(c)	45 36	91 62	32 21	0·8435	0·4128
	4. Brazil, Pôrto Alegre	Whites	Salzano *et al.* 1967	P C	100(c) 333(c)	24 102	53 161	23 70	0·7152	1·6297
					688				0·9825	0·0244
				χ_3^2 for homogeneity of areas						2·7873
Tuberculoid	1. Philippines, Cebu		Lechat *et al.* 1968	P C	222 429	76 128	111 237	35 64	1·2241	1·3129
	2. Brazil, Curitiba	Whites	Salzano *et al.* 1967	P C	81(c) 120(c)	20 39	42 61	19 20	0·6810	1·4146
	3. Brazil, Florianópolis	Whites	Salzano *et al.* 1967	P C	20(c) 119(c)	5 36	13 62	2 21	0·7685	0·2262
	4. Brazil, Pôrto Alegre	Whites	Salzano *et al.* 1967	P C	40(c) 333(c)	11 102	20 161	9 70	0·8590	0·1655
					363				1·0167	0·0143
				χ_3^2 for homogeneity of areas						3·1049
Indeterminate	1. Brazil, Curitiba	Whites	Salzano *et al.* 1967	P C	66(c) 120(c)	22 39	25 61	19 20	1·0385	0·0134
	2. Brazil, Florianópolis	Whites	Salzano *et al.* 1967	P C	23(c) 119(c)	5 36	10 62	8 21	0·6404	0·6722
	3. Brazil, Pôrto Alegre	Whites	Salzano *et al.* 1967	P C	11(c) 333(c)	2 102	4 161	5 70	0·5033	0·7540
					100				0·8553	0·3519
				χ_2^2 for homogeneity of areas						1·0878

TABLE 2 THE MN BLOOD GROUP SYSTEM (*cont.*)

	Place	Additional details	Authors		Number	MM	MN	NN	MM/MN+NN Relative incidence	MM/MN+NN χ_1^2 for difference from unity
Unspecified types	1. Moçambique, Nampula	Macua	Spielmann *et al.* 1970	P	126	31	75	20	0·9945	0·0004
				C	170	42	92	36		
	2. New Guinea, Mount Hagen		Simmons *et al.* 1968	P	94	0	8	86		
			MacLennan *et al.* 1960 M2	C	473	0	34	439		
SYPHILIS	1. Belgium, Liège		Moureau & Firket 1934	P	250(c)	75	128	47	1·0559	0·1433
				C	3100	895	1561	644		
	2. India, Dehra Dun, Rourkela		Seth 1969	P	132	53	56	23	0·8518	0·4985
				C	202	89	81	32		
	3. U.S.A., Brooklyn	General paresis	Herman & Derby 1937	P	273	85	130	58	1·0589	0·1674
				C	1905	570	950	385		
					655				1·0208	0·0505
				χ_2^2 for homogeneity of areas						0·7587
WORM INFESTATIONS										
FILARIASIS	S. India, Rourkela		Anand 1965	P	603	262	240	101	0·9402	0·2524
				C	487	219	203	65		
NEOPLASMS										
MALIGNANT NEOPLASMS										
OESOPHAGUS	United Kingdom, London		Walther *et al.* 1956	P	20	9	10	1	1·9632	2·2072
			Ikin *et al.* 1952 M2	C	1166	343	567	256		
STOMACH	1. United Kingdom, London		Walther *et al.* 1956	P	86	32	35	19	1·4219	2·2985
			Ikin *et al.* 1952 M2	C	1166	343	567	256		
	2. Japan	Japanese	Desai & Creger 1964	P	233	72	125	36	1·0001	0·0000
			Furuhata *et al.* 1954 M2	C	46449	14352	22714	9383		
	3. U.S.A.	Whites	Desai & Creger 1964	P	105	38	55	12	1·8159	6·8089
			Wiener 1969 M2	C	500	119	242	139		
	4. U.S.A., Iowa		Buckwalter & Tweed 1962	P	170	40	104	26	0·8382	0·8900
				C	2186	587	1208	391		
					594				1·1180	1·4398
				χ_3^2 for homogeneity of areas						8·5576
CAECUM, COLON, RECTUM	United Kingdom, London		Walther *et al.* 1956	P	182	52	95	35	0·9598	0·0543
			Ikin *et al.* 1952 M2	C	1166	343	567	256		
BILE DUCTS, GALL-BLADDER	United Kingdom, London		Walther *et al.* 1956	P	18	4	7	7	0·6855	0·4378
			Ikin *et al.* 1952 M2	C	1166	343	567	256		
PANCREAS	United Kingdom, London		Walther *et al.* 1956	P	13	5	5	3	1·4996	0·4989
			Ikin *et al.* 1952 M2	C	1166	343	567	256		
VOCAL CORDS, LARYNX	United Kingdom, London		Walther *et al.* 1956	P	10	6	2	2	3·5991	3·8978
			Ikin *et al.* 1952 M2	C	1166	343	567	256		
LUNG	Czechoslovakia, Praha		Jakoubková & Májský 1965	P	63	18	37	8	0·7927	0·6606
				C	1142	383	563	196		
BRONCHUS	United Kingdom, London		Walther *et al.* 1956	P	182	57	96	29	1·0941	0·2727
			Ikin *et al.* 1952 M2	C	1166	343	567	256		
RODENT ULCER, EPITHELIOMA	United Kingdom, London		Walther *et al.* 1956	P	20	5	13	2	0·7998	0·1843
			Ikin *et al.* 1952 M2	C	1166	343	567	256		

TABLE 2 THE MN BLOOD GROUP SYSTEM (*cont.*)

	Place	Additional details	Authors		Number	MM	MN	NN	MM/MN+NN Relative incidence	MM/MN+NN χ_1^2 for difference from unity
NEOPLASMS (*cont.*)										
MALIGNANT NEOPLASMS (*cont.*)										
Breast	1. Czechoslovakia, Praha		Jakoubková & Májský 1965	P	76	21	39	16	0·7567	1·1151
				C	1142	383	563	196		
	2. Finland, Helsinki	(s) MNS	Morosini *et al.* 1972	P	199	78	92	29	0·9124	0·3852
				C	5536	2292	2530	714		
	3. United Kingdom, London		Walther *et al.* 1956	P	136	33	63	40	0·7687	1·5669
			Ikin *et al.* 1952 M2	C	1166	343	567	256		
	4. United Kingdom, Oxford		Morosini *et al.* 1972	P	100	24	56	20	0·8538	0·2367
				C	100	27	50	23		
	5. U.S.A., Boston	Whites	Boston Collaborative Drug Surveillance Programme 1971	P	150	44	81	25	0·9533	0·0570
			Dublin *et al.* 1964	C	600	182	305	113		
					661				0·8662	2·4209
				χ_4^2 for homogeneity of areas						0·9399
Cervix Uteri	Czechoslovakia		Milunič ová *et al.* 1969[a]	P	85	29	35	21	1·0262	0·0119
			Kout 1959 M2	C	1142	383	563	196		
Corpus Uteri	Czechoslovakia		Miluničová *et al.* 1969	P	142	47	78	17	0·9804	0·0109
			Kout 1959 M2	C	1142	383	563	196		
Uterus incl. Cervix	United Kingdom, London		Walther *et al.* 1956	P	44	13	21	10	1·0062	0·0003
			Ikin *et al.* 1952 M2	C	1166	343	567	256		
Ovary	1. Czechoslovakia		Miluničová *et al.* 1969	P	50	12	26	12	0·6258	1·9343
			Kout 1959 M2	C	1142	383	563	196		
	2. United Kingdom, London		Walther *et al.* 1956	P	31	11	13	7	1·3197	0·5305
			Ikin *et al.* 1952 M2	C	1166	343	567	256		
					81				0·8684	0·3123
				χ_1^2 for homogeneity of areas						2·1525
Prostate	United Kingdom, London		Walther *et al.* 1956	P	44	14	23	7	1·1197	0·1174
			Ikin *et al.* 1952 M2	C	1166	343	567	256		
Kidney	United Kingdom, London		Walther *et al.* 1956	P	17	6	9	2	1·3088	0·2767
			Ikin *et al.* 1952 M2	C	1166	343	567	256		
Bladder	United Kingdom, London		Walther *et al.* 1956	P	25	5	14	6	0·5999	1·0278
			Ikin *et al.* 1952 M2	C	1166	343	567	256		
NEOPLASMS OF NERVOUS SYSTEM										
Brain Cancer	United Kingdom, London		Walther *et al.* 1956	P	13	4	7	2	1·0664	0·0113
			Ikin *et al.* 1952 M2	C	1166	343	567	256		
NEOPLASMS OF LYMPHATIC AND HAEMATOPOIETIC TISSUE										
Hodgkin's Disease	1. Italy, Cagliari		Adamo 1961[a, c]	P	10	2	8	0	0·2130	3·7083
			Aru 1951 M2	C	200	108	78	14		
	2. Netherlands, Leiden	(s) MNS	Does *et al.* 1972	P	45	19	13	13	3·6538	6·3958
				C	42	7	28	7		
	3. United Kingdom, London		Walther *et al.* 1956	P	10	4	5	1	1·5996	0·5244
			Ikin *et al.* 1952 M2	C	1166	343	567	256		
	4. United Kingdom, London		Kay & Shorter 1956	P	49	15	26	8	1·0586	0·0323
			Ikin *et al.* 1952 M2	C	1166	343	567	256		
					114				1·2693	1·0068
				χ_3^2 for homogeneity of areas						9·6541

TABLE 2 THE MN BLOOD GROUP SYSTEM (*cont.*)

	Place	Additional details	Authors		Number	MM	MN	NN	MM/MN+NN Relative incidence	MM/MN+NN χ_1^2 for difference from unity
LYMPHOSARCOMA	Italy, Cagliari		Adamo 1961[a, c]	P	17	12	5	0	2·0444	1·6852
			Aru 1951 M2	C	200	108	78	14		
MYELOID LEUKAEMIA	1. Italy, Cagliari	Acute	Adamo 1961[a, c]	P	9	8	1	0	6·8148	3·2161
			Aru 1951 M2	C	200	108	78	14		
	2. Italy, Cagliari	Chronic	Adamo 1961[a, c]	P	10	7	2	1	1·9877	0·9508
			Aru 1951 M2	C	200	108	78	14		
	3. United Kingdom, London		Kay & Shorter 1956	P	31	8	16	7	0·8346	0·1894
			Ikin *et al.* 1952 M2	C	1166	343	567	256		
					50				1·2613	0·4671
				χ_2^2 for homogeneity of areas						3·8892
LEUKAEMIAS, UNSPECIFIED	1. United Kingdom, London		Walther *et al.* 1956	P	44	7	30	7	0·4539	3·5845
			Ikin *et al.* 1952 M2	C	1166	343	567	256		
	2. U.S.A., Michigan	Whites	Gershowitz & Neel 1965	P	170	41	95	34	0·7592	2·1478
				C	1508	445	750	313		
	3. Brazil, Rio Grande do Sul	Whites	Ayres *et al.* 1966	P	51(c)	11	36	4	0·6228	1·7244
				C	333(c)	102	161	70		
					265				0·6820	6·1154
				χ_2^2 for homogeneity of areas						1·3413
ILL-DEFINED MALIGNANT NEOPLASMS										
SARCOMAS	United Kingdom, London		Walther *et al.* 1956	P	20	8	9	3	1·5996	1·0386
			Ikin *et al.* 1952 M2	C	1166	343	567	256		
CANCERS	Belgium, Liège		Moureau & Firket 1934	P	200(c)	57	102	41	0·9820	0·0126
				C	3100(c)	895	1561	644		
CANCERS OTHER THAN BREAST AND LUNG	Czechoslovakia, Praha		Jakoubková & Májský 1965	P	79	25	43	11	0·9175	0·1188
				C	1142	383	563	196		
ENDOCRINE AND METABOLIC DISEASES										
DIABETES MELLITUS	1. Czechoslovakia, Praha	(s) A	Miluničová & Dominec 1966	P	121	42	60	19	1·0536	0·0674
			Kout 1959 M2	C	1142	383	563	196		
	2. Norway, Oslo		Berg, K. *et al.* 1967	P	180	49	90	41	0·9571	0·0649
				C	3089	868	1565	656		
	3. Poland, Wrocław	Juveniles	Wartenberg & Wąsikowa 1971	P	145	44	74	27	0·8063	1·0044
				C	325	114	160	51		
	4. United Kingdom, Oxford	(s) A, S	McConnell *et al.* 1956	P	500	123	265	112	0·7828	4·0212
			Ikin *et al.* 1952 M2	C	1166	343	567	256		
	5. United Kingdom, Belfast	(s) A, S	Macafee 1962	P	453	135	231	87	1·0047	0·0006
				C	202	60	102	40		
	6. Canada, Toronto		Simpson *et al.* 1962	P	101	28	44	29	0·9679	0·0200
				C	1279	363	634	282		
	7. U.S.A., Iowa		Buckwalter & Tweed 1962	P	1153	302	614	237	0·9667	0·1684
				C	2186	587	1208	391		
					2653				0·9248	2·0884
				χ_6^2 for homogeneity of areas						3·2585
HAEMOCHROMATOSIS	Australia, Sydney	(s) MNS	Bradley & Walsh 1965	P	54	18	27	9	1·2949	0·5617
			Kooptzoff & Walsh 1957	C	140	39	67	34		

TABLE 2 **THE MN BLOOD GROUP SYSTEM** *(cont.)*

	Place	Additional details	Authors		Number	MM	MN	NN	MM/MN+NN Relative incidence	MM/MN+NN χ_1^2 for difference from unity
DISEASES OF THE BLOOD										
PERNICIOUS ANAEMIA	1. United Kingdom, England	(s) MNS	Callender *et al.* 1957	P	201	49	104	48	0·6286	4·1285
				C	177	60	82	35		
	2. U.S.A., Chicago	Whites	Ladenson *et al.* 1949	P	119	40	55	24	1·2689	1·2304
			Wiener *et al.* 1944 M2	C	582	166	289	127		
	3. U.S.A., Chicago	Negroes	Ladenson *et al.* 1949	P	41	12	20	9	1·1783	0·1912
			Wiener *et al.* 1945 M2	C	227	59	100	68		
					361				0·9480	0·1367
				χ_2^2 for homogeneity of areas						5·4134
MENTAL DISORDERS										
SENILE DEMENTIA	United Kingdom, England		Thomas & Hewitt 1939	P	94	32	41	21	1·1479	0·3179
				C	374	116	181	77		
SCHIZOPHRENIA	1. Czechoslovakia, Bohemia	Paranoid; (s) ABO	Prokop *et al.* 1938	P	356(c)	104	193	59	1·0377	0·0924
			Raška *et al.* 1948 M2	C	4038	1149	2022	867		
	2. Czechoslovakia, Bohemia	Other than paranoid; (s) ABO	Prokop *et al.* 1938	P	711(c)	156	397	158	0·7067	12·7776
			Raška *et al.* 1948 M2	C	4038	1149	2022	867		
	3. Italy, Arezzo		Marzi & Turchini 1952	P	105(c)	34	52	19	0·8816	0·2604
			Chiodi 1949 M2	C	250	88	111	51		
	4. United Kingdom, England		Thomas & Hewitt 1939	P	67	23	32	12	1·1626	0·2885
				C	374	116	181	77		
	5. United Kingdom, England	Delusional insanity	Thomas & Hewitt 1939	P	65	20	31	14	0·9885	0·0016
				C	374	116	181	77		
	6. United Kingdom, Chorley, Leyland, Preston		Masters 1967	P	87	24	47	16	0·9141	0·1309
			Ikin *et al.* 1952 M2	C	1166	343	567	256		
	7. U.S.A., Brooklyn	Catatonic	Herman & Derby 1937	P	209	56	96	57	0·8572	0·8822
				C	1905	570	950	385		
	8. U.S.A., Brooklyn	Paranoid	Herman & Derby 1937	P	218	57	123	38	0·8292	1·3360
				C	1905	570	950	385		
	9. U.S.A., Brooklyn	Simple hebephrenic	Herman & Derby 1937	P	81	30	33	18	1·3777	1·8518
				C	1905	570	950	385		
					1899				0·8754	5·7433
				χ_8^2 for homogeneity of areas						11·8781
MANIC-DEPRESSIVE PSYCHOSES	1. United Kingdom, England		Thomas & Hewitt 1939	P	257	78	126	53	0·9692	0·0317
				C	374	116	181	77		
	2. United Kingdom, Chorley, Leyland, Preston		Masters 1967	P	35	11	17	7	1·0997	0·0661
			Ikin *et al.* 1952 M2	C	1166	343	567	256		
	3. U.S.A., Brooklyn		Herman & Derby 1937	P	188	62	85	41	1·1525	0·7579
				C	1905	570	950	385		
					480				1·0671	0·3264
				χ_2^2 for homogeneity of areas						0·5293
DYSTHYMIA	Italy, Arezzo		Marzi & Turchini 1952	P	95	33	44	18	0·9798	0·0065
			Chiodi 1949 M2	C	250	88	111	51		
INVOLUTIONAL PSYCHOSES	U.S.A., Brooklyn		Herman & Derby 1937	P	160	49	84	27	1·0339	0·0348
				C	1905	570	950	385		
ALCOHOLISM	U.S.A., Brooklyn		Herman & Derby 1937	P	78	18	40	20	0·7026	1·6668
				C	1905	570	950	385		
PHRENASTHENIA	Italy, Arezzo		Marzi & Turchini 1952	P	100(c)	32	48	20	0·8663	0·3244
			Chiodi 1949 M2	C	250	88	111	51		
MENTAL DISEASES, UNSPECIFIED	Belgium, Liège		Moureau & Firket 1934	P	250(c)	81	121	48	1·1808	1·3931
				C	3100(c)	895	1561	644		

TABLE 2 THE MN BLOOD GROUP SYSTEM (*cont.*)

	Place	Additional details	Authors		Number	MM	MN	NN	MM/MN+NN Relative incidence	MM/MN+NN χ^2_1 for difference from unity
DISEASES OF THE NERVOUS SYSTEM										
MULTIPLE SCLEROSIS	1. Germany, Essen	(s) MNSs	Bertrams & Kuwert 1976	P	802	250	403	149	0·9580	0·1770
				C	1000	321	488	191		
	2. United Kingdom, Newcastle upon Tyne		MacDonald *et al.* 1976	P	136	31	67	38	0·7086	1·5375
				C	136	40	61	35		
	3. United Kingdom, Newcastle upon Tyne		Roberts 1976	P	188	66	77	45	1·2984	1·1625
				C	136	40	61	35		
					1126				0·9677	0·1359
				χ^2_2 for homogeneity of areas						2·7411
EPILEPSY	1. U.S.A., Brooklyn	With psychosis	Herman & Derby 1937	P	35	9	15	11	0·8107	0·2895
				C	1905	570	950	385		
	2. Australia	Whites	Simmons *et al.* 1944	P	22	6	13	3	0·8505	0·1121
				C	1000	306	477	217		
					57				0·8262	0·3957
				χ^2_1 for homogeneity of areas						0·0059
KURU	1. New Guinea, Eastern Highlands	North Fore	Simmons *et al.* 1972	P	94	0	11	83		
				C	428	1	17	410		
	2. New Guinea, Eastern Highlands	South Fore	Simmons *et al.* 1972	P	158	0	11	147		
				C	1086	2	65	1019		
	3. New Guinea, Eastern Highlands	Other than Fore	Simmons *et al.* 1972	P	48	0	5	43		
				C	1168	3	99	1066		
	4. New Guinea, Eastern Highlands	Fore	Simmons *et al.* 1961	P	192	0	15	177		
				C	356	0	18	338		
					492					
AMYOTROPHIC LATERAL SCLEROSIS	U.S.A., Maryland		Myrianthopoulos & Leyshon 1967	P	346	104	163	79	1·1191	0·4499
				C	346	96	182	68		
DISEASES OF THE CIRCULATORY SYSTEM										
RHEUMATIC FEVER	1. U.S.A., Boston		Dublin *et al.* 1964	P	606	200	293	113	1·1314	0·9927
				C	600	182	305	113		
	2. U.S.A., Iowa		Buckwalter *et al.* 1962	P	540	128	284	128	0·8463	2·2159
				C	2186	587	1208	391		
	3. U.S.A., Michigan	Whites	Gershowitz & Neel 1965	P	104	25	52	27	0·7559	1·4018
				C	1508	445	750	313		
	4. Australia, Sydney		Walsh & Kooptzoff 1956	P	260	88	123	49	1·3250	1·5020
				C	140	39	67	34		
					1510				0·9733	0·1327
				χ^2_3 for homogeneity of areas						5·9797
HYPERTENSION	Czechoslovakia		Mikolášek & Miluničová 1967	P	383	138	171	74	1·3973	9·6960
				C	23000	6608	11732	4660		
CORONARY OCCLUSION WITHOUT INFARCTION	Poland, Kraków		Jaegermann 1964	P	87	30	41	16	0·9659	0·0236
			Socha 1966	C	15599	5502	7558	2539		
MYOCARDIAL INFARCTION	1. Poland, Kraków	Post-mortem	Jaegermann 1964	P	104	37	56	11	1·0134	0·0041
			Socha 1966	C	15599	5502	7558	2539		
	2. Israel; born in Austria, Hungary, Romania	Jewish men over 40; (s) G	Medalie *et al.* 1971	P	74(a)	22	38	14	0·8813	0·2365
				C	1631	529	787	315		

TABLE 2 THE MN BLOOD GROUP SYSTEM (*cont.*)

	Place	Additional details	Authors		Number	MM	MN	NN	MM/MN+NN Relative incidence	MM/MN+NN χ_1^2 for difference from unity
DISEASES OF THE CIRCULATORY SYSTEM (*cont.*)										
MYOCARDIAL INFARCTION (*cont.*)										
	3. Israel; born in Germany	Jewish men over 40	Medalie *et al.* 1971	P	25(a)	4	14	7	0·4595	1·9660
				C	488	143	240	105		
	4. Israel; born in Poland	Jewish men over 40	Medalie *et al.* 1971	P	63(a)	26	29	8	1·5894	3·0999
				C	1233	378	607	248		
	5. Israel; born in Bulgaria, Jugoslavia	Jewish men over 40; (s) G	Medalie *et al.* 1971	P	17(a)	8	6	3	2·0019	1·9373
				C	374	115	188	71		
	6. Israel; born in U.S.S.R.	Jewish men over 40	Medalie *et al.* 1971	P	36(a)	12	20	4	0·9275	0·0427
				C	551	193	264	94		
	7. Israel; born in Turkey, Israel, Syria	Jewish men over 40; (s) G	Medalie *et al.* 1971	P	85(a)	28	40	17	0·9176	0·1327
				C	1804	629	826	349		
	8. Israel; born in Iraq	Jewish men over 40	Medalie *et al.* 1971	P	38(a)	12	14	12	0·9035	0·0818
				C	1118	378	502	238		
	9. Israel; born in Egypt	Jewish men over 40	Medalie *et al.* 1971	P	17(a)	6	5	6	1·0220	0·0018
				C	523	182	251	90		
	10. Israel; born in Morocco	Jewish men over 40	Medalie *et al.* 1971	P	12(a)	4	7	1	0·7278	0·2622
				C	415	169	190	56		
					471				1·0175	0·0300
				χ_9^2 for homogeneity of areas						7·7350
CEREBRAL ARTERIOSCLEROSIS	U.S.A., Brooklyn	With psychosis	Herman & Derby 1937	P	224	62	112	50	0·8964	0·4826
				C	1905	570	950	385		
DISEASES OF THE DIGESTIVE SYSTEM										
ULCERATIVE COLITIS	U.S.A., Connecticut	(s) MNSs	Thayer & Bove 1965	P	169	62	80	27	1·2542	1·4775
			Wiener 1969 M2	C	500	158	249	93		
GASTRIC ULCER	U.S.A., Iowa		Buckwalter & Tweed 1962	P	348	90	199	59	0·9502	0·1504
				C	2186	587	1208	391		
DUODENAL ULCER	1. United Kingdom, Chorley, Leyland, Preston		Masters 1967	P	26	11	11	4	1·7596	1·9746
			Ikin *et al.* 1952 M2	C	1166	343	567	256		
	2. U.S.A., Iowa		Buckwalter & Tweed 1962	P	1030	273	581	176	0·9824	0·0432
				C	2186	587	1208	391		
					1056				1·0075	0·0079
				χ_1^2 for homogeneity of areas						2·0099
DISEASES OF THE GENITO-URINARY SYSTEM										
NEPHRITIS-NEPHROSIS	U.S.A., Michigan	Whites	Gershowitz & Neel 1965	P	70	27	35	8	1·4999	2·5891
				C	1508	445	750	313		
RENAL LITHIASIS	N. India		Anand 1964[a]	P	187	80	87	20	1·0681	0·0988
				C	187	77	90	20		
MENOPAUSAL METRORRHAGIA	Czechoslovakia		Miluničová *et al.* 1969[a]	P	170	68	67	35	1·3211	2·7274
			Kout 1959 M2	C	1142	383	563	196		
DISEASES OF THE SKIN										
PSORIASIS	1. Germany, Giessen, Kassel, Marburg		Wendt 1968	P	401	148	184	69	1·4497	8·2041
				C	800	230	417	153		
	2. Italy, Napoli		Villano & Santoianni 1972	P	40	18	16	6	1·9091	1·9001
				C	40	12	20	8		
	3. Sweden, Northern	(s) MNSs	Beckman *et al.* 1974	P	115	48	46	21	1·3817	2·0392
				C	287	98	137	52		
					556				1·4552	11·7548
				χ_2^2 for homogeneity of areas						0·3885

TABLE 2 **THE MN BLOOD GROUP SYSTEM** (*cont.*)

	Place	Additional details	Authors		Number	MM	MN	NN	MM/MN+NN Relative incidence	MM/MN+NN χ_1^2 for difference from unity
DISEASES OF THE MUSCULOSKELETAL SYSTEM										
ARTICULAR RHEUMATISM, ACUTE	France, Paris		Pham-Huu-Trung *et al.* 1961	P	222	72	106	44	0·9309	0·0771
				C	97	33	47	17		
ANKYLOSING SPONDYLITIS	Norway, Oslo		Kornstad *et al.* 1968	P	200	63	101	36	1·0649	0·1685
				C	16542	4989	8115	3438		
CONGENITAL ANOMALIES										
HYDROCEPHALUS	U.S.A., Michigan	Whites	Gershowitz & Neel 1965	P	145	36	82	27	0·7889	1·4000
				C	1508	445	750	313		
CONGENITAL HEART DISEASE	1. U.S.A., Cook County	Negro children	Lev *et al.* 1967	P	580	136	280	164	0·6892	3·0309
				C	130	40	53	37		
	2. U.S.A., Michigan	Whites	Gershowitz & Neel 1965	P	122	39	63	20	1·1224	0·3263
				C	1508	445	750	313		
					702				0·8916	0·6101
					χ_1^2 for homogeneity of areas					2·7472
OSTEOGENESIS IMPERFECTA	Sweden		Smårs *et al.* 1961	P	152	48	80	24	0·8871	0·2859
				C	225	77	108	40		
DOWN'S SYNDROME	1. Germany, Hamburg		Manitz 1932	P	26	2	18	6	0·2009	4·7516
			Hoppe 1957 M2	C	10000	2932	5008	2060		
	2. United Kingdom, London	(s) MNS	Lang-Brown *et al.* 1952–3	P	144	41	72	31	1·0097	0·0022
				C	580	164	292	124		
	3. U.S.A., Michigan	(s) MNS	Shaw & Gershowitz 1962	P	370	102	186	82	0·7828	1·9706
				C	269	88	127	54		
	4. U.S.A., Michigan	(s) MNSs	Shaw & Gershowitz 1963	P	206	61	96	49	0·8653	0·5211
			Shaw & Gershowitz 1962	C	269	88	127	54		
	5. Australia	Whites	Simmons *et al.* 1944	P	24	7	12	5	0·9339	0·0227
				C	1000	306	477	217		
					770				0·8459	2·4627
					χ_4^2 for homogeneity of areas					4·8055
ALLERGIES										
ECZEMA	Germany, Berlin		Dorn 1959	P	192	73	96	23	1·1908	0·7638
				C	250	85	126	39		
ASTHMA	1. Italy, Cagliari	Bronchial	Adamo 1961[b]	P	50	30	16	4	1·2778	0·5807
			Aru 1951 M2	C	200	108	78	14		
	2. N. India, Delhi		Anand 1964[b]	P	545	263	197	85	1·0380	0·1006
				C	617	292	245	80		
					595				1·0638	0·3132
					χ_1^2 for homogeneity of areas					0·3681
ALLERGIES OTHER THAN ECZEMA	Germany, Berlin		Dorn 1959	P	176	58	91	27	0·9541	0·0506
				C	250	85	126	39		
ALLERGIES, UNSPECIFIED	Mexico, Distrito Federal	Mestizos	Salázar-Mallén *et al.* 1969	P	100	44	39	17	0·7549	0·9808
				C	100	51	44	5		

TABLE 3
THE RHESUS BLOOD GROUP SYSTEM

	Place	Additional details	Authors		Number	D+	D−	D+/D− Relative incidence	D+/D− χ_1^2 for difference from unity
INFECTIVE AND PARASITIC DISEASES									
BACTERIAL INFECTIONS									
TYPHOID FEVER	Poland, Warszawa	Children	Paciorkiewicz 1970	P	445(c)	326	119	0·5729	24·7874
				C	6626(c)	5480	1146		
PARATYPHOID FEVER	Poland, Warszawa	A, B, and C; children	Paciorkiewicz 1970	P	237(c)	175	62	0·5903	12·1368
				C	6626(c)	5480	1146		
BACILLARY DYSENTERY	Poland, Warszawa	Children	Paciorkiewicz 1970	P	124(c)	99	25	0·8281	0·6952
				C	6626(c)	5480	1146		
GONORRHOEA	United Kingdom, Newcastle upon Tyne	(s) S	Schofield 1966	P	374	299	75	0·9099	0·5290
			Kopeć 1970	C	36621	29816	6805		
WHOOPING COUGH	Poland, Warszawa	Children	Paciorkiewicz 1970	P	684(c)	551	133	0·8664	1·9806
				C	6626(c)	5480	1146		
DIPHTHERIA	Poland, Warszawa	Children	Paciorkiewicz 1970	P	672(c)	550	122	0·9428	0·3137
				C	6626(c)	5480	1146		
SCARLET FEVER	Poland, Warszawa	Children	Paciorkiewicz 1970	P	697(c)	566	131	0·9035	0·9840
				C	6626(c)	5480	1146		
STAPHYLOCOCCI, CARRIERS/NON-CARRIERS	United Kingdom, London	Male surgical patients	White & Shooter 1962	+	*596(c)*	*488*	*108*	*1·0269*	*0·0274*
				−	*459(c)*	*374*	*85*		
TETANUS	Poland, Warszawa	Children	Paciorkiewicz 1970	P	57(c)	47	10	0·9829	0·0024
				C	6626(c)	5480	1146		
TUBERCULOSIS									
Pulmonary Tuberculosis	1. Czechoslovakia, Praha	Males; (s) A	Miluničová & Dominec 1966	P	106	87	19	1·0360	0·0175
			Miluničová & Sottner 1965 M2	C	878	716	162		
	2. Denmark, Köbenhavn		Viskum 1973	P	609	512	97	1·0129	0·0129
			Andersen 1955	C	14304	12001	2303		
	3. United Kingdom, Glasgow	(s) S	Campbell 1956	P	400	330	70	0·9613	0·0840
				C	5898	4899	999		
	4. N. India, Patiala		Sanghvi *et al.* 1974	P	500	457	43	0·3999	27·9426
			Jolly *et al.* 1969 M2	C	6204	5979	225		
	5. Australia, Sydney		Kooptzoff & Walsh 1967	P	470	390	80	1·1684	0·6647
				C	300	242	58		
					2085			0·8783	3·4846
				χ_4^2 for homogeneity of areas					25·2370
Tuberculous Meningitis	Poland, Warszawa	Children	Paciorkiewicz 1970	P	38(c)	28	10	0·5855	2·0944
				C	6626(c)	5480	1146		
Tuberculosis of Bones and Joints	United Kingdom, Glasgow	(s) S	Campbell 1956	P	87	63	24	0·5353	6·6485
				C	5898	4899	999		
Tuberculosis of Genito-Urinary System	United Kingdom, Glasgow		Campbell 1956	P	122	90	32	0·5735	7·0947
				C	5898	4899	999		
Tuberculosis, Sites Unspecified	Germany, Göttingen		Jörgensen & Kallenbach 1968	P	1034	865	169	0·8890	1·6530
				C	6122	5216	906		

TABLE 3 THE RHESUS BLOOD GROUP SYSTEM (*cont.*)

	Place	Additional details	Authors		Number	D+	D−	D+/D− Relative incidence	D+/D− χ_1^2 for difference from unity
SARCOIDOSIS	1. Denmark, København		Viskum 1973	P	52	46	6	1·4712	0·7891
			Andersen 1955	C	14304	12001	2303		
	2. Germany, Göttingen		Jörgensen & Kallenbach 1968	P	495	416	79	0·9147	0·4865
				C	6122	5216	906		
	3. United Kingdom, London		Citron 1956	P	65	54	11	1·0016	0·0000
				C	419	348	71		
	4. United Kingdom, London		Cudkowicz 1956	P	32	11	21	0·1096	33·5983
				C	1000	827	173		
	5. United Kingdom, London		Smellie 1956	P	80	68	12	1·1987	0·3327
			Discombe 1954 M2	C	10000	8254	1746		
					724			0·8324	3·0742
				χ_4^2 for homogeneity of areas					32·1323
LEPROSY									
Lepromatous	1. Philippines, Cebu		Lechat *et al.* 1968	P	250	245	5	0·3451	2·0974
				C	429	426	3		
	2. Ghana		Yankah 1965	P	196	183	13	0·9385	0·0323
				C	400	375	25		
	3. Senegal, Dakar	Mainly Bambara	Languillon *et al.* 1973	P	135	129	6	2·8043	2·9307
				C	52	46	6		
	4. Brazil	White Brazilians	Beiguelman 1963	P	441(c)	405	36	1·6470	5·0109
			Salzano *et al.* 1967	C	462	403	59		
	5. Brazil	Of Italian origin	Beiguelman 1963	P	525(c)	474	51	1·3607	2·3052
			Salzano *et al.* 1967	C	462	403	59		
	6. Brazil	Of Portuguese origin	Beiguelman 1963	P	92(c)	86	6	2·0984	2·7789
			Salzano *et al.* 1967	C	462	403	59		
	7. Brazil	Of Spanish origin	Beiguelman 1963	P	100(c)	88	12	1·0736	0·0443
			Salzano *et al.* 1967	C	462	403	59		
	8. Brazil	Whites of mixed Brazilian, Italian, Portuguese, or Spanish origin	Beiguelman 1963	P	203(c)	182	21	1·2688	0·7819
			Salzano *et al.* 1967	C	462	403	59		
	9. Brazil	Whites of other origin than those mentioned	Beiguelman 1963	P	89(c)	75	14	0·7843	0·5666
			Salzano *et al.* 1963	C	462	403	59		
	10. Brazil, Central	Whites	Cesarino-Netto 1952	P	91	80	11	1·1530	0·1846
			Novais 1953 M2	C	1330	1148	182		
	11. Brazil, Curitiba	Whites	Salzano *et al.* 1967	P	224	192	32	0·9903	0·0009
				C	120	103	17		
	12. Brazil, Florianópolis	Whites	Salzano *et al.* 1967	P	168	135	33	0·5900	2·4417
				C	119	104	15		
	13. Brazil, Pôrto Alegre	Whites	Salzano *et al.* 1967	P	162	139	23	0·8325	0·3620
				C	223	196	27		
					2676			1·1440	2·3964
				χ_{12}^2 for homogeneity of areas					17·1410
Tuberculoid	1. Philippines, Cebu		Lechat *et al.* 1968	P	223	221	2	0·7782	0·0749
				C	429	426	3		
	2. Ghana		Yankah 1965	P	204	190	14	0·9048	0·0839
				C	400	375	25		
	3. Senegal, Dakar	Mainly Bambara	Languillon *et al.* 1973	P	90	85	5	2·2174	1·5847
				C	52	46	6		
	4. Brazil	White Brazilians	Beiguelman 1963	P	135(c)	121	14	1·2653	0·5588
			Salzano *et al.* 1967	C	462	403	59		

TABLE 3 THE RHESUS BLOOD GROUP SYSTEM (*cont.*)

	Place	Additional details	Authors		Number	D+	D−	D+/D− Relative incidence	D+/D− χ_1^2 for difference from unity
INFECTIVE AND PARASITIC DISEASES (*cont.*)									
BACTERIAL INFECTIONS (*cont.*)									
LEPROSY (*cont.*)									
Tuberculoid (*cont.*)									
	5. Brazil	Of Italian origin	Beiguelman 1963 Salzano *et al.* 1967	P C	132(c) 462	118 403	14 59	1·2340	0·4449
	6. Brazil	Of Portuguese origin	Beiguelman 1963 Salzano *et al.* 1967	P C	27(c) 462	25 403	2 59	1·8300	0·6528
	7. Brazil	Of Spanish origin	Beiguelman 1963 Salzano *et al.* 1967	P C	32(c) 462	30 403	2 59	2·1960	1·1196
	8. Brazil	Whites of mixed Brazilian, Italian, Portuguese, or Spanish origin	Beiguelman 1963 Salzano *et al.* 1967	P C	56(c) 462	52 403	4 59	1·9032	1·4345
	9. Brazil	Whites of other origin than those mentioned	Beiguelman 1963 Salzano *et al.* 1967	P C	27(c) 462	25 403	2 59	1·8300	0·6528
	10. Brazil, Curitiba	Whites	Salzano *et al.* 1967	P C	32 120	26 103	6 17	0·7152	0·4105
	11. Brazil, Florianópolis	Whites	Salzano *et al.* 1967	P C	20 119	19 104	1 15	2·7404	0·9002
	12. Brazil, Pôrto Alegre	Whites	Salzano *et al.* 1967	P C	19 223	18 196	1 27	2·4796	0·7512
					997			1·2846	2·9178
				χ_{11}^2 for homogeneity of areas					5·7511
Indeterminate	1. Brazil, Curitiba	Whites	Salzano *et al.* 1967	P C	43 120	38 103	5 17	1·2544	0·1742
	2. Brazil, Florianópolis	Whites	Salzano *et al.* 1967	P C	23 119	20 104	3 15	0·9615	0·0033
	3. Brazil, Pôrto Alegre	Whites	Salzano *et al.* 1967	P C	12 223	12 196	0 27		
					66			1·1399	0·0010
				χ_1^2 for homogeneity of areas					0·1765
Unspecified or Mixed	1. Greece	239 lepromatous, 55 tuberculoid, 6 indeterminate	Markianos *et al.* 1957	P C	300 4851	275 4392	25 459	1·1496	0·4221
	2. Moçambique, Pula	Macua	Spielmann *et al.* 1970	P C	126 171	126 171	0 0		
	3. Venezuela, Aragua	Creoles	Lechat *et al.* 1967	P C	16(c) 163(c)	16 152	0 11		
	4. Venezuela, Aragua	Germans	Lechat *et al.* 1967	P C	53(c) 123(c)	51 116	2 7	1·5388	0·2768
	5. New Guinea, Mount Hagen		Simmons *et al.* 1968	P C	94 473	93 473	1 0		
					353			1·1713	0·5803
				χ_1^2 for homogeneity of areas					0·1186

TABLE 3 THE RHESUS BLOOD GROUP SYSTEM (*cont.*)

	Place	Additional details	Authors		Number	D+	D−	D+/D− Relative incidence	D+/D− χ_1^2 for difference from unity
SYPHILIS									
Cardiovascular	1. United Kingdom, Newcastle upon Tyne	Aortitis and/or aneurysms of aorta; (s) S	Schofield 1966	P	95	72	23	0·7145	1·9643
			Kopeć 1970	C	36621	29816	6805		
	2. United Kingdom, Newcastle upon Tyne	Aortic incompetence; (s) S	Schofield 1966	P	124	99	25	0·9038	0·2035
			Kopeć 1970	C	36621	29816	6805		
					219			0·8100	1·6553
				χ_1^2 for homogeneity of areas					0·5125
Other than cardiovascular	United Kingdom, Newcastle upon Tyne	(s) S	Schofield 1966	P	1207	969	238	0·9292	0·9949
			Kopeć 1970	C	36621	29816	6805		
Mental disorders due to syphilis	Italy, Vercelli		Giuli 1959	P	35	28	7	0·6948	0·7107
				C	1000	852	148		
Unspecified	India, Dehra Dun, Rourkela		Seth 1969	P	132	118	14	1·0302	0·0067
				C	202	180	22		
SEPTICAEMIA	Poland, Warszawa	Children	Paciorkiewicz 1970	P	45(c)	39	6	1·3593	0·4873
				C	6626(c)	5480	1146		
BACTERIAL MENINGITIS	Poland, Warszawa	Children	Paciorkiewicz 1970	P	86(c)	70	16	0·9149	0·1016
				C	6626(c)	5480	1146		
SEPTIC ANGINA	Poland, Warszawa	Children	Paciorkiewicz 1970	P	322(c)	255	67	0·7959	2·6179
				C	6626(c)	5480	1146		
LUNG ABSCESSES	Italy, Milano		Mor & Sforza 1960	P	156	138	18	1·4386	1·6994
				C	500	421	79		
VIRAL INFECTIONS									
POLIOMYELITIS	1. Germany, Schwerin		Kreil 1966	P	317	250	67	0·8844	0·7614
				C	7093	5734	1359		
	2. Poland, Warszawa	Children	Paciorkiewicz 1970	P	187(c)	157	30	1·0944	0·1997
				C	6626(c)	5480	1146		
					504			0·9483	0·2116
				χ_1^2 for homogeneity of areas					0·7496
REACTIONS TO SMALLPOX VACCINATION	Irish Republic, Dublin	Students	Bourke *et al.* 1965	+	*612*	*477*	*135*	*0·8574*	*0·5023*
				−	*169*	*136*	*33*		
CHICKENPOX	Poland, Warszawa	Children	Paciorkiewicz 1970	P	371(c)	295	76	0·8117	2·4716
				C	6626(c)	5480	1146		
MEASLES	Poland, Warszawa	Children	Paciorkiewicz 1970	P	1836(c)	1476	360	0·8574	5·2472
				C	6626(c)	5480	1146		
INFECTIOUS HEPATITIS	1. Czechoslovakia, Praha		Veselý 1969[a]	P	440	382	58	1·2323	1·6499
				C	1142(c)	962	180		
	2. Poland, Warszawa	Children	Paciorkiewicz 1970	P	728(c)	599	129	0·9710	0·0824
				C	6626(c)	5480	1146		
					1168			1·0390	0·1947
				χ_1^2 for homogeneity of areas					1·5376
MUMPS	Poland, Warszawa	Children	Paciorkiewicz 1970	P	403(c)	302	101	0·6253	15·4514
				C	6626(c)	5480	1146		
INFECTIOUS MONONUCLEOSIS	Poland, Warszawa	Children	Paciorkiewicz 1970	P	274(c)	202	72	0·5867	14·2919
				C	6626(c)	5480	1146		
VIRAL MENINGITIS	Poland, Warszawa	Children	Paciorkiewicz 1970	P	129(c)	95	34	0·5843	7·0427
				C	6626(c)	5480	1146		

TABLE 3 **THE RHESUS BLOOD GROUP SYSTEM** (*cont.*)

	Place	Additional details	Authors		Number	D+	D−	D+/D− Relative incidence	D+/D− χ_1^2 for difference from unity
INFECTIVE AND PARASITIC DISEASES (*cont.*)									
WORM INFESTATIONS									
Filariasis	S. India, Rourkela		Anand 1965	P	281	252	29	1·1724	0·4168
				C	429	378	51		
NEOPLASMS									
MALIGNANT NEOPLASMS									
Oesophagus	1. France, Haut-Languedoc		Larrouy 1960	P	129	114	15	1·6920	3·3651
			Khérumian & Lorfeuvre 1966 M2	C	994	813	181		
	2. Italy, Milano		Mor & Sforza 1960	P	70	58	12	0·9070	0·0825
				C	500	421	79		
	3. United Kingdom		Aird *et al.* 1960	P	511	418	93	0·9503	0·1874
			Kopeć 1970	C	10038	8286	1752		
	4. United Kingdom, London, Leytonstone		Walther *et al.* 1956	P	20	16	4	0·8044	0·1498
			Kopeć 1970	C	1953	1626	327		
	5. United Kingdom, Belfast	(s) S, A	Macafee 1962	P	61	47	14	0·6074	2·6611
				C	11363	9622	1741		
					791			0·9619	0·1613
				χ_4^2 for homogeneity of areas					6·2846
Stomach	1. Austria, Wien	(s) S, ABO	Speiser 1956	P	1146	949	197	0·9965	0·0018
				C	10000	8286	1714		
	2. Denmark, Köbenhavn		Jordal 1956	P	334	291	43	1·3488	3·1965
			Gürtler & Henningsen 1954 M2	C	5500	4586	914		
	3. France, Haut-Languedoc		Larrouy 1960	P	182	157	25	1·3981	2·1142
			Khérumian & Lorfeuvre 1966 M2	C	994	813	181		
	4. Iceland		Bjarnason *et al.* 1973	P	323	270	53	0·9134	0·3588
				C	26717	22655	4062		
	5. Italy, Aquila		Curtoni & Morgante 1964	P	170(c)	147	23	0·9877	0·0030
				C	8920(c)	7726	1194		
	6. Italy, Milano		Mor & Sforza 1960	P	470	386	84	0·8623	0·7434
				C	500	421	79		
	7. Poland, Katowice		Machalski *et al.* 1968	P	144	115	29	0·9438	0·0614
				C	567(c)	458	109		
	8. Poland, Lower Silesia		Sagan *et al.* 1957	P	71	58	13	0·8963	0·1233
				C	2397	1996	401		
	9. United Kingdom, London, Leytonstone		Walther *et al.* 1956	P	97	83	14	1·1923	0·3549
			Kopeć 1970	C	1953	1626	327		
	10. United Kingdom, Belfast	(s) S, A	Macafee 1962	P	474	403	71	1·0270	0·0412
				C	11363	9622	1741		
	11. Japan		Desai & Creger 1964	P	236	232	4	0·2272	4·3455
			Furuhata *et al.* 1954 M2	C	1025	1021	4		
	12. U.S.A.	Whites	Desai & Creger 1964	P	105	82	23	0·5901	4·9651
			Tisdall & Garland 1945 M2	C	22133	18990	3143		
	13. U.S.A., Iowa		Buckwalter & Tweed 1962	P	170	135	35	0·7702	1·7362
				C	2181	1818	363		
	14. Brazil, São Paulo		Ribeiro 1963	P	77	71	6	1·2307	0·2341
				C	3588	3250	338		
	15. New Zealand, Auckland		Cotter *et al.* 1961	P	377(c)	316	61	0·9941	0·0017
				C	12428(c)	10427	2001		
					4376			0·9810	0·1828
				χ_{14}^2 for homogeneity of areas					18·0985

TABLE 3 THE RHESUS BLOOD GROUP SYSTEM (*cont.*)

	Place	Additional details	Authors		Number	D+	D−	D+/D− Relative incidence	D+/D− χ^2_1 for difference from unity
COLON	1. Austria, Wien	(s) S, ABO	Speiser 1958[a]	P	204	159	45	0·7599	2·1310
				C	1000	823	177		
	2. Denmark, København		Jordal 1956	P	284	240	44	1·0871	0·2473
			Gürtler & Henningsen 1954 M2	C	5500	4586	914		
	3. France, Haut-Languedoc		Larrouy 1960	P	264	225	39	1·2844	1·7006
			Khérumian & Lorfeuvre 1966 M2	C	994	813	181		
	4. United Kingdom, Belfast	(s) S, A	Macafee 1962	P	361	298	63	0·8559	1·2167
				C	11363	9622	1741		
					1113			0·9596	0·2404
				χ^2_3 for homogeneity of areas					5·0553
RECTUM	1. Austria, Wien	(s) S, ABO	Speiser 1958[a]	P	891	751	140	1·1537	1·3323
				C	1000	823	177		
	2. Denmark, København		Jordal 1956	P	715	614	101	1·2116	2·8689
			Gürtler & Henningsen 1954 M2	C	5500	4586	914		
	3. United Kingdom, Belfast	(s) S, A	Macafee 1962	P	249	202	47	0·7777	2·3504
				C	11363	9622	1741		
					1855			1·0863	1·2351
				χ^2_2 for homogeneity of areas					5·3165
COLON OR RECTUM	1. Italy, Milano		Mor & Sforza 1960	P	168	137	31	0·8293	0·6419
				C	500	421	79		
	2. United Kingdom		Aird *et al.* 1954	P	1129	910	219	0·8786	2·6357
			Kopeć 1970	C	10038	8286	1752		
	3. United Kingdom, London, Leytonstone		Walther *et al.* 1956	P	185	151	34	0·8932	0·3216
			Kopeć 1970	C	1953	1626	327		
					1482			0·8758	3·5333
				χ^2_2 for homogeneity of areas					0·0658
INTESTINES	Iceland		Bjarnason *et al.* 1973	P	108	90	18	0·8965	0·1783
				C	26717	22655	4062		
LIVER	1. France, Haut-Languedoc		Larrouy 1960	P	16	16	0		
			Khérumian & Lorfeuvre 1966 M2	C	994	813	181		
	2. Senegal, Dakar		Sankalé *et al.* 1968	P	120	115	5	1·7302	1·4310
				C	11363	10568	795		
GALL-BLADDER	Austria, Wien	(s) S, ABO	Speiser 1958[a]	P	54	46	8	1·2366	0·2937
				C	1000	823	177		
GALL-BLADDER, BILE DUCTS	United Kingdom, London, Leytonstone		Walther *et al.* 1956	P	18	17	1	3·4188	1·4223
			Kopeć 1970	C	1953	1626	327		
PANCREAS	1. France, Haut-Languedoc		Larrouy 1960	P	31	28	3	2·0779	1·4233
			Khérumian & Lorveuvre 1966 M2	C	994	813	181		
	2. United Kingdom		Aird *et al.* 1960	P	498	416	82	1·0727	0·3219
			Kopeć 1970	C	10038	8286	1752		
	3. United Kingdom, London, Leytonstone		Walther *et al.* 1956	P	13	8	5	0·3218	3·9120
			Kopeć 1970	C	1953	1626	327		
	4. United Kingdom, Belfast	(s) S, A	Macafee 1962	P	117	98	19	0·9333	0·0751
				C	11363	9622	1741		
					659			1·0233	0·0459
				χ^2_3 for homogeneity of areas					5·6864

TABLE 3 **THE RHESUS BLOOD GROUP SYSTEM** (*cont.*)

	Place	Additional details	Authors		Number	D+	D−	D+/D− Relative incidence	D+/D− χ^2_1 for difference from unity
NEOPLASMS (*cont.*)									
MALIGNANT NEOPLASMS (*cont.*)									
LIVER, GALL-BLADDER, BILE DUCTS, PANCREAS	Iceland		Bjarnason *et al.* 1973	P	63	56	7	1·4344	0·8082
				C	26717	22655	4062		
THYROID GLAND	Czechoslovakia	(s) S	Miluničová & Hájek 1966	P	150	129	21	1·1570	0·3433
			Kout 1959 M2	C	1142	961	181		
LARYNX	1. France, Haut-Languedoc		Larrouy 1960	P	36	28	8	0·7792	0·3716
			Khérumian & Lorfeuvre 1966 M2	C	994	813	181		
	2. United Kingdom, London, Leytonstone		Walther *et al.* 1956	P	10	9	1	1·8100	0·3158
			Kopeć 1970	C	1953	1626	327		
					46			0·8699	0·1335
				χ^2_1 for homogeneity of areas					0·5539
BRONCHUS	1. Austria, Wien	(s) S, ABO	Speiser 1958[a]	P	2640	2212	428	1·1115	1·1579
				C	1000	823	177		
	2. Denmark, Köbenhavn		Viskum 1973	P	466	392	74	1·0166	0·0163
			Andersen 1955	C	14304	12001	2303		
	3. United Kingdom		Aird *et al.* 1954	P	636	533	103	1·0942	0·6596
			Kopeć 1970	C	10038	8286	1752		
	4. United Kingdom, London, Leytonstone		Walther *et al.* 1956	P	184	144	40	0·7240	2·9289
			Kopeć 1970	C	1953	1626	327		
					3926			1·0380	0·3808
				χ^2_3 for homogeneity of areas					4·3818
LUNG	1. Czechoslovakia, Praha		Jakoubková & Májský 1965	P	63	51	12	0·8005	0·4523
				C	1142	961	181		
	2. France, Haut-Languedoc		Larrouy 1960	P	117	101	16	1·4054	1·4630
			Khérumian & Lorfeuvre 1966 M2	C	994	813	181		
	3. Italy, Milano		Mor & Sforza 1960	P	354	299	55	1·0201	0·0109
				C	500	421	79		
	4. Italy, Milano	(s) ABO	Orlandi & Tosi 1962	P	300	262	38	0·9287	0·1601
			Vajani 1961 M2	C	2342	2064	278		
	5. Italy, Napoli		Percesepe *et al.* 1959	P	90	82	8	0·8431	0·1759
				C	500	462	38		
	6. United Kingdom, Liverpool B.T.C. Region		McConnell *et al.* 1955	P	716	627	89	1·0056	0·0022
				C	665	5822	831		
	7. United Kingdom, Liverpool		McConnell *et al.* 1954	P	555	486	69	1·5882	9·2208
				C	1000	816	184		
	8. United Kingdom, Swansea		Ashley 1969	P	2019	1699	320	1·0542	0·6248
				C	9652	8053	1599		
	9. United Kingdom, Belfast	(s) S, A	Macafee 1962	P	166	134	32	0·7577	1·9548
				C	11363	9622	1741		
	10. Australia, Sydney		Rennie & Haber 1961	P	218	182	36	0·9465	0·0486
			Lai 1966 M2	C	260	219	41		
					4598			1·0528	1·2268
				χ^2_9 for homogeneity of areas					12·8865
RESPIRATORY SYSTEM	Iceland		Bjarnason *et al.* 1973	P	76	65	11	1·0595	0·0313
				C	26717	22655	4062		
OSTEOMA	Germany, Göttingen		Jörgensen & Kallenbach 1968	P	224	199	25	1·3826	2·2660
				C	6122	5216	906		

TABLE 3 **THE RHESUS BLOOD GROUP SYSTEM** *(cont.)*

	Place	Additional details	Authors		Number	D+	D−	D+/D−: Relative incidence	D+/D−: χ_1^2 for difference from unity
SKIN									
Melanoma	1. Germany, Göttingen		Jörgensen & Kallenbach 1968	P	84	75	9	1·4475	1·0877
				C	6122	5216	906		
Melanoma	2. Germany, Göttingen		Jörgensen & Lal 1972	P	164	146	18	1·3975	1·5159
				C	694	592	102		
Rodent Ulcer, Epithelioma	3. United Kingdom, London, Leytonstone		Walther *et al.* 1956	P	20	17	3	1·1396	0·0431
			Kopeć 1970	C	1953	1626	327		
					268			1·3838	2·5341
			χ_2^2 for homogeneity of areas						0·1126
BREAST	1. Austria, Wien	Females; (s) ABO	Speiser 1958[b]	P	573	491	82	1·2878	3·0321
				C	1000	823	177		
	2. Czechoslovakia, Praha		Jakoubková & Májský 1965	P	76	57	19	0·5650	4·2466
				C	1142	961	181		
	3. France, Haut-Languedoc		Larrouy 1960	P	77	60	17	0·7858	0·7068
			Khérumian & Lorfeuvre 1966 M2	P	994	813	181		
	4. Iceland		Bjarnason *et al.* 1973	P	105	89	16	0·9973	0·0001
				C	26717	22655	4062		
	5. Italy, Milano		Mor & Sforza 1960	P	88	71	17	0·7837	0·6754
				C	500	421	79		
	6. Poland, Gdańsk		Domaradzka-Woźniak 1964	P	271	234	37	1·1511	0·5888
				C	3286	2780	506		
	7. Poland, Lower Silesia		Sagan *et al.* 1957	P	56	51	5	2·0492	2·3123
				C	2397	1996	401		
	8. United Kingdom	Females	Aird *et al.* 1954	P	945	773	172	0·9503	0·3338
			Kopeć 1970	C	10038	8286	1752		
	9. United Kingdom, London, Leytonstone	Females	Walther *et al.* 1956	P	137	122	15	1·6357	3·0828
			Kopeć 1970	C	1953	1626	327		
	10. United Kingdom, Belfast	Females; (s) A	Macafee 1962	P	373	317	56	1·0242	0·0265
				C	11363	9622	1741		
					2701			1·0223	0·1557
			χ_9^2 for homogeneity of areas						14·8496
CERVIX UTERI	1. Czechoslovakia		Miluničová *et al.* 1969[a]	P	85	72	13	1·0431	0·0183
			Kout 1959 M2	C	1142	961	181		
	2. France, Haut-Languedoc		Larrouy 1960	P	240	209	31	1·5010	3·7657
			Khérumian & Lorfeuvre 1966 M2	C	994	813	181		
	3. Germany, Essen	Epithelial	Verhagen 1951	P	54	48	6	1·9437	2·2475
			Prokop *et al.* 1961	C	706	568	138		
	4. Italy, Varese	(s) ABO	Carrera 1963	P	40	34	6	1·2271	0·2064
				C	1000	822	178		
	5. Norway		Bergsjö & Kolstad 1962[b]	P	741	599	142	0·8824	0·9964
				C	1000	827	173		
	6. Poland, Gdańsk		Domaradzka-Woźniak 1964	P	1368	1202	166	1·3180	8·2923
				C	3286	2780	506		
	7. United Kingdom, London, Leytonstone		Walther *et al.* 1956	P	45	37	8	0·9301	0·0337
			Kopeć 1970	C	1953	1626	327		
	8. U.S.A., San Francisco Bay	(s) ABO	Rotkin 1965	P	353	295	58	0·8198	0·8904
				C	353	304	49		
					2926			1·1361	3·9848
			χ_7^2 for homogeneity of areas						12·4659

TABLE 3 THE RHESUS BLOOD GROUP SYSTEM (*cont.*)

	Place	Additional details	Authors		Number	D+	D−	D+/D− Relative incidence	D+/D− χ_1^2 for difference from unity
NEOPLASMS (*cont.*)									
MALIGNANT NEOPLASMS (*cont.*)									
CORPUS UTERI	1. Czechoslovakia		Miluničová *et al.* 1969[a]	P	142	114	28	0·7668	1·3806
			Kout 1959 M2	C	1142	961	181		
	2. France, Haut-Languedoc		Larrouy 1960	P	45	40	5	1·7811	1·4376
			Khérumian & Lorfeuvre 1966 M2	C	994	813	181		
	3. Italy, Varese	(s) ABO	Carrera 1963	P	61	58	3	4·1865	5·7365
				C	1000	822	178		
	4. Norway		Bergsjö & Kolstad 1962[b]	P	493	422	71	1·2434	2·0237
				C	1000	827	173		
	5. United Kingdom, Belfast	(s) A	Macafee 1962	P	53	46	7	1·1890	0·1814
				C	11363	9622	1741		
					794			1·1668	1·7952
				χ_4^2 for homogeneity of areas					8·9644
UTERUS	1. Austria, Wien	(s) ABO	Speiser 1958[b]	P	1561	1279	282	0·9754	0·0553
				C	1000	823	177		
	2. Iceland		Bjarnason *et al.* 1973	P	136	117	19	1·1041	0·1595
				C	26717	22655	4062		
	3. Italy, Lazio		Liotta *et al.* 1957	P	179	158	21	1·0455	0·0360
				C	10008	8787	1221		
	4. Italy, Pisa		Baisi 1959	P	150	135	15	2·0562	6·7108
				C	1968	1602	366		
	5. Poland, Lower Silesia		Sagan *et al.* 1957	P	263	220	43	1·0279	0·0245
				C	2397(c)	1996	401		
					2289			1·0634	0·6393
				χ_4^2 for homogeneity of areas					6·3470
OVARY	1. Austria, Wien	(s) ABO	Speiser 1958[b]	P	318	268	50	1·1528	0·6605
				C	1000	823	177		
	2. Czechoslovakia		Miluničová *et al.* 1969[a]	P	50	47	3	2·9507	3·2418
			Kout 1959 M2	C	1142	961	181		
	3. France, Haut-Languedoc		Larrouy 1960	P	25	20	5	0·8905	0·0524
			Khérumian & Lorfeuvre 1966 M2	C	994	813	181		
	4. Norway		Bergsjö & Kolstad 1962[b]	P	397	327	70	0·9772	0·0218
				C	1000	827	173		
	5. United Kingdom, London, Leytonstone		Walther *et al.* 1956	P	33	28	5	1·1262	0·0590
			Kopeć 1970	C	1953	1626	327		
					823			1·0829	0·5368
				χ_4^2 for homogeneity of areas					3·4986
VAGINA	Austria, Wien	(s) ABO	Speiser 1958[b]	P	77	62	15	0·8889	0·1546
				C	1000	823	177		
VULVA	1. Austria, Wien	(s) ABO	Speiser 1958[b]	P	74	62	12	1·1112	0·1045
				C	1000	823	177		
	2. United Kingdom, Belfast	(s) A	Macafee 1962	P	75	59	16	0·6672	2·0435
				C	11363	9622	1741		
					226			0·8307	0·7526
				χ_1^2 for homogeneity of areas					1·3953

TABLE 3 THE RHESUS BLOOD GROUP SYSTEM (*cont.*)

	Place	Additional details	Authors		Number	D+	D−	D+/D− Relative incidence	D+/D− χ_1^2 for difference from unity
UNSPECIFIED FEMALE GENITAL ORGANS	1. Germany, Berlin		Hoffbauer 1961	P	605	498	107	0·9941	0·0030
				C	15818	13034	2784		
	2. Germany, Berlin		Mosler 1961	P	464	392	72	1·2681	3·1000
				C	3716	3014	702		
	3. Germany, Bonn		Prokop *et al.* 1961	P	645	547	98	1·3561	4·4103
				C	706	568	138		
	4. Germany, Erfurt		Schuberth 1961	P	212	174	38	0·9733	0·0219
				C	5807	4789	1018		
	5. Germany, Frankfurt am Main		Schwenzer 1961	P	192	157	35	0·9714	0·0220
				C	2000	1644	356		
	6. Germany, Freiburg in Breisgau		Preisler & Matthes 1961	P	803	740	63	2·0848	28·3682
				C	4332	3679	653		
	7. Germany, Halle an der Saale		Mazur & Alex 1961	P	435	347	88	0·8785	1·0108
				C	2854	2334	520		
	8. Germany, Heidelberg		Krah *et al.* 1961	P	500	412	88	1·1167	0·8203
				C	6117	4939	1178		
	9. Germany, Karl-Marx Stadt		Scheffler 1961	P	915	755	160	1·0562	0·3818
				C	25063	20479	4584		
	10. Germany, Leipzig		Zuber & Andreas 1961	P	2000	1604	396	0·9016	1·9988
				C	3021	2471	550		
					6771			1·0722	3·5819
				χ_9^2 for homogeneity of areas					36·5553
PROSTATE	1. Germany, Göttingen		Jörgensen & Kallenbach 1968	P	130	111	19	1·0148	0·0034
				C	6122	5216	906		
	2. United Kingdom, London		Bourke & Griffin 1962	P	224(c)	180	44	0·8510	0·8982
				C	10000	8278	1722		
	3. United Kingdom, London, Leytonstone		Walther *et al.* 1956 Kopeć 1970	P	45	33	12	0·5530	2·9907
				C	1953	1626	327		
					399			0·8384	1·8301
				χ_2^2 for homogeneity of areas					2·0622
KIDNEY	1. France, Haut-Languedoc		Larrouy 1960 Khérumian & Lorfeuvre 1966 M2	P	23	21	2	2·3376	1·3006
				C	994	813	181		
	2. Iceland		Bjarnason *et al.* 1973	P	65	62	3	3·7055	4·9052
				C	26717	22655	4062		
	3. United Kingdom, London, Leytonstone		Walther *et al.* 1956 Kopeć 1970	P	17	15	2	1·5083	0·2962
				C	1953	1626	327		
					105			2·5464	5·6056
				χ_2^2 for homogeneity of areas					0·8964
URINARY BLADDER	1. Austria, Wien	(s) S, ABO	Speiser 1958[a]	P	131	100	31	0·6938	2·7214
				C	1000	823	177		
	2. United Kingdom, London, Leytonstone		Walther *et al.* 1956 Kopeć 1970	P	25	23	2	2·3127	1·2848
				C	1953	1626	327		
					156			0·7661	1·5748
				χ_1^2 for homogeneity of areas					2·4313
NEOPLASMS OF NERVOUS SYSTEM									
RETINOBLASTOMAS	United Kingdom, Manchester	Children	Campbell *et al.* 1961	P	13	10	3	0·7653	0·1648
				C	10384	8445	1939		
ASTROCYTOMAS	United Kingdom, Manchester		Pearce & Yates 1965	P	295	239	56	0·9761	0·0258
				C	12184	9916	2268		

TABLE 3 THE RHESUS BLOOD GROUP SYSTEM (*cont.*)

	Place	Additional details	Authors		Number	D+	D−	D+/D− Relative incidence	D+/D− χ_1^2 for difference from unity
NEOPLASMS (*cont.*)									
NEOPLASMS OF NERVOUS SYSTEM (*cont.*)									
Glioblastomas	United Kingdom, Manchester		Pearce & Yates 1965	P	212	174	38	1·0473	0·0655
				C	12184	9916	2268		
Ependymomas	United Kingdom, Manchester		Pearce & Yates 1965	P	50	43	7	1·4050	0·6938
				C	12184	9916	2268		
Oligodendrogliomas	United Kingdom, Manchester		Pearce & Yates 1965	P	17	16	1	3·6595	1·5833
				C	12184	9916	2268		
Medulloblastomas	United Kingdom, Manchester		Pearce & Yates 1965	P	52	43	9	1·0928	0·0584
				C	12184	9916	2268		
Meningiomas	United Kingdom, Manchester		Pearce & Yates 1965	P	224	182	42	0·9911	0·0027
				C	12184	9916	2268		
Neurilemmomas	United Kingdom, Manchester		Pearce & Yates 1965	P	89	69	20	0·7891	0·8628
				C	12184	9916	2268		
Malignant Neoplasms of Brain	United Kingdom, London, Leytonstone		Walther *et al.* 1956 Kopeć 1970	P	13	9	4	0·4525	1·7238
				C	1953	1626	327		
Brain Tumours	Austria, Wien	(s) S, ABO	Speiser 1958[a]	P	1264	1062	202	1·1307	1·1828
				C	1000	823	177		
Neoplasms of Sympathetic System	United Kingdom, Manchester		Campbell *et al.* 1961	P	31	25	6	0·9567	0·0095
				C	10384	8445	1939		
Vascular Neoplasms of C.N.S.	United Kingdom, Manchester		Pearce & Yates 1965	P	68	57	11	1·1852	0·2649
				C	12184	9916	2268		
NEOPLASMS OF LYMPHATIC AND HAEMATOPOIETIC TISSUE									
Lymphosarcomas	Italy, Cagliari		Adamo 1961[a, c] Aru 1951 M2	P	17	17	0		
				C	200	180	20		
Reticulosarcomas	Italy, Cagliari		Adamo 1961[a, c] Aru 1951 M2	P	5	5	0		
				C	200	180	20		
Hodgkin's Disease, Lymphogranulomas	1. Czechoslovakia, Praha	Lympho-granuloma	Májský 1964 Kout 1959 M2	P	85	70	15	0·8732	0·2101
				C	1142(c)	962	180		
	2. Italy, Cagliari	Lympho-granuloma	Adamo 1961[a, c] Aru 1951 M2	P	10	10	0		
				C	200	180	20		
	3. Netherlands, Leiden	Hodgkin's disease	Does *et al.* 1972	P	46	39	7	0·5865	0·6402
				C	42	38	4		
	4. Poland, Kraków	Lympho-granuloma; (s) S, A	Cichecka 1965	P	160	125	35	0·7843	1·6000
				C	21581	17695	3886		
	5. United Kingdom, London	Hodgkin's disease	Kay & Shorter 1956 Discombe & Meyer 1952 M2	P	73	53	20	0·5513	5·0983
				C	10000	8278	1722		
	6. United Kingdom, London, Leytonstone	Hodgkin's disease	Walther *et al.* 1956 Kopeć 1970	P	11	8	3	0·5363	0·8403
				C	1953	1626	327		
					375			0·7148	6·4621
				χ_4^2 for homogeneity of areas					1·9268
Reticuloses	1. Czechoslovakia, Praha		Májský 1964 Kout 1959 M2	P	43	37	6	1·1538	0·1022
				C	1142(c)	962	180		
	2. Poland, Kraków	(s) S, A	Cichecka 1965	P	102	90	12	1·6471	2·6278
				C	21581	17695	3886		
					145			1·4692	2·3007
				χ_1^2 for homogeneity of areas					0·4293

TABLE 3 THE RHESUS BLOOD GROUP SYSTEM (*cont.*)

	Place	Additional details	Authors		Number	D+	D−	D+/D− Relative incidence	D+/D− χ_1^2 for difference from unity
MYELOMAS	Czechoslovakia, Praha		Májský 1964	P	49	36	13	0·5182	3·8842
			Kout 1959 M2	C	1142(c)	962	180		
LYMPHATIC LEUKAEMIAS, CHRONIC	1. Czechoslovakia, Praha		Májský 1964	P	73	61	12	0·9511	0·0236
			Kout 1959 M2	C	1142(c)	962	180		
	2. Poland, Kraków		Gurda & Turowska 1970	P	76	66	10	1·4494	1·1931
				C	21581	17695	3886		
					149			1·1640	0·4166
				χ_1^2 for homogeneity of areas					0·8001
LYMPHATIC LEUKAEMIAS, UNSPECIFIED	Poland, Kraków	(s) S	Cichecka 1965	P	148	131	17	1·6923	4·1450
				C	21581	17695	3886		
MYELOID LEUKAEMIAS, ACUTE	1. Italy, Cagliari		Adamo 1961[a, c]	P	9	9	0		
			Aru 1951 M2	C	200	180	20		
	2. Poland, Kraków	(s) S, A	Cichecka 1965	P	301	249	52	1·0516	0·1074
				C	21581	17695	3886		
					301				
MYELOID LEUKAEMIAS, CHRONIC	1. Czechoslovakia, Praha		Májský 1964	P	75	65	10	1·2162	0·3141
			Kout 1959 M2	C	1142(c)	962	180		
	2. Poland, Kraków	(s) S, A	Cichecka 1965	P	175	145	30	1·0614	0·0877
				C	21581	17695	3886		
	3. Poland, Kraków		Gurda & Turowska 1970	P	45	41	4	2·2510	2·3965
				C	21581	17695	3886		
					295			1·1796	0·9959
				χ_2^2 for homogeneity of areas					1·8024
MYELOID LEUKAEMIAS, UNSPECIFIED	United Kingdom, London		Kay & Shorter 1956	P	40	34	6	1·1788	0·1375
			Discombe & Meyer 1952 M2	C	10000	8278	1722		
ERYTHROLEUKAEMIA	Poland, Kraków		Cichecka 1965	P	15	13	2	1·4275	0·2194
				C	21581	17695	3886		
LEUKAEMIAS, ACUTE	1. Czechoslovakia, Praha		Májský 1964	P	122	96	26	0·6909	2·4653
			Kout 1959 M2	C	1142(c)	962	180		
	2. Germany, Göttingen		Jörgensen & Kallenbach 1968	P	78	67	11	1·0580	0·0296
				C	6122	5216	906		
	3. Poland, Kraków		Gurda & Turowska 1970	P	51	38	13	0·6419	1·8974
				C	21581	17695	3886		
					251			0·7546	2·9336
				χ_2^2 for homogeneity of areas					1·4587
LEUKAEMIAS, CHRONIC	Germany, Göttingen		Jörgensen & Kallenbach 1968	P	104	88	16	0·9553	0·0278
				C	6122	5216	906		
LEUKAEMIAS, UNSPECIFIED	1. United Kingdom, London, Leytonstone	Includes lympho-sarcoma	Walther *et al.* 1956	P	46	38	8	0·9553	0·0135
			Kopeć 1970	C	1953	1626	327		
	2. United Kingdom, Manchester	Children	Campbell *et al.* 1961	P	102	82	20	0·9414	0·0581
				C	10384	8445	1939		
	3. U.S.A., Boston		Steinberg 1960	P	450(c)	390	60	0·8724	0·5293
			Dublin *et al.* 1964	C	600	529	71		
	4. U.S.A., Chicago		Best *et al.* 1949	P	30	23	7	0·9234	0·0294
			Davidson & Toharsky 1942 M2	C	196	153	43		

TABLE 3 **THE RHESUS BLOOD GROUP SYSTEM** *(cont.)*

	Place	Additional details	Authors		Number	D+	D−	D+/D− Relative incidence	D+/D− χ_1^2 for difference from unity
NEOPLASMS *(cont.)*									
NEOPLASMS OF LYMPHATIC AND HAEMATOPOIETIC TISSUE *(cont.)*									
LEUKAEMIAS, UNSPECIFIED *(cont.)*									
	5. U.S.A., Michigan	Whites	Gershowitz & Neel 1965	P	170	143	27	1·1465	0·3850
				C	1506	1238	268		
	6. U.S.A., New York City	Gentiles; (s) S, A, ABO	De George 1970	P	374	306	68	0·9783	0·0061
			Rife & Schonfeld 1944 M2	C	112	92	20		
	7. Brazil, Rio Grande do Sul	Whites	Ayres *et al.* 1966	P	51(c)	44	7	1·3518	0·4014
				C	113(c)	93	20		
					1223			0·9826	0·0287
					χ_6^2 for homogeneity of areas				1·3941
POLYCYTHAEMIA VERA	1. Czechoslovakia, Praha		Májský 1964	P	16	14	2	1·3098	0·1260
			Kout 1959 M2	C	1142(c)	962	180		
	2. Poland, Kraków	(s) S	Cichecka 1965	P	18	10	8	0·4941	2·7478
				C	21581	17695	3886		
					34			0·6234	1·6215
					χ_1^2 for homogeneity of areas				1·2522
MYELOFIBROSIS	Poland, Kraków	(s) S, A	Cichecka 1965	P	11	9	2	0·9882	0·0002
				C	21581	17695	3886		
UNSPECIFIED NEOPLASMS OF LYMPHATIC AND HAEMATOPOIETIC TISSUE	Iceland		Bjarnason *et al.* 1973	P	91	77	14	0·9861	0·0023
				C	26717	22655	4062		
SARCOMAS									
	United Kingdom, London, Leytonstone		Walther *et al.* 1956	P	21	19	2	1·9105	0·7534
			Kopeć 1970	C	1953	1626	327		
MALIGNANT NEOPLASMS DEFINED AS CANCERS OF MIXED OR UNSPECIFIED SITES									
OTHER THAN BREAST AND LUNG	Czechoslovakia, Praha		Jakoubková & Májský 1965	P	79	62	17	0·6869	1·7302
				C	1142	961	181		
UNSPECIFIED	Italy, Milano		Mor & Sforza 1960	P	292	247	45	1·0300	0·0211
				C	500	421	79		
					371			0·8988	0·4152
					χ_1^2 for homogeneity of areas				1·3361
MALIGNANT NEOPLASMS OF UNSPECIFIED SITES									
	Greece	(s) S	Hatzesoterios 1959	P	1470	1337	133	1·0506	0·2281
			Markianos *et al.* 1957	C	4851	4392	459		
VARIOUS									
SALIVARY GLAND TUMOURS	United Kingdom, Manchester	Benign and malignant	Garrett *et al.* 1971	P	407(c)	347	60	1·2161	1·5932
				C	1554(c)	1284	270		
FIBROMAS OF UTERUS	Italy, Varese	(s) ABO	Carrera 1963	P	229	200	29	1·4934	3·4728
				C	1000	822	178		
PITUITARY TUMOURS	United Kingdom, Manchester		Pearce & Yates 1965	P	144	119	25	1·0887	0·1476
				C	12184	9916	2268		
OSTEOMAS	Germany, Göttingen		Jörgensen & Kallenbach 1968	P	197	171	26	1·1424	0·3886
				C	6122	5216	906		

TABLE 3 THE RHESUS BLOOD GROUP SYSTEM (*cont.*)

	Place	Additional details	Authors		Number	D+	D−	D+/D− Relative incidence	D+/D− χ_1^2 for difference from unity
ENDOCRINE AND METABOLIC DISEASES									
THYROTOXICOSIS	United Kingdom, Belfast	(s) S, A	Macafee 1962	P C	208 11363	174 9622	34 1741	0·9260	0·1650
GOITRE	Italy, Milano		Mor & Sforza 1960	P C	308 500	244 421	64 79	0·7154	3·2269
DIABETES MELLITUS	1. Austria, Wien	(s) S, ABO	Speiser 1958[a]	P C	239 1000	203 823	36 177	1·2127	0·9402
	2. Czechoslovakia, Praha	Males; (s) A	Milunčová & Dominec 1966 Milunčová & Sottner 1965 M2	P C	121 878	97 716	24 162	0·9145	0·1343
	3. Denmark, Köbenhavn	(s) S	Andersen & Lauritzen 1960	P C	992 4319(c)	823 3517	169 802	1·1105	1·2678
	4. Denmark	Females	Klebe & Nielsen 1972 Andersen & Lauritzen 1960	P C	652 4319	547 3517	105 802	1·1880	2·3026
	5. Germany, Rügen	Females	Worm 1954 Wiedow & Kreil 1970 M2	P C	218(c) 8864	179 7303	39 1561	0·9810	0·0114
	6. Poland, Wrocław	Children	Wartenberg & Wąsikowa 1971	P C	145 325	117 259	28 66	1·0648	0·0623
	7. San Marino	(s) S	Dominici 1965	P C	92 3350	77 2787	15 563	1·0370	0·0161
	8. Switzerland, Genève		Zeytinoglu 1957	P C	393 23790	322 19695	71 4095	0·9430	0·1972
	9. United Kingdom, Oxford	(s) S, A	McConnell *et al.* 1956 Kopeć 1970	P C	500 11662	401 9631	99 2031	0·8542	1·8833
	10. United Kingdom, Glasgow		Craig & Wang 1955	P C	817 1518	684 1255	133 263	1·0777	0·4128
	11. N. India, Chandigarh		Jolly *et al.* 1969	P C	818 6204	786 5979	32 225	0·9243	0·1667
	12. Canada, Toronto	Juveniles	Simpson *et al.* 1962	P C	100 36042	85 30279	15 5763	1·0785	0·0727
	13. U.S.A., Iowa		Buckwalter & Tweed 1962	P C	1153 2181	943 1818	210 363	0·8966	1·3048
					6240			1·0105	0·0705
				χ_{12}^2 for homogeneity of areas					8·7017
DIABETES, KIMMELSTIEL-WILSON SYNDROME	Switzerland, Genève		Zeytinoglu 1957	P C	39 23790	33 19695	6 4095	1·1436	0·0912
TOXAEMIA OF PREGNANCY	U.S.S.R., Leningrad	(s) ABO	Golovachev & Bokarius 1972	P C	2234 5889	1913 5010	321 879	1·0456	0·3995
HAEMOCHROMATOSIS	1. Belgium, Bruxelles		Cornil & Pirart 1961 Hubinont 1949 M2	P C	24 1419	18 1177	6 242	0·6168	1·0275
	2. Australia, Sydney		Bradley & Walsh 1965 Lai 1966 M2	P C	56 260	50 219	6 41	1·5601	0·9174
					80			0·9930	0·0005
				χ_1^2 for homogeneity of areas					1·9445
DISEASES OF THE BLOOD									
PERNICIOUS ANAEMIA	1. Austria, Wien	(s) S, ABO	Speiser 1958[a]	P C	202 1000	164 823	38 177	0·9282	0·1414
	2. Poland, Katowice		Machalski *et al.* 1968	P C	81 567	63 458	18 109	0·8330	0·4035

TABLE 3 THE RHESUS BLOOD GROUP SYSTEM (*cont.*)

	Place	Additional details	Authors		Number	D+	D−	D+/D− Relative incidence	D+/D− χ^2_1 for difference from unity
DISEASES OF THE BLOOD (*cont.*)									
PERNICIOUS ANAEMIA (*cont.*)									
	3. Poland, Kraków	(s) S	Cichecka 1965	P	57	43	14	0·6745	1·6321
				C	21581	17695	3886		
	4. United Kingdom, England		Callender *et al.* 1957	P	201	165	36	0·9586	0·0474
				C	1798	1487	311		
	5. U.S.A., Chicago	Whites	Ladenson *et al.* 1949	P	119	107	12	1·4758	1·6278
			Tisdall & Garland 1945 M2	C	22133	18990	3143		
	6. U.S.A., Chicago	Negroes	Ladenson *et al.* 1949	P	41	39	2	2·1412	1·0254
			Tisdall & Garland 1945 M2	C	283	255	28		
					701			0·9568	0·1695
				χ^2_5 for homogeneity of areas					4·7082
HAEMOLYTIC ANAEMIA									
Congenital	Poland, Kraków	(s) S, A	Cichecka 1965	P	33	25	8	0·6863	0·8573
				C	21581	17695	3886		
Acquired	1. Austria, Wien		Lal & Speiser 1957	P	97	76	21	0·7486	1·3634
				C	10000	8286	1714		
	2. United Kingdom, Sheffield		Dunsford & Owen 1960	P	127(c)	104	23	0·9814	0·0065
				C	6000(c)	4930	1070		
					224			0·8644	0·7365
				χ^2_1 for homogeneity of areas					0·6335
COOLEY'S ANAEMIA	India	Bengali Hindu	Das Gupta *et al.* 1955	P	43	34	9	0·2099	3·6472
				C	38	36	2		
APLASTIC ANAEMIA	Poland, Kraków	(s) S, A	Cichecka 1965	P	63	53	10	1·1639	0·1934
				C	21581	17695	3886		
HAEMOPHILIA	1. Czechoslovakia, Praha		Májský 1964	P	30	27	3	1·6840	0·7205
			Kout 1959 M2	C	1142(c)	962	180		
	2. Poland, Kraków	(s) S, A	Cichecka 1965	P	51	45	6	1·6471	1·3161
				C	21581	17695	3886		
					81			1·6593	2·0357
				χ^2_1 for homogeneity of areas					0·0009
IDIOPATHIC THROMOBCYTOPENIC PURPURA	1. Poland, Kraków	Schönlein-Henoch syndrome: children	Cichecka 1965	P	112	95	17	1·2272	0·6019
				C	21581	17695	3886		
	2. Poland, Kraków	Werlhof's disease; (s) S, A	Cichecka 1965	P	61	48	13	0·8109	0·4482
				C	21581	17695	3886		
					173			1·0332	0·0262
				χ^2_1 for homogeneity of areas					1·0239
MENTAL DISORDERS									
SENILE DEMENTIA	1. Greece, Makedhonia and Thraki		Zervopoulos *et al.* 1967	P	39	33	6	0·7795	0·3118
				C	4479	3923	556		
	2. Italy, Vercelli		Giuli 1959	P	57	40	17	0·4087	8·7244
				C	1000	852	148		
					96			0·5011	7·6028
				χ^2_1 for homogeneity of areas					1·4335

TABLE 3 THE RHESUS BLOOD GROUP SYSTEM (*cont.*)

	Place	Additional details	Authors		Number	D+	D−	D+/D− Relative incidence	D+/D− χ_1^2 for difference from unity
POSTENCEPHALITIC PSYCHOSES	Italy, Vercelli		Giuli 1959	P C	12 1000	7 852	5 148	0·2432	5·6989
SCHIZOPHRENIA	1. Czechoslovakia, Nitra		Miššík 1962	P C	257 1000	222 821	35 179	1·3829	2·6354
	2. Greece, Makedhonia and Thraki	Catatonic	Zervopoulos *et al.* 1967	P C	38 4479	32 3923	6 556	0·7559	0·3917
	3. Greece, Makedhonia and Thraki	Hebephrenic	Zervopoulos *et al.* 1967	P C	215 4479	190 3923	25 556	1·0771	0·1167
	4. Greece, Makedhonia and Thraki	Paranoid	Zervopoulos *et al.* 1967	P C	192 4479	175 3923	17 556	1·4590	2·1426
	5. Greece, Makedhonia and Thraki	Simple	Zervopoulos *et al.* 1967	P C	97 4479	86 3923	11 556	1·1081	0·1007
	6. Italy, Vercelli		Giuli 1959	P C	291 1000	233 852	58 148	0·6978	4·3932
	7. Poland, Kraków		Turowska *et al.* 1968 Jaegermann & Próchnicka 1966 M2	P C	197(c) 2919	154 2400	43 519	0·7745	2·0352
	8. United Kingdom, Chorley, Leyland, Preston		Masters 1967 Kopeć 1970	P C	87 859	74 710	13 149	1·1946	0·3207
					1374			0·9776	0·0773
				χ_7^2 for homogeneity of areas					12·0589
MANIC-DEPRESSIVE PSYCHOSES	1. Czechoslovakia, Nitra		Miššík 1962	P C	35 1000	30 821	5 179	1·3082	0·3005
	2. Greece, Makedhonia and Thraki		Zervopoulos *et al.* 1967	P C	40 4479	33 3923	7 556	0·6681	0·9281
	3. United Kingdom, Chorley, Leyland, Preston		Masters 1967 Kopeć 1970	P C	35 859	27 710	8 149	0·7083	0·6992
					110			0·8156	0·6543
				χ_2^2 for homogeneity of areas					1·2735
VARIOUS PSYCHOSES	1. Czechoslovakia, Nitra	Involutional	Miššík 1962	P C	71 1000	61 821	10 179	1·3300	0·6600
	2. Czechoslovakia, Nitra	Various	Miššík 1962	P C	42 1000	37 821	5 179	1·6134	0·9785
	3. Italy, Vercelli	Affective	Giuli 1959	P C	172 1000	145 852	27 148	0·9329	0·0931
					285			1·1000	0·2880
				χ_2^2 for homogeneity of areas					1·4436
PSYCHOPATHY	Czechoslovakia, Nitra		Miššík 1962	P C	26 1000	23 821	3 179	1·6715	0·6880
NEUROSES	Czechoslovakia, Nitra		Miššík 1962	P C	46 1000	39 821	7 179	1·2147	0·2158
ALCOHOLISM	1. Czechoslovakia, Nitra		Miššík 1962	P C	77 1000	65 821	12 179	1·1810	0·2622
	2. Italy, Vercelli		Giuli 1959	P C	65 1000	49 852	16 148	0·5320	4·3852
					142			0·7693	1·4085
				χ_1^2 for homogeneity of areas					3·2388

TABLE 3 **THE RHESUS BLOOD GROUP SYSTEM** *(cont.)*

	Place	Additional details	Authors		Number	D+	D−	D+/D− Relative incidence	D+/D− χ_1^2 for difference from unity
MENTAL DISORDERS *(cont.)*									
MENTAL RETARDATION	1. Czechoslovakia, Nitra	Oligophrenia	Miššík 1962	P	29	23	6	0·8358	0·1484
				C	1000	821	179		
	2. Greece, Makedhonia and Thraki	Mental deficiency	Zervopoulos *et al.* 1967	P	125	111	14	1·1237	0·1649
				C	4479	3923	556		
	3. Italy, Ferrara	Children; phrenasthenia	Caselli 1955	P	105	91	14	1·0000	0·0000
				C	60	52	8		
	4. Italy, Vercelli	Oligophrenia, phrenasthenia	Giuli 1959	P	130	92	38	0·4206	16·6295
				C	1000	852	148		
					389			0·6507	7·9982
				χ_3^2 for homogeneity of areas					8·9445
DISEASES OF THE NERVOUS SYSTEM									
MULTIPLE SCLEROSIS	1. Germany, Essen	(s) $Rh_{CC^{w}DEce}$	Bertrams & Kuwert 1976	P	802	660	142	1·3048	4·8899
				C	990	773	217		
	2. United Kingdom, Newcastle upon Tyne	(s) Rh_{CDEce}	MacDonald *et al.* 1976	P	127	92	35	0·4532	6·3875
				C	136	116	20		
	3. United Kingdom, Newcastle upon Tyne	(s) Rh_{CDEce}	Roberts 1976	P	185	145	40	0·6250	2·4404
				C	136	116	20		
	4. U.S.A., Boston		Alexander *et al.* 1950	P	111	90	21	0·5752	4·0939
			Dublin *et al.* 1964	C	600	529	71		
					1225			0·9783	0·0499
				χ_3^2 for homogeneity of areas					17·7618
EPILEPSY	1. Greece, Makedhonia and Thraki		Zervopoulos *et al.* 1967	P	79	71	8	1·2578	0·3728
				C	4479	3923	556		
	2. Italy, Vercelli		Giuli 1959	P	38	33	5	1·1465	0·0784
				C	1000	852	148		
	3. United Kingdom, Berkshire, Oxfordshire	Females	Fedrick 1972	P	164	139	25	1·1280	0·3037
				C	12902	10726	2176		
	4. Australia		Simmons *et al.* 1944	P	22	19	3	1·2621	0·1396
				C	3641(c)	3036	605		
					303			1·1652	0·8135
				χ_3^2 for homogeneity of areas					0·0811
MOTOR NEURONE DISEASE	U.S.A., Maryland	Amyotrophic lateral sclerosis	Myrianthopoulos & Leyshon 1967	P	346	292	54	0·8921	0·2850
				C	346	297	49		
DISEASES OF THE CIRCULATORY SYSTEM									
RHEUMATIC FEVER	1. Poland, Katowice		Machalski *et al.* 1968	P	206	153	53	0·6870	3·8330
				C	567	458	109		
	2. U.S.A., Iowa		Buckwalter *et al.* 1962	P	538	451	87	1·0351	0·0698
				C	2181	1818	263		
	3. U.S.A., Michigan		Gershowitz & Neel 1965	P	104	86	18	1·0343	0·0158
				C	1506	1238	268		
	4. Australia, Sydney		Walsh & Kooptzoff 1956	P	260	217	43	1·2095	0·7347
				C	300	242	58		
					1108			0·9685	0·1235
				χ_3^2 for homogeneity of areas					4·5299

TABLE 3 **THE RHESUS BLOOD GROUP SYSTEM** *(cont.)*

	Place	Additional details	Authors		Number	D+	D−	D+/D− Relative incidence	D+/D− χ_1^2 for difference from unity
RHEUMATIC HEART DISEASE	1. United Kingdom, Bristol	(s) Isolated mitral, isolated aortic, and multi-valvular	David 1970 Kopeć 1970	P C	165 9921	141 8193	24 1728	1·2391	0·9293
	2. United Kingdom, Cardiff	Carditis, mitral stenosis	Hooper 1960 Kopeć 1970	P C	213 1053	174 868	39 185	0·9509	0·0668
	3. United Kingdom, Belfast	Mitral stenosis; (s) S	Macafee 1962	P C	431 11363	362 9622	69 1741	0·9493	0·1511
	4. U.S.A., Boston		Dublin *et al.* 1964	P C	606 600	514 529	92 71	0·7499	2·8785
					1415			0·9304	0·7142
				χ_3^2 for homogeneity of areas					3·3115
HYPERTENSION	1. Austria, Wien	(s) S, ABO	Speiser 1958[a]	P C	250 1000	219 823	31 177	1·5193	4·0046
	2. Czechoslovakia		Mikolášek & Miluničová 1967	P C	383 176000	308 145957	75 30043	0·8453	1·6645
	3. United Kingdom, Scotland	(s) S	Maxwell & Maxwell 1955	P C	1247 1518	1034 1255	213 263	1·0173	0·0287
					1880			1·0075	0·0101
				χ_2^2 for homogeneity of areas					5·6876
CORONARY OCCLUSION	Denmark, Köbenhavn		Gjørup 1963	P C	846 14304	697 12001	149 2303	0·8977	1·3448
ANGINA PECTORIS, ACUTE CORONARY INSUFFICIENCY, CARDIAC INFARCTION	Irish Republic, Dublin		Maurer *et al.* 1969	P C	446 117287	364 97457	82 19830	0·9032	0·6905
MYOCARDIAL INFARCTION	1. Finland		Kalliomäki & Saarimaa 1962	P C	359 1600	308 1348	51 252	1·1290	0·5340
	2. Greece, Athínai		Koidakis *et al.* 1970 Païdoussis 1967 M2	P C	182 2017	157 1822	25 195	0·6721	3·0335
	3. Poland, Lublin	(s) ABO	Szczepański & Jach 1973	P C	1279 1100	1071 815	208 285	1·8006	33·0122
	4. Israel	Jewish men over 40, born in Austria, Hungary, Romania; (s) G	Medalie *et al.* 1971 (a)	P C	74 1632	68 1511	6 121	0·9076	0·0494
	5. Israel	Jewish men over 40, born in Germany	Medalie *et al.* 1971	P C	25(a) 488	22 442	3 46	0·7632	0·1813
	6. Israel	Jewish men over 40, born in Poland	Medalie *et al.* 1971	P C	65(a) 1233	60 1122	5 111	1·1872	0·1299
	7. Israel	Jewish men over 40, born in Bulgaria, Jugoslavia; (s) G	Medalie *et al.* 1971	P C	17(a) 374	12 346	5 28	0·1942	8·3418
	8. Israel	Jewish men over 40, born in the U.S.S.R.	Medalie *et al.* 1971	P C	36(a) 551	33 503	3 48	1·0497	0·0061

TABLE 3 THE RHESUS BLOOD GROUP SYSTEM (*cont.*)

	Place	Additional details	Authors		Number	D+	D−	D+/D− Relative incidence	D+/D− χ^2_1 for difference from unity
DISEASES OF THE CIRCULATORY SYSTEM (*cont.*)									
MYOCARDIAL INFARCTION (*cont.*)									
	9. Israel	Jewish men over 40, born in Israel, Turkey, Syria	Medalie *et al.* 1971	P	85(a)	78	7	0·9745	0·0041
				C	1803	1658	145		
	10. Israel	Jewish men over 40, born in Iraq	Medalie *et al.* 1971	P	38(a)	37	1	2·8845	1·0788
				C	1120	1039	81		
	11. Israel	Jewish men over 40, born in Egypt	Medalie *et al.* 1971	P	17(a)	15	2	0·6889	0·2347
				C	523	479	44		
	12. Israel	Jewish men over 40, born in Morocco	Medalie *et al.* 1971	P	12(a)	11	1	1·1765	0·0236
				C	414	374	40		
	13. Malaya, Singapore	Malays	Saha *et al.* 1973	P	42	42	0		
				C	148	148	0		
	14. Malaya, Singapore	Chinese	Saha *et al.* 1973	P	169	169	0		
				C	237	235	2		
	15. Malaya, Singapore	Indians	Saha *et al.* 1973	P	143	136	7	0·8831	0·0606
				C	230	220	10		
	16. U.S.A.	Males under 40; (s) ABO	Gertler & White 1954	P	80	71	9	1·9722	2·7407
				C	145	116	29		
					2412			1·3141	14·0470
				χ^2_{13} for homogeneity of areas					35·3837
ARTERIOSCLEROTIC HEART DISEASE	Denmark, København		Viskum 1973	P	253	216	37	1·1203	0·4010
			Andersen 1955	C	14304	12001	2303		
ATHEROMATOSIS	Poland, Katowice		Machalski *et al.* 1968	P	213	174	39	1·0618	0·0841
				C	567	458	109		
CEREBRO-VASCULAR DISEASES	Italy, Piemonte	147 thromboses, 15 embolisms, 6 cerebral haemorrhages; (s) S	Morato *et al.* 1969	P	168	150	18	1·4620	1·8754
			Garrone & Bocci 1951 M2	C	536	456	80		
SUPERFICIAL PUERPERAL THROMBOPHLEBITIS	United Kingdom, Aberdeen	(s) ABO	Allan & Stewart 1971	P	607	480	127	0·8594	2·2519
				C	27093	22074	5019		
ARTERITIS	Italy, Milano		Mor & Sforza 1960	P	128	112	16	1·3135	0·8602
				C	500	421	79		
DISEASES OF THE RESPIRATORY SYSTEM									
BRONCHOPNEUMONIA	Denmark, København		Viskum 1973	P	177	152	25	1·1668	0·5050
			Andersen 1955	C	14304	12001	2303		
CHRONIC BRONCHITIS	Denmark, København		Viskum 1973	P	347	282	65	0·8326	1·7268
			Andersen 1955	C	14304	12001	2303		
SPONTANEOUS PNEUMOTHORAX	Denmark, København		Viskum 1973	P	85	73	12	1·1674	0·2456
			Andersen 1955	C	14304	12001	2303		
DISEASES OF THE DIGESTIVE SYSTEM									
DENTAL CARIES	Germany, Göttingen		Jörgensen & Kallenbach 1968	P	251	225	26	1·5031	3·7579
				C	6122	5216	906		
PERIODONTOSIS	France, Bordeau	(s) S, ABO	Toussaint & Mériaux 1970	P	1784	1482	302	0·9771	0·0864
				C	3216	2682	534		

TABLE 3 **THE RHESUS BLOOD GROUP SYSTEM** (*cont.*)

	Place	Additional details	Authors		Number	D+	D−	D+/D− Relative incidence	D+/D− χ^2_1 for difference from unity
ULCERATIVE COLITIS	1. Czechoslovakia, Praha		Veselý 1969[a]	P	57	50	7	1·3365	0·4965
				C	1142(c)	962	180		
	2. United Kingdom, West Midlands		Winstone *et al.* 1960	P	277	230	47	1·0632	0·1457
				C	39084(c)	32108	6976		
	3. U.S.A., Connecticut	25% Jewish	Thayer & Bove 1965	P	170	150	20	1·2413	0·8193
			Tisdall & Garland 1945 M2	C	22133	18990	3143		
					504			1·1350	0·9978
					χ^2_2 for homogeneity of areas				0·4636
CIRRHOSIS OF LIVER	1. Austria, Wien	(s) S, ABO	Speiser 1958[a]	P	355	300	55	1·1731	0·8980
				C	1000	823	177		
	2. Czechoslovakia, Bohemia		Kordač 1965	P	304	251	53	0·9716	0·0362
				C	80518	66811	13707		
	3. Czechoslovakia, Praha		Veselý 1969[a]	P	142	112	30	0·6985	2·6343
				C	1142(c)	962	180		
					801			0·9705	0·0890
					χ^2_2 for homogeneity of areas				3·4795
CHOLELITHIASIS	1. Czechoslovakia, Praha		Veselý 1969[b]	P	680	559	121	0·8644	1·2752
				C	1142(c)	962	180		
	2. Denmark, Köbenhavn		Jordal 1956	P	413	359	54	1·3250	3·5014
			Gürtler & Henningsen 1954 M2	C	5500	4586	914		
	3. Denmark, Köbenhavn		Kjølbye & Lykkegaard Nielsen 1959	P	1291	1080	211	0·9822	0·0519
				C	14304	12001	2303		
	4. Germany, Berlin		Schmauss *et al.* 1968	P	3082(c)	2559	523	1·0446	0·6893
				C	15154	12488	2666		
	5. Germany, Göttingen		Jörgensen & Kallenbach 1968	P	396	332	64	0·9010	0·5447
				C	6122	5216	906		
	6. Italy, Milano		Mor & Sforza 1960	P	553	483	70	1·2948	2·1261
				C	500	421	79		
	7. Poland, Katowice		Machalski *et al.* 1968	P	472	378	94	0·9570	0·0783
				C	567	458	109		
					6887			1·0240	0·4228
					χ^2_6 for homogeneity of areas				7·8441
PANCREATITIS	Czechoslovakia, Praha		Veselý 1969[b]	P	167	128	39	0·6141	5·9389
				C	1142(c)	962	180		
GASTRIC ULCERS	1. Austria, Wien	(s) S, ABO	Speiser 1956	P	1028	868	160	1·1222	1·6394
				C	10000	8286	1714		
	2. Czechoslovakia, Praha		Kubičková & Veselý 1966	P	406	329	77	0·8047	2·0887
				C	1142	961	181		
	3. Denmark, Köbenhavn		Jordal 1956	P	415	349	66	1·0539	0·1425
			Gürtler & Henningsen 1954 M2	C	5500	4586	914		
	4. Italy, Aquila		Curtoni & Morgante 1964	P	210(c)	183	27	1·0475	0·0495
				C	8920(c)	7726	1194		
	5. Italy, Milano		Mor & Sforza 1960	P	285	255	30	1·5950	4·1688
				C	500	421	79		
	6. Italy, Roma		Misiti *et al.* 1968	P	26	24	2	1·6765	0·4902
			Siciliano & Mittiga 1954 M2	C	3100	2720	380		
	7. Poland, Katowice		Machalski *et al.* 1968	P	235	192	43	1·0627	0·0927
				C	567	458	109		

TABLE 3 **THE RHESUS BLOOD GROUP SYSTEM** (*cont.*)

		Place	Additional details	Authors		Number	D+	D−	D+/D− Relative incidence	D+/D− χ_1^2 for difference from unity
DISEASES OF THE DIGESTIVE SYSTEM (*cont.*)										
GASTRIC ULCERS (*cont.*)										
	8.	Poland, Lower Silesia		Sagan *et al.* 1957	P	67	59	8	1·4817	1·0664
					C	2397	1996	401		
	9.	United Kingdom, Oxford	With metaplasia	Glober *et al.* 1972	P	54(c)	41	13	0·6651	1·6321
				Kopeć 1970	C	11662	9631	2031		
	10.	United Kingdom, Oxford	Without metaplasia	Glober *et al.* 1972	P	40(c)	34	6	1·1950	0·1614
				Kopeć 1970	C	11662	9631	2031		
	11.	United Kingdom, Belfast	(s) S, A	Macafee 1962	P	319	255	64	0·7209	5·2939
					C	11363	9622	1741		
	12.	U.S.A., Iowa		Buckwalter 1962	P	348(c)	294	54	1·0871	0·2764
					C	2181(c)	1818	363		
						3433			1·0165	0·1071
						χ_{11}^2 for homogeneity of areas				16·9948
DUODENAL ULCERS	1.	Austria, Wien	(s) S, ABO	Speiser 1956	P	1160	961	199	0·9989	0·0002
					C	10000	8286	1714		
	2.	Czechoslovakia, Praha		Kubičková & Veselý 1966	P	934	768	166	0·8714	1·3645
					C	1142	961	181		
	3.	Denmark, Köbenhavn		Jordal 1956	P	1223	1039	184	1·1254	1·8066
				Gürtler & Henningsen 1954 M2	C	5500	4586	914		
	4.	Italy, Aquila		Curtoni & Morgante 1964	P	473(c)	405	68	0·9204	0·3788
					C	8920(c)	7726	1194		
	5.	Italy, Milano		Mor & Sforza 1960	P	437	378	59	1·2022	0·9795
					C	500	421	79		
	6.	Italy, Roma		Misiti *et al.* 1968	P	316	274	42	0·9114	0·2825
				Siciliano & Mittiga 1954 M2	C	3100	2720	380		
	7.	Poland, Katowice		Machalski *et al.* 1968	P	481	413	68	1·4454	4·7651
					C	567	458	109		
	8.	Poland, Lower Silesia		Sagan *et al.* 1957	P	77	72	5	2·8930	5·2031
					C	2397	1996	401		
	9.	Spain	Basques	Goti Iturriaga & Velasco Alonso 1965	P	95(c)	68	27	1·0038	0·0002
					C	386(c)	276	110		
	10.	Spain	Non-Basques	Goti Iturriaga & Velasco Alonso 1965	P	143(c)	111	32	0·8479	0·4604
					C	336(c)	270	66		
	11.	United Kingdom, Chorley, Leyland, Preston		Masters 1967	P	26	21	5	0·8814	0·0623
				Kopeć 1970	C	859	710	149		
	12.	United Kingdom, South Tees-side	(s) S, ABO	Grahame 1961	P	722	651	71	2·1108	28·5630
				Kopeć 1970	C	1678	1364	314		
	13.	U.S.A., Iowa		Buckwalter 1962	P	1029	883	146	1·2075	3·1525
					C	2181	1818	363		
						7116			1·1122	7·7053
						χ_{12}^2 for homogeneity of areas				39·3134
BOTH GASTRIC AND DUODENAL ULCERS PRESENT		Czechoslovakia, Praha		Kubičková & Veselý 1966	P	112	96	16	1·1301	0·1881
					C	1142	961	181		
PEPTIC ULCERS, SITE UNSPECIFIED	1.	United Kingdom		Aird *et al.* 1954	P	2618	2196	422	1·1003	2·5978
				Kopeć 1970	C	10038	8286	1752		
	2.	United Kingdom, Glasgow		Peebles Brown *et al.* 1956	P	1606	1319	287	0·9372	0·7728
					C	5898	4899	999		
						4224			1·0332	0·4982
						χ_1^2 for homogeneity of areas				2·8724

TABLE 3 THE RHESUS BLOOD GROUP SYSTEM (*cont.*)

	Place	Additional details	Authors		Number	D+	D−	D+/D− Relative incidence	D+/D− χ^2_1 for difference from unity
DISEASES OF THE GENITO-URINARY SYSTEM									
NEPHROSES	Austria, Wien	(s) S, ABO	Speiser 1958[a]	P	141	120	21	1·2290	0·6766
				C	1000	823	177		
NEPHRITIS	Austria, Wien	(s) S, ABO	Speiser 1958[a]	P	232	196	36	1·1709	0·6264
				C	1000	823	177		
NEPHRITIS-NEPHROSIS	U.S.A., Michigan	White children	Gershowitz & Neel 1965	P	70	61	9	1·4143*	0·9092
				C	1506	1246	260		
CALCULUS OF KIDNEY	1. Czechoslovakia, Praha		Veselý 1969[c]	P	383	311	72	0·8082	1·9132
				C	1142(c)	962	180		
	2. Germany, Göttingen		Jörgensen & Kallenbach 1968	P	280	240	40	1·0422	0·0560
				C	6122	5216	906		
	3. Italy, Milano		Mor & Sforza 1960	P	164	136	28	0·9114	0·1480
				C	500	421	79		
	4. N. India		Anand 1964[a]	P	187	167	20	1·1133	0·1072
				C	187	165	22		
					1014			0·9222	0·6665
					χ^2_3 for homogeneity of areas				1·5580
NON-GONOCOCCAL URETHRITIS	United Kingdom, Newcastle upon Tyne	(s) S	Schofield 1966	P	345	275	70	0·8966	0·6577
			Kopeć 1970	C	36621	29816	6805		
HYPERPLASIA OF PROSTATE	1. Germany, Göttingen		Jörgensen & Kallenbach 1968	P	1097	896	201	0·7743	8·8591
				C	6122	5216	906		
	2. Italy, Aquila		Curtoni & Morgante 1964	P	180(c)	164	16	1·5841	3·0417
				C	8920(c)	7726	1194		
	3. Italy, Milano		Mor & Sfroza 1960	P	105	85	20	0·7975	0·6666
				C	500	421	79		
	4. United Kingdom, London		Bourke & Griffin 1962	P	271(c)	219	52	0·8761	0·7143
				C	10000	8278	1722		
					1653			0·8364	6·4954
					χ^2_3 for homogeneity of areas				6·7865
MENOPAUSAL METRORRHAGIA	Czechoslovakia		Miluničová *et al.* 1969[a]	P	170	130	40	0·6121	6·1365
			Kout 1959 M2	C	1142	961	181		
DISEASES OF THE SKIN									
PSORIASIS VULGARIS	1. Germany, Giessen, Kassel, Marburg		Wendt 1968	P	403	346	57	1·2322	1·4885
				C	806	670	136		
	2. Germany, Göttingen		Jörgensen & Kallenbach 1968	P	206	168	38	0·7679	2·0776
				C	6122	5216	906		
	3. Northern Sweden		Beckman *et al.* 1974	P	122	102	20	0·8833	0·1878
				C	359	306	53		
					731			0·9709	0·0666
					χ^2_2 for homogeneity of areas				3·6874
DISEASES OF THE MUSCULOSKELETAL SYSTEM									
RHEUMATOID ARTHRITIS	1. Norway, Oslo		Grönvik Kornstad *et al.* 1965	P	217	191	26	1·3416	1·9617
				C	24051	20337	3714		
	2. Romania, Bucureşti		Stoia *et al.* 1969	P	411	369	42	1·5502	7·1625
				C	24829	21105	3724		
					628			1·4677	8·8297
					χ^2_1 for homogeneity of areas				0·2945

TABLE 3 **THE RHESUS BLOOD GROUP SYSTEM** (*cont.*)

	Place	Additional details	Authors		Number	D+	D−	D+/D− Relative incidence	D+/D− χ_1^2 for difference from unity
DISEASES OF THE MUSCULOSKELETAL SYSTEM (*cont.*)									
ANKYLOSING SPONDYLITIS	Norway, Oslo		Grönvik Kornstad *et al.* 1968	P C	200 24051	174 20337	26 3714	1·2222	0·9040
ARTICULAR RHEUMATISM	France, Paris	Acute	Pham-Huu-Trung *et al.* 1961	P C	222 97	186 85	36 12	0·7294	0·7762
PERTHES' DISEASE	United Kingdom, Glasgow		Cameron & Izatt 1962	P C	142 4632	106 3837	36 795	0·6101	6·3056
DUPUYTREN'S DISEASE	Norway, Bergen		Mikkelsen 1967 Kornstad 1959 M2	P C	80 2750	66 2335	14 415	0·8379	0·3499
FRACTURES OF FEMORAL NECK	Germany, Göttingen		Jörgensen & Kallenbach 1968	P C	226 6122	200 5216	26 906	1·3361	1·8761
CONGENITAL ANOMALIES									
SPINA BIFIDA CYSTICA	N. India, Chandigarh		Sidana *et al.* 1970	P C	72 6204	71 5979	1 225	2·6719	0·9481
HYDROCEPHALUS	U.S.A., Michigan	Whites	Gershowitz & Neel 1965	P C	145 1506	123 1256	22 250	1·1128	0·1958
CONGENITAL HEART DEFECTS									
Tetralogy of Fallot	1. Germany, Göttingen		Jörgensen & Kallenbach 1968	P C	316 6122	269 5216	47 906	0·9941	0·0013
	2. United Kingdom, Bristol		David 1970 Kopeć 1970	P C	84 9921	65 8193	19 1728	0·7215	1·5503
					400			0·9102	0·4705
				χ_1^2 for homogeneity of areas					1·0811
Ventricular Septal Defect	1. Germany, Göttingen		Jörgensen & Kallenbach 1968	P C	612 6122	508 5216	104 906	0·8484	2·0976
	2. United Kingdom, Bristol		David 1970 Kopeć 1970	P C	112 9921	91 8193	21 1728	0·9139	0·1365
					724			0·8598	2·1575
				χ_1^2 for homogeneity of areas					0·0766
Atrial Septal Defect	1. Germany, Göttingen		Jörgensen & Kallenbach 1968	P C	296 6122	247 5216	49 906	0·8756	0·6858
	2. United Kingdom, Bristol		David 1970 Kopeć 1970	P C	114 9921	90 8193	24 1728	0·7909	1·0289
					410			0·8471	1·5842
				χ_1^2 for homogeneity of areas					0·1305
Aortic Stenosis	1. Germany, Göttingen		Jörgensen & Kallenbach 1968	P C	242 6122	209 5216	33 906	1·1000	0·2497
	2. Germany, Göttingen	Stenosis of aortic isthmus	Jörgensen & Kallenbach 1968	P C	127 6122	110 5216	17 906	1·1239	0·1968
	3. United Kingdom, Bristol		David 1970 Kopeć 1970	P C	19 9921	17 8193	2 1728	1·7927	0·6090
					388			1·1301	0·6545
				χ_2^2 for homogeneity of areas					0·4010

TABLE 3 **THE RHESUS BLOOD GROUP SYSTEM** (*cont.*)

	Place	Additional details	Authors		Number	D+	D−	D+/D− Relative incidence	D+/D− χ^2_1 for difference from unity
Pulmonary Stenosis	1. Germany, Göttingen		Jörgensen & Kallenbach 1968	P	211	178	33	0·9369	0·1141
				C	6122	5216	906		
	2. United Kingdom, Bristol		David 1970	P	52	44	8	1·1600	0·1484
			Kopeć 1970	C	9921	8193	1728		
					263			0·9779	0·0168
				χ^2_1 for homogeneity of areas					0·2457
Defect not specified	1. N. India, Chandigarh		Sidana *et al.* 1970	P	105	95	10	0·3575	9·1894
				C	6204	5979	225		
	2. U.S.A., Cook County	Negro children	Lev *et al.* 1967	P	200	188	12	0·3701	2·2987
				C	130	127	3		
	3. U.S.A., Michigan	Whites	Gershowitz & Neel 1965	P	122	104	18	1·2508	0·7182
				C	1506	1238	268		
					427			0·7285	2·5457
				χ^2_2 for homogeneity of areas					9·6606
CLEFT LIP OR PALATE	1. Germany, Göttingen		Jörgensen & Kallenbach 1968	P	565	471	94	0·8703	1·3722
				C	6122	5216	906		
	2. Poland, Wrocław	Children	Handzel & Nowakowski 1961	P	90	76	14	1·2241	0·4814
			Grodecka *et al.* 1958 M2	C	20000	16320	3680		
	3. N. India, Chandigarh		Sidana *et al.* 1970	P	35	34	1	1·2795	0·0587
				C	6204	5979	225		
					690			0·9171	0·6285
				χ^2_2 for homogeneity of areas					1·2839
PYLORIC STENOSIS	1. Germany, Göttingen	Pylorospasm	Jörgensen & Kallenbach 1961	P	198	162	36	0·7816	1·7221
				C	6122	5216	906		
	2. United Kingdom, Northern Ireland	Infantile hypertrophic	Dodge 1971	P	486	392	94	0·9822	0·0183
				C	1495(c)	1210	285		
					684			0·9105	0·7515
				χ^2_1 for homogeneity of areas					0·9889
MALFORMATIONS									
Osteogenesis Imperfecta	Sweden		Smårs *et al.* 1961	P	152	131	21	1·4738	1·7909
				C	225	182	43		
Ano-Rectal Defects	N. India, Chandigarh		Sidana *et al.* 1970	P	26	26	0		
				C	6204	5979	225		
Hypospadias	N. India, Chandigarh		Sidana *et al.* 1970	P	23	21	2	0·3951	1·5613
				C	6204	5979	225		
DOWN'S SYNDROME	1. United Kingdom, London		Lang-Brown *et al.* 1952–3	P	144	121	23	1·1104	0·1882
				C	1073	886	187		
	2. U.S.A., Michigan, Ohio		Shaw & Gershowitz 1962	P	370	314	56	1·0947	0·3163
				C	1506	1260	246		
	3. U.S.A., Michigan		Shaw & Gershowitz 1963	P	207	167	40	0·8151	1·1657
				C	1506	1260	246		
	4. U.S.A., Polk	Whites	Kaplan, S. *et al.* 1964	P	290	248	42	0·9773	0·0187
			Tisdall & Garland 1945 M2	C	22133	18990	3143		
	5. Australia	Whites	Simmons *et al.* 1944	P	24	19	5	0·7572	0·3037
				C	3641(c)	3036	605		
					1035			0·9814	0·0436
				χ^2_4 for homogeneity of areas					1·9490

TABLE 3 **THE RHESUS BLOOD GROUP SYSTEM** *(cont.)*

	Place	Additional details	Authors		Number	D+	D−	D+/D− Relative incidence	D+/D− χ_1^2 for difference from unity
ALLERGIES									
ECZEMA	Germany, Berlin		Dorn 1959	P	192	160	32	1·3131	1·2012
				C	250	198	52		
ASTHMA	1. Denmark, Köbenhavn	Bronchial	Viskum 1973	P	39	34	5	1·3049	0·3081
			Andersen 1955	C	14304	12001	2303		
	2. Germany, Göttingen	Exogeneous-allergic	Jörgensen & Kallenbach 1968	P	125	97	28	0·6017	5·4527
				C	6122	5216	906		
	3. Germany, Göttingen	Infection-allergic	Jörgensen & Kallenbach 1968	P	57	47	10	0·8164	0·3359
				C	6122	5216	906		
	4. Germany, Göttingen	Atopic	Jörgensen & Kallenbach 1968	P	137	106	31	0·5939	6·3158
				C	6122	5216	906		
	5. Germany, Göttingen	Asthmatic group	Jörgensen & Kallenbach 1968	P	374	308	66	0·8106	2·2401
				C	6122	5216	906		
	6. Germany, Göttingen	Unclassifiable	Jörgensen & Kallenbach 1968	P	133	115	18	1·1097	0·1642
				C	6122	5216	906		
	7. Italy, Cagliari	Bronchial	Adamo 1961[b]	P	50	50	0		
			Aru 1951 M2	C	200	180	20		
	8. N. India, Delhi		Anand 1964[b]	P	545	487	58	1·2869	1·9078
				C	617	535	82		
	9. U.S.A., Colorado	(s) ABO	Charney 1969	P	206	171	35	1·0023	0·0001
				C	3648	3027	621		
					1616			0·8715	3·4118
				χ_7^2 for homogeneity of areas					13·3129
HAY FEVER	1. Germany, Göttingen	Allergic rhinitis	Jörgensen & Kallenbach 1968	P	141	103	38	0·4708	15·2054
				C	6122	5216	906		
	2. Germany, Göttingen	Pollinosis	Jörgensen & Kallenbach 1968	P	119	88	31	0·4931	11·1335
				C	6122	5216	906		
	3. U.S.A., Colorado	Allergic rhinitis; (s) ABO	Charney 1969	P	211	176	35	1·0316	0·0268
				C	3648	3027	621		
					471			0·6330	16·0349
				χ_2^2 for homogeneity of areas					10·3308
ASTHMA AND/OR HAY FEVER		(s) S, ABO	Vanarsdell & Motulsky 1959	Present	*717*	*587*	*130*	*0·9358*	*0·3898*
				Absent	*3670*	*3040*	*630*		
UNSPECIFIED ALLERGIES	1. Germany, Berlin	Other than eczema	Dorn 1959	P	176	145	31	1·2284	0·6672
				C	250	198	52		
	2. Germany, Göttingen	Atopic group	Jörgensen & Kallenbach 1968	P	205	161	44	0·6356	6·7954
				C	6122	5216	906		
	3. Mexico, Distrito Federal	Mestizos	Salázar-Mallén *et al.* 1969	P	100	91	9	0·4213	1·9534
				C	100	96	4		
					481			0·7616	3·8149
				χ_2^2 for homogeneity of areas					5·6011

TABLE 4
THE ABH SECRETOR SYSTEM

	Place	Additional details	Authors		Number	Secretors	Non-secretors	Secretors/Non-secretors: Relative incidence	Secretors/Non-secretors: χ_1^2 for difference from unity
INFECTIVE AND PARASITIC DISEASES									
BACTERIAL INFECTIONS									
HAEMOLYTIC STREPTOCOCCUS A									
Chronic infection	Romania, Timişoara	School-children; (s) ABO	Radivoievici *et al.* 1972	P	100	65	35	0·3804	8·1365
				C	100	83	17		
Throat carrier status	1. Netherlands	Recruits	Haverkorn & Goslings 1969	Carriers	*144*	*103*	*41*	*0·6692*	*4·1392*
				Non-carriers	*1236*	*976*	*260*		
	2. Netherlands	School-children	Haverkorn & Goslings 1969	Carriers	*55*	*45*	*10*	*1·4717*	*1·0107*
				Non-carriers	*211*	*159*	*52*		
	3. Netherlands, Voorhout		Haverkorn & Goslings 1969	Carriers	*111*	*82*	*29*	*0·6030*	*4·0567*
				Non-carriers	*421*	*347*	*74*		
					310/1868			*0·7222*	*5·1122*
				χ_2^2 for homogeneity of areas					*4·0944*
PULMONARY TUBERCULOSIS	Czechoslovakia, Praha	Males; (s) A	Miluničová & Dominec 1966; Kout 1959 M2	P	106	85	21	1·2004	0·4391
				C	341	263	78		
LEPROSY									
Lepromatous	N. India, Varanasi		Sehgal & Dube 1967[a]	P	42	32	10	1·3714	0·6922
				C	370	259	111		
Non-Lepromatous	N. India, Varanasi		Sehgal & Dube 1967[a]	P	170	111	59	0·8063	1·1939
				C	370	259	111		
					212			0·9025	0·3440
				χ_1^2 for homogeneity of areas					1·5421
SYPHILIS	India, Dehra Dun, Rourkela		Seth 1969	P	132	114	18	0·8945	0·1129
				C	202	177	25		
WORM INFESTATIONS									
BILHARZIAL HEPATIC FIBROSIS	Egypt, Alexandria	(s) ABO	Sadek *et al.* 1965	P	14	10	4	1·1250	0·0322
				C	58	40	18		
FILARIASIS	S. India, Rourkela		Anand 1965	P	178	153	25	0·9905	0·0010
				C	201	173	28		
NEOPLASMS									
MALIGNANT NEOPLASMS									
SALIVARY GLANDS	United Kingdom, Manchester	(s) histo-logically	Garrett *et al.* 1971	P	47	38	9	1·3571	0·6485
				C	851	644	207		
OESOPHAGUS	United Kingdom, London, Leytonstone		Walther *et al.* 1956; Doll *et al.* 1961	P	19	19	0		
				C	610	481	129		
STOMACH	1. Germany, Erlangen, Nürnberg		Berg, G. *et al.* 1967	P	46	39	7	1·1143	0·0406
				C	60	50	10		
	2. United Kingdom, Liverpool		McConnell 1959	P	200	150	50	0·9673	0·0335
				C	849	642	207		

TABLE 4 THE ABH SECRETOR SYSTEM (*cont.*)

	Place	Additional details	Authors		Number	Secretors	Non-secretors	Secretors/Non-secretors: Relative incidence	Secretors/Non-secretors: χ_1^2 for difference from unity
NEOPLASMS (*cont.*)									
MALIGNANT NEOPLASMS (*cont.*)									
STOMACH (*cont.*)									
	3. United Kingdom, London, Leytonstone		Walther *et al.* 1956	P	75	62	13	1·2791	0·5888
			Doll *et al.* 1961	C	610	481	129		
	4. United Kingdom, London	(s) S, ABO	Doll *et al.* 1961	P	105	78	27	0·7748	1·0910
				C	610	481	129		
	5. Japan	Japanese; (s) ABO	Desai & Creger 1964	P	210	186	24	1·9945	5·7448
				C	171	136	35		
	6. U.S.A., California	Whites; (s) ABO	Desai & Creger 1964	P	97	79	18	1·5433	1·7049
				C	123	91	32		
	7. U.S.A., Iowa	(s) S, A_1A_2BO	Newman *et al.* 1961	P	118	92	26	1·0568	0·0567
				C	1261	971	290		
					851			1·1138	1·1597
				χ_6^2 for homogeneity of areas					8·1006
CAECUM, COLON, RECTUM	United Kingdom, London, Leytonstone		Walther *et al.* 1956	P	172	133	39	0·9146	0·1854
			Doll *et al.* 1961	C	610	481	129		
BILE DUCTS, GALL-BLADDER	United Kingdom, London, Leytonstone		Walther *et al.* 1956	P	15	12	3	1·0728	0·0116
			Doll *et al.* 1961	C	610	481	129		
PANCREAS	United Kingdom, London, Leytonstone		Walther *et al.* 1956	P	12	11	1	2·9501	1·0633
			Doll *et al.* 1961	C	610	481	129		
LARYNX, VOCAL CORDS	United Kingdom, London, Leytonstone		Walther *et al.* 1956	P	10	9	1	0·9831	0·0003
			Doll *et al.* 1961	C	610	481	129		
BRONCHUS	United Kingdom, London, Leytonstone		Walther *et al.* 1956	P	161	129	32	1·0811	0·1247
			Doll *et al.* 1961	C	610	481	129		
LUNG	U.S.A., Boston		Krant *et al.* 1968	P	61	47	14	1·2061	0·3465
			Dublin *et al.* 1964	C	594	437	157		
					222			1·1203	0·3914
				χ_1^2 for homogeneity of areas					0·0798
EAR, NOSE, THROAT REGION	Germany, Berlin		Kaiser-Meinhardt 1962	P	65	62	3	3·6773	4·5459
				C	331	281	50		
RODENT ULCER, EPITHELIOMA	United Kingdom, London, Leytonstone		Walther *et al.* 1956	P	20	14	6	0·6258	0·8863
			Doll *et al.* 1961	C	610	481	129		
BREAST	1. United Kingdom, London, Leytonstone	Females	Walther *et al.* 1956	P	133	109	24	1·2180	0·6412
			Doll *et al.* 1961	C	610	481	129		
	2. United Kingdom, Dundee, Edinburgh		Bremner 1961	P	258	176	82	0·6054	6·7531
				C	300	234	66		
	3. Egypt, Alexandria		Sadek *et al.* 1965	P	20	12	8	0·6750	0·5347
				C	58	40	18		
	4. U.S.A., Boston		Krant *et al.* 1968	P	47	34	13	0·9396	0·0337
			Dublin *et al.* 1964	C	594	437	157		
					458			0·8039	2·6432
				χ_3^2 for homogeneity of areas					5·3196

TABLE 4 THE ABH SECRETOR SYSTEM (*cont.*)

	Place	Additional details	Authors		Number	Secretors	Non-secretors	Secretors/Non-secretors: Relative incidence	Secretors/Non-secretors: χ_1^2 for difference from unity
UTERUS	1. Czechoslovakia		Miluničová *et al.* 1969[b]	P	142	119	23	1·5345	2·6763
			Kout 1959 M2	C	341	263	78		
	2. United Kingdom, London, Leytonstone		Walther *et al.* 1956	P	43	36	7	1·3793	0·5729
			Doll *et al.* 1961	C	610	481	129		
					185			1·4901	0·5242
				χ_1^2 for homogeneity of areas					2·7250
OVARIES	1. Czechoslovakia		Miluničová *et al.* 1969[b]	P	50	43	7	1·8218	1·9690
			Kout 1959 M2	C	341	263	78		
	2. United Kingdom, London, Leytonstone		Walther *et al.* 1956	P	32	24	8	0·8046	0·2679
			Doll *et al.* 1961	C	610	481	129		
					82			1·2021	0·3775
				χ_1^2 for homogeneity of areas					1·8594
PROSTATE	United Kingdom, London, Leytonstone		Walther *et al.* 1956	P	41	34	7	1·3026	0·3839
			Doll *et al.* 1961	C	610	481	129		
KIDNEY	United Kingdom, London, Leytonstone		Walther *et al.* 1956	P	16	13	3	1·1622	0·0538
			Doll *et al.* 1961	C	610	481	129		
URINARY BLADDER	1. United Kingdom, London Leytonstone		Walther *et al.* 1956	P	24	16	8	0·5364	1·9663
			Doll *et al.* 1961	C	610	481	129		
	2. Egypt, Alexandria		Sadek *et al.* 1965	P	19	14	5	1·2600	0·1517
				C	58	40	18		
					43			0·7290	0·7903
				χ_1^2 for homogeneity of areas					1·3277
BRAIN	United Kingdom, London, Leytonstone		Walther *et al.* 1956	P	12	11	1	2·9501	1·0633
			Doll *et al.* 1961	C	610	481	129		
CANCERS, SITE UNSPECIFIED	United Kingdom, Sheffield		Green & Dunsford 1954	P	325	255	70	1·2410	1·1702
			Callender *et al.* 1957	C	244	182	62		
SARCOMAS, SITE UNSPECIFIED	United Kingdom, London, Leytonstone		Walther *et al.* 1956	P	20	14	6	0·6258	0·8863
			Doll *et al.* 1961	C	610	481	129		
NEOPLASMS OF LYMPHATIC AND HAEMATOPOIETIC TISSUE									
HODGKIN'S DISEASE	United Kingdom, London, Leytonstone		Walther *et al.* 1956	P	11	7	4	0·4693	1·4210
			Doll *et al.* 1961	C	610	481	129		
LEUKAEMIAS	1. United Kingdom, London, Leytonstone		Walther *et al.* 1956	P	40	31	9	0·9238	0·0410
			Doll *et al.* 1961	C	610	481	129		
	2. U.S.A., Michigan	Whites	Gershowitz & Neel 1965	P	159	117	42	0·8439	0·7978
				C	1501	1152	349		
	3. Brazil, Rio Grande do Sul	Whites	Ayres *et al.* 1966	P	28(c)	23	5	1·2545	0·1129
				C	28(c)	22	6		
					227			0·8784	0·6119
				χ_2^2 for homogeneity of areas					0·3398

TABLE 4 THE ABH SECRETOR SYSTEM (*cont.*)

	Place	Additional details	Authors		Number	Secretors	Non-secretors	Secretors/Non-secretors: Relative incidence	Secretors/Non-secretors: χ_1^2 for difference from unity
NEOPLASMS (*cont.*)									
BENIGN NEOPLASMS									
ADENOLYMPHOMA	United Kingdom, Manchester		Garrett *et al.* 1971	P	21	13	8	0·5223	2·0250
				C	851	644	207		
MIXED SALIVARY ADENOMAS	United Kingdom, Manchester		Garrett *et al.* 1971	P	208	161	47	1·1011	0·2737
				C	851	644	207		
ENDOCRINE AND METABOLIC DISEASES									
NON-TOXIC GOITRE									
Single adenoma	United Kingdom, Liverpool	(s) ABO	Kitchin *et al.* 1959	P	34	23	11	0·7893	0·3532
				C	208	151	57		
Multiple adenoma	United Kingdom, Liverpool	(s) ABO	Kitchin *et al.* 1959	P	179	135	44	1·1582	0·3972
				C	208	151	57		
THYROTOXICOSIS									
Primary diffuse goitre	United Kingdom, Liverpool	(s) ABO	Kitchin *et al.* 1959	P	104	70	34	0·7772	0·9365
				C	208	151	57		
Secondary multiple adenoma	United Kingdom, Liverpool	(s) ABO	Kitchin *et al.* 1959	P	24	21	3	2·6424	2·3306
				C	208	151	57		
DIABETES MELLITUS	1. Czechoslovakia, Praha	Males; (s) A	Miluničová & Dominec 1966 Kout 1959 M2	P	121	102	19	1·5922	2·7360
				C	341	263	78		
	2. Germany, Erlangen, Nürnberg		Berg *et al.* 1967[a]	P	49	43	6	1·4333	0·4182
				C	60	50	10		
	3. Poland, Kołobrzeg		Grabowska 1969	P	1394	1234	160	1·9615	23·5911
				C	508	405	103		
	4. United Kingdom, London	(s) S, ABO	Doll *et al.* 1961	P	102	85	17	1·3410	1·0703
				C	610	481	129		
	5. United Kingdom, Belfast		Macafee 1964[b]	P	616	387	229	0·9333	0·2949
				C	475	306	169		
	6. U.S.A., Iowa	(s) ABO	Buckwalter 1964	P	768	601	167	1·0748	0·4292
				C	1261	971	290		
					3178			1·2348	9·9920
				χ_5^2 for homogeneity of areas					18·5477
CELIAC DISEASE	1. United Kingdom, Birmingham	(s) ABO	Langman *et al.* 1969	P	50	43	7	1·7666	1·8412
				C	591	459	132		
	2. United Kingdom, London	(s) ABO	Langman *et al.* 1969	P	92	67	25	0·7707	1·0486
				C	591	459	132		
					142			0·9633	0·0296
				χ_1^2 for homogeneity of areas					2·8603
DISEASES OF THE BLOOD									
PERNICIOUS ANAEMIA	1. United Kingdom, England	(s) Le	Callender *et al.* 1957	P	244	176	68	0·8817	0·3773
				C	244	182	62		
	2. U.S.A., Boston	(s) S, ABO	Hoskins *et al.* 1965	P	112	90	22	1·2280	0·7219
				C	3032(c)	2332	700		
	3. U.S.A., Chicago	Whites	Ladenson *et al.* 1949 Newman *et al.* 1961	P	85	66	19	1·0375	0·0187
				C	1261	971	290		
	4. U.S.A., Chicago	Negroes	Ladenson *et al.* 1949 Miller *et al.* 1954 M2	P	21	12	9	0·5167	1·8230
				C	111	80	31		
					462			0·9710	0·0510
				χ_3^2 for homogeneity of areas					2·8899

TABLE 4 THE ABH SECRETOR SYSTEM (*cont.*)

	Place	Additional details	Authors		Number	Secretors	Non-secretors	Secretors/Non-secretors: Relative incidence	Secretors/Non-secretors: χ^2_1 for difference from unity
MENTAL DISORDERS									
SCHIZOPHRENIA	U.S.A., Biloxi	(s) ABO	Lafferty *et al.* 1960	P	110	88	22	1·7143	2·7817
				C	100	70	30		
ALCOHOLISM	1. United Kingdom	English; (s) ABO	Camps *et al.* 1969	P	403(a)	280	123	0·7306	3·1950
				C	284	215	69		
	2. United Kingdom	Scottish; (s) ABO	Camps *et al.* 1969	P	263(a)	162	101	0·6676	6·3845
				C	507	358	149		
	3. United Kingdom	Irish; (s) ABO	Camps *et al.* 1969	P	175(a)	116	59	0·8638	0·7047
				C	973	676	297		
					841			0·7446	9·0812
				χ^2_2 for homogeneity of areas					1·2030
DISEASES OF THE NERVOUS SYSTEM AND SENSE ORGANS									
MULTIPLE SCLEROSIS	1. United Kingdom, Newcastle upon Tyne		MacDonald *et al.* 1976	P	97	69	28	0·7187	0·9763
				C	93	72	21		
	2. United Kingdom, Newcastle upon Tyne		Roberts 1976	P	177	129	48	0·7838	0·6584
				C	93	72	21		
					274			0·7541	1·5974
				χ^2_1 for homogeneity of areas					0·0373
AMYOTROPHIC LATERAL SCLEROSIS	U.S.A., Maryland		Myrianthopoulis & Leyshon 1967	P	319	256	63	1·2244	1·0605
				C	298	229	69		
UVEITIS	Japan, Tokyo	(s) ABO	Oda 1971	P	239	149	90	0·5519	4·9666
				C	100	75	25		
PRIMARY GLAUCOMA	N. India, Sitapur	56 wide angle, 39 narrow angle, 5 could not be classified; (s) ABO	Garg & Pahwa 1965	P	100	31	69	0·1821	50·8841
			Tyagi *et al.* 1968 M2	C	475	338	137		
DISEASES OF THE CIRCULATORY SYSTEM									
RHEUMATIC FEVER	1. Irish Republic, Dublin		Glynn & Holborow 1961	P	29	17	12	0·8657	0·0720
				C	29	18	11		
	2. Netherlands		Haverkorn & Goslings 1969	P	133	102	31	0·8923	0·2905
				C	2250	1770	480		
	3. United Kingdom, Slough	Children	Glynn *et al.* 1959	P	553	393	160	0·7283	5·8204
				C	669	516	153		
	4. United Kingdom, Belfast		Glynn & Holborow 1961	P	36	19	17	0·3193	4·7879
				C	36	28	8		
	5. U.S.A., Iowa	(s) A_1A_2BO	Buckwalter *et al.* 1962	P	376	279	97	0·8590	1·2567
				C	1261	971	290		
	6. U.S.A., Michigan	Whites	Gershowitz & Neel 1965	P	102	70	32	0·6627	3·4356
				C	1501	1152	349		
	7. U.S.A., New York		Glynn & Holborow 1961	P	79	56	23	0·8747	0·2559
			Dublin *et al.* 1964	C	594	437	157		
					1308			0·7787	11·0406
				χ^2_6 for homogeneity of areas					4·8783

TABLE 4 THE ABH SECRETOR SYSTEM (*cont.*)

	Place	Additional details	Authors		Number	Secretors	Non-secretors	Secretors/Non-secretors: Relative incidence	Secretors/Non-secretors: χ_1^2 for difference from unity
DISEASES OF THE CIRCULATORY SYSTEM (*cont.*)									
RHEUMATIC HEART DISEASE	1. Netherlands	Mitral stenosis	Haverkorn & Goslings 1969	P	375	298	77	1·0495	0·1230
				C	2250	1770	480		
	2. United Kingdom, Liverpool	Carditis	Clarke *et al.* 1960	P	263	190	73	0·8366	1·2559
				C	851	644	207		
	3. U.S.A., Boston	(s) Le	Dublin *et al.* 1964	P	600	420	180	0·8383	1·8749
				C	594	437	157		
					1238			0·9055	1·5011
					χ_2^2 for homogeneity of areas				1·7529
HYPERTENSION	Czechoslovakia	Diastolic pressure ⩾ 110 mmHg; (s) ABO	Mikolášek & Miluničová 1967	P	383	312	71	1·3033	2·0689
				C	341	263	78		
OCCLUSIVE PERIPHERAL ARTERIOSCLEROSIS	United Kingdom, Leeds, York	Males; (s) ABO	Hall *et al.* 1971	P	66	36	30	0·3851	11·3453
			Lincoln & Dodd 1972 M2	C	284	215	69		
DISEASES OF THE RESPIRATORY SYSTEM									
BRONCHITIS	Germany, Erlangen, Nürnberg	Chronic or recurrent	Berg, G. *et al.* 1967	P	48	40	8	1·0000	0·0000
				C	60	50	10		
DISEASES OF THE DIGESTIVE SYSTEM									
GASTRITIS	Egypt, Alexandria	(s) ABO	Sadek *et al.* 1965	P	26	12	14	0·3857	3·8567
				C	58	40	18		
PANCREATITIS	Germany, Erlangen, Nürnberg	Acute or chronic	Berg, G. *et al.* 1967	P	27	22	5	0·8800	0·0447
				C	60	50	10		
ULCERATIVE COLITIS	1. United Kingdom, Liverpool		Winstone *et al.* 1960	P	163	117	46	0·8136	1·0279
				C	491(c)	372	119		
	2. United Kingdom, Oxford		Smith & Truelove 1961	P	101	77	24	1·0929	0·1036
			Callender *et al.* 1957	C	244	182	62		
					264			0·9026	0·3913
					χ_1^2 for homogeneity of areas				0·7403
APHTHOUS ULCERS	United Kingdom, Liverpool		McConnell 1959	P	156	119	37	1·0370	0·0316
				C	849	642	207		
GASTRIC ULCERS	1. Czechoslovakia, Praha		Kubičková & Veselý 1966	P	171	125	46	0·8059	1·0042
			Kout 1959 M2	C	341	263	78		
	2. Germany, Erlangen, Nürnberg		Berg, G. *et al.* 1967	P	78	57	21	0·5429	2·0156
				C	60	50	10		
	3. Poland		Belec *et al.* 1971	P	196	91	105	0·2153	99·7159
			Socha 1966 M2	C	2000	1602	398		
	4. Romania		Fodor & Urcan 1966	P	94	70	24	0·8922	0·1606
				C	222	170	52		
	5. Spain, Viscaya	Basques	Goti Iturriaga & Velasco Alonso 1965	P	19	11	8	0·3153	5·7186
				C	386	314	72		
	6. Spain, Viscaya	Non-Basques	Goti Iturriaga & Velasco Alonso 1965	P	21	13	8	0·5246	1·9085
				C	336	254	82		
	7. United Kingdom, Liverpool		McConnell 1966	P	404	288	116	0·7939	3·7154
				C	2435	1845	590		

TABLE 4 THE ABH SECRETOR SYSTEM (*cont.*)

	Place	Additional details	Authors		Number	Secretors	Non-secretors	Secretors/Non-secretors: Relative incidence	Secretors/Non-secretors: χ_1^2 for difference from unity
	8. United Kingdom, London	(s) S, ABO	Doll *et al.* 1961	P	202	139	63	0·5917	8·3690
				C	610	481	129		
	9. United Kingdom, Glasgow		Wallace *et al.* 1958	P	47	30	17	0·6279	2·1148
				C	503	371	132		
	10. U.S.A., Iowa	(s) S, A_1A_2BO	Newman *et al.* 1961	P	184	137	47	0·8706	0·5813
				C	1261	971	290		
					1416			0·5867	65·5866
				χ_9^2 for homogeneity of areas					59·7173
Bleeding	United Kingdom, London	(s) S, ABO	Langman & Doll 1965	P	92	61	31	0·5277	6·9856
			Doll *et al.* 1961	C	610	481	129		
Not Bleeding	United Kingdom, London	(s) S, ABO	Langman & Doll 1965	P	269	202	67	0·8086	1·5198
			Doll *et al.* 1961	C	610	481	129		
Bleeding/Not bleeding	United Kingdom, London	(s) S, ABO	Langman & Doll 1965	Bleeding	*92*	*61*	*31*	*0·6527*	*2·6568*
				Not bleeding	*269*	*202*	*67*		
STOMAL ULCERS	1. United Kingdom, London	(s) S, ABO	Doll *et al.* 1961	P	83	42	41	0·2747	28·7633
				C	610	481	129		
	2. United Kingdom, London	(s) ABO	Langman *et al.* 1967	P	176	99	77	0·3448	34·4383
			Doll *et al.* 1961	C	610	481	129		
	3. United Kingdom, Glasgow		Wallace *et al.* 1958	P	52	31	21	0·5252	4·5997
				C	503	371	132		
					311			0·3493	64·9569
				χ_2^2 for homogeneity of areas					2·8443
DUODENAL ULCERS	1. Czechoslovakia, Praha		Kubičková & Veselý 1966	P	461	300	161	0·5526	13·4415
			Kout 1959 M2	C	341	263	78		
	2. Germany, Erlangen, Nürnberg		Berg, G. *et al.* 1967	P	92	62	30	0·4133	4·6062
				C	60	50	10		
	3. Poland		Belec *et al.* 1971	P	804	583	221	0·6554	19·0396
			Socha 1966 M2	C	2000	1602	398		
	4. Romania		Fodor & Urcan 1966	P	352	225	127	0·5419	10·0271
				C	222	170	52		
	5. Spain	Basques; (s) ABO	Goti Iturriaga & Velasco Alonso 1965	P	95	74	21	0·8080	0·5811
				C	386	314	72		
	6. Spain	Non-Basques; (s) ABO	Goti Iturriaga & Velasco Alonso 1965	P	143	108	35	0·9962	0·0003
				C	336	254	82		
	7. United Kingdom, Liverpool	(s) S	McConnell 1966	P	1540	997	543	0·5871	55·8161
				C	2435	1845	590		
	8. United Kingdom, Liverpool	Perforated; (s) ABO	Evans *et al.* 1968	P	60	33	27	0·3908	12·6845
			Horwich *et al.* 1966	C	2435	1845	590		
	9. United Kingdom, London	(s) S, ABO	Doll *et al.* 1961	P	369	233	136	0·4595	28·1608
				C	610	481	129		
	10. United Kingdom, London	(s) ABO	Langman *et al.* 1967	P	611	285	226	0·4569	36·4106
			Doll *et al.* 1961	C	610	481	129		
	11. United Kingdom, Glasgow		Wallace *et al.* 1958	P	310	192	118	0·5789	12·4722
				C	503	371	132		
	12. Egypt, Alexandria	(s) ABO	Sadek *et al.* 1965	P	47	20	27	0·3333	7·2017
				C	58	40	18		
	13. Nigeria	Yoruba	Ball 1962	P	172	108	64	0·5725	7·3163
				C	300	224	76		
	14. U.S.A., Iowa	(s) S, A_1A_2BO	Newman 1961	P	479	326	153	0·6364	14·5077
				C	1261	971	290		
	15. U.S.A., Los Angeles	25% Negroes	Ventzke & Grossman 1962	P	100	51	49	0·3320	26·5653
			Vanarsdel & Motulsky 1959	C	947	718	229		
			Cepellini *et al.* 1959 M2						
					5635			0·5668	222·4635
				χ_{14}^2 for homogeneity of areas					26·3675

TABLE 4 THE ABH SECRETOR SYSTEM (*cont.*)

	Place	Additional details	Authors		Number	Secretors	Non-secretors	Secretors/Non-secretors: Relative incidence	Secretors/Non-secretors: χ_1^2 for difference from unity
DISEASES OF THE DIGESTIVE SYSTEM (*cont.*)									
DUODENAL ULCERS (*cont.*)									
Bleeding	1. United Kingdom, Liverpool and SW. Lancashire	(s) S, ABO	Horwich *et al.* 1966	P C	128 2435	81 1845	47 590	0·5511	9·8999
	2. United Kingdom, London	(s) ABO	Langman & Doll 1965 Doll *et al.* 1961	P C	120 610	78 481	42 129	0·4981	10·4571
	3. United Kingdom, Newcastle upon Tyne		Pringle *et al.* 1964	P C	75 301	44 230	31 71	0·4381	9·2750
					323			0·5066	29·1417
				χ_2^2 for homogeneity of areas					0·4903
Not bleeding	1. United Kingdom, Liverpool and SW. Lancashire	(s) S, ABO	Horwich *et al.* 1966	P C	674 2435	437 1845	237 590	0·5896	31·9265
	2. United Kingdom, London	(s) ABO	Langman & Doll 1965 Doll *et al.* 1961	P C	359 610	220 481	139 129	0·4245	34·0440
	3. United Kingdom, Newcastle upon Tyne		Pringle *et al.* 1964	P C	100 301	72 230	28 71	0·7938	0·7839
					1133			0·5542	61·1182
				χ_2^2 for homogeneity of areas					5·6362
Bleeding/Not bleeding	1. United Kingdom, Liverpool and SW. Lancashire	(s) S, ABO	Horwich *et al.* 1966	Bleeding Not bleeding	*128* *674*	*81* *437*	*47* *237*	*0·9347*	*0·1138*
	2. United Kingdom, London	(s) ABO	Langman & Doll 1965	Bleeding Not bleeding	*120* *359*	*78* *220*	*42* *139*	*1·1734*	*0·5290*
	3. United Kingdom, Newcastle upon Tyne		Pringle *et al.* 1964	Bleeding Not bleeding	*75* *100*	*44* *72*	*31* *28*	*0·5520*	*3·3767*
					323/1133			*0·9290*	*0·2987*
				χ_2^2 for homogeneity of areas					*3·7208*
BOTH DUODENAL AND GASTRIC ULCERS PRESENT	Czechoslovakia, Praha		Kubičková & Veselý 1966 Kout 1959 M2	P C	52 341	37 263	15 78	0·7316	0·8857
PEPTIC ULCERS, SITE UNSPECIFIED	Venezuela, Maracai	84% duodenal; (s) S, ABO	Arias & Bermúdez 1963	P C	81 202	49 109	32 93	1·3065	0·9984
DISEASES OF THE GENITO-URINARY SYSTEM									
NEPHRITIS-NEPHROSIS	U.S.A., Michigan	Whites	Gershowitz & Neel 1965	P C	69 1501	57 1152	12 349	1·4390	1·2663
MENOPAUSAL METRORRHAGIA	Czechoslovakia		Miluničová *et al.* 1969[a] Kout 1959 M2	P C	170 341	146 263	24 78	1·8042	5·3459
DISEASES OF THE SKIN									
VITILIGO	1. N. India, Calcutta		Dutta *et al.* 1969	P C	247 438	170 321	77 117	0·8047	1·5462
	2. N. India, Varanasi		Sehgal & Dube 1967[b]	P C	76 370	65 259	11 111	2·5325	7·2455
					323			1·0167	0·0113
				χ_1^2 for homogeneity of areas					8·7804

TABLE 4 **THE ABH SECRETOR SYSTEM** *(cont.)*

	Place	Additional details	Authors		Number	Secretors	Non-secretors	Secretors/Non-secretors: Relative incidence	Secretors/Non-secretors: χ_1^2 for difference from unity
CONGENITAL ANOMALIES									
HYDROCEPHALUS	U.S.A., Michigan	Whites	Gershowitz & Neel 1965	P	138	100	38	0·7972	1·2821
				C	1501	1152	349		
CONGENITAL HEART DISEASE	U.S.A., Michigan	Whites	Gershowitz & Neel 1965	P	116	88	28	0·9521	0·0474
				C	1501	1152	349		
PYLORIC STENOSIS	United Kingdom, Northern Ireland	Infantile hypertrophic	Dodge 1971	P	465	362	103	1·2706	2·5929
				C	531	390	141		
				χ_1^2 for homogeneity of areas					0·0254
DOWN'S SYNDROME	1. United Kingdom, Liverpool	(s) S, ABO	Evans *et al.* 1966	P	82	69	13	1·6487	2·5783
			McConnell 1966	C	1000	763	237		
	2. U.S.A., Michigan		Shaw & Gershowitz 1962	P	367	282	85	1·0051	0·0014
				C	1501	1152	349		
	3. U.S.A., Michigan		Shaw & Gershowitz 1963	P	207	147	60	0·7422	3·2666
				C	1501	1152	349		
					656			0·9459	0·3076
				χ_2^2 for homogeneity of areas					5·5387
ALLERGIES									
ASTHMA	United Kingdom, Liverpool		McConnell 1959	P	250(c)	191	59	1·0438	0·0643
				C	849(c)	642	207		
ASTHMA AND/OR HAY FEVER	Australia, Melbourne	(s) S	Denborough & Downing 1968	P	404	306	98	0·8141	1·3765
				C	353	280	73		
ASTHMA OR HAY FEVER	U.S.A., Seattle	Whites; (s) S, ABO	Vanarsdel & Motulsky 1959	Present	*789*	*619*	*170*	*1·2089*	*3·6855*
				Absent	*2355*	*1768*	*587*		

TABLE 5
THE PLASMA HAPTOGLOBIN SYSTEM

	Place	Additional details	Authors		Number	Hp 1-1	Hp 2-1	Hp 2-2	Hp 0	Hp 2-2/Hp 1-1+ Hp 2-1		Hp 0/Hp 1-1+ Hp 2-1+Hp 2-2	
										Relative incidence	χ_1^2 for difference from unity	Relative incidence	χ_1^2 for difference from unity
INFECTIVE AND PARASITIC DISEASES													
BACTERIAL INFECTIONS													
TUBERCULOSIS													
Pulmonary	1. Germany, Southern Niedersachsen		Jörgensen & Rübberdt 1968	P	684	113	353	218	0	0·8509	1·9880		
				C	685	114	328	243	0				
	2. Hungary, Budapest		Hevér 1969	P	1351	158	589	604	0	1·2047	6·8019		
				C	1977	250	933	794	0				
					2035					1·0929	2·1517		
				χ_1^2 for homogeneity of areas							6·6381		
Of bones and joints	Hungary, Budapest		Hevér 1969	P	519	64	213	242	0	1·3017	7·0588		
				C	1977	250	933	794	0				
SARCOIDOSIS	Germany, Göttingen		Jörgensen 1965	P	392	66	189	137	0	0·9933	0·0038		
				C	5088	839	2463	1786	0				
LEPROSY													
Lepromatous	1. N. India, Bankura, Purulia		Walter *et al.* 1972	P	310	8	71	231	0	1·3675	3·3885		
				C	386	13	110	263	0				
	2. S. India, near Vellore		Horton & Povey 1964	P	133	1	21	98	13	0·9608	0·0192	0·8141	0·3536
				C	281	4	40	204	33				
					443					1·2486	2·2968		
				χ_1^2 for homogeneity of areas							1·1109		
Tuberculoid	S. India, near Vellore		Horton & Povey 1964	P	102	2	13	75	12	1·0784	0·0532	1·0020	0·0000
				C	281	4	40	204	33				
Dimorphous	S. India, near Vellore		Horton & Povey 1964	P	46	1	6	31	8	0·9552	0·0104	1·5821	1·1337
				C	281	4	40	204	33				
Non-lepromatous	N. India, Bankura, Purulia		Walter *et al.* 1972	P	291	9	80	202	0	1·0615	0·1266		
				C	386	13	110	263	0				
Unspecified types	1. Moçambique	Macua	Walter *et al.* 1970	P	125(c)	51	59	15	0	0·5377	3·4513		
				C	173(c)	65	73	35	0				
	2. Brazil, Curitiba	Whites	Schwantes *et al.* 1967	P	299(c)	55	144	98	2	1·2167	0·6793	0·3973	0·8420
				C	120(c)	21	63	34	2				
	3. Brazil, Florianópolis	Whites	Schwantes *et al.* 1967	P	212(c)	49	111	49	3	0·6044	3·8227	0·2703	3·3316
				C	119(c)	21	54	38	6				
	4. Brazil, Pôrto Alegre	Whites	Schwantes *et al.* 1967	P	424(c)	71	210	131	12	0·6501	6·8838		
				C	261(c)	43	109	109	0				
					1060					0·7221	8·4666	0·3077	4·0764
				χ_3^2 for homogeneity of areas							6·3705		
					(511)	χ_1^2 for homogeneity of areas							0·0972
VIRAL INFECTIONS													
POLIOMYELITIS	Poland, Kraków	Children	Kobielowa *et al.* 1962	P	161	24	54	83	0	1·7350	11·6861		
				C	3809	561	1800	1448	0				
INFECTIOUS HEPATITIS	Hungary, Budapest		Hevér 1969	P	162	18	85	59	0	0·8535	0·8731		
				C	1977	250	933	794	0				

TABLE 5 **THE PLASMA HAPTOGLOBIN SYSTEM** (*cont.*)

	Place	Additional details	Authors		Number	Hp 1-1	Hp 2-1	Hp 2-2	Hp 0	Hp 2-2/Hp 1-1+Hp 2-1 Relative incidence	Hp 2-2/Hp 1-1+Hp 2-1 χ_1^2 for difference from unity	Hp 0/Hp 1-1+Hp 2-1+Hp 2-2 Relative incidence	Hp 0/Hp 1-1+Hp 2-1+Hp 2-2 χ_1^2 for difference from unity
NEOPLASMS													
MALIGNANT NEOPLASMS													
OESOPHAGUS	Germany, Düsseldorf		Pietrek & Kindler 1971	P	16	1	13	2	0	0·2527	3·3014		
				C	2345	336	1162	847	0				
STOMACH	1. Germany, Düsseldorf		Pietrek & Kindler 1971	P	21	3	8	10	0	1·6078	1·1699		
				C	2345	336	1162	847	0				
	2. Australia, New South Wales	(s) S	Larkin 1967	P	22	4	9	9	0	1·1683	0·1222		
				C	430	65	205	160					
					43					1·3735	1·0311		
				χ_1^2 for homogeneity of areas							0·2610		
COLON, CAECUM, RECTUM	Australia, New South Wales	(s) S	Larkin 1967	P	52	7	24	21	0	1·1431	0·1992		
				C	430	65	205	160	0				
BRONCHUS	Australia, New South Wales	(s) S	Larkin 1967	P	21	6	10	5	0	0·5273	1·5029		
				C	430	65	205	160	0				
LUNG	Germany, Düsseldorf		Pietrek & Kindler 1971	P	28	4	13	11	0	1·1444	0·1200		
				C	2345	336	1162	847	0				
BREAST	Australia, New South Wales		Larkin 1967	P	144	21	66	57	0	1·1056	0·2585		
				C	430	65	205	160	0				
CERVIX UTERI	1. Czechoslovakia		Miluničová *et al.* 1969[d]	P	85	16	41	28	0	0·7148	1·9149		
			Kout & Baitsch 1963 M2	C	739	109	329	301	0				
	2. Germany, Marburg		Ihm & Wendt 1966	P	184	20	96	68	0	1·1998	1·1571		
				C	847	143	426	278	0				
	3. Australia, New South Wales		Larkin 1967	P	30	1	15	14	0	1·4766	1·0556		
				C	430	65	205	160	0				
					299					1·0587	0·1916		
				χ_2^2 for homogeneity of areas							3·9361		
CORPUS UTERI	Czechoslovakia		Miluničová *et al.* 1969[d]	P	140	16	69	55	0	0·9416	0·1020		
			Kout & Baitsch 1963 M2	C	739	109	329	301	0				
OVARIES	Czechoslovakia		Miluničová *et al.* 1969[d]	P	50	7	21	22	0	1·1433	0·2068		
			Kout & Baitsch 1963 M2	C	739	109	329	301	0				
VULVA	Czechoslovakia		Miluničová *et al.* 1969[d]	P	14	2	7	5	0	0·8084	0·1428		
			Kout & Baitsch 1963 M2	C	739	109	329	301	0				
MELANOMAS	1. Germany, Göttingen		Jörgensen & Lal 1972	P	164	28	84	52	0	0·8445	0·8270		
				C	685	114	328	243	0				
	2. Australia, New South Wales	(s) S	Larkin 1967	P	83	9	37	37	0	1·3573	1·5897		
				C	430	65	205	160	0				
					247					1·0068	0·0021		
				χ_1^2 for homogeneity of areas							2·4146		
OTHER THAN OESOPHAGUS, STOMACH, LUNG	Germany, Düsseldorf		Pietrek & Kindler 1971	P	43	4	27	12	0	0·6846	1·2224		
				C	2345	336	1162	847	0				
SITE UNSPECIFIED	Hungary, Budapest		Hevér 1966	P	25	6	11	8	0	0·7011	0·6780		
				C	1977	250	933	794	0				

TABLE 5 **THE PLASMA HAPTOGLOBIN SYSTEM** (*cont.*)

	Place	Additional details	Authors		Number	Hp 1-1	Hp 2-1	Hp 2-2	Hp 0	Hp 2-2/Hp 1-1+Hp 2-1		Hp 0/Hp 1-1+Hp 2-1+Hp 2-2	
										Relative incidence	χ_1^2 for difference from unity	Relative incidence	χ_1^2 for difference from unity
NEOPLASMS (*cont.*)													
NEOPLASMS OF LYMPHATIC AND HAEMATOPOIETIC TISSUE													
RETICULOSES	Australia, New South Wales	(s) S	Larkin 1967	P	36	7	17	12	0	0·8436	0·2139		
				C	430	65	205	160	0				
MYELOID LEUKAEMIA Acute	1. United Kingdom, Newcastle upon Tyne		Latner & Zaki 1960	P	6	2	2	2	0	0·7500	0·0931		
				C	30	3	15	12	0				
	2. U.S.A., Bethesda		Peacock 1966	P	19	3	11	5	0	0·4690	1·9587		
				C	192(c)	24	85	83	0				
					25					0·5268	1·8661		
				χ_1^2 for homogeneity of areas							0·1857		
Chronic	1. United Kingdom, Newcastle upon Tyne		Latner & Zaki 1960	P	10	4	4	2	0	0·3750	1·2761		
				C	30	3	15	12	0				
	2. U.S.A., Bethesda		Peacock 1966	P	24	4	14	6	0	0·4378	2·8033		
				C	192(c)	24	85	83	0				
					34					0·4219	4·0510		
				χ_1^2 for homogeneity of areas							0·0284		
LYMPHATIC LEUKAEMIA Acute	U.S.A., Bethesda		Peacock 1966	P	36	11	19	6	0	0·2627	8·0796		
				C	192(c)	24	85	83	0				
Chronic	United Kingdom, Newcastle upon Tyne		Latner & Zaki 1960	P	10	5	2	3	0	0·6429	0·3174		
				C	30	3	15	12	0				
BENIGN NEOPLASMS													
	Hungary, Budapest		Hevér 1966	P	41	2	15	24	0	2·1034	5·3891		
				C	1977	250	933	794	0				
ENDOCRINE AND METABOLIC DISEASES													
DIABETES MELLITUS	1. Germany, Niedersachsen		Jörgensen & Hopfer, U. 1967	P	216	32	105	79	0	1·0489	0·0865		
				C	685	114	328	243	0				
	2. Canada, Toronto		Simpson *et al.* 1962	P	98	13	39	46	0	1·5329	3·5248		
				C	399	51	202	146	0				
					314					1·1920	1·7677		
				χ_1^2 for homogeneity of areas							1·8435		
PHENYLKETONURIA	U.S.A., Dixon		Hsia *et al.* 1969	P	68	8	30	30	0	1·7023	2·6853		
				C	101	18	51	32	0				
CYSTIC FIBROSIS OF PANCREAS	U.S.A., Dixon		Hsia *et al.* 1969	P	75	17	34	24	0	1·0147	0·0020		
				C	101	18	51	32	0				
MENTAL DISORDERS													
SCHIZOPHRENIA	1. Germany, Rostock		Göhler & Göhler 1963	P	65	10	26	29	0	1·5034	2·5050		
				C	1072	183	515	374	0				
	2. Canada, London		Lovegrove & Nicholls 1965	P	198	32	115	51	0	1·0472	0·0417		
				C	217	33	130	54	0				
					263					1·2256	1·4334		
				χ_1^2 for homogeneity of areas							1·1133		

TABLE 5 **THE PLASMA HAPTOGLOBIN SYSTEM** (*cont.*)

	Place	Additional details	Authors		Number	Hp 1-1	Hp 2-1	Hp 2-2	Hp 0	Hp 2-2/Hp 1-1+Hp 2-1		Hp 0/Hp 1-1+Hp 2-1+Hp 2-2	
										Relative incidence	χ_1^2 for difference from unity	Relative incidence	χ_1^2 for difference from unity
Manic-depressive Psychoses	Germany, Rostock		Göhler & Göhler 1963	P	22	2	10	10	0	1·5553	1·0406		
				C	1072	183	515	374	0				
Symptomatic Psychoses	Germany, Rostock		Göhler & Göhler 1963	P	25	4	11	10	0	1·2442	0·2796		
				C	1072	183	515	374	0				
Psychopathy	Germany, Rostock		Göhler & Göhler 1963	P	109	16	57	36	0	0·9204	0·1510		
				C	1072	183	515	374	0				
Oligophrenia	Germany, Rostock		Göhler & Göhler 1963	P	30	3	18	9	0	0·7998	0·3063		
				C	1072	183	515	374	0				
DISEASES OF THE NERVOUS SYSTEM													
Multiple Sclerosis	1. Germany, Essen		Bertrams & Kuwert 1976	P	799(c)	136	386	277	0	0·8725	2·6991		
				C	3107(c)	475	1457	1175	0				
	2. United Kingdom, Newcastle upon Tyne		MacDonald *et al.* 1976	P	136	13	74	49	0	1·3517	1·3490		
				C	136	24	72	40	0				
	3. United Kingdom, Newcastle upon Tyne		Roberts 1976	P	84	8	44	32	0	1·4769	1·7708		
				C	136	24	72	40	0				
					1019					0·9391	0·6765		
					χ_2^2 for homogeneity of areas						5·1424		
Epilepsy	1. Germany, Rostock		Göhler & Göhler 1963	P	68	10	32	26	0	1·1553	0·3141		
				C	1072	183	515	374	0				
	2. United Kingdom, England		Rundle *et al.* 1972	P	409	59	185	165	0	1·4108	3·3204		
			Harris *et al.* 1959 M2	C	179	33	88	58	0				
					477					1·3156	3·2435		
					χ_1^2 for homogeneity of areas						0·3910		
Kuru	New Guinea, Highlands	Fore	Curtain *et al.* 1961	P	73	28	26	19	0	1·2063	0·2154		
				C	62	31	17	14	0				
DISEASES OF THE CIRCULATORY SYSTEM													
Rheumatic Fever	U.S.A., Boston		Murray *et al.* 1966	P	405	45	183	167	10	1·1032	0·4673	10·2785	4·9123
				C	407	51	193	162	1				
Hypertension	Czechoslovakia		Mikolášek & Miluničová 1967	P	383	57	180	145	1	1·1265	0·7995		
				C	662	113	316	233	0				
Cardiac Infarction	Germany, Marburg		Ihm & Wendt 1966	P	458	84	201	173	0	1·2424	3·2175		
				C	847	143	426	278	0				
Cerebral Sclerosis	Germany, Dresden	(s) A, S	Thomas & Hofmann 1967	P	298	53	146	99	0	1·1273	0·8264		
				C	2100	413	1044	643	0				
DISEASES OF THE DIGESTIVE SYSTEM													
Cholelithiasis	Germany, Marburg		Ihm & Wendt 1966	P	101	17	45	39	0	1·2875	1·3549		
				C	847	143	426	278	0				
Ulcerative Colitis	Australia, New South Wales	(s) S	Larkin 1967	P	26	4	9	13	0	1·6875	1·6715		
				C	430	65	205	160	0				
Gastric Ulcer	Germany, Marburg		Ihm & Wendt 1966	P	99	14	47	38	0	1·2750	1·2283		
				C	847	143	426	278	0				

TABLE 5 **THE PLASMA HAPTOGLOBIN SYSTEM** (*cont.*)

		Place	Additional details	Authors		Number	Hp 1-1	Hp 2-1	Hp 2-2	Hp 0	Hp 2-2/Hp 1-1+Hp 2-1		Hp 0/Hp 1-1+Hp 2-1+Hp 2-2	
											Relative incidence	χ_1^2 for difference from unity	Relative incidence	χ_1^2 for difference from unity
DISEASES OF THE GENITO-URINARY SYSTEM														
Menopausal Metrorrhagia		Czechoslovakia		Miluničová *et al.* 1969[a]	P	169	21	82	66	0	0·9324	0·1607		
				Kout & Baitsch 1963 M2	C	739	109	329	301	0				
DISEASES OF THE SKIN														
Neurodermatitis		Germany, Marburg		Ihm & Wendt 1966	P	64	7	28	29	0	1·6959	4·0785		
					C	847	143	426	278	0				
Lupus Erythematosus		Germany, Berlin		Stäps *et al.* 1961	P	121	16	69	36	0	0·6876	3·2912		
					C	1380	201	653	526	0				
Psoriasis Vulgaris	1.	Germany, Berlin		Stäps *et al.* 1961	P	110	23	54	33	0	0·6958	2·8370		
					C	1380	201	653	526	0				
	2.	Germany, Giessen, Kassel, Marburg		Wendt 1968	P	423	62	210	151	0	1·1459	1·2116		
					C	907	156	455	296	0				
	3.	Germany, Southern Niedersachsen		Jörgensen & Hopfer, U. 1967	P	203	30	91	82	0	1·2327	1·6304		
					C	685	114	328	243	0				
	4.	Sweden, Northern		Beckman *et al.* 1974	P	122	22	45	55	0	1·2859	1·8100		
					C	2297	311	1091	895	0				
						858					1·1109	1·6894		
					χ_3^2 for homogeneity of areas							5·7996		
DISEASES OF THE MUSCULOSKELETAL SYSTEM														
Rheumatoid Arthritis	1.	Sweden		Nettelbladt & Sunblad 1967	P	150(c)	16	62	72	0	1·3731	3·2573		
					C	1000	153	445	402	0				
	2.	U.S.A., Bethesda	Juvenile	Peacock & Alepa 1966	P	50	7	26	17	0	0·8831	0·1641		
					C	855	124	416	315	0				
						200					1·2314	1·8632		
					χ_1^2 for homogeneity of areas							1·5582		
CONGENITAL ANOMALIES														
Down's Syndrome	1.	United Kingdom, England	English	Hutton & Smith 1964	P	100	18	48	31	3	0·9764	0·0097	2·0155	0·9576
					C	397	55	209	127	6				
	2.	U.S.A., Dixon		Hsia *et al.* 1969	P	79	18	36	25	0	0·9983	0·0000		
					C	101	18	51	32	0				
						179					0·9842	0·0067		
					χ_1^2 for homogeneity of areas							0·0030		

TABLE 6
THE PHENYLTHIOCARBAMIDE TASTING SYSTEM

	Place	Additional details	Authors		Number	Tasters	Non-tasters	Tasters/Non-tasters	
								Relative incidence	χ^2_1 for difference from unity
INFECTIVE AND PARASITIC DISEASES									
BACTERIAL INFECTIONS									
TUBERCULOSIS									
Pulmonary	1. Czechoslovakia	Males; filter paper	Milunіčová *et al.* 1969[c]	P	50	36	14	0·8996	0·1013
				C	463	343	120		
	2. Czechoslovakia, Praha	Males; (s) A	Milunіčová & Dominec 1966	P	106	80	26	1·0765	0·0877
				C	463	343	120		
					156			1·0092	0·0021
				χ^2_1 for homogeneity of areas					0·1869
Site Unspecified	1. Sweden, Götaland	Single solution	Åkesson 1959	P	128	88	40	1·0732	0·0678
				C	122	82	40		
	2. Brazil	Males; threshold	Saldanha 1956	P	289	250	39	5·4945	31·7072
				C	66	35	30		
	3. Brazil	Females; threshold	Saldanha 1956	P	207	176	31	1·4557	1·3993
				C	98	78	20		
					624			1·9673	15·7635
				χ^2_2 for homogeneity of areas					17·4108
LEPROSY									
Lepromatous	1. S. India, Godavari District	Males; threshold	Busi 1972	P	217	177	40	1·2424	0·9774
				C	333	260	73		
	2. S. India, Godavari District	Females; threshold	Busi 1972	P	75	65	10	2·1985	3·5765
				C	91	68	23		
	3. Brazil	White males of old-Brazilian stock; single solution	Beiguelman 1962 Beiguelman 1964	P	203	163	40	1·3367	2·3057
				C	1000	753	247		
	4. Brazil	White females of old-Brazilian stock; single solution	Beiguelman 1962 Beiguelman 1964	P	93	77	16	1·6217	2·8906
				C	1000	753	247		
	5. Brazil	White males of European origin; (s) country of origin; single solution	Beiguelman 1962 Beiguelman 1964	P	482	384	98	1·2853	3·4682
				C	1000	753	247		
	6. Brazil	White females of European origin; (s) country of origin; single solution	Beiguelman 1962 Beiguelman 1964	P	388	310	78	1·3036	3·2790
				C	1000	753	247		
					1458			1·3400	14·3847
				χ^2_5 for homogeneity of areas					2·1127
Almost all lepromatous	1. Brazil, São Paulo	White males; threshold	Beiguelman 1964	P	600	483	117	1·3541	5·7466
				C	1000	753	247		
	2. Brazil, São Paulo	White females; threshold	Beiguelman 1964	P	300	240	60	1·3121	2·8140
				C	1000	753	247		
					900			1·3380	8·5370
				χ^2_1 for homogeneity of areas					0·0236

TABLE 6 THE PHENYLTHIOCARBAMIDE TASTING SYSTEM (*cont.*)

	Place	Additional details	Authors		Number	Tasters	Non-tasters	Tasters/Non-tasters: Relative incidence	Tasters/Non-tasters: χ_1^2 for difference from unity
INFECTIVE AND PARASITIC DISEASES (*cont.*)									
BACTERIAL INFECTIONS (*cont.*)									
LEPROSY (*cont.*)									
Tuberculoid	1. S. India, Godavari District	Males; threshold	Busi 1972	P	106	88	18	1·3726	1·1878
				C	333	260	73		
	2. S. India, Godavari District	Females; threshold	Busi 1972	P	18	15	3	1·6912	0·6026
				C	91	68	23		
	3. Brazil	White males of old-Brazilian stock; single solution	Beiguelman 1962	P	63	50	13	1·2616	0·5279
			Beiguelman 1964	C	1000	753	247		
	4. Brazil	White females of old-Brazilian stock; single solution	Beiguelman 1962	P	62	50	12	1·3668	0·8984
			Beiguelman 1964	C	1000	753	247		
	5. Brazil	White males of European origin; (s) country of origin; single solution	Beiguelman 1962	P	143	123	20	2·0173	7·7526
			Beiguelman 1964	C	1000	753	247		
	6. Brazil	White females of European origin; (s) country of origin; single solution	Beiguelman 1962	P	125	101	24	1·3804	1·8251
			Beiguelman 1964	C	1000	753	247		
					517			1·4970	10·7948
				χ_5^2 for homogeneity of areas					1·9996
BOTH LEPROSY AND TUBERCULOSIS	Brazil, São Paulo	Whites; threshold	Beiguelman 1964	P	58	51	7	2·3899	4·5225
				C	1000	753	247		
WORM INFESTATIONS									
FILARIASIS	1. S. India, Godavari District	Males; threshold	Busi 1972	P	110	85	25	1·6485	1·7282
				C	49	33	16		
	2. S. India, Godavari District	Females; threshold	Busi 1972	P	151	127	24	1·0148	0·0016
				C	87	73	14		
					261			1·2822	0·8863
				χ_1^2 for homogeneity of areas					0·8435
MALIGNANT NEOPLASMS									
DIGESTIVE TRACT	1. Czechoslovakia	Males; filter paper	Miluničová *et al.* 1969[c]	P	43	34	9	1·3217	0·5124
				C	463	343	120		
	2. Czechoslovakia	Females; filter paper	Miluničová *et al.* 1969[c]	P	40	35	5	1·7237	1·2160
				C	415	333	82		
					83			1·4634	1·5501
				χ_1^2 for homogeneity of areas					0·1783
LUNG	Czechoslovakia	Males; filter paper	Miluničová *et al.* 1969[c]	P	58	43	15	1·0029	0·0001
				C	463	343	120		
BREAST	Czechoslovakia	Females; filter paper	Miluničová *et al.* 1969[c]	P	71	66	5	3·2505	6·0324
				C	415	333	82		
CERVIX UTERI	Czechoslovakia	Filter paper	Miluničová *et al.* 1969[a]	P	85	79	6	3·2422	7·1128
				C	415	333	82		
CORPUS UTERI	Czechoslovakia	Filter paper	Miluničová *et al.* 1969[a]	P	142	135	7	4·7490	14·6691
				C	415	333	82		
OVARIES	Czechoslovakia	Filter paper	Miluničová *et al.* 1969[a]	P	50	47	3	3·8579	4·9291
				C	415	333	82		

TABLE 6 THE PHENYLTHIOCARBAMIDE TASTING SYSTEM (*cont.*)

	Place	Additional details	Authors		Number	Tasters	Non-tasters	Tasters/Non-tasters: Relative incidence	Tasters/Non-tasters: χ_1^2 for difference from unity
PROSTATE	Czechoslovakia	Filter paper	Miluničová *et al.* 1969[c]	P	40	29	11	0·9223	0·0478
				C	463	343	120		
THYROID GLAND	1. Czechoslovakia	Males; filter paper	Miluničová & Hájek 1966	P	26	22	4	1·9242	1·3966
				C	463	343	120		
	2. Czechoslovakia	Females; filter paper	Miluničová & Hájek 1966	P	124	113	11	2·5296	7·4915
				C	415	333	82		
					150			2·3477	8·7106
				χ_1^2 for homogeneity of areas					0·1775
ENDOCRINE AND METABOLIC DISEASES									
NON-TOXIC GOITRE									
Diffuse	1. Japan, Hiroshima	Simple; Japanese females; filter paper	Hollingsworth 1963	P	79	59	20	0·7314	0·9014
				C	151	121	30		
	2. Brazil, Pôrto Alegre	White females; threshold	Araújo *et al.* 1972	P	50	42	8	1·3713	0·5394
				C	169(c)	134	35		
	3. Brazil, Pôrto Alegre	Negro females; threshold	Araújo *et al.* 1972	P	15	13	2	1·6596	0·3766
				C	59	47	12		
					144			0·9736	0·0115
				χ_2^2 for homogeneity of areas					1·8059
Nodular	1. Italy, Roma	Males; (s) mononodular, polynodular; threshold	Fedeli 1959	P	30	15	15	0·5278	1·9108
				C	55	36	19		
	2. Italy, Roma	Females; (s) mononodular, polynodular; threshold	Fedeli 1959	P	229	147	82	0·7004	2·9754
				C	210	151	59		
	3. United Kingdom	Male adults; threshold	Fraser 1963	P	29	20	9	1·0228	0·0029
			Harris & Kalmus 1949 M2	C	441	302	139		
	4. United Kingdom, Liverpool	Females; mononodular; threshold	Kitchin *et al.* 1959	P	38	26	12	0·8466	0·1909
				C	210	151	59		
	5. United Kingdom, Liverpool	Males; polynodular; threshold	Kitchin *et al.* 1959	P	25	10	15	0·3518	4·4163
				C	55	36	19		
	6. United Kingdom, Liverpool	Females; polynodular; threshold	Kitchin *et al.* 1959	P	191	121	70	0·6754	3·3397
				C	210	151	59		
	7. Israel	Ashkenazi children; males; threshold; (s) G	Brand 1963	P	104	83	21	0·2080	20·2773
				C	340	323	17		
	8. Israel	Ashkenazi children; females; threshold; (s) G	Brand 1963	P	184	145	39	0·1748	29·7182
				C	334	319	15		
	9. Japan, Hiroshima	Japanese females; filter paper	Hollingsworth 1963	P	52	42	10	1·0413	0·0099
				C	151	121	30		
	10. Brazil, Pôrto Alegre	White males; (s) mononodular, polynodular; threshold	Araújo *et al.* 1972	P	14	11	3	1·2941	0·1024
				C	23	17	6		
	11. Brazil, Pôrto Alegre	White females; (s) mononodular, polynodular; threshold	Araújo *et al.* 1972	P	81	59	22	0·7005	1·2876
				C	169	134	35		
	12. Brazil, Pôrto Alegre	Negro females; (s) mononodular, polynodular; threshold	Araújo *et al.* 1972	P	21	15	6	0·6383	0·5964
				C	59	47	12		
					998			0·5691	33·4625
				χ_{11}^2 for homogeneity of areas					31·3653
TOXIC GOITRE									
Diffuse	1. Denmark	Males; threshold	Persson *et al.* 1972	P	22	15	7	1·0305	0·0039
				C	194	131	63		
	2. Denmark	Females; threshold	Persson *et al.* 1972	P	86	57	29	1·0201	0·0044
				C	120	79	41		
	3. Italy, Roma	Males; threshold	Fedeli 1959	P	18	15	3	2·6389	2·4751
				C	55	36	19		

TABLE 6 THE PHENYLTHIOCARBAMIDE TASTING SYSTEM (*cont.*)

	Place	Additional details	Authors		Number	Tasters	Non-tasters	Tasters/Non-tasters: Relative incidence	Tasters/Non-tasters: χ_1^2 for difference from unity
ENDOCRINE AND METABOLIC DISEASES (*cont.*)									
TOXIC GOITRE (*cont.*)									
Diffuse (*cont.*)									
	4. Italy, Roma	Females; threshold	Fedeli 1959	P	107	89	18	1·9319	4·7987
				C	210	151	59		
	5. United Kingdom	Males; threshold	Fraser 1963	P	17	11	6	0·8438	0·1076
			Harris & Kalmus 1949 M2	C	441	302	139		
	6. United Kingdom, Liverpool	Males; threshold	Kitchin *et al.* 1959	P	18	15	3	2·6389	1·9599
				C	55	36	19		
	7. United Kingdom, Liverpool	Females; threshold	Kitchin *et al.* 1959	P	107	89	18	1·9319	4·7987
				C	210	151	59		
	8. United Kingdom, London	Threshold	Harris *et al.* 1949	P	218	151	67	1·0239	0·0185
				C	541	372	169		
	9. Brazil, Pôrto Alegre	White females; threshold	Araújo *et al.* 1972	P	10	8	2	1·0448	0·0506
				C	169	134	35		
					603			1·2913	5·2780
				χ_8^2 for homogeneity of areas					8·9394
Nodular	1. Italy, Roma	Females; (s) mononodular, polynodular; threshold	Fedeli 1959	P	28	19	9	0·8249	0·1979
				C	210	151	59		
	2. United Kingdom, Liverpool	Females; threshold	Kitchin *et al.* 1959	P	27	18	9	0·7815	0·3197
				C	210	151	59		
	3. Brazil, Pôrto Alegre	White females; threshold	Araújo *et al.* 1972	P	18	14	4	0·9142	0·0225
				C	169	134	35		
					73			0·8251	0·4952
				χ_2^2 for homogeneity of areas					0·0449
Unspecified	1. Romania, Bătrîna	Excessive activity of thyroid without goitre; crystals	Tibera-Dumitru 1963	P	110	93	17	1·7699	1·7165
				C	45	34	11		
	2. Romania, Bătrîna	Excessive activity of thyroid with goitre; crystals	Tibera-Dumitru 1963	P	85	74	11	2·1765	2·6912
				C	45	34	11		
	3. Romania, Galda de Jos	Excessive activity of thyroid without goitre; crystals	Tibera-Dumitru 1963	P	31	27	4	0·7181	0·2758
				C	104	94	10		
	4. Romania, Galda de Jos	Excessive activity of thyroid with goitre; crystals	Tibera-Dumitru 1963	P	72	64	8	0·8511	0·1035
				C	104	94	10		
	5. Romania, Nucşoara	Excessive activity of thyroid without goitre; crystals	Tibera-Dumitru 1963	P	58	43	15	0·8919	0·0714
				C	59	45	14		
	6. Romania, Nucşoara	Excessive activity of thyroid with goitre; crystals	Tibera-Dumitru 1963	P	106	86	20	1·3378	0·5454
				C	59	45	14		
	7. Romania, Poiana	Excessive activity of thyroid without goitre; crystals	Tibera-Dumitru 1963	P	62	56	6	0·7235	0·3584
				C	139	129	10		
	8. Romania, Poiana	Excessive activity of thyroid with goitre; crystals	Tibera-Dumitru 1963	P	76	71	5	1·1008	0·0286
				C	139	129	10		
	9. Japan, Hiroshima	Japanese females; filter paper	Hollingsworth 1963	P	24	20	4	1·2397	0·1350
				C	151	121	30		
					624			1·1752	0·9786
				χ_8^2 for homogeneity of areas					4·9471
NODULAR GOITRE	1. United Kingdom, London	61% non-toxic; threshold	Harris *et al.* 1949	P	134	79	55	0·6525	4·6197
				C	541	372	169		
	2. Brazil	Migrants from NE. Brazil; threshold	Azevêdo *et al.* 1965	P	46	34	12	0·4686	5·0038
				C	3988	3422	566		
	3. Chile, Pedregoso Valley	Pevenche; threshold	Covarrubias *et al.* 1965	P	73(c)	70	3	0·9333	0·0034
				C	26(c)	25	1		
					253			0·6051	8·7790
				χ_2^2 for homogeneity of areas					0·8479

TABLE 6 THE PHENYLTHIOCARBAMIDE TASTING SYSTEM (*cont.*)

	Place	Additional details	Authors		Number	Tasters	Non-tasters	Tasters/Non-tasters: Relative incidence	Tasters/Non-tasters: χ^2_1 for difference from unity
DIFFUSE GOITRE	1. Brazil	Migrants from NE. Brazil; threshold	Azevêdo *et al.* 1965	P	143	122	21	0·9609	0·0275
				C	3988	3422	566		
	2. Brazil, Minas Gerais		Memória 1958	P	210	190	20	2·0567	4·5939
				C	118	97	21		
	3. Chile, Pedregoso Valley	Pevenche; threshold	Covarrubias *et al.* 1965	P	59	58	1	2·3200	0·3443
				C	26	25	1		
					412			1·2573	1·3946
				χ^2_2 for homogeneity of areas					3·5711
ENDEMIC GOITRE	1. Greece, Central	Males; threshold	Malamos *et al.* 1966	P	241	185	56	1·1450	0·5664
				C	575	427	148		
	2. Greece, Central	Females; threshold	Malamos *et al.* 1966	P	577	459	118	1·0312	0·0407
				C	482	381	101		
	3. Italy, Frosinone	Males; threshold	Luca & Cramarossa 1965	P	40	28	12	0·6187	0·3094
				C	167	132	35		
	4. Italy, Frosinone	Females; threshold	Luca & Cramarossa 1965	P	96	78	18	0·8580	0·1827
				C	121	101	20		
	5. United Kingdom, Derbyshire	Males; threshold	Cartwright & Sunderland 1967	P	32	23½	8½	1·1121	0·0627
				C	251	179	72		
	6. United Kingdom, Derbyshire	Females; threshold	Cartwright & Sunderland 1967	P	99	57	42	0·5411	7·4991
				C	549	392½	156½		
	7. Peru, Pasco	Indian males; mostly simple non-toxic	Paolucci *et al.* 1971	P	33	33	0		
				C	72	68	4		
	8. Peru, Pasco	Indian females; mostly simple non-toxic	Paolucci *et al.* 1971	P	34	34	0		
				C	32	32	0		
					1085			0·9126	0·9509
				χ^2_5 for homogeneity of areas					7·7101
HYPOTHYROIDISM	1. Romania, Bătrîna	Insufficient activity of thyroid without goitre; crystals	Tiberia-Dumitru 1963	P	77	63	14	1·4559	0·6795
				C	45	34	11		
	2. Romania, Bătrîna	Insufficient activity of thyroid with goitre; crystals	Tibera-Dumitru 1963	P	50	41	9	1·4739	0·5881
				C	45	34	11		
	3. Romania, Galda de Jos	Insufficient activity of thyroid without goitre; crystals	Tibera-Dumitru 1963	P	88	72	16	0·4787	2·9013
				C	104	94	10		
	4. Romania, Galda de Jos	Insufficient activity of thyroid with goitre; crystals	Tibera-Dumitru 1963	P	225	200	25	0·8511	0·1671
				C	104	94	10		
	5. Romania, Nucşoara	Insufficient activity of thyroid without goitre; crystals	Tibera-Dumitru 1963	P	94	66	28	0·7333	0·6656
				C	59	45	14		
	6. Romania, Nucşoara	Insufficient activity of thyroid with goitre; crystals	Tibera-Dumitru 1963	P	131	99	32	0·9625	0·0108
				C	59	45	14		
	7. Romania, Poiana	Insufficient activity of thyroid without goitre; crystals	Tibera-Dumitru 1963	P	206	187	19	0·7630	0·4417
				C	139	129	10		
	8. Romania, Poiana	Insufficient activity of thyroid with goitre; crystals	Tibera-Dumitru 1963	P	185	174	11	1·2262	0·2035
				C	139	129	10		
	9. United Kingdom, Birmingham, Oxford, Reading	Anatomical; children; (s) A, S; threshold	Fraser 1970	P	54	21	33	0·2929	17·0516
			Harris & Kalmus 1949 M2	C	441	302	139		
	10. United Kingdom, Birmingham, Oxford, Reading	Metabolic; children; (s) A, S; threshold	Fraser 1970	P	21	12	9	0·6137	1·1633
			Harris & Kalmus 1949 M2	C	441	302	139		
	11. United Kingdom, London	Pendred's syndrome; threshold	Thould & Scowen 1964	P	23	19	4	2·1863	1·9541
			Harris & Kalmus 1949 M2	C	441	302	139		
	12. U.S.A., Seattle	Athyreotic; threshold	Shephard & Gartler 1960	P	27	18	9	0·5577	1·6179
				C	133	104	29		
					1181			0·7377	6·5269
				χ^2_{11} for homogeneity of areas					20·9177

TABLE 6 **THE PHENYLTHIOCARBAMIDE TASTING SYSTEM** (*cont.*)

		Place	Additional details	Authors		Number	Tasters	Non-tasters	Tasters/Non-tasters Relative incidence	χ_1^2 for difference from unity
ENDOCRINE AND METABOLIC DISEASES (*cont.*)										
DIABETES MELLITUS	1.	Czechoslovakia, Praha	Males; filter paper	Sottner 1964	P	222	145	77	0·6982	3·1742
					C	244	178	66		
	2.	Czechoslovakia, Praha	Females; filter paper	Sottner 1964	P	303	236	67	1·1439	0·4496
					C	257	194	63		
	3.	Czechoslovakia, Praha	Males; (s) A	Miluničová & Dominec 1966	P	121	74	47	0·5838	5·2138
				Sottner 1964	C	244	178	66		
	4.	Sweden, Götaland	Single solution	Åkesson 1959	P	106	76	30	1·2358	0·5355
					C	122	82	40		
	5.	United Kingdom, Devon	Males; single solution; (s) A	Harper 1975	P	211	163	48	1·3755	1·4349
					C	111	79	32		
	6.	United Kingdom, Devon	Females; single solution; (s) A	Harper 1975	P	240	207	33	0·3485	1·9742
					C	38	36	2		
	7.	United Kingdom, London	Threshold	Harris *et al.* 1949	P	103	72	31	1·0552	0·0526
					C	541	372	169		
	8.	U.S.A., Los Angeles	Non-Jewish; filter paper	Terry & Segall 1947	P	87	55	32	0·6757	1·9270
					C	163	117	46		
	9.	U.S.A., Los Angeles	Jewish; filter paper	Terry & Segall 1947	P	124	69	55	0·3787	12·8506
					C	138	106	32		
	10.	U.S.A., Los Angeles	Negroes; filter paper	Terry & Segall 1947	P	11	11	0		
					C	157	125	32		
	11.	Jamaica	Wholly or partly of Negro origin; filter paper	Terry 1950	P	121	99	22	0·3782	12·1699
					C	632	583	49		
						1638			0·7709	10·3328
					χ_9^2 for homogeneity of areas					29·4495
CYSTIC FIBROSIS		U.S.A., Albany		Manlapas *et al.* 1965	P	54	24	30	0·3846	10·1662
					C	308	208	100		
DISEASES OF THE BLOOD										
PERNICIOUS ANAEMIA		United Kingdom, England	Single solution	Callender *et al.* 1957	P	261	199	62	1·2660	1·3641
					C	251	180	71		
MENTAL DISORDERS										
SCHIZOPHRENIA		Brazil, Paraná	White males; threshold	Freire-Maia *et al.* 1968	P	55(c)	29	26	0·3937	6·7214
					C	92	68	24		
OTHER THAN SCHIZOPHRENIA		Brazil, Paraná	White males; threshold	Freire-Maia *et al.* 1968	P	84(c)	48	36	0·4706	5·4123
					C	92	68	24		
UNSPECIFIED		Brazil, Paraná	White females; threshold	Freire-Maia *et al.* 1968	P	205(c)	151	54	0·9869	0·0212
					C	92	68	24		
DISEASES OF THE NERVOUS SYSTEM AND SENSE ORGANS										
GLAUCOMA Primary, open-angle	1.	United Kingdom, London	Males; threshold	Kalmus & Lewkonia 1973	P	144	84	60	0·6444	4·9435
					C	441	302	139		
	2.	United Kingdom, London	Females; threshold	Kalmus & Lewkonia 1973	P	87	61	26	1·0055	0·0003
					C	100	70	30		
	3.	Japan, Chiba		Suzuki *et al.* 1966	P	30(c)	25	5	1·5625	0·5365
					C	42(c)	32	10		
	4.	Japan, Tokyo	Threshold	Takahashi 1969	P	107	76	31	0·5089	8·1600
					C	669	554	115		
	5.	Japan, Tokyo	Open-angle suspect; threshold	Takahashi 1969	P	78	63	15	0·8718	0·2022
					C	669	554	115		

TABLE 6 THE PHENYLTHIOCARBAMIDE TASTING SYSTEM (*cont.*)

	Place	Additional details	Authors		Number	Tasters	Non-tasters	Tasters/Non-tasters: Relative incidence	Tasters/Non-tasters: χ_1^2 for difference from unity
	6. U.S.A.	Whites; threshold	Becker & Morton 1964[a]	P	211	100	111	0·3467	39·0170
				C	511	369	142		
	7. U.S.A.	Negroes; threshold	Becker & Morton 1964[a]	P	89	56	33	0·3370	13·0060
				C	169	141	28		
					746			0·5256	46·5316
				χ_6^2 for homogeneity of areas					19·3339
Primary, angle-closure	1. United Kingdom, London	Males; threshold	Kalmus & Lewkonia 1973	P	22	15	7	0·9863	0·0009
				C	441	302	139		
	2. United Kingdom, London	Females; threshold	Kalmus & Lewkonia 1973	P	38	25	13	0·8242	0·2273
				C	100	70	30		
	3. Japan, Chiba		Suzuki *et al.* 1966	P	40(c)	32	8	1·2500	0·1732
				C	42(c)	32	10		
	4. Japan, Tokyo	Threshold	Takahashi 1969	P	43	39	4	2·0239	1·7372
				C	669	554	115		
	5. U.S.A.	Whites; threshold	Becker & Morton 1964[a]	P	155	129	26	1·9093	7·4739
				C	511	369	142		
	6. U.S.A.	Negroes; threshold	Becker & Morton 1964[a]	P	30	30	0		
				C	169	141	28		
					298			1·4657	5·1839
				χ_4^2 for homogeneity of areas					4·4285
Secondary	1. United Kingdom, London	Males; threshold	Kalmus & Lewkonia 1973	P	26	16	10	0·7364	0·5411
				C	441	302	139		
	2. United Kingdom, London	Females; threshold	Kalmus & Lewkonia 1973	P	22	14	8	0·7500	0·3391
				C	100	70	30		
	3. Japan, Tokyo	Threshold	Takahashi 1969	P	55	46	9	1·0610	0·0244
				C	669	554	115		
	4. U.S.A.	Whites; threshold	Becker & Morton 1964[a]	P	46	33	13	0·9769	0·0047
				C	511	369	142		
	5. U.S.A.	Negroes; threshold	Becker & Morton 1964[a]	P	36	30	6	0·9929	0·0002
				C	169	141	28		
					185			0·9106	0·2588
				χ_4^2 for homogeneity of areas					0·6507
BUPHTHALMOS	Japan, Tokyo	Threshold	Takahashi 1969	P	51	49	2	5·0857	4·9826
				C	669	554	115		
KERATOCONUS	Japan, Tokyo	Threshold	Takahashi 1969	P	105	75	30	0·5190	7·5263
				C	669	554	115		
DISEASES OF THE GENITO-URINARY SYSTEM									
HYPERPLASIA OF PROSTATE	Czechoslovakia	Filter paper	Miluničová *et al.* 1969[c]	P	48	37	11	1·1768	0·2051
				C	463	343	120		
MENOPAUSAL METRORRHAGIA	Czechoslovakia	Filter paper	Miluničová *et al.* 1969[a]	P	170	154	16	2·3701	8·8449
				C	415	333	82		
DISEASES OF THE SKIN									
PSORIASIS	Spain, Barcelona		Giménez Camarasa 1968	P	76(c)	61	15	1·1478	0·1588
			Pons 1960 M2	C	159	124	35		

TABULAR SUMMARIES OF ASSOCIATIONS BETWEEN POLYMORPHISMS AND DISEASES

TABLE 1A
THE ABO BLOOD GROUP SYSTEM

	A/O					B/O				
	Number of patients	Number of studies (N)	Combined incidence	χ_1^2 for difference from unity	χ_{N-1}^2 for homogeneity of areas	Number of patients	Number of studies (N)	Combined incidence	χ_1^2 for difference from unity	χ_{N-1}^2 for homogeneity of areas
INFECTIVE AND PARASITIC DISEASES										
BACTERIAL INFECTIONS										
Typhoid Fever	956	5	0·8670	3·2053	9·8275	956	5	0·9381	0·3884	16·0478
Paratyphoid Fever	237	1	0·7022	5·5459		237	1	0·5993	6·7906	
Unspecified Salmonella Infections	51	3	1·0349	0·0094	0·9268	45	2	1·6915	1·9160	0·0259
Shigella Flexneri Dysentery	1050	1	1·0244	0·1174		1050	1	0·9380	0·4017	
Unspecified Bacillary Dysentery	124	1	1·3932	2·0855		124	1	1·3617	1·3048	
Escherichia Coli Infections	999	5	0·9318	0·8934	7·6991	999	5	1·2375	5·0315	6·9672
Enteritis in Infants										
No evidence of Escherichia coli	1316	1	1·1103	2·9081		1316	1	0·9933	0·0046	
No mention of pathogenesis	871	2	1·0051	0·0034	3·8279	871	2	1·1561	1·4973	3·1774
Gonorrhoea	608	3	1·0650	0·4953	1·5350	608	3	0·9684	0·0541	0·9403
Brucellosis	165	1	0·9034	0·2809		165	1	0·9556	0·0331	
Whooping Cough	807	3	0·8905	1·7252	0·9482	793	2	0·9698	0·0792	7·6748
Diphtheria										
Patients/controls	2727	3	1·0000	0·0000	1·5694	2727	3	1·0682	0·5588	6·7809
Schick test for susceptibility, +/−	*991/1410*	*5*	*1·0342*	*0·1297*	*4·0551*	*991/1410*	*5*	*0·9535*	*0·1371*	*3·3968*
Scarlet Fever										
Patients/controls	3374	10	0·8766	8·9465	31·7173	3374	10	1·0317	0·2569	40·4825
Dick test for susceptibility, +/−	*447/742*	*1*	*1·4601*	*6·9503*		*447/742*	*1*	*1·4611*	*4·9912*	
Infection with Haemolytic Streptococcus A	100	1	1·4797	1·4549		100	1	0·8922	0·0659	
Staphylococcal Infections										
Patients/controls	603	3	0·9031	1·1755	1·5701	603	3	1·0125	0·0079	2·5849
Carriers/non-carriers	*1875/2178*	*3*	*0·8692*	*4·2896*	*1·7863*	*1875/2178*	*3*	*0·7779*	*4·4321*	*4·2944*
Coccal Infections	100	1	0·9383	0·0636		100	1	1·1588	0·3179	
Tetanus	82	2	0·7550	1·1388	0·0188	82	2	0·7238	0·8631	0·7657
Tuberculosis										
Pulmonary	24966	42	0·9311	15·0460	84·1581	24966	42	0·9779	1·1040	104·1899
With haemoptysis	637	3	0·8578	2·7747	1·1955	637	3	0·8910	0·6054	3·8364
Without haemoptysis	1146	3	1·2318	8·4706	4·5878	1146	3	0·9963	0·0010	0·0488
With/without haemoptysis	*637/1146*	*3*	*0·6883*	*11·4157*	*4·0492*	*637/1146*	*3*	*0·8525*	*0·8299*	*3·4246*
Tuberculous meningitis	38	1	0·7740	0·4891		38	1	0·7332	0·4568	
Of intestines and peritoneum	180	3	1·4101	3·6945	0·8132	150	2	1·6296	4·8574	0·0000
Of bones and joints	886	3	0·9714	0·0735	1·6603	886	3	1·2327	3·5191	3·9651
Of genito-urinary system	436	5	1·0529	0·2226	2·0628	436	5	0·7022	3·6420	3·3576
Of skin	48	2	1·1887	0·2678	1·2573	48	2	1·0553	0·1551	0·5877
Of lymphatic system	69	1	0·7691	0·8386		69	1	0·8090	0·4257	
Sites unspecified	10329	27	1·1719	32·8466	86·7265	10329	27	1·1923	24·1848	51·3663
	38735	90	1·0058	0·1628	247·0227	38705	89	1·0300	2·8331	203·4700

TABULAR SUMMARIES. TABLE 1A **THE ABO BLOOD GROUP SYSTEM** *(cont.)*

	A/O					B/O				
	Number of patients	Number of studies (N)	Combined incidence	χ_1^2 for difference from unity	χ_{N-1}^2 for homogeneity of areas	Number of patients	Number of studies (N)	Combined incidence	χ_1^2 for difference from unity	χ_{N-1}^2 for homogeneity of areas
SARCOIDOSIS	910	5	1·1865	4·5654	8·8234	910	5	0·9921	0·0001	5·5933
LEPROSY										
Lepromatous	8013	34	1·0330	1·0941	44·0509	8013	34	0·9845	0·1864	41·1867
Tuberculoid	2863	27	0·9223	2·6033	20·6191	2852	26	0·9434	0·9600	25·1558
Indeterminate	93	3	1·0043	0·0003	1·2527	93	3	1·1198	0·0616	3·4197
Dimorphous	728	5	1·1307	1·2939	4·5790	728	5	1·0383	0·1177	3·3359
Non-lepromatous	2807	8	1·1915	8·4992	10·1636	2807	8	0·8620	6·5679	33·0010
Unspecified types	4220	23	1·0788	3·5021	38·4401	4220	23	1·0852	3·2925	35·3426
	18724	100	1·0450	4·7025	128·8080	18713	99	1·0155	0·4275	152·2004
SYPHILIS										
Cardiovascular	219	2	1·0293	0·0407	2·2049	219	2	0·7001	1·5689	0·7595
Cerebrospinal	341	2	1·5741	10·5917	0·4444	341	2	1·2996	2·5573	4·0593
Tabes dorsalis	277	2	0·7686	3·1127	0·5453	277	2	1·0832	0·2368	6·2064
Cerebrospinal and tabes dorsalis	29	1	1·8962	1·9419		29	1	0·2352	1·8196	
Progressive paralysis	1991	19	1·0686	1·4596	22·2964	1991	19	1·3055	13·8502	54·5737
Mental disorders due to syphilis	102	2	1·0563	0·0702	0·1754	102	2	0·2644	4·9782	0·0814
Tertiary	160	1	1·1279	0·3657		160	1	1·1975	0·6803	
Treated, Wassermann reaction positive	1701	7	1·4855	32·1094	17·6806	1593	6	1·5557	27·4198	1·7022
Treated, Wassermann reaction negative	3197	7	0·9677	0·3779	14·9570	3197	7	0·9557	0·4761	11·4978
Treated, Wassermann reaction positive/negative	*1700/3177*	*7*	*1·5960*	*38·6249*	*12·2272*	*1592/3039*	*6*	*1·6287*	*29·0075*	*10·8016*
Not stated whether treated, Wassermann reaction positive	3590	4	1·0976	5·4578	34·5822	3590	4	1·0061	0·0101	11·6049
Not stated whether treated, Wassermann reaction negative	1191	1	0·9895	0·0132		1191	1	0·7084	9·9792	
Not stated whether treated, Wassermann reaction positive/negative	*175/1191*	*1*	*1·4302*	*3·2608*		*175/1191*	*1*	*1·3522*	*1·5398*	
Not stated whether treated, Wassermann reaction not stated	5343	16	0·9818	0·0003	8·7482	5343	16	1·0911	4·0015	10·0569
	18141	64	1·0635	10·3151	146·8605	18033	63	1·0862	10·6876	157·4324
YAWS, PRESENT/ABSENT	*114/1262*	*2*	*0·8289*	*0·5894*	*1·5782*	*114/1262*	*2*	*0·8767*	*0·1654*	*2·2760*
SEPTICAEMIA	86	2	1·2571	0·7763	0·5612	86	2	1·4173	1·2382	2·9714
BACTERIAL MENINGITIS	86	1	0·5439	5·5895		86	1	0·7644	0·8611	
SEPTIC ANGINA	322	1	1·0115	0·0072		322	1	1·0267	0·0264	
LUNG ABSCESSES	156	1	0·6650	4·2301		156	1	0·5682	2·6747	
IMPETIGO, FOLLICULITIS, FURUNCULOSIS	57	1	0·7208	1·1862						
INFECTIOUS DERMATITIS	58	1	1·1668	0·2909						

RICKETTSIAL INFECTIONS

BARTONELLOSIS	41	1	1·0581	0·0225		41	1	0·8718	0·0645	
TYPHUS	28	1	0·8772	0·1033		28	1	0·7775	0·1532	

VIRAL INFECTIONS

POLIOMYELITIS										
Patients/controls	2221	10	0·9217	2·3684	21·2700	2199	9	0·9357	0·6626	16·6546
Paralytic/abortive	*1838/1681*	*5*	*0·8224*	*3·7963*	*6·9546*	*1838/1681*	*5*	*0·6991*	*5·5962*	*13·4146*
SMALLPOX										
Patients/controls	22	1	1·3645	0·4690		22	1	0·8063	0·0748	
Survivors/controls	1455	5	1·2704	7·9365	59·6848	1455	5	1·1035	1·4348	14·8955
Fatal/controls	410	3	2·2697	27·2704	71·0507	410	3	0·8955	0·3804	1·7227
Fatal/survivors	*410/798*	*3*	*0·8955*	*0·3804*	*7·5849*	*410/798*	*3*	*0·6806*	*4·6771*	*5·6104*
Confluent/controls	375	2	0·6965	3·8245	0·1412	375	2	0·5507	12·3275	0·1109
Discrete/controls	554	2	0·6890	6·8802	2·5541	554	2	0·6271	13·5355	8·8135
Confluent/discrete	*375/554*	*2*	*1·2255*	*1·3268*	*2·4692*	*375/554*	*2*	*1·2202*	*1·4357*	*5·5518*
Reactions to vaccination +/−	*956/341*	*2*	*1·6040*	*7·0793*	*52·6096*	*956/341*	*2*	*0·8416*	*0·8704*	*0·1121*
CHICKENPOX	1290	5	1·0783	1·4298	0·4395	1290	5	0·9498	0·2856	3·5209
MEASLES	2030	3	0·8820	4·4960	5·0721	2030	5	0·9300	1·0069	2·3146
INFECTIOUS HEPATITIS	3168	9	1·0072	0·0265	17·0034	3168	9	1·0266	0·1976	29·6204
SERUM HEPATITIS, transfusions with/without	*252/4888*	*3*	*1·0464*	*0·0932*	*8·7927*	*252/4888*	*3*	*0·8656*	*0·4088*	*6·1642*
SERUM HEPATITIS, Australia antigens, carriers/non-carriers	*347/8864*	*3*	*1·0214*	*0·0281*	*5·9634*	*347/8864*	*3*	*0·9701*	*0·0029*	*0·7011*

	A/O					B/O				
	Number of patients	Number of studies (N)	Combined incidence	χ_1^2 for difference from unity	χ_{N-1}^2 for homogeneity of areas	Number of patients	Number of studies (N)	Combined incidence	χ_1^2 for difference from unity	χ_{N-1}^2 for homogeneity of areas
INFECTIVE AND PARASITIC DISEASES *(cont.)*										
VIRAL INFECTIONS *(cont.)*										
Mumps	403	1	0·8054	3·3185		403	1	0·6794	6·3181	
Infectious Mononucleosis	274	1	0·8059	2·2091		274	1	0·8585	0·7648	
Trachoma	26	1	7·8788	7·7306		26	1	1·7333	0·2725	
Viral Meningitis	129	1	1·0388	0·0309		129	1	1·3645	1·6686	
Warts	402	1	0·8442	2·0901						
Infection with Adenovirus	667	3	1·2687	8·0272	0·0841	667	3	1·1314	0·7057	0·6279
Infection with Coxsackie A21	125	3	0·8372	0·9031	1·7048	125	3	0·4842	2·8832	0·1788
Influenza 1918	34	1	0·3883	5·1895		34	1	0·3155	2·4103	
Infection with Influenza A_1	129	3	0·8987	0·3257	0·0047	129	3	0·7765	0·5007	0·3822
Infection with Influenza A_2	701	3	0·6715	22·8695	2·1364	701	3	0·9568	0·1070	3·9724
Infection with Influenza B	63	3	1·0136	0·0023	7·6322	57	2	0·8623	0·0748	0·6465
Influenza A/Sing/57 antibodies: strong/weak inhibition of haemagglutination	*515/1026*	*2*	*0·8088*	*3·4676*	*0·0847*					
Influenza A2/Sing/1/57 antibodies: positive/negative inhibition of haemagglutination	*389/126*	*1*	*0·4215*	*16·9162*						
Influenza A/HK/68 antibodies: strong/weak inhibition of haemagglutination	*637/904*	*2*	*0·8897*	*0·9602*	*0·5158*					
Influenza A_1 antibodies: strong/weak inhibition of haemagglutination	*885/615*	*1*	*0·4418*	*47·9748*		*885/615*	*1*	*0·8812*	*0·4953*	
Influenza A_2 antibodies: strong/weak inhibition of haemagglutination	*1057/443*	*1*	*0·3574*	*67·8538*		*1057/443*	*1*	*0·7566*	*2·0043*	
FUNGAL INFECTIONS										
Trichophytosis	28	1	0·6461	0·9949		28	1	0·6533	0·7007	
Fungal Infections of Skin	259	2	1·0304	0·0384	0·1319	59	1	1·1588	0·6231	
PROTOZOAL INFECTIONS										
Malaria	3643	7	1·3092	19·3035	39·5270	3643	7	1·0104	0·0600	14·8593
Parasites present/absent	*163/641*	*1*	*0·8314*	*0·7550*		*163/641*	*1*	*1·0164*	*0·0045*	
Other than Malaria	53	1	0·4648	3·5469		53	1	0·6943	1·1501	
WORM INFESTATIONS										
Bilharzial Hepatic Fibrosis	353	2	4·0488	65·9812	8·3671	353	2	2·1905	16·4104	1·7198
Hydatid Cyst	355	2	1·0727	0·3264	0·3094	355	2	1·2951	2·0895	0·0502
Tape Worm Anaemia	197	1	1·3716	2·6346		197	1	1·6259	4·1514	
Loiasis	314	1	1·0061	0·0018		314	1	1·0709	0·2434	
Filariasis	603	1	0·9438	0·1297		603	1	1·0186	0·0155	
Ascariasis	74	1	1·3475	1·0780		74	1	1·2621	0·5116	
Helminthiasis	206	2	0·9612	0·0457	0·0259	206	2	1·2079	0·9479	2·6104
ARTHROPOD INFESTATIONS										
Pediculosis and Scabies	30	1	1·2224	0·2545						
NEOPLASMS										
MALIGNANT NEOPLASMS										
Lip	580	2	1·1987	3·9526	1·6724	580	2	0·8054	1·5101	1·0473
Tongue	404	5	1·2799	3·8044	3·8951	404	5	1·3298	3·7092	3·0415
Gum	63	2	1·1191	0·0981	1·0606	63	2	1·2569	0·5675	0·3680
Buccal Mucosa	401	2	1·0165	0·0152	0·0746	401	2	0·8502	1·6554	5·5838
Cheek	334	2	1·6171	6·1075	0·0131	334	2	1·4923	4·5161	10·2573
	1202	11	1·2154	5·8383	9·2298	1202	11	1·1189	1·8628	27·8360

TABULAR SUMMARIES. TABLE 1A **THE ABO BLOOD GROUP SYSTEM** (*cont.*)

	A/O					B/O				
	Number of patients	Number of studies (N)	Combined incidence	χ_1^2 for difference from unity	χ_{N-1}^2 for homogeneity of areas	Number of patients	Number of studies (N)	Combined incidence	χ_1^2 for difference from unity	χ_{N-1}^2 for homogeneity of areas
Buccal Cavity	200	5	1·0503	0·0749	6·7396	200	5	1·1791	0·6431	2·6433
Nasopharynx	483	8	0·9082	0·6791	14·7613	483	8	1·0190	0·0246	8·2262
Oropharynx	78	2	1·2981	0·7617	2·2176	78	2	2·1824	6·2002	0·5252
Hypopharynx	198	2	0·7715	2·1337	0·8148	198	2	1·4096	2·4728	3·0503
Pharynx	24	1	0·4299	2·7398		24	1	2·3590	2·6205	
Tonsils	40	2	0·9164	0·0474	0·1523	40	2	1·2572	0·2736	4·5085
	340	7	0·8422	1·5618	7·3055	340	7	1·6262	9·4193	10·2317
Buccal Cavity, Larynx	46	1	2·0268	4·5329		46	1	0·6851	0·4381	
Salivary Glands	393	8	1·5547	16·1503	19·2231	382	7	1·3740	3·3422	4·3538
Oesophagus	2705	31	1·0994	4·6547	25·7427	2705	31	1·2876	16·1100	23·9797
Stomach										
Cardia	1295	7	1·0584	0·7386	7·4841	1269	6	0·9016	1·3331	14·8215
Fundus	104	1	0·6540	3·6132		104	1	0·9244	0·0591	
Aditus, fundus	52	1	0·8408	0·3055		52	1	0·9441	0·0201	
Corpus	2300	8	1·1455	7·3818	16·2560	2279	7	0·8759	3·9121	9·3746
Cardia, corpus	220	1	1·6047	10·5315		220	1	1·1603	0·3391	
Antrum	1080	3	1·0840	1·4107	0·2641	1080	3	0·9181	0·6119	1·9290
Prepyloric	90	1	1·4613	2·7792		90	1	1·0602	0·0197	
Pylorus	2851	3	1·1841	11·5021	1·4603	2851	3	0·8669	5·3785	4·1481
Antrum, pylorus	1734	3	1·1909	9·1756	3·8837	1734	3	0·9483	0·4930	6·4432
Cardia, antrum, pylorus	49	1	0·9832	0·0029		49	1	0·6290	0·5830	
Other than cardia and prepyloric	293	1	1·4778	9·6940		293	1	0·7337	1·3276	
Whole body or site uncertain	144	1	1·2251	1·3352		144	1	0·5808	1·8419	
Other than cardia, corpus, antrum, or pylorus	72	1	1·1780	0·3312		72	1	1·0759	0·0485	
Part unspecified	53155	129	1·2228	369·4846	273·1223	53130	128	1·0780	23·6766	215·4786
	63439	161	1·2120	402·7567	327·9742	63367	158	1·0422	8·7637	283·0752
Small Intestine	62	1	1·2259	0·3916		62	1	1·8037	2·5851	
Colon	1653	11	1·1512	6·4386	20·1251	1653	11	1·1372	2·1938	12·3745
Rectum	2685	9	1·0675	1·8667	8·7948	2685	9	0·9766	0·1081	9·0406
Colon, Rectum	5325	11	1·0852	6·5481	6·7240	5325	11	0·9521	0·9656	9·5849
Large Intestine	607	4	0·9306	0·5161	3·4722	607	4	1·0290	0·0485	2·7955
	10270	35	1·0833	11·7687	42·7169	10270	35	0·9931	0·0381	37·0734
Anus, Rectum	17	1	1·0740	0·0188		17	1	0·8410	0·0473	
Intestinal Tract	1220	6	1·2061	7·7551	11·6989	1220	6	1·0978	0·8779	7·1321
Oesophagus, Intestinal Tract	238	2	1·2481	2·6133	1·3264	238	2	0·8701	0·2955	0·2574
Gastro-intestinal Tract	1033	2	0·9544	0·2658	2·2201	1033	2	1·1451	0·8807	0·0021
Liver	394	4	1·0979	0·5543	5·8217	394	4	1·0981	0·4988	16·8248
Liver, Bile Ducts	266	2	0·9984	0·0001	0·0181	266	2	1·1269	0·3791	0·1556
	660	6	1·0522	0·2977	6·0965	660	6	1·1072	0·8657	16·9927
Gall-bladder	154	2	1·1571	0·6376	0·1069	154	2	1·1173	0·1935	0·1082
Bile Ducts	94	2	1·2980	0·9950	3·4204	94	2	1·9234	5·0218	6·3581
Gall-bladder, Bile Ducts	18	1	0·5230	1·3918		18	1	1·3459	0·1453	
	266	5	1·1344	0·7613	5·7904	266	5	1·4054	3·3731	8·4537
Pancreas	1394	16	1·1572	6·1144	20·7671	1381	15	1·2841	6·9039	25·5382
Liver, Bile Ducts, Gall-bladder, Pancreas	119	1	1·2523	1·1758		119	1	1·2931	0·7367	
Thyroid Gland	204	2	0·9204	0·2269	5·0987	204	2	0·9124	0·1644	3·0441
Larynx	1611	10	0·9916	0·0584	11·6227	1575	9	0·9375	0·5818	6·4337
Bronchus, Lung										
Bronchus	8183	11	1·0668	4·5329	13·8145	8183	11	1·0412	0·7727	7·2160
Lung	7904	24	1·0271	1·0105	65·4986	7904	24	0·9560	1·0661	33·1720
Bronchus, lung	327	1	1·6361	14·5066		327	1	1·4255	3·0064	
	16414	36	1·0551	7·3680	91·9951	16414	36	1·0039	0·0152	45·2180
Respiratory System	141	1	1·2947	1·8321		141	1	1·5120	2·4974	
Bone	216	4	1·1287	0·5411	10·0909	216	4	1·5225	4·3603	5·3781

	A/O					B/O				
	Number of patients	Number of studies (N)	Combined incidence	χ_1^2 for difference from unity	χ_{N-1}^2 for homogeneity of areas	Number of patients	Number of studies (N)	Combined incidence	χ_1^2 for difference from unity	χ_{N-1}^2 for homogeneity of areas
NEOPLASMS (*cont.*)										
MALIGNANT NEOPLASMS (*cont.*)										
Skin	429	5	0·6617	12·1785	3·8117	386	4	0·7803	1·8698	3·4780
Breast	12190	46	1·0736	11·3362	54·4588	12190	46	1·0243	0·5890	75·1499
Cervix Uteri	23255	41	1·0914	28·6839	123·8022	23255	41	1·0187	0·6845	45·5931
Corpus Uteri	4541	24	1·0573	2·7257	41·6504	4541	24	0·9840	0·1000	39·7476
Endometrial Adenocarcinoma	115	1	1·3191	1·6624		115	1	1·0863	0·0572	
	4656	25	1·0625	3·3124	42·7612	4656	25	0·9861	0·0773	39·8275
Malignant Melanoma of Uterus	192	1	0·9197	0·2080		192	1	1·1199	0·1993	
Choriocarcinoma	314	1	1·2403	1·5578		314	1	1·2667	0·7568	
Uterus (Precise Site Unspecified)	6066	20	1·1596	19·9261	34·2954	6066	20	1·1343	7·0094	17·4304
Ovary	3175	24	1·2257	25·2147	21·0116	3175	24	1·0908	1·8988	34·5643
Vagina	789	11	0·9969	0·0015	9·8629	789	11	0·9153	0·5220	14·5742
Vulva	199	4	1·3884	4·2043	1·9503	199	4	1·1065	0·1613	0·6465
Uterus, Ovary	767	3	1·2095	5·2380	8·6956	767	3	1·1494	1·3903	3·8529
Corpus Uteri, Ovary, Vagina, Vulva	58	1	1·8208	2·7085		58	1	1·4652	1·1262	
Tube, Vagina, Vulva	26	1	0·8049	0·2565		26	1	0·9764	0·0014	
Unspecified Female Genital Organs	1686	8	1·0635	1·1486	9·7723	1686	8	1·1267	1·9659	11·3249
Prostate	1467	9	1·1756	7·8693	21·3610	1467	9	1·0140	0·0139	4·0701
Seminal Vesicle	57	1	0·7912	0·2516		57	1	1·6246	1·6269	
Penis	83	2	1·4591	0·6963	3·0557	83	2	1·7930	3·4230	3·4338
Kidney	717	9	1·1232	1·7349	10·3556	700	8	1·1105	0·6941	8·1293
Bladder	787	9	1·3359	11·2958	14·3752	787	9	1·3823	6·8479	10·0705
Bladder, Prostate	12	1	4·0536	3·1194		12	1	2·3979	0·7611	
NEOPLASMS OF THE NERVOUS SYSTEM										
Retinoblastomas	13	1	2·8012	2·2259		13	1	3·8342	2·1636	
Glial Tumours										
Gliomas	157	3	1·4972	5·5510	3·0836	157	3	1·0256	0·0063	1·3097
Astrocytomas	2658	7	1·1620	11·1056	6·8117	2658	7	1·0308	0·1616	2·0160
Glioblastomas	844	4	1·1013	1·7179	1·3587	844	4	1·0409	0·0972	5·1216
Ependymomas	178	3	1·1020	0·3701	0·0971	178	3	0·9170	0·0880	0·8271
Oligodendrogliomas	122	2	1·0982	0·2225	0·2532	122	2	1·2711	0·4548	3·5180
	3959	19	1·1549	16·0858	14·4856	3959	19	1·0341	0·2972	13·3031
Medulloblastomas	215	4	1·3125	3·4047	4·1852	215	4	1·1383	0·2200	4·9035
Meningiomas	1380	5	1·0655	1·0344	1·3395	1380	5	1·3124	7·4417	7·1179
Neuromas	483	5	1·1796	2·7485	9·1030	483	5	0·9343	0·1409	0·4788
Malignant Neorogenous Neoplasms	81	1	1·0273	0·0095		81	1	1·0320	0·0097	
Malignant Neoplasms of Brain	74	2	0·8761	0·2594	0·4468	74	2	1·3024	0·4863	0·2995
Metastatic Neoplasms of Brain	65	1	1·1725	0·3720		65	1	0·6813	0·5148	
Benign Neoplasms of Brain	143	2	1·9132	13·0577	2·6640	143	2	0·9755	0·0056	0·4031
Neoplasms of Brain	1669	4	1·0557	0·4609	0·5888	1669	4	1·0449	0·1615	0·7549
Neoplasms of Sympathetic System	30	1	1·6371	1·5372		30	1	1·0457	0·0034	
Vascular Neoplasms of Central Nervous System	107	1	0·9967	0·0003		107	1	0·8681	0·1316	
NEOPLASMS OF LYMPHATIC AND HAEMATOPOIETIC TISSUE										
Hodgkin's Disease, Lymphogranuloma	1651	13	0·8998	3·3228	14·3602	1640	12	0·9452	0·5235	11·6779
Lymphosarcomas	101	2	2·0265	9·0663	4·9568	84	1	2·2230	7·6050	
Reticulosarcomas	166	1	1·6010	5·5814		166	1	1·1758	0·4467	
Lymphosarcomas, Reticulosarcomas	50	1	1·2316	0·3047		50	1	2·1035	3·9710	
Reticulo-endothelial Neoplasms	37	1	0·8846	0·1207		37	1	1·2108	0·1203	
Reticuloses	145	2	1·4181	3·0219	0·6165	145	2	1·2234	0·6672	0·5302
Lymphomas	130	2	1·0804	0·1001	0·1074	130	2	1·0061	0·0007	1·2135
Unspecified Neoplasms	233	2	1·2163	1·6693	2·3632	233	2	1·8570	10·0873	0·7644
	862	11	1·3556	13·2782	14·6301	845	10	1·4596	14·3575	11·0488

TABULAR SUMMARIES. TABLE 1A **THE ABO BLOOD GROUP SYSTEM** *(cont.)*

	A/O					B/O				
	Number of patients	Number of studies (N)	Combined incidence	χ^2_1 for difference from unity	χ^2_{N-1} for homogeneity of areas	Number of patients	Number of studies (N)	Combined incidence	χ^2_1 for difference from unity	χ^2_{N-1} for homogeneity of areas
MYELOID LEUKAEMIAS										
Acute	850	4	0·8442	4·5636	1·4172	850	4	1·1046	0·9547	1·6161
Chronic	811	9	1·2897	9·1541	12·2292	801	8	1·2551	4·0879	8·2881
Unspecified	123	2	1·3236	1·9463	0·1007	123	2	1·3578	0·9856	0·4430
	1784	15	1·0503	0·7841	28·6270	1774	14	1·1180	5·0996	11·2758
LYMPHATIC LEUKAEMIAS										
Acute	103	1	1·2655	1·1788		103	1	1·3530	0·9331	
Chronic	617	7	0·9636	0·1547	10·5632	606	6	0·9688	0·0653	7·7671
Unspecified	240	3	0·8863	0·6590	3·0060	240	3	0·8297	0·8056	1·0173
	960	11	0·9745	0·1196	15·4421	949	10	0·9671	0·1099	10·4785
MONOCYTIC LEUKAEMIAS										
Chronic	15	1	1·0465	0·0061		15	1	0·9375	0·0035	
Unspecified	44	1	0·6267	2·0877		44	1	0·2935	2·7870	
	59	2	0·7075	1·4992	0·5946	59	2	0·4222	2·0074	0·7832
LEUKAEMIAS										
Acute	1644	11	1·1208	3·4913	12·9505	1644	11	1·0465	0·2738	10·5284
Chronic	711	3	1·0172	0·0402	9·1499	711	3	0·9944	0·0016	1·6981
Unspecified	3092	17	1·0698	1·8569	23·4070	3092	17	1·2198	7·2679	21·3821
	5447	31	1·0880	4·4942	46·4016	5447	31	1·1225	4·8898	36·2621
POLYCYTHAEMIA VERA	560	5	0·9525	0·2655	3·3182	560	5	1·1141	0·5852	6·0730
MYELOFIBROSIS	42	2	1·5348	1·1270	0·4284	42	2	1·3587	0·4623	0·0472
MYELOMAS	202	3	1·2525	2·0461	2·2630	202	3	1·0932	0·1566	0·4013
ERYTHROLEUKAEMIA	15	1	0·4847	0·9830		15	1	2·2059	1·8244	
ILL-DEFINED MALIGNANT NEOPLASMS										
SARCOMAS	219	5	1·0020	0·0002	2·8882	204	4	1·3800	1·8846	2·7838
MALIGNANT NEOPLASMS DEFINED AS CANCERS OF MIXED OR UNSPECIFIED SITES	9707	20	1·0310	1·5577	32·4363	9707	20	1·0279	0·4981	32·0984
MALIGNANT NEOPLASMS OF UNSPECIFIED SITES	3955	11	1·0514	1·6599	8·3922	3955	11	1·0123	0·0515	22·9768
MALIGNANT NEOPLASMS, SITE SPECIFIED BY EXCLUSION	4038	7	1·0674	3·6249	4·2363	4038	7	1·0199	0·0197	6·3333
BENIGN NEOPLASMS										
SALIVARY GLANDS	891	5	1·5554	33·2950	44·0606	891	5	1·0598	0·2050	1·6899
NASOPHARYNGEAL	38	1	1·1041	0·0683		38	1	1·1371	0·0678	
DIGESTIVE SYSTEM	67	1	0·9879	0·0017		67	1	1·0199	0·0036	
ABDOMINAL	88	1	1·8712	6·3233		88	1	1·9271	4·3985	
POLYPS OF COLON	391	3	0·9613	0·1086	9·3002	391	3	0·8975	0·4020	2·8834
FEMUR	27	1	0·8465	0·1042		27	1	2·0923	2·3348	
BREAST	80	1	0·9677	0·0160		80	1	1·4778	1·5459	
UTERUS	5472	13	1·1662	20·0232	46·8492	5472	13	1·0732	2·2060	13·2478
OVARY	1071	4	1·2360	8·1867	2·2549	1071	4	1·2673	8·1867	8·3638
TESTIS	34	1	1·3544	0·4799		34	1	1·7436	1·1585	
BLADDER	41	1	0·8465	0·1666		41	1	0·8718	0·0645	
NEOPLASMS OF PITUITARY										
ADENOMAS, CHROMOPHOBE	1269	12	0·9572	0·4923	11·0117	1269	12	1·0792	0·5946	4·3050
ADENOMAS, OTHER THAN CHROMOPHOBE	33	1	0·4751	3·0382		33	1	1·2932	0·2489	
UNSPECIFIED	337	2	1·0993	0·6573	0·0183	337	2	1·0094	0·0019	0·5600
NEOPLASMS OF UNDEFINED OR MIXED CHARACTER										
SALIVARY GLANDS	73	1	3·3137	22·0000		73	1	0·9822	0·0008	
ALIMENTARY TRACT	83	1	1·6013	2·8621		83	1	5·0174	20·7767	
SPLEEN	148	1	0·9159	0·2288		148	1	0·8320	0·3342	
FEMALE GENITAL ORGANS, BENIGN OR MALIGNANT	567	1	1·3247	7·8111		567	1	1·2403	3·0824	
NEPHROGENITAL RIDGE	26	1	0·4943	2·4553		26	1	0·3383	1·1078	
EPITHELIAL	58	2	1·1666	0·1171	11·6909	58	2	1·0623	0·0213	0·0848
OTHER THAN CANCER, BENIGN OR MALIGNANT	65	1	0·6660	2·0039		65	1	1·7045	1·9604	

	A/O					B/O				
	Number of patients	Number of studies (N)	Combined incidence	χ^2_1 for difference from unity	χ^2_{N-1} for homogeneity of areas	Number of patients	Number of studies (N)	Combined incidence	χ^2_1 for difference from unity	χ^2_{N-1} for homogeneity of areas
ENDOCRINE AND METABOLIC DISEASES										
NON-TOXIC GOITRE	315	3	1·1075	0·4586	5·1281	281	2	1·1432	0·3616	0·3338
THYROTOXICOSIS	1950	13	0·8929	4·4328	24·2405	1925	12	0·9535	0·3828	8·6644
GOITRE	3923	19	0·9931	0·0270	28·8267	3899	18	0·8919	3·8723	10·3831
CRETINISM	77	1	1·2729	0·9935		77	1	0·2673	3·2114	
DIABETES MELLITUS	23735	43	1·0727	18·8268	80·9002	23735	43	1·0487	4·1313	112·8194
Patients under 20 years (included in 23735)	826	7	0·8804	2·6722	14·7791	826	7	0·8022	2·9512	6·3067
Patients over 20 years (included in 23735)	11372	19	1·0804	11·0011	42·0009	11372	19	1·1170	9·9464	42·3546
Patients under 20/patients over 20	*580/2805*	*6*	*0·9052*	*0·8748*	*4·9438*	*580/2805*	*6*	*0·9146*	*0·2367*	*9·9760*
Patients under 30/patients over 30	*155/1058*	*2*	*0·8366*	*0·8705*	*1·6209*	*155/1058*	*2*	*0·6597*	*1·5872*	*0·4162*
Patients under 40/patients over 40	*449/1381*	*2*	*0·6902*	*9·2780*	*0·8577*	*449/1381*	*2*	*0·5797*	*8·5006*	*0·0015*
Younger patients/older patients	*1184/5244*	*10*	*0·8095*	*8·1755*	*10·2702*	*1184/5244*	*10*	*0·7212*	*7·2103*	*13·5079*
Males/females	*6136/8102*	*22*	*1·0803*	*3·9863*	*27·5233*	*6136/8102*	*22*	*0·9722*	*0·2576*	*22·1146*
DIABETES, KIMMELSTIEL-WILSON SYNDROME	39	1	5·3130	12·0002		39	1	1·9859	0·6718	
TOXAEMIA OF PREGNANCY	4869	8	0·9903	0·0710	14·3192	4869	8	0·9954	0·0052	14·1201
PELLAGRA	20	1	0·9383	0·0141		20	1	0·9460	0·0090	
RICKETS	557	1	0·9470	0·2883		557	1	1·1471	0·9110	
CELIAC DISEASE	209	3	1·0466	0·0943	7·9380	186	2	1·0765	0·0721	0·6911
NON-TROPICAL SPRUE	28	1	0·4550	3·1803		28	1	0·2016	2·4315	
HAEMOCHROMATOSIS	80	2	0·9887	0·0023	1·2366	80	2	0·6672	0·7193	0·3680
SPASMOPHILIA	100	1	0·9937	0·0008		100	1	0·8259	0·2918	
HYPOGAMMAGLOBULINAEMIA	194	2	0·8717	0·7240	12·1028	194	2	0·6429	2·2052	0·0000
DISEASES OF THE BLOOD										
HYPOCHROMIC ANAEMIA	898	5	1·1074	1·4895	11·7829	898	5	0·9675	0·1157	6·8216
PERNICIOUS ANAEMIA	3446	24	1·2524	32·3099	27·0572	3446	24	1·1929	7·8940	25·7411
MACROCYTIC ANAEMIA	47	2	0·8064	0·3619	0·1402	30	1	1·4530	0·5460	
HAEMOLYTIC ANAEMIA										
Congenital	90	3	1·0202	0·0068	1·6558	90	3	1·1436	0·1992	0·3902
Acquired	479	6	0·8234	3·4099	11·6311	479	6	0·8176	1·5863	5·9826
Unspecified	88	2	0·9494	0·0449	0·4448	88	2	1·0807	0·0396	0·4625
HAEMOLYTIC JAUNDICE	58	1	0·7674	0·8407		58	1	0·5625	0·8680	
APLASTIC ANAEMIA	108	3	0·8853	0·2856	1·4129	108	2	0·8730	0·2045	0·1715
SECONDARY ANAEMIA	385	2	0·7865	3·4987	0·4486	385	2	0·9423	0·1340	0·1886
CHRONIC ANAEMIA	41	1	0·5520	1·4494		41	1	1·8194	2·1248	
NUTRITIONAL ANAEMIA	44	1	1·1543	0·1415		44	1	1·6643	1·3773	
POSTINFECTIVE ANAEMIA	50	1	0·8465	0·1666		50	1	2·1794	4·2815	
ANAEMIA DUE TO RENAL INSUFFICIENCY	23	1	2·9022	4·2373		23	1	3·7362	5·0657	
HAEMOPHILIA	231	4	0·9071	0·0040	4·0620	231	4	0·8491	0·6504	1·0674
IDIOPATHIC THROMBOCYTOPENIC PURPURA	334	5	1·2925	3·5637	8·5171	334	5	1·2535	1·6668	12·7846
HAEMOPHILIA AND PURPURA	40	1	0·8813	0·1335		40	1	1·1842	0·0902	
TROPICAL EOSINOPHILIA	780	4	2·2173	43·0102	1·5784	780	4	1·7541	21·9835	6·7384
MENTAL DISORDERS										
PSYCHOSES										
Senile dementia	747	12	1·0376	0·1791	13·8702	747	12	1·1352	0·9787	19·1356
Postencephalitic	12	1	1·6831	0·6430		12	1	1·6615	0·3392	
Schizophrenia	12608	43	1·0172	0·4983	68·7037	12608	43	1·1663	20·7444	153·2420
Manic-depressive	1856	22	0·8880	4·5266	32·2696	1856	22	1·0483	0·3488	20·9544
Paranoia	218	4	0·8197	1·4405	0·9489	201	3	0·8916	0·2810	5·1366
Arteriosclerotic	271	1	0·7543	4·5739		271	1	1·0637	0·0959	
Confusional	184	3	1·0832	0·2304	0·1751	184	3	1·2737	0·8690	4·1135
Involutional	338	3	0·9383	0·2536	0·0636	338	3	1·2574	1·9649	0·5771
Symptomatic	21	1	0·4715	2·1024		21	1	0·8904	0·0444	
Unspecified*	353	3				353	3			

* For details see elsewhere.

TABULAR SUMMARIES. TABLE 1A **THE ABO BLOOD GROUP SYSTEM** *(cont.)*

	A/O					B/O				
	Number of patients	Number of studies (N)	Combined incidence	χ^2_1 for difference from unity	χ^2_{N-1} for homogeneity of areas	Number of patients	Number of studies (N)	Combined incidence	χ^2_1 for difference from unity	χ^2_{N-1} for homogeneity of areas
NEUROSES										
Psychopathy	781	7	1·1993	4·3101	10·8341	781	7	1·1761	1·9710	13·8366
Anxiety	51	1	1·2381	0·3998		51	1	1·9986	2·0747	
Depressive	229	2	1·1040	0·3949	1·7350	229	2	1·2234	0·5907	0·2821
Hysteria	151	3	1·1616	0·6024	8·2099	151	3	0·7435	1·0647	5·2005
Neurasthenia	111	2	0·6068	3·5773	1·1791	111	2	0·9164	0·0597	0·0111
Unspecified	46	1	1·4590	0·8688		46	1	2·3856	4·0832	
ALCOHOLISM	1392	11	1·0339	0·2275	15·8093	1392	11	0·9733	0·6750	6·1025
MENTAL RETARDATION	2281	22	0·9671	0·4547	13·0681	2281	22	1·0784	1·0376	45·8923

DISEASES OF THE NERVOUS SYSTEM AND SENSE ORGANS

	A/O Number of patients	A/O Number of studies (N)	A/O Combined incidence	A/O χ^2_1	A/O χ^2_{N-1}	B/O Number of patients	B/O Number of studies (N)	B/O Combined incidence	B/O χ^2_1	B/O χ^2_{N-1}
MUSCULAR DYSTROPHY	49	1	0·9326	0·0525		49	1	0·5636	0·8797	
HUNTINGTON'S CHOREA	70	1	1·9928	6·3685		70	1	2·1821	3·7855	
MULTIPLE SCLEROSIS	2242	13	0·8903	5·0069	16·1521	2227	12	0·8860	2·0302	9·7323
PARKINSON'S DISEASE	481	3	0·7651	6·7363	1·1767	481	3	1·1145	0·5173	6·6507
EPILEPSY	3072	29	1·0231	0·2844	45·2545	3049	28	1·2168	10·4511	49·4607
KURU	492	4	0·9609	0·1189	3·8278	492	4	1·2615	2·5956	0·2614
MOTOR NEURONE DISEASE	386	2	1·1409	0·7384	0·7569	386	2	1·7439	7·3409	2·6061
BLEPHARITIS	28	1	1·5758	0·5708		28	1	1·1556	0·0328	
UVEITIS	239	1	0·8761	0·2058		239	1	0·8854	0·1365	
REFRACTIVE ERRORS OF EYE										
Hyperopia	312	2	1·5732	4·7871	0·4407	312	2	1·3909	1·6582	0·0769
Myopia	519	3	2·5515	67·8905	11·1256	519	3	2·6200	41·3025	7·0005
Astigmatism	98	1	1·5634	2·1775		98	1	1·5451	1·4212	
Difference of refraction	159	1	1·1539	0·3328		159	1	0·9061	0·0956	
CATARACT	182	2	0·8795	0·5736	5·8522	182	2	0·6141	2·7243	0·1386
GLAUCOMA	336	5	1·4114	6·6127	11·8608	336	5	1·0254	0·0164	3·3753

DISEASES OF THE CIRCULATORY SYSTEM

	A/O Number of patients	A/O Number of studies (N)	A/O Combined incidence	A/O χ^2_1	A/O χ^2_{N-1}	B/O Number of patients	B/O Number of studies (N)	B/O Combined incidence	B/O χ^2_1	B/O χ^2_{N-1}
RHEUMATIC FEVER	3144	10	1·1376	9·0415	3·8124	3144	10	1·1012	2·3314	11·7101
RHEUMATIC HEART DISEASE	5103	22	1·2306	36·5332	37·4200	5103	22	1·2845	24·6475	22·4303
MALIGNANT HYPERTENSION	180	2	0·6011	6·6006	0·8658	180	2	0·6063	4·0227	0·0877
HYPERTENSION	4710	13	0·9994	0·0003	9·3636	4710	13	1·0327	0·4002	18·9073
HYPOTENSION	65	1	1·3563	0·9276		65	1	1·5520	0·8833	
ANGINA PECTORIS, CORONARY OCCLUSION WITHOUT INFARCTION	1631	12	1·0548	0·9098	21·1611	1631	12	1·0120	0·0204	8·1536
MYOCARDIAL INFARCTION	7124	37	1·2927	76·2639	61·0888	7112	36	1·1882	18·0048	58·2656
MYOCARDIAL INFARCTION, CORONARY INSUFFICIENCY, ANGINA PECTORIS, PRESENT/ABSENT	*273/3852*	*1*	*0·8339*	*1·7573*		*273/3852*	*1*	*0·9601*	*0·0391*	
MYOCARDISM	143	1	1·6115	5·5792		143	1	0·9290	0·0592	
INTRACEREBRAL ARTERIOVENOUS ANEURISM	150	1	0·6245	6·4053		150	1	1·1977	0·5103	
CEREBRAL STROKE	649	1	0·9815	0·0418		649	1	0·9257	0·4064	
ARTERIOSCLEROSIS	3282	12	1·2058	20·7369	27·1408	3282	12	1·1282	4·3078	10·8413
ATHEROSCLEROSIS, WITH OCCLUSION/WITHOUT OCCLUSION	*506/129*	*1*	*1·8061*	*7·4449*		*506/129*	*1*	*1·0372*	*0·0132*	
BUERGER'S DISEASE	66	1	2·2810	6·5100		66	1	0·5865	1·1660	
ARTERIOSCLEROTIC HEART DISEASE	253	1	0·9297	0·2907		253	1	0·6381	3·2323	
ACROCYANOSIS	43	1	1·3671	0·7659		43	1	2·0147	1·7878	
THROMBOSIS AND EMBOLISM	2691	10	1·2299	22·0826	9·8827	2691	10	1·1351	3·1639	15·5959
THROMBOEMBOLISM IN PREGNANT OR PUERPERAL WOMEN	931	6	1·5147	32·1817	5·3093	931	6	1·3820	7·9972	6·4489
THROMBOEMBOLISM IN WOMEN ON ORAL CONTRACEPTIVES	236	4	2·9649	40·4703	1·7265	236	4	3·0746	24·4424	0·5556
ARTERITIS	128	1	1·2146	0·7699		128	1	1·7003	2·9292	
VARICOSE VEINS OF LOWER EXTREMITIES	307	1	1·0874	0·3528		307	1	1·4216	3·0953	
HAEMORRHAGES	2478	10	0·7486	31·8088	24·2277	2478	1	0·8011	10·6987	31·2857

DISEASES OF THE RESPIRATORY SYSTEM

	A/O Number of patients	A/O Number of studies (N)	A/O Combined incidence	A/O χ^2_1	A/O χ^2_{N-1}	B/O Number of patients	B/O Number of studies (N)	B/O Combined incidence	B/O χ^2_1	B/O χ^2_{N-1}
RESPIRATORY INFECTIONS	798	2	1·1608	3·0692	0·3028	798	2	1·1766	1·7618	0·3524
BRONCHOPNEUMONIA	496	3	1·2893	6·3612	9·9294	496	3	1·4608	6·4216	2·8407
PNEUMONIA	695	4	0·9099	1·0145	0·9210	695	4	1·1125	0·6955	7·5280
BRONCHITIS	1001	5	0·8828	3·0467	1·5971	1001	5	0·9189	0·6185	1·7055
EMPHYSEMA	242	2	1·1398	0·7798	0·6002	242	2	1·1132	0·2947	1·2596

	A/O					B/O				
	Number of patients	Number of studies (N)	Combined incidence	χ_1^2 for difference from unity	χ_{N-1}^2 for homogeneity of areas	Number of patients	Number of studies (N)	Combined incidence	χ_1^2 for difference from unity	χ_{N-1}^2 for homogeneity of areas
DISEASES OF THE RESPIRATORY SYSTEM (*cont.*)										
Atrophic Ozenous Rhinitis	20	1	0·3087	3·3624		20	1	0·4752	0·9577	
Pleurisy	332	3	1·2847	3·4822	1·6036	332	3	1·1685	0·7921	1·3898
Spontaneous Pneumothorax	85	1	1·0366	0·0218		85	1	1·5144	1·5802	
Bronchiectasis	78	1	1·0851	0·1158		78	1	0·7348	0·4129	
DISEASES OF THE DIGESTIVE SYSTEM										
Dental Caries	251	1	1·2657	2·0893		251	1	1·3413	1·3750	
Dental Caries, Extensive/None at All	*36/24*	*1*	*0·8148*	*0·1230*		*36/24*	*1*	*0·6111*	*0·2983*	
Periodontosis	1784	1	1·0044	0·0050		1784	1	1·1894	2·3195	
Gastritis	343	3	1·3064	4·0939	3·3612	343	3	0·9690	0·0337	13·2265
Appendicitis	4025	6	0·9863	0·1190	9·9344	4025	6	0·9744	0·2823	12·2370
Hernia of Abdominal Cavity	169	1	0·9982	0·0001		169	1	0·9868	0·0039	
Hernia of Unspecified Sites	80	1	1·2401	0·6764		80	1	1·3619	0·8367	
Intestinal Obstruction	262	1	1·3495	3·6199		262	1	1·4233	4·1542	
Ulcerative Colitis	1092	6	1·0030	0·0021	4·8234	1092	6	1·1445	1·5674	9·4350
Anal Fissure and Fistula	107	1	1·3331	1·4931		107	1	0·7479	0·8772	
Peritonitis	61	1	0·8299	0·3726		61	1	0·8286	0·2879	
Diseases of Intestines and Peritoneum Besides Peritonitis	121	1	1·0046	0·0005		121	1	0·3740	9·1353	
Cirrhosis of Liver	2837+?	18	1·2372	24·8769	30·1399	2837+?	14	1·1811	6·6605	12·3764
Cholelithiasis	14660	21	1·1468	43·8033	63·1423	14660	21	1·0079	0·0722	50·1931
Cholecystitis	1582	5	1·3409	20·8809	23·9491	1582	5	1·0916	1·1141	24·1700
Cholelithiasis, Cholecystitis	1343	3	1·1092	2·4876	1·9265	1343	3	1·0462	0·2018	6·0708
Diseases of Gall-bladder and Biliary Ducts	1436	4	1·1742	6·6769	10·9396	1436	4	1·1396	2·0578	5·6925
Jaundice	173	1	1·3572	2·8953		173	1	1·7578	3·9599	
Diseases of the Pancreas	244	3	0·9799	0·0156	1·1321	244	3	1·1578	0·5129	2·3986
Gastric Ulcers	30391	88	0·8692	107·4638	191·9718	30140	86	0·8726	49·6415	186·0383
Bleeding	600	4	0·7440	10·7511	0·7548	600	4	0·5401	12·9784	1·8284
Not bleeding	890	3	1·0194	0·0672	0·9917	890	3	0·9563	0·1435	3·8485
Bleeding/not bleeding	*523/890*	*3*	*0·7312*	*6·5626*	*0·1510*	*523/890*	*3*	*0·5004*	*9·5220*	*0·0196*
Stomal Ulcers	374	3	0·5271	29·1885	0·6194	374	3	0·4822	10·5410	0·7685
Bleeding	63	1	0·5425	4·7090		63	1	0·8122	0·2227	
Not bleeding	152	1	0·7276	3·3962		152	1	0·4841	3·8103	
Bleeding/not bleeding	*63/152*	*1*	*0·7456*	*0·7962*		*63/152*	*1*	*1·6776*	*0·8119*	
Duodenal Ulcers	37160	83	0·7315	624·0396	150·5906	37134	82	0·8001	161·4559	156·5601
Bleeding	2648	7	0·6963	66·7506	6·6027	2648	7	0·6439	37·6534	4·6390
Not bleeding	4348	6	0·8639	16·6472	5·7648	4348	6	0·8349	10·3739	6·4679
Bleeding/not bleeding	*2214/4348*	*6*	*0·7856*	*16·4062*	*1·3009*	*2214/4348*	*6*	*0·7650*	*7·7812*	*8·0640*
Ulcers to the Right of the Gastric Angulus	1058	5	0·6675	34·5016	10·5070	1058	5	0·6677	11·1520	4·4249
Both Gastric and Duodenal Ulcers Present	4148	19	0·7011	96·9575	42·1506	4148	19	0·7970	18·0034	43·5442
Peptic Ulcers, Site Unspecified	6296	27	0·7971	56·5238	34·8836	6296	27	0·7336	43·8080	44·4411
DISEASES OF THE GENITO-URINARY SYSTEM										
Diseases of Kidney										
Nephrosis	141	1	0·9621	0·0379		141	1	0·9239	0·0744	
Nephritis	232	1	1·1452	0·6771		232	1	1·2865	1·2478	
Nephritis, chronic	72	1	0·6688	1·8242		72	1	1·1866	0·3473	
Infections of kidney	59	1	1·1302	0·1688		59	1	0·7713	0·4775	
Nephritis-nephrosis	70	1	0·8309	0·5054		70	1	0·7963	0·2558	
Unspecified	62	1	0·5940	3·4271		62	1	0·6081	0·8480	
Contracted kidney	159	1	0·8941	0·3913		159	1	0·8355	0·3411	
Calculus of Urinary System	4270	10	1·0667	2·4667	31·4462	4270	10	0·9857	0·0560	23·5036
Non-Gonococcal Uretritis	345	1	1·1750	1·9414		345	1	1·1397	0·4633	
Hyperplasia of the Prostate	3701	13	1·0507	1·4061	9·9603	3701	13	1·0605	0·8878	7·3102
Other Diseases of Male Genital Organs										
Azoospermia	50	1	0·2019	10·9967		50	1	0·3467	10·2555	
Other than hyperplasia of prostate	49	1	1·3331	0·7484		49	1	0·7479	0·4394	
Diseases of Female Genital Organs										
Salpingitis	28	1	2·0674	2·2414		28	1	1·8869	1·0889	
Salpingitis, oophoritis	184	1	1·0067	0·0013		184	1	1·1809	0·7138	
Infective diseases of uterus, vagina, vulva	131	1	1·1146	0·2563		131	1	1·0428	0·0290	
Uterovaginal prolapse	72	1	1·1855	0·3663		72	1	0·8924	0·1106	

	A/O					B/O				
	Number of patients	Number of studies (N)	Combined incidence	χ^2_1 for difference from unity	χ^2_{N-1} for homogeneity of areas	Number of patients	Number of studies (N)	Combined incidence	χ^2_1 for difference from unity	χ^2_{N-1} for homogeneity of areas
DISORDERS OF MENSTRUATION										
Menopausal metrorrhagia	170	1	0·8493	0·7399		170	1	0·8402	0·4755	
Menorrhagia	466	1	0·8118	3·9645		466	1	1·1764	0·9875	
Unspecified	87	1	0·9625	0·0214		87	1	0·8514	0·2727	
ECTOPIC PREGNANCY	113	1	1·4852	2·3586		113	1	2·0451	7·2504	

PERINATAL DISORDERS

	A/O					B/O				
	Number of patients	Number of studies (N)	Combined incidence	χ^2_1 for difference from unity	χ^2_{N-1} for homogeneity of areas	Number of patients	Number of studies (N)	Combined incidence	χ^2_1 for difference from unity	χ^2_{N-1} for homogeneity of areas
ABORTION										
Mothers/controls	4559	11	0·8716	13·3433	24·3153	4559	11	0·7812	17·3482	12·8740
Fetuses/controls	133	2	1·2425	1·1556	4·2821	133	2	1·6852	3·0885	3·1867
Mothers of normal/mothers of abnormal fetuses	*116/139*	*1*	*0·8123*	*0·5779*		*116/139*	*1*	*1·4400*	*0·6044*	
Fetuses normal/abnormal	*42/21*	*1*	*5·0000*	*7·0067*						
Abortions/live births (mothers)	*2913/153923*	*4*	*0·8992*	*5·9937*	*5·9393*	*2913/153923*	*4*	*0·8198*	*8·5799*	*1·9872*
PREMATURE INFANTS	1634	5	1·1554	4·9175	4·3808	1634	5	1·2994	7·3783	4·1502
Premature/full term infants	*822/1390*	*3*	*1·1697*	*1·1528*	*1·5877*	*822/1390*	*3*	*1·1503*	*0·7121*	*5·5703*
POST-TERM INFANTS	52	1	0·4368	5·9456		52	1	1·5234	1·3262	

DISEASES OF THE SKIN

	A/O					B/O				
	Number of patients	Number of studies (N)	Combined incidence	χ^2_1 for difference from unity	χ^2_{N-1} for homogeneity of areas	Number of patients	Number of studies (N)	Combined incidence	χ^2_1 for difference from unity	χ^2_{N-1} for homogeneity of areas
ANGIODERMATITIS	50	1	1·5821	2·2129		50	1	0·6592	0·6724	
SEBORRHOEIC DERMATITIS	67	2	1·1814	0·3448	0·0341	67	2	2·3678	6·3449	0·2827
SOLAR DERMATITIS	20	1	0·4692	1·9018		20	1	0·6622	0·5638	
DERMATITIS MEDICAMENTOSA	15	1	1·0660	0·0098		15	1	1·1976	0·0649	
DERMATITIS, UNSPECIFIED	25	1	0·6202	0·7770		25	1	1·9813	1·7223	
ROSACEA	78	1	1·1262	0·2083						
LUPUS ERYTHEMATOSUS	153	3	0·8574	4·3985	2·5340	120	2	0·8414	0·5181	2·0125
PSORIASIS	2102	13	0·9140	2·6607	37·1356	1871	12	0·9022	1·4766	22·4752
PITYRIASIS ROSEA	24	1	0·8334	0·1543						
LICHEN PLANUS	68	2	1·2308	0·5285	3·7432	51	1	1·0128	0·0012	
PRURIGO	135	2	0·7336	2·0065	6·8042	135	2	1·0193	0·0078	1·8809
LICHEN SIMPLEX CHRONICUS	58	1	0·8890	0·1432						
PRURITUS	22	1	1·2501	0·2552						
ALOPECIA	119	2	1·3054	1·6418	1·3774	40	1	0·7984	0·2419	
ACNE VULGARIS	504	2	1·3118	4·6190	2·2124	300	1	0·8663	0·4510	
JUVENILE ACNE	26	1	1·0008	0·0000		26	1	3·1136	4·2083	
ACNE VULGARIS AND SEBORRHOEA	100	1	0·9383	0·0636		100	1	1·0760	0·0756	
ULCER OF SKIN	57	1	1·2964	0·7884						
VITILIGO	1247	8	0·9476	0·4037	27·2305	1247	8	1·1164	2·3175	16·9374
FRECKLES	70	1	0·3284	12·7047		70	1	0·3973	7·7651	

DISEASES OF THE MUSCULOSKELETAL SYSTEM AND CONNECTIVE TISSUE

	A/O					B/O				
	Number of patients	Number of studies (N)	Combined incidence	χ^2_1 for difference from unity	χ^2_{N-1} for homogeneity of areas	Number of patients	Number of studies (N)	Combined incidence	χ^2_1 for difference from unity	χ^2_{N-1} for homogeneity of areas
RHEUMATOID ARTHRITIS	2960	7	0·7274	51·1159	122·4388	2960	7	0·7959	17·6577	63·6195
ANKYLOSING SPONDYLITIS	352	2	1·0750	0·3190	0·8666	352	2	1·1804	1·1822	0·0000
DEGENERATIVE OSTEO-ARTHRITIS	120	1	0·8498	0·5414		120	1	1·0299	0·0136	
ARTHRITIS, UNSPECIFIED	49	1	1·2404	0·4372		49	1	0·8491	0·1149	
URIC ACID DIATHESIS	30	1	0·9158	0·0399		30	1	1·3736	0·3150	
OSTEOMYELITIS, PERIOSTITIS	123	1	1·1748	0·5489		123	1	0·9854	0·0033	
PERTHES' DISEASE	142	1	1·1417	0·5083		142	1	1·0248	0·0073	
DUPUYTREN'S DISEASE	80	1	0·9677	0·0185		80	1	1·1370	0·0940	
BONE FRACTURES	2649	6	1·1153	6·2543	14·3659	2649	6	1·1180	2·5837	0·9406

CONGENITAL ANOMALIES

	A/O					B/O				
	Number of patients	Number of studies (N)	Combined incidence	χ^2_1 for difference from unity	χ^2_{N-1} for homogeneity of areas	Number of patients	Number of studies (N)	Combined incidence	χ^2_1 for difference from unity	χ^2_{N-1} for homogeneity of areas
SPINA BIFIDA CYSTICA	72	1	1·0027	0·0001		72	1	0·7706	0·8222	
HYDROCEPHALUS	145	1	1·2741	1·7143		145	1	0·8759	0·1513	
DEAF-MUTISM	425	3	0·9045	0·7821	10·7562	425	3	0·8515	0·8454	0·5229
CONGENITAL HEART DEFECTS										
Tetralogy of Fallot	400	2	0·9499	0·1616	0·2398	400	2	1·4872	4·5665	0·3921
Ventricular septal defect	834	3	0·9642	0·1526	4·2101	834	3	0·9849	0·0094	2·2820
Atrial septal defect	596	3	0·8874	1·5898	1·8103	596	3	0·7713	2·0493	3·7518
Aortic stenosis	388	3	0·9049	0·6563	0·3967	388	3	0·8941	0·2995	0·3181
Pulmonary stenosis	263	2	1·3643	4·3652	0·0086	263	2	1·1409	0·2762	0·4453
Defect not specified	1781	8	1·0512	0·7143	5·4618	1781	8	0·9463	0·3505	5·2963
CLEFT PALATE OR LIP	690	3	0·9795	0·0357	3·5296	690	3	1·1931	1·4015	0·8117
PYLORIC STENOSIS	756	3	0·7658	8·2226	10·1987	756	3	1·1217	0·7355	0·5996

TABULAR SUMMARIES. TABLE 1A **THE ABO BLOOD GROUP SYSTEM** (*cont.*)

	A/O					B/O				
	Number of patients	Number of studies (N)	Combined incidence	χ^2_1 for difference from unity	χ^2_{N-1} for homogeneity of areas	Number of patients	Number of studies (N)	Combined incidence	χ^2_1 for difference from unity	χ^2_{N-1} for homogeneity of areas
CONGENITAL ANOMALIES (*cont.*)										
MALFORMATIONS										
Of digestive system	249	1	0·8694	0·8995		249	1	0·6031	7·0795	
Ano-rectal	26	1	1·2378	0·1918		26	1	0·6243	0·8707	
Malposition of uterus	210	1	1·1346	0·5279		210	1	1·1884	0·7987	
Hypospadias	23	1	1·3926	0·2733		23	1	1·7659	1·1080	
Of urinary tract	470	1	1·0158	0·0208		470	1	0·8115	1·2465	
Of genito-urinary system	71	1	0·7560	0·8346		71	1	1·0975	0·0870	
Dislocation of hip	140	1	0·9660	0·0294		140	1	2·0157	9·6194	
Osteo-articular	83	1	1·4488	2·1300		83	1	0·7198	0·7068	
Osteogenesis imperfecta	152	1	0·7732	1·2646		152	1	1·6296	1·8296	
Of bone and joint	117	1	1·5835	3·8000		117	1	1·3022	0·9353	
Naevi	37	1	1·0001	0·0000						
Xeroderma pigmentosum	24	1	0·1564	8·8259		24	1	0·2207	5·8486	
Other than osteo-articular	45	1	0·6508	1·4153		45	1	1·0161	0·0015	
Unspecified	23	1	1·4359	0·5073		23	1	1·5564	0·4687	
DOWN'S SYNDROME	3457	17	1·0550	1·5826	18·3273	3415	16	1·0087	0·0189	19·8171
ALLERGIES										
ECZEMA	883	7	1·0318	0·1254	13·0889	831	6	0·9709	0·0743	10·5831
URTICARIA	259	4	1·0047	0·0010	1·1599	259	4	1·1937	1·0159	0·9213
DERMATITIS	170	2	0·9269	0·1726	0·0034	82	1	1·2225	0·4951	
DERMATOSES	260	1	3·3752	52·7909		260	1	1·7579	6·3809	
ASTHMA	1684	8	1·1286	3·7198	19·5079	1684	8	1·4671	20·2960	15·7367
HAY FEVER	320	2	0·9435	0·2195	2·0980	320	2	1·2641	1·4858	0·8977
ASTHMA AND/OR HAY FEVER	435	1	0·8877	0·6541		435	1	1·3379	1·3897	
Present/absent	*926/4731*	*1*	*1·0723*	*0·8128*		*926/4731*	*1*	*0·9922*	*0·0040*	
UNSPECIFIED OR MIXED ALLERGIES	776	3	0·9687	0·1042	0·5020	776	3	1·0709	0·3744	0·5934

TABLE 1A.1 Selected examples of the combined incidence AB/O, with A/O and B/O (extracted from Table 1A) shown for comparison

			A/O	B/O	AB/O		
	Number of patients	Number of sets (N)	Combined incidence	Combined incidence	Combined incidence	χ^2_1 for difference from unity	χ^2_{N-1} for homogeneity of areas
Cancer of oesophagus	2657	29	1·0994	1·2876	1·2588	5·2382	33·6102
Cancer of stomach	63241	157	1·2120	1·0422	1·1030	24·5806	218·3919
Cancer of cervix uteri	23161	40	1·0914	1·0187	1·0504	2·1446	110·1424
Pernicious anaemia	3446	24	1·2524	1·2170	1·5656	27·4010	26·7122
Rheumatic heart disease	5060	21	1·2306	1·2845	1·5016	30·2498	17·4017
Myocardial infarction	7124	37	1·2927	1·1882	1·3434	25·7716	38·1574
Haemorrhages	2446	9	0·7486	0·8011	1·2407	4·3314	56·9916
Cholelithiasis	14660	21	1·1468	1·0079	1·1642	15·5471	32·3237
Rheumatoid arthritis	2960	7	0·7274	0·7959	0·7465	12·8048	19·6979
Asthma	1684	8	1·1286	1·4671	1·2968	4·2454	3·9485

The numbers of specimens and sets refer to AB/O, and may be slightly lower than for A/O or B/O owing to the very occasional absence of AB (and sometimes of B) in the sets of disease data.

TABLE 2A
THE MN BLOOD GROUP SYSTEM

	MM/MN+NN				
	Number of patients	Number of studies (N)	Combined incidence	χ_1^2 for difference for unity	χ_{N-1}^2 for homogeneity of areas
INFECTIVE AND PARASITIC DISEASES					
BACTERIAL INFECTIONS					
TUBERCULOSIS					
Pulmonary	576	2	1·0153	0·0101	0·3412
Sites unspecified	250	1	1·0359	0·0598	
	826	3	1·0261	0·0607	0·3504
LEPROSY					
Lepromatous	688	4	0·9825	0·0244	2·7873
Tuberculoid	363	4	1·0167	0·0143	3·1049
Indeterminate	100	3	0·8553	0·3519	1·0878
Unspecified types	126	1	0·9945	0·0004	
	1277	12	0·9822	0·0511	7·3199
SYPHILIS	655	3	1·0208	0·0505	0·7587
WORM INFESTATIONS					
FILARIASIS	603	1	0·9402	0·2524	
NEOPLASMS					
MALIGNANT NEOPLASMS					
OESOPHAGUS	20	1	1·9632	2·2072	
STOMACH	594	4	1·1180	1·4398	8·5576
CAECUM, COLON, RECTUM	182	1	0·9598	0·0543	
BILE DUCTS, GALL-BLADDER	18	1	0·6855	0·4378	
PANCREAS	13	1	1·4996	0·4989	
VOCAL CHORDS, LARYNX	10	1	3·5991	3·8978	
LUNG	63	1	0·7927	0·6606	
BRONCHUS	182	1	1·0941	0·2727	
RODENT ULCER, EPITHELIOMA	20	1	0·7998	0·1843	
BREAST	661	5	0·8662	2·4209	0·9399
CERVIX UTERI	85	1	1·0262	0·0119	
CORPUS UTERI	142	1	0·9804	0·0109	
UTERUS	44	1	1·0062	0·0003	
OVARY	81	2	0·8684	0·3123	2·1525
PROSTATE	44	1	1·1197	0·1174	
KIDNEY	17	1	1·3088	0·2767	
BLADDER	25	1	0·5999	1·0278	
NEOPLASMS OF THE NERVOUS SYSTEM					
BRAIN CANCER	13	1	1·0664	0·0113	
NEOPLASMS OF LYMPHATIC AND HAEMATOPOIETIC TISSUE					
HODGKIN'S DISEASE	114	4	1·2693	1·0068	9·6541
LYMPHOSARCOMA	17	1	2·0444	1·6852	
MYELOID LEUKAEMIA	50	3	1·2613	0·4671	3·8892
UNSPECIFIED LEUKAEMIAS	265	3	0·6820	6·1154	1·3413
ILL-DEFINED MALIGNANT NEOPLASMS					
SARCOMAS	20	1	1·5996	1·0386	
CANCERS	200	1	0·9820	0·0126	
CANCERS OTHER THAN BREAST AND LUNG	79	1	0·9175	0·1188	

TABULAR SUMMARIES. TABLE 2A **THE MN BLOOD GROUP SYSTEM** *(cont.)*

	MM/MN+NN				
	Number of patients	Number of studies (N)	Combined incidence	χ_1^2 for difference from unity	χ_{N-1}^2 for homogeneity of areas
ENDOCRINE AND METABOLIC DISEASES					
Diabetes Mellitus	2653	7	0·9248	2·0884	3·2585
Haemachromatosis	54	1	1·2949	0·5617	
DISEASES OF THE BLOOD					
Pernicious Anaemia	361	3	0·9480	0·1367	5·4134
MENTAL DISORDERS					
Senile Dementia	94	1	1·1479	0·3179	
Schizophrenia	1899	9	0·8754	5·7433	11·8781
Manic-depressive Psychoses	480	3	1·0671	0·3264	0·5293
Dysthymia	95	1	0·9798	0·0065	
Involutional Psychoses	160	1	1·0339	0·0348	
Alcoholism	78	1	0·7026	1·6668	
Phrenasthenia	100	1	0·8663	0·3244	
Unspecified Mental Diseases	250	1	1·1808	1·3931	
DISEASES OF THE NERVOUS SYSTEM					
Multiple Sclerosis	1126	3	0·9677	0·1359	2·7411
Epilepsy	57	2	0·8262	0·3957	0·0059
Amyotrophic Lateral Sclerosis	346	1	1·1191	0·4499	
DISEASES OF THE CIRCULATORY SYSTEM					
Rheumatic Fever	1510	4	0·9733	0·1327	5·9797
Hypertension	383	1	1·3973	9·6960	
Coronary Occlusion without Infarction	87	1	0·9659	0·0236	
Myocardial Infarction	471	10	1·0175	0·0300	7·7350
Cerebral Arteriosclerosis	224	1	0·8964	0·4826	
DISEASES OF THE DIGESTIVE SYSTEM					
Ulcerative Colitis	169	1	1·2542	1·4772	
Gastric Ulcer	348	1	0·9502	0·1504	
Duodenal Ulcer	1056	2	1·0075	0·0079	2·0099
DISEASES OF THE GENITO-URINARY SYSTEM					
Nephritis-Nephrosis	70	1	1·4999	2·5891	
Renal Lithiasis	187	1	1·0681	0·0988	
Menopausal Metrorrhagia	170	1	1·3211	2·7274	
DISEASES OF THE SKIN					
Psoriasis	556	3	1·4552	11·7548	0·3885
DISEASES OF THE MUSCULOSKELETAL SYSTEM					
Articular Rheumatism	222	1	0·9309	0·0771	
Ankylosing Spondylitis	200	1	1·0649	0·1685	
CONGENITAL ANOMALIES					
Hydrocephalus	145	1	0·7889	1·4000	
Congenital Heart Disease	702	2	0·8916	0·6101	2·7472
Osteogenesis Imperfecta	152	1	0·8871	0·2859	
Down's Syndrome	770	5	0·8459	2·4627	4·8055
ALLERGIES					
Eczema	192	1	1·1908	0·7638	
Asthma	595	2	1·0638	0·3132	0·3681
Allergies other than Eczema	176	1	0·9541	0·0506	
Unspecified Allergies	100	1	0·7549	0·9808	

TABLE 3A
THE RHESUS BLOOD GROUP SYSTEM

	D+/D−				
	Number of patients	Number of studies (N)	Combined incidence	χ_1^2 for difference from unity	χ_{N-1}^2 for homogeneity of areas
INFECTIVE AND PARASITIC DISEASES					
BACTERIAL INFECTIONS					
Typhoid Fever	445	1	0·5729	24·7874	
Paratyphoid Fever	237	1	0·5903	12·1368	
Bacillary Dysentery, Unspecified	124	1	0·8281	0·6952	
Gonorrhoea	374	1	0·9099	0·5290	
Whooping Cough	684	1	0·8664	1·9806	
Diphtheria	672	1	0·9428	0·3137	
Scarlet Fever	697	1	0·9035	0·9840	
Staphylococci Carriers/Non-Carriers	*596/459*	*1*	*1·0269*	*0·0274*	
Tetanus	57	1	0·9829	0·0024	
Tuberculosis					
Pulmonary	2085	5	0·8783	3·4846	25·2370
Tuberculous meningitis	38	1	0·5855	2·0944	
Of bones and joints	87	1	0·5353	6·6485	
Of genito-urinary system	122	1	0·5735	7·0947	
Sites unspecified	1034	1	0·8890	1·6530	
	3366	9	0·8331	12·4541	33·7581
Sarcoidosis	724	5	0·8324	3·0742	32·1323
Leprosy					
Lepromatous	2676	13	1·1440	2·3964	17·1410
Tuberculoid	997	12	1·2846	2·9178	5·7511
Indeterminate	66	2	1·1399	0·0010	0·1765
Unspecified types	353	2	1·1713	0·5803	0·1186
	4092	29	1·1771	5·5207	23·5620
Syphilis					
Cardiovascular	219	2	0·8100	1·6553	0·5125
Other than cardiovascular	1207	1	0·9292	0·9949	
Mental disorders due to syphilis	35	1	0·6948	0·7107	
Unspecified	132	1	1·0302	0·0067	
	1593	5	0·9062	2·2780	1·6021
Septicaemia	45	1	1·3593	0·4873	
Bacterial Meningitis	86	1	0·9149	0·1016	
Septic Angina	322	1	0·7959	2·6179	
Lung Abscesses	156	1	1·4386	1·6994	
VIRAL INFECTIONS					
Poliomyelitis	504	2	0·9483	0·2116	0·7496
Reactions to Smallpox Vaccination +/−	*612/169*	*1*	*0·8574*	*0·5023*	
Chickenpox	371	1	0·8117	2·4716	
Measles	1836	1	0·8574	5·2472	
Infectious Hepatitis	1168	2	1·0390	0·1947	1·5376
Mumps	403	1	0·6253	15·4514	
Infectious Mononucleosis	274	1	0·5867	14·2919	
Viral Meningitis	129	1	0·5843	7·0427	
WORM INFESTATIONS					
Filariasis	281	1	1·1724	0·4168	

	D+/D−				
	Number of patients	Number of studies (N)	Combined incidence	χ^2_1 for difference from unity	χ^2_{N-1} for homogeneity of areas
NEOPLASMS					
MALIGNANT NEOPLASMS					
Oesophagus	791	5	0·9619	0·1613	6·2846
Stomach	4376	15	0·9810	0·1828	18·0985
Colon	1113	4	0·9596	0·2404	5·0553
Rectum	1855	3	1·0863	1·2351	5·3165
Colon, Rectum	1482	3	0·8758	3·5333	0·0658
Intestines	108	1	0·8965	0·1783	
Liver	120	1	1·7302	1·4310	
Gall-bladder	54	1	1·2366	0·2937	
Gall-bladder, Bile Ducts	18	1	3·4188	1·4223	
Pancreas	659	4	1·0233	0·0459	5·6864
Liver, Gall-bladder, Bile Ducts, Pancreas	63	1	1·4344	0·8082	
Thyroid Gland	150	1	1·1570	0·3433	
Larynx	46	2	0·8699	0·1335	0·5539
Bronchus	3926	4	1·0380	0·3808	4·3818
Lung	4598	10	1·0528	1·2268	12·8865
Respiratory System	76	1	1·0595	0·0313	
Osteoma	224	1	1·3826	2·2660	
Skin	268	3	1·3838	2·5341	0·1126
Breast	2701	10	1·0223	0·1557	14·8496
Cervix Uteri	2926	8	1·1361	3·9848	12·4659
Corpus Uteri	794	5	1·1668	1·7952	8·9644
Uterus	2289	5	1·0634	0·6393	6·3470
Ovary	823	5	1·0829	0·5368	3·4986
Vagina	77	1	0·8889	0·1546	
Vulva	226	2	0·8307	0·7526	1·3953
Unspecified Female Genital Organs	6771	10	1·0722	3·5819	36·5553
Prostate	399	3	0·8384	1·8301	2·0622
Kidney	105	3	2·5464	5·6056	0·8964
Urinary Bladder	156	2	0·7661	1·5748	2·4313
NEOPLASMS OF THE NERVOUS SYSTEM					
Retinoblastomas	13	1	0·7653	0·1648	
Glial Tumours					
Astrocytomas	295	1	0·9761	0·0258	
Glioblastomas	212	1	1·0473	0·0655	
Ependymomas	50	1	1·4050	0·6938	
Oligodendrogliomas	17	1	3·6595	1·5833	
	575	4	1·0451	0·1591	2·2093
Medulloblastomas	52	1	1·0928	0·0584	
Meningiomas	224	1	0·9911	0·0027	
Neurilemomas	89	1	0·7891	0·8628	
Malignant Neoplasms of Brain	13	1	0·4525	1·7238	
Neoplasms of Brain	1264	1	1·1307	1·1828	
Neoplasms of Sympathetic System	31	1	0·9567	0·0095	
Vascular Neoplasms of Central Nervous System	68	1	1·1852	0·2649	
NEOPLASMS OF LYMPHATIC AND HAEMATOPOIETIC TISSUE					
Hodgkin's Disease, Lymphogranulomas	375	5	0·7148	6·4621	1·9268
Reticuloses	145	2	1·4692	2·3007	0·4293
Myelomas	49	1	0·5182	3·8842	
Lymphatic Leukaemias, Chronic	149	2	1·1640	0·4166	0·8001
Lymphatic Leukaemias, Unspecified	148	1	1·6923	4·1450	
Myeloid Leukaemias, Acute	301	1	1·0516	0·1074	
Myeloid Leukaemias, Chronic	295	3	1·1796	0·9959	1·8024
Myeloid Leukaemias, Unspecified	40	1	1·1788	0·1375	
Erythroleukaemia	15	1	1·4275	0·2194	
Leukaemias, Acute	251	3	0·7546	2·9336	1·4587
Leukaemias, Chronic	104	1	0·9553	0·0278	
Leukaemias, Unspecified	1223	7	0·9826	0·0287	1·3941
Polycythaemia Vera	34	2	0·6234	1·6215	1·2522
Myelofibrosis	11	1	0·9882	0·0002	
Unspecified Neoplasms of Lymphatic and Haematopoietic Tissue	91	1	0·9861	0·0023	

TABULAR SUMMARIES. TABLE 3A **THE RHESUS BLOOD GROUP SYSTEM** *(cont.)*

	D+/D−				
	Number of patients	Number of studies (N)	Combined incidence	χ_1^2 for difference from unity	χ_{N-1}^2 for homogeneity of areas
ILL-DEFINED MALIGNANT NEOPLASMS					
Sarcomas	21	1	1·9105	0·7534	
Malignant Neoplasms Defined as Cancers of Mixed or Unspecified Sites	371	2	0·8988	0·4152	1·3361
Malignant Neoplasms of Unspecified Sites	1470	1	1·0506	0·2281	
VARIOUS NEOPLASMS					
Salivary Gland Tumours	407	1	1·2161	1·5932	
Fibromas of Uterus	229	1	1·4934	3·4728	
Pituitary Tumours	144	1	1·0887	0·1476	
Osteomas	197	1	1·1424	0·3886	
ENDOCRINE AND METABOLIC DISEASES					
Thyrotoxicosis	208	1	0·9260	0·1650	
Goitre	308	1	0·7154	3·2269	
Diabetes Mellitus	6240	13	1·0105	0·0705	8·7017
Diabetes, Kimmelstiel–Wilson Syndrome	39	1	1·1436	0·0912	
Toxaemia of Pregnancy	2234	1	1·0456	0·3995	
Haemochromatosis	80	2	0·9930	0·0005	1·9445
DISEASES OF THE BLOOD					
Pernicious Anaemia	701	6	0·9568	0·1695	4·7082
Haemolytic Anaemia	224	3	0·8644	0·7365	0·6335
Cooley's Anaemia	43	1	0·2099	3·6472	
Aplastic Anaemia	63	1	1·1639	0·1934	
Haemophilia	81	2	1·6593	2·0357	0·0009
Idiopathic Thrombocytopenic Purpura	173	2	1·0332	0·0262	1·0239
MENTAL DISORDERS					
Psychoses					
Senile dementia	96	2	0·5011	7·6028	1·4335
Postencephalitic	12	1	0·2432	5·6989	
Schizophrenia	1374	8	0·9776	0·0773	12·0589
Manic depressive	110	3	0·8156	0·6543	1·2735
Various	285	3	1·1000	0·2880	1·4436
Neuroses					
Psychopathy	26	1	1·6715	0·6880	
Various	46	1	1·2147	0·2158	
Alcoholism	142	2	0·7693	1·4085	3·4085
Mental Retardation	389	4	0·6507	7·9982	8·9445
DISEASES OF THE NERVOUS SYSTEM					
Multiple Sclerosis	1225	4	0·9783	0·0499	17·7618
Epilepsy	303	4	1·1652	0·8135	0·0811
Motor Neurone Disease	346	1	0·8921	0·2850	
DISEASES OF THE CIRCULATORY SYSTEM					
Rheumatic Fever	1108	4	0·9685	0·1235	4·5299
Rheumatic Heart Disease	1415	4	0·9304	0·7142	3·3115
Hypertension	1880	3	1·0075	0·0101	5·6876
Coronary Occlusion	846	1	0·8977	1·3448	
Angina Pectoris, Acute Coronary Insufficiency, Cardiac Infarction	446	1	0·9032	0·6905	
Myocardial Infarction	2412	14	1·3141	14·0470	35·3837
Arteriosclerotic Heart Disease	253	1	1·1203	0·4010	
Atheromatosis	213	1	1·0618	0·0841	
Cerebro-Vascular Diseases	168	1	1·4620	1·8754	
Superficial Puerperal Thrombophlebitis	607	1	0·8594	2·2519	
Arteritis	128	1	1·3135	0·8602	
DISEASES OF THE RESPIRATORY SYSTEM					
Bronchopneumonia	177	1	1·1668	0·5050	
Chronic Bronchitis	347	1	0·8326	1·7268	
Spontaneous Pneumothorax	85	1	1·1674	0·2456	

TABULAR SUMMARIES. TABLE 3A **THE RHESUS BLOOD GROUP SYSTEM** *(cont.)*

	D+/D−				
	Number of patients	Number of studies (N)	Combined incidence	χ_1^2 for difference from unity	χ_{N-1}^2 for homogeneity of areas
DISEASES OF THE DIGESTIVE SYSTEM					
Cirrhosis of Liver	801	3	0·9705	0·0890	3·4795
Cholelithiasis	6887	7	1·0240	0·4228	7·8441
Pancreatitis	167	1	0·6141	5·9389	
Gastric Ulcers	3433	12	1·0165	0·1071	16·9948
Duodenal Ulcers	7116	13	1·1122	7·7053	39·3134
Both Gastric and Duodenal Ulcers Present	112	1	1·1301	0·1881	
Peptic Ulcers, Site Unspecified	4224	2	1·0332	0·4982	2·8724
DISEASES OF THE GENITO-URINARY SYSTEM					
Diseases of Kidney					
Nephroses	141	1	1·2290	0·6766	
Nephritis	232	1	1·1709	0·6264	
Nephritis-Nephrosis	70	1	1·4143	0·9092	
Calculus of Kidney	1014	4	0·9222	0·6665	1·5580
Non-Gonococcal Urethritis	345	1	0·8966	0·6577	
Hyperplasia of the Prostate	1653	4	0·8364	6·4954	6·7865
Menopausal Metrorrhagia	170	1	0·6121	6·1365	
DISEASES OF THE SKIN					
Psoriasis Vulgaris	731	3	0·9709	0·0666	3·6874
DISEASES OF THE MUSCULOSKELETAL SYSTEM					
Rheumatoid Arthritis	628	2	1·4677	8·8297	0·2945
Ankylosing Spondylitis	200	1	1·2222	0·9040	
Articular Rheumatism	222	1	0·7294	0·7762	
Perthes' Disease	142	1	0·6101	6·3056	
Dupuytren's Disease	80	1	0·8379	0·3499	
Fractures of Femoral Neck	226	1	1·3361	1·8761	
CONGENITAL ANOMALIES					
Spina Bifida Cystica	72	1	2·6719	0·9481	
Hydrocephalus	145	1	1·1128	0·1958	
Congenital Heart Defects					
Tetralogy of Fallot	400	2	0·9102	0·4705	1·0811
Ventricular septal defect	724	2	0·8598	2·1575	0·0766
Atrial septal defect	410	2	0·8471	1·5842	0·1305
Aortic stenosis	388	3	1·1301	0·6545	0·4010
Pulmonary stenosis	263	2	0·9779	0·0168	0·2457
Defect not specified	427	3	0·7285	2·5457	9·6606
Cleft Lip or Palate	690	3	0·9171	0·6285	1·2839
Pyloric Stenosis	684	2	0·9105	0·7515	0·9889
Malformations					
Osteogenesis imperfecta	152	1	1·4738	1·7909	
Hypospadias	23	1	0·3951	1·5613	
Down's Syndrome	1035	5	0·9814	0·0436	1·9490
ALLERGIES					
Eczema	192	1	1·3131	1·2012	
Asthma	1616	8	0·8715	3·4118	13·3129
Hay Fever	471	3	0·6330	16·0349	10·3308
Asthma and/or Hay Fever, Present/Absent	*717/3670*	*1*	*0·9358*	*0·3898*	
Unspecified Allergies	481	3	0·7616	3·8149	5·6011

TABLE 4A
THE ABH SECRETOR SYSTEM

	Secretors/non-secretors				
	Number of patients	Number of studies (N)	Combined incidence	χ_1^2 for difference from unity	χ_{N-1}^2 for homogeneity of areas
INFECTIVE AND PARASITIC DISEASES					
BACTERIAL INFECTIONS					
HAEMOLYTIC STREPTOCOCCUS A					
Chronic infection	100	1	0·3804	8·1365	
Throat carrier status, carriers/non-carriers	*310/1868*	*3*	*0·7222*	*5·1122*	*4·0944*
PULMONARY TUBERCULOSIS	106	1	1·2004	0·4391	
LEPROSY					
Lepromatous	42	1	1·3714	0·6922	
Non-lepromatous	170	1	0·8063	1·1939	
	212	2	0·9025	0·3440	1·5421
SYPHILIS	132	1	0·8945	0·1129	
WORM INFESTATIONS					
BILHARZIAL HEPATIC FIBROSIS	14	1	1·1250	0·0322	
FILARIASIS	178	1	0·9905	0·0010	
NEOPLASMS					
MALIGNANT NEOPLASMS					
SALIVARY GLANDS	47	1	1·3571	0·6485	
STOMACH	851	7	1·1138	1·1597	8·1006
CAECUM, COLON, RECTUM	172	1	0·9146	0·1854	
BILE DUCTS, GALL-BLADDER	15	1	1·0728	0·0116	
PANCREAS	12	1	2·9501	1·0633	
LARYNX, VOCAL CHORDS	10	1	0·9831	0·0003	
BRONCHUS	161	1	1·0811	0·1247	
LUNG	222	2	1·1203	0·3914	0·0798
EAR, NOSE, THROAT REGION	65	1	3·6773	4·5459	
SKIN	20	1	0·6258	0·8863	
BREAST	458	4	0·8039	2·6432	5·3196
UTERUS	185	2	1·4901	0·5242	2·7250
OVARIES	82	2	1·2021	0·3775	1·8594
PROSTATE	41	1	1·3026	0·3839	
KIDNEY	16	1	1·1622	0·0538	
URINARY BLADDER	43	2	0·7290	0·7903	1·3277
BRAIN	12	1	2·9501	1·0633	
CANCERS, SITE UNSPECIFIED	325	1	1·2410	1·1702	
SARCOMAS, SITE UNSPECIFIED	20	1	0·6258	0·8863	
NEOPLASMS OF LYMPHATIC AND HAEMATOPOIETIC TISSUE					
HODGKIN'S DISEASE	11	1	0·4693	1·4210	
LEUKAEMIAS	227	3	0·8784	0·6119	0·3398
BENIGN NEOPLASMS					
ADENOLYMPHOMA	21	1	0·5223	2·0250	
MIXED SALIVARY ADENOMAS	208	1	1·1011	0·2737	
ENDOCRINE AND METABOLIC DISEASES					
NON-TOXIC GOITRE					
Single adenoma	34	1	0·7893	0·3532	
Multiple adenoma	179	1	1·1582	0·3972	
THYROTOXICOSIS					
Primary, diffuse goitre	104	1	0·7772	0·9365	
Secondary, multiple adenoma	24	1	2·6424	2·3306	
DIABETES MELLITUS	3178	6	1·2348	9·9920	18·5477
CELIAC DISEASE	142	2	0·9633	0·0296	2·8603

TABULAR SUMMARIES. TABLE 4A **THE ABH SECRETOR SYSTEM** (*cont.*)

	Secretors/non-secretors				
	Number of patients	Number of studies (N)	Combined incidence	χ_1^2 for difference from unity	χ_{N-1}^2 for homogeneity of areas
DISEASES OF THE BLOOD					
Pernicious Anaemia	462	4	0·9710	0·0510	2·8899
MENTAL DISORDERS					
Schizophrenia	110	1	1·7143	2·7817	
Alcoholism	841	3	0·7446	9·0812	1·2030
DISEASES OF THE NERVOUS SYSTEM AND SENSE ORGANS					
Multiple Sclerosis	274	2	0·7541	1·5974	0·0373
Amyotrophic Lateral Sclerosis	319	1	1·2244	1·0605	
Uveitis	239	1	0·5519	4·9666	
Primary Glaucoma	100	1	0·1821	50·8841	
DISEASES OF THE CIRCULATORY SYSTEM					
Rheumatic Fever	1308	7	0·7787	11·0406	4·8783
Rheumatic Heart Disease	1238	3	0·9055	1·5011	1·7529
Hypertension	383	1	1·3033	2·0689	
Occlusive Peripheral Arteriosclerosis	66	1	0·3851	11·3453	
DISEASES OF THE RESPIRATORY SYSTEM					
Bronchitis	48	1	1·0000	0·0000	
DISEASES OF THE DIGESTIVE SYSTEM					
Gastritis	26	1	0·3857	3·8567	
Pancreatitis	27	1	0·8800	0·0447	
Ulcerative Colitis	264	2	0·9026	0·3913	0·7403
Aphthous Ulcers	156	1	1·0370	0·0316	
Gastric Ulcers	1416	10	0·5867	65·5866	59·7173
Bleeding	92	1	0·5277	6·9856	
Not bleeding	269	1	0·8086	1·5198	
Bleeding/not bleeding	*92/269*	*1*	*0·6527*	*2·6568*	
Stomal Ulcers	311	3	0·3493	64·9569	2·8443
Duodenal Ulcers	5635	15	0·5668	222·4635	26·3675
Bleeding	323	3	0·5066	29·1417	0·4903
Not bleeding	1133	3	0·5542	61·1182	5·6362
Bleeding/not bleeding	*323/1133*	*3*	*0·9290*	*0·2987*	*3·7208*
Both Duodenal and Gastric Ulcers Present	52	1	0·7316	0·8857	
Peptic Ulcers, Site Unspecified	81	1	1·3065	0·9984	
DISEASES OF THE GENITO-URINARY SYSTEM					
Nephritis-Nephrosis	69	1	1·4390	1·2663	
Menopausal Metrorrhagia	170	1	1·8042	5·3459	
DISEASES OF THE SKIN					
Vitiligo	323	2	1·0167	0·0113	8·7804
CONGENITAL ANOMALIES					
Hydrocephalus	138	1	0·7972	1·2821	
Congenital Heart Disease	116	1	0·9521	0·0474	
Pyloric Stenosis	753	2	1·2904	5·0892	0·0254
Down's Syndrome	656	3	0·9459	0·3076	5·5387
ALLERGIES					
Asthma	250	1	1·0438	0·0643	
Asthma and/or Hay Fever	404	1	0·8141	1·3765	
Asthma or Hay Fever, Present/Absent	*789/2355*	*1*	*1·2089*	*3·6855*	

TABLE 5A
THE PLASMA HAPTOGLOBIN SYSTEM

	Hp2-2/Hp1-1 + Hp2-1					Hp0/Hp1-1 + Hp2-1 + Hp2-2				
	Number of patients	Number of studies (N)	Combined incidence	χ^2_1 for difference from unity	χ^2_{N-1} for homogeneity of areas	Number of patients	Number of studies (N)	Combined incidence	χ^2_1 for difference from unity	χ^2_{N-1} for homogeneity of areas
INFECTIVE AND PARASITIC DISEASES										
BACTERIAL INFECTIONS										
TUBERCULOSIS										
Pulmonary	2035	2	1·0929	2·1517	6·6381					
Of bones and joints	519	1	1·3017	7·0588						
	2554	3	1·1461	6·9512	8·8974					
SARCOIDOSIS	392	1	0·9933	0·0038						
LEPROSY										
Lepromatous	443	2	1·2486	2·2968	1·1109	133	1	0·8141	0·3536	
Tuberculoid	102	1	1·0784	0·0532		102	1	1·0020	0·0000	
Dimorphous	46	1	0·9552	0·0104		46	1	1·5821	1·1337	
Non-lepromatous	291	1	1·0615	0·1266						
Unspecified types	1060	4	0·7221	8·4666	6·3705	511	2	0·3077	4·0764	0·0972
	1942	9	0·9299	0·9250	17·5100	792	5	0·8957	0·2965	5·3644
VIRAL INFECTIONS										
POLIOMYELITIS	161	1	1·7350	11·6861						
INFECTIOUS HEPATITIS	162	1	0·8535	0·8731						
NEOPLASMS										
MALIGNANT NEOPLASMS										
OESOPHAGUS	16	1	0·2527	3·3014						
STOMACH	43	2	1·3735	1·0311	0·2610					
CAECUM, COLON, RECTUM	52	1	1·1431	0·1992						
BRONCHUS	21	1	0·5273	1·5029						
LUNG	28	1	1·1444	0·1200						
BREAST	144	1	1·1056	0·2585						
CERVIX UTERI	299	3	1·0587	0·1916	3·9361					
CORPUS UTERI	140	1	0·9416	0·1020						
OVARIES	50	1	1·1433	0·2068						
VULVA	14	1	0·8084	0·1428						
MELANOMAS	247	2	1·0068	0·0021	2·4146					
OTHER THAN OESOPHAGUS, STOMACH, LUNG	43	1	0·6846	1·2224						
SITE UNSPECIFIED	25	1	0·7011	0·6780						
NEOPLASMS OF LYMPHATIC AND HAEMOTOPOIETIC TISSUE										
RETICULOSES	36	1	0·8436	0·2139						
MYELOID LEUKAEMIA, ACUTE	25	2	0·5268	1·8661	0·1857					
MYELOID LEUKAEMIA, CHRONIC	34	2	0·4219	4·0510						
	59	4	0·4667	5·7953	0·3359					
LYMPHATIC LEUKAEMIA, ACUTE	36	1	0·2627	8·0796						
LYMPHATIC LEUKAEMIA, CHRONIC	10	1	0·6429	0·3174						
	46	2	0·3330	7·4342	0·9628					
BENIGN NEOPLASMS	41	1	2·1034	5·3891						

TABULAR SUMMARIES. TABLE 5A **THE PLASMA HAPTOGLOBIN SYSTEM** (*cont.*)

	Hp2-2/Hp1-1+Hp2-1					Hp0/Hp1-1+Hp2-1+Hp2-2				
	Number of patients	Number of studies (N)	Combined incidence	χ_1^2 for difference from unity	χ_{N-1}^2 for homogeneity of areas	Number of patients	Number of studies (N)	Combined incidence	χ_1^2 for difference from unity	χ_{N-1}^2 for homogeneity of areas
ENDOCRINE AND METABOLIC DISEASES										
Diabetes Mellitus	314	2	1·1920	1·7677	1·8435					
Phenylketonuria	68	1	1·7023	2·6853						
Cystic Fibrosis of Pancreas	75	1	1·0147	0·0020						
MENTAL DISORDERS										
Schizophrenia	263	2	1·2256	1·4334	1·1133					
Manic-depressive Psychoses	25	1	1·2442	0·2796						
Psychopathy	109	1	0·9204	0·1510						
Oligophrenia	30	1	0·7998	0·3063						
DISEASES OF THE NERVOUS SYSTEM										
Multiple Sclerosis	1019	3	0·9391	0·6765	5·1424					
Epilepsy	477	2	1·3156	3·2435	0·3910					
Kuru	73	1	1·2063	0·2154						
DISEASES OF THE CIRCULATORY SYSTEM										
Rheumatic Fever	405	1	1·1032	0·4673		405	1	10·2785	4·9123	
Hypertension	383	1	1·1265	0·7995						
Cardiac Infarction	458	1	1·2424	3·2175						
Cerebral Sclerosis	298	1	1·1273	0·8264						
DISEASES OF THE DIGESTIVE SYSTEM										
Cholelithiasis	101	1	1·2875	1·3549						
Ulcerative Colitis	26	1	1·6875	1·6715						
Gastric Ulcer	99	1	1·2750	1·2283						
DISEASES OF THE GENITO-URINARY SYSTEM										
Menopausal Metrorrhagia	169	1	0·9324	0·1607						
DISEASES OF THE SKIN										
Neurodermatitis	64	1	1·6959	4·0785						
Lupus Erythematosus	121	1	0·6876	3·2912						
Psoriasis	858	4	1·1109	1·6894	5·7996					
DISEASES OF THE MUSCULOSKELETAL SYSTEM										
Rheumatoid Arthritis	200	2	1·2314	1·8632	1·5582					
CONGENITAL ANOMALIES										
Down's Syndrome	179	2	0·9842	0·0067	0·0030	100	1	2·0155	0·9576	

TABLE 6A
THE PHENYLTHIOCARBAMIDE TASTING SYSTEM

	Tasters/non tasters				
	Number of patients	Number of studies (N)	Combined incidence	χ^2_1 for difference from unity	χ^2_{N-1} for homogeneity of areas
INFECTIVE AND PARASITIC DISEASES					
BACTERIAL INFECTIONS					
TUBERCULOSIS					
Pulmonary	156	2	1·0092	0·0021	0·1869
Site unspecified	624	2	1·9673	15·7635	17·4108
LEPROSY					
Lepromatous	1458	6	1·3400	14·3847	2·1127
Mainly lepromatous	900	2	1·3380	8·5370	0·0236
Tuberculoid	517	6	1·4970	10·7948	1·9996
LEPROSY AND TUBERCULOSIS (BOTH PRESENT)	58	1	2·3899	4·5225	
WORM INFESTATIONS					
FILARIASIS	261	2	1·2822	0·8863	0·8435
MALIGNANT NEOPLASMS					
DIGESTIVE TRACT	83	2	1·4634	1·5501	0·1783
LUNG	58	1	1·0029	0·0001	
BREAST	71	1	3·2505	6·0324	
CERVIX UTERI	85	1	3·2422	7·1128	
CORPUS UTERI	142	1	4·7490	14·6691	
OVARIES	50	1	3·8579	4·9291	
PROSTATE	40	1	0·9223	0·0478	
THYROID GLAND	150	2	2·3477	8·7106	0·1775
ENDOCRINE AND METABOLIC DISEASES					
NON-TOXIC GOITRE					
Diffuse	144	3	0·9736	0·0115	1·8059
Nodular	998	12	0·5691	33·4625	31·3653
TOXIC GOITRE					
Diffuse	603	9	1·2913	5·2780	8·9394
Nodular	73	3	0·8251	0·4952	0·0449
Unspecified	624	9	1·1752	0·9786	4·9471
NODULAR GOITRE	253	3	0·6051	8·7790	0·8479
DIFFUSE GOITRE	412	3	1·2573	1·3946	3·5711
ENDEMIC GOITRE	1085	8	0·9126	0·9509	7·7101
HYPOTHYROIDISM	1181	12	0·7377	6·5269	20·9177
DIABETES MELLITUS	1638	10	0·7709	10·3328	29·4495
CYSTIC FIBROSIS	54	1	0·3846	10·1662	
DISEASES OF THE BLOOD					
PERNICIOUS ANAEMIA	261	1	1·2660	1·3641	
MENTAL DISORDERS					
SCHIZOPHRENIA	55	1	0·3937	6·7214	
OTHER THAN SCHIZOPHRENIA	84	1	0·4706	5·4123	
UNSPECIFIED	205	1	0·9869	0·0212	

TABULAR SUMMARIES. TABLE 6A **THE PHENYLTHIOCARBAMIDE TASTING SYSTEM** (*cont.*)

	Tasters/non tasters				
	Number of patients	Number of studies (N)	Combined incidence	χ_1^2 for difference from unity	χ_{N-1}^2 for homogeneity of areas
DISEASES OF THE NERVOUS SYSTEM AND SENSE ORGANS					
Glaucoma					
Primary, open-angle	746	7	0·5256	46·5316	19·3339
Primary, angle-closure	298	6	1·4657	5·1839	4·4285
Secondary	185	5	0·9106	0·2588	0·6507
Buphthalmos	51	1	5·0857	4·9826	
Keratoconus	105	1	0·5190	7·5263	
DISEASES OF THE GENITO-URINARY SYSTEM					
Hyperplasia of Prostate	48	1	1·1768	0·2051	
Menopausal Metrorrhagia	170	1	2·3701	8·8449	
DISEASES OF THE SKIN					
Psoriasis	76	1	1·1478	0·1588	

APPENDIX

ASSOCIATIONS BETWEEN HLA AND DISEASE

REPORT FROM THE HLA AND DISEASE REGISTRY OF COPENHAGEN, 1976

LARS P. RYDER *and* ARNE SVEJGAARD
with the assistance of
ELLY ANDERSEN *and* ELISABETH SCHACHT

The HLA and Disease Registry of Copenhagen (sponsored by WHO),
Tissue-typing Laboratory of the Blood-Grouping Department,
State University Hospital (Rigshospitalet) of Copenhagen,
Blegdamsvej 9, DK-2100, Copenhagen Ø, Denmark

First published by the authors, Copenhagen, 1976

INTRODUCTION

THE Registry on HLA and Disease in Copenhagen was started in 1972–3 when it became clear that many different groups all over the world were going to put considerable efforts in studying HLA in a variety of diseases. It was anticipated that if steps were not taken to facilitate and speed up the information between groups on a world-wide basis, a considerable amount of unnecessary duplication of work would be done. Moreover, it was feared that the tendency primarily to publish positive findings might give a distorted picture of the true situation. Accordingly, it was decided to establish at least one international registry which should attempt to collect all published data on such studies and to which investigators could send as yet unpublished data. Naturally, the Registry is prepared on request to inform colleagues as to the present state of association(s) for a given disease. At intervals, the Registry should publish the essence of the data in the Registry.

This, then, is the first report from the Registry, and it has been prepared in connection with the First International Symposium on HLA and Disease, held in Paris, June 1976. We are greatly indebted to our colleagues from all over the world for submitting data to us and for the many contacts which the journal *Tissue Antigens* has enabled us to establish. The Registry could not have been established and run without grants from the Danish Medical Research Council, the Danish Blood Donor Foundation, the Danish Rheumatoid Association, and, most recently, from WHO.

ASCERTAINMENT AND TREATMENT OF DATA IN THIS REPORT

The bulk of the material in the Registry has been obtained from the international literature and has been ascertained both through screening of common international journals, Current Contents, and as pre- or reprints sent to us. A minor part of the data has been submitted to the Registry without being published by the investigators. However, most of the data submitted has later been published. It has been the general policy of the Registry to advocate publication by the investigators because the Registry may not be known to all colleagues all over the world, and new and original observations should, of course, always be published as soon as possible.

In this report, we have dealt only with association data in *unrelated patients*. Although some family data are available both in the literature and in the Registry, we have not had the time to analyze them in detail. Only the frequencies of *HLA-A and B antigens* have been treated systematically because very few data on C and D antigens have been reported. Combined calculations have been done only on Caucasians (in fact only Europeans or American, Australian, and New Zealand Whites) because there are not enough data on other ethnic groups to allow combinations. We are well aware that even Caucasians are not a homogeneous group in terms of HLA, other genes, or environment, but we have not been able to make too many subdivisions. Mixed populations (e.g. patient groups consisting of both American Blacks and Whites) have not been included when it has not been indicated how the antigen frequencies were in the two groups. Nevertheless, non-Caucasian data are quoted in the report: they are clearly of the greatest interest.

We have attempted to include all data known to us at about April 1976, and in some cases we have included more recent data. We cannot be sure to know all published data, and we hope that colleagues will contact us during the congress if they fail to find their material.

Rather often, the same data have been published more than once, and we have then used the reference giving the most detailed information (in terms of HLA) which is not necessarily the original or first publication of the investigators: we have tried to be complete, rather than historical, and we wish to apologize when the first and original observations are not in the list of references.

Very often, different groups have used different *diagnostic criteria*, which has caused quite a bit of trouble. Whenever possible we have attempted to take such differences into account, but mostly we have found it impossible and have ended up by pooling all available data; thus, there are bound to be some differences between the various sources of data, and occasionally, such differences betray themselves by significant heterogeneities (cf. below).

Various investigators have not used the same criteria for *subdividing* patients suffering from a given disease; for example, diabetes mellitus has been subdivided both according to age-at-onset and to insulin dependency, and for the need of simplicity, we have been forced to distinguish between juvenile and/or insulin-dependent diabetes on the one hand and maturity onset on the other.

In a few cases we have had to omit data because control data were not given. In other cases the number of controls have not been indicated which is invalidating for the calculations of statistical significance. Whenever possible we have in such situations used control data previously published by the same group. Not infrequently, the exact antigen frequencies (per cent) given in the papers cannot be obtained from the total number of patients studied without assuming some patients only being 'half positive'. In these cases we have used the nearest integer as the number of positive patients.

Another problem has been the continuous 'splitting' of antigens (e.g. HLA-A10 to Aw25 and Aw26). When the authors have given data for both the supertypic, say HLA-A10, and the subtypic, Aw25 and Aw26 antigens, we have included data for all three, but the supertypic antigen has not been used when only the subtypic was given. The HLA-Aw19 complex has been particularly difficult, but again we have followed the above rules.

Calculations have been done according to the method of Woolf as modified by Haldane (for details, see Ryder and Svejgaard, 'Histocompatibility Associated Disease', in *T and B Lymphocytes in Immune Responses*, eds. F. Loor and G. E. Roelants (in press), and Svejgaard *et al.*, 'HL-A Antigens and Disease. Statistical and Genetical Considerations', *Tissue Antigens*, **4**, 95, 1974). The cross-product ratio of the four entries of a 2×2 table is an estimate of the *relative risk* which is the risk of developing a disease when an antigen is present in an individual relative to the risk when it is lacking. This only holds for diseases of low frequency in the population, and, thus, for all diseases studied so far. A relative risk higher than one is seen when an antigen is more frequent (positive association) in the patients than in the controls, whereas risks below unity reflects decreased frequencies (negative association) in the patients. Combined estimates of relative risks can be made from different sources of data (i.e. different 2×2 tables for a given antigen) by special formula. A more accurate estimate of the relative risk is thus obtained, and it becomes easier to evaluate the statistical significance.

The *statistical significance* is usually obtained as a chi square value which can be 'divided' in two parts: (i) one is a chi square with one degree of freedom (d.f.) and estimates the significance for the relative risk being different from one (i.e. that there is an association); (ii) the other chi square has n-1 d.f. (n being the number of studies) and concerns the possibility that there may be significant *heterogeneity* between the n risks obtained in the individual studies. Significant heterogeneity may reflect, e.g. the use of different diagnostic criteria, different definitions of the antigen, or it may, of course, reflect true differences in the risks which again could be due to differences in other genetic or in environmental factors.

Explanations for tables

The diseases are given under the following groups: rheumatology, neurology, dermatology, endocrinology, gastroenterology, allergology, immunopathology, malignant diseases, and other diseases in that order. Allocation of a disease to a certain group is not always completely logical (e.g. rheumatic heart disease to rheumatology).

For each disease (indicated by an extended WHO code number, and the name) data are given for the antigens which showed significant associations and/or significant heterogeneity (P-values less than 4×10^{-4} in the combined calculations estimated from chi square values; this is an arbitrary limit taking into account the number of antigens studied). Occasionally, other 'interesting' antigens are also given. The HLA-A antigens are given first and then the B antigens. If not otherwise indicated, the data concern Caucasians. Below, an example is given.

(1) HLA	(2) Ref. No.	(3) Pos.	(4) Ptt. (%)	(5) Total	(6) Pos.	(7) Ctr. (%)	(8) Total	(9) Rel. risk X (Haldane)
Disease WHO Code: 712.490		**Ankylosing spondylitis**						
HLA-A2	1	33	(62·3)	53	78	(51·3)	152	1·55
	2	51	(68·0)	75	43	(57·3)	75	1·57
	5	24	(60·0)	40	435	(48·0)	906	1·61
	6	14	(53·8)	26	199	(50·0)	398	1·16
	7	32	(64·0)	50	159	(53·9)	295	1·50
	8	8	(47·1)	17	285	(47·7)	597	0·98
	10	48	(60·0)	80	203	(50·8)	400	1·45
	11	42	(67·7)	62	491	(49·1)	1000	2·15
	13	29	(61·7)	47	147	(48·0)	306	1·72
	15	17	(48·6)	35	124	(47·0)	264	1·07
	16	32	(64·0)	50	240	(50·2)	478	1·74
	17	18	(66·7)	27	281	(52·0)	540	1·80
(10) Combined:		(P = 3·0E-06)		562			5411	1·55
(11) 95% confidence interval:								(1·29:1·86)
(12) Heterogeneity: (P > 0·05)								

(1) = HLA antigen.
(2) = Reference number for the disease in question. The references are given immediately below the disease; to save space, only the first author and the data of the journal is given.
(3) = Number of patients carrying the antigen in the corresponding study.
(4) = Percentage of patients carrying the antigen.
(5) = Total number of patients studied.
(6), (7), and (8) = (3), (4), and (5), but for the controls.
(9) = The relative risk in the corresponding study.
(10) = 'Combined': the P-value for the statistical significance of the association, total numbers of patients and controls, combined estimate of relative risk (in column (9)). When only one study is given, Fisher's exact P-value for the association is given in this place.
P-values are given in floating-point notation; e.g. P = 3·0E-06 means $P = 3{\cdot}0 \times 10^{-6}$. No P-values have been multiplied with the number of comparisons.
(11) = Estimated 95 per cent confidence limits for the combined relative risk.
(12) = Statistical significance of the heterogeneity between the relative risk of the individual studies.

RHEUMATOLOGY

HLA	Ref. No.	Pos.	Ptt. (%)	Total	Pos.	Ctr. (%)	Total	Rel. risk X (Haldane)
Disease WHO Code: 712.490		**Ankylosing spondylitis**						
HLA-A2	1	33	(62·3)	53	78	(51·3)	152	1·55
	2	51	(68·0)	75	43	(57·3)	75	1·57
	5	24	(60·0)	40	435	(48·0)	906	1·61
	6	14	(53·8)	26	199	(50·0)	398	1·16
	7	32	(64·0)	50	159	(53·9)	295	1·50
	8	8	(47·1)	17	285	(47·7)	597	0·98
	10	48	(60·0)	80	203	(50·8)	400	1·45
	11	42	(67·7)	62	491	(49·1)	1000	2·15
	13	29	(61·7)	47	147	(48·0)	306	1·72
	15	17	(48·6)	35	124	(47·0)	264	1·07
	16	32	(64·0)	50	240	(50·2)	478	1·74
	17	18	(66·7)	27	281	(52·0)	540	1·80
Combined:		(P = 3·0E-06)		562			5411	1·55
95% confidence interval:								(1·29:1·86)
Heterogeneity: (P > 0·05)								

HLA	Ref. No.	Pos.	Ptt. (%)	Total	Pos.	Ctr. (%)	Total	Rel. risk X (Haldane)
HLA-B7	1	4	(7·5)	53	32	(21·1)	152	0·34
	2	13	(17·3)	75	18	(24·0)	75	0·67
	5	1	(2·5)	40	227	(25·1)	906	0·11
	6	0	(0·0)	26	12	(3·0)	398	0·58
	7	6	(12·0)	50	74	(25·1)	295	0·43
	8	2	(11·8)	17	177	(29·6)	597	0·38
	10	9	(11·3)	80	109	(27·3)	400	0·35
	11	20	(32·3)	62	187	(18·7)	1000	2·09
	13	3	(6·4)	47	70	(22·9)	306	0·26
	15	2	(5·7)	35	42	(15·9)	264	0·39
	16	5	(10·0)	50	115	(24·1)	478	0·38
	17	4	(14·8)	27	130	(24·1)	540	0·60
Combined:		(P = 4·4E–05)		562			5411	0·58
95% confidence interval:								(0·45:0·75)
Heterogeneity: (P = 3·9E–04)								
HLA-B8	1	6	(11·3)	53	17	(11·2)	152	1·06
	2	8	(10·7)	75	21	(28·0)	75	0·32
	5	6	(15·0)	40	190	(21·0)	906	0·71
	6	0	(0·0)	26	12	(3·0)	398	0·58
	7	6	(12·0)	50	60	(20·3)	295	0·57
	8	5	(29·4)	17	186	(31·2)	597	0·97
	10	8	(10·0)	80	88	(22·0)	400	0·41
	11	7	(11·3)	62	141	(14·1)	1000	0·82
	13	8	(17·0)	47	71	(23·2)	306	0·71
	15	2	(5·7)	35	43	(16·3)	264	0·38
	16	3	(6·0)	50	77	(16·1)	478	0·38
	17	0	(0·0)	27	92	(17·0)	540	0·09
Combined:		(P = 5·3E–05)		562			5411	0·57
95% confidence interval:								(0·44:0·75)
Heterogeneity: (P > 0·05)								
HLA-B27	1	43	(81·1)	53	6	(3·9)	152	93·37
	2	72	(96·0)	75	3	(4·0)	75	429·08
	3	28	(90·3)	31	17	(8·5)	200	85·38
	4	74	(86·0)	86	61	(8·0)	764	68·18
	5	35	(87·5)	40	72	(7·9)	906	74·29
	6	20	(76·9)	26	20	(5·0)	398	58·23
	7	45	(90·0)	50	27	(9·2)	295	80·77
	8	14	(82·4)	17	53	(8·9)	597	42·16
	9	63	(94·0)	67	17	(9·8)	174	127·00
	11	60	(96·8)	62	67	(6·7)	1000	334·68
	12	35	(100·0)	35	11	(12·4)	89	484·65
	13	43	(91·5)	47	24	(7·8)	306	111·46
	14	106	(84·1)	126	12	(12·0)	100	36·78
	15	32	(91·4)	35	23	(8·7)	264	95·43
	16	47	(94·0)	50	45	(9·4)	478	129·30
	17	26	(96·3)	27	49	(9·1)	540	175·42
Combined:		(P < 1·0E–10)		827			6338	87·78
95% confidence interval:								(68·20:112·99)
Heterogeneity: (P > 0·05)								

ANKYLOSING SPONDYLITIS (HAIDA INDIANS—BRITISH COLUMBIA)

HLA	Ref. No.	Pos.	Ptt. (%)	Total	Pos.	Ctr. (%)	Total	Rel. risk X (Haldane)
HLA-B27	50	17	(100·0)	17	112	(50·5)	222	34·38
Fisher: P = 1·7E–05								

ANKYLOSING SPONDYLITIS (BELLA COOLA INDIANS—BRITISH COLUMBIA)

HLA	Ref. No.	Pos.	Ptt. (%)	Total	Pos.	Ctr. (%)	Total	Rel. risk X (Haldane)
HLA-B27	50	3	(100·0)	3	33	(25·6)	129	20·16
Fisher: P = 1·9E–02								

ANKYLOSING SPONDYLITIS (JAPANESE)

HLA	Ref. No.	Pos.	Ptt. (%)	Total	Pos.	Ctr. (%)	Total	Rel. risk X (Haldane)
HLA-B27	51	18	(66·7)	27	0	(0·0)	78	305·74
Fisher: P = 1·0E–10								

References

1. Amor, *Nouv. Pres. Med.* **3,** 1373, 1974.
2. Brewerton, *Lancet*, **ii,** 904, 1973.
3. Deuxchaisnes, *Lancet*, **ii,** 1238, 1974.
4. Keuning, quoted in Ceppellini and Rood, *Seminars in Hematology*, **11,** 233, 1974.
5. Schlosstein, *New Engl. J. Med.* **288,** 704, 1973.

6. Marcolongo, *Nouv. Pres. Med.* **3,** 2023, 1974.
7. Russell, *J. Rheum.* **1,** 203, 1974.
8. Dick, *Tissue Antigens*, **5,** 26, 1975.
9. Sachs, *Tissue Antigens*, **5,** 120, 1975.
10. Rood, *Trpl. Rev.* **22,** 75, 1975.
11. Veys, *Tissue Antigens*, 1976, in press.
12. Calin, *Lancet*, **i,** 874, 1974.
13. Cross, *Aust. N.Z. J. Med.* **5,** 108, 1975.
14. Möller, *Histocompatibility Testing*, 1975.
15. Sany, *Rev. Rheum.* **42,** 451, 1975.
16. Truog, *Histocompatibility Testing*, 788, 1975.
17. Mills, *JAMA*, **231,** 268, 1975.
50. Gofton, *J. Rheum.* **2,** 314, 1975.
51. Sonozaki, *Tissue Antigens*, **5,** 131, 1975.

HLA	Ref. No.	Pos.	Ptt. (%)	Total	Pos.	Ctr. (%)	Total	Rel. risk X (Haldane)
Disease WHO code: 136.010	**Reiter's syndrome**							
HLA-B27	1	56	(91·8)	61	46	(14·1)	326	61·97
	2	37	(80·4)	46	6	(3·9)	152	88·97
	3	47	(74·6)	63	2	(6·1)	33	36·27
	4	6	(100·0)	6	24	(7·8)	306	149·90
	5	23	(95·8)	24	149	(8·0)	1863	179·67
	6	34	(68·0)	50	15	(7·7)	194	24·21
	7	31	(64·6)	48	172	(8·2)	2103	20·15
	8	17	(73·9)	23	49	(9·1)	540	26·73
Combined:		(P < 1·0E–10)		321			5517	35·89
95% confidence interval:								(25·77:49·98)
Heterogeneity: (P = 2·7E–02)								

References

1. Aho, *Arthr. & Rheum.* **17,** 521, 1974 and *Rheum. Dis.* **34,** suppl. 29, 1975.
2. Amor, *Nouv. Pres. Med.* **3,** 1373, 1974.
3. Brewerton, *Sem. in Arthr. and Rheum.* **4,** 191, 1975.
4. Cross, *Aust. N.Z. J. Med.* **5,** 108, 1975.
5. Morris, *New Engl. J. Med.* **290a,** 554, 1974.
6. Woodrow, *Tissue Antigens*, **4,** 533, 1974.
7. Zachariae, *Scand. J. Rheum.* **4,** 13, 1975.
8. Mills, *JAMA*, **231,** 268, 1975.

HLA	Ref. No.	Pos.	Ptt. (%)	Total	Pos.	Ctr. (%)	Total	Rel. risk X (Haldane)
Disease WHO code: 714.991	**Yersinia arthritis**							
HLA-A2	1	44	(89·8)	49	179	(54·9)	326	6·65
	2	12	(63·2)	19	1055	(53·6)	1967	1·44
Combined:		(P = 3·6E–04)		68			2293	3·11
95% confidence interval:								(1·67:5·81)
Heterogeneity: (P = 1·6E–02)								
HLA-B27	1	43	(87·8)	49	46	(14·1)	326	40·37
	2	11	(57·9)	19	170	(8·6)	1967	14·26
Combined:		(P < 1·0E–10)		68			2293	24·33
95% confidence interval:								(13·18:44·90)
Heterogeneity: (P > 0·05)								

References

1. Aho, *Arthr. & Rheum.* **17,** 521, 1974.
2. Copenhagen material (in the Registry).

HLA	Ref. No.	Pos.	Ptt. (%)	Total	Pos.	Ctr. (%)	Total	Rel. risk X (Haldane)
Disease WHO code: 714.992	**Salmonella arthritis**							
HLA-B27	1	3	(60·0)	5	125	(8·1)	1541	15·80
	2	9	(69·2)	13	45	(10·1)	446	18·63
Combined:		(P = 3·6E–10)		18			1987	17·57
95% confidence interval:								(7·17:43·10)
Heterogeneity: (P > 0·05)								

References

1. Friis, *Lancet*, **ii,** 1350, 1974.
2. Håkansson, *Tissue Antigens*, **6,** 366, 1975.

HLA	Ref. No.	Pos.	Ptt. (%)	Total	Pos.	Ctr. (%)	Total	Rel. risk X (Haldane)
Disease WHO code: 696.091		**Psoriasis arthropathica—Peripheral**						
HLA-B13	2	4	(9·1)	44	8	(5·3)	152	1·89
	3	2	(11·8)	17	25	(7·7)	326	1·91
	4	1	(5·9)	17	10	(3·9)	254	2·12
	5	5	(11·6)	43	12	(4·5)	264	2·89
Combined:		(P = 9·5E–03)		121			996	2·23
95% confidence interval:								(1·22:4·10)
Heterogeneity: (P > 0·05)								
HLA-B27	1	11	(23·4)	47	3	(4·0)	75	6·53
	2	3	(6·8)	44	6	(3·9)	152	1·90
	3	4	(23·5)	17	46	(14·1)	326	2·01
	4	3	(17·6)	17	15	(5·9)	254	3·73
	5	5	(11·6)	43	23	(8·7)	264	1·47
Combined:		(P = 3·5E–04)		168			1071	2·50
95% confidence interval:								(1·51:4·13)
Heterogeneity: (P > 0·05)								
HLA-Bw17	2	10	(22·7)	44	9	(5·9)	152	4·60
	3	1	(5·9)	17	12	(3·7)	326	2·29
	4	6	(35·3)	17	23	(9·1)	254	5·57
	5	13	(30·2)	43	11	(4·2)	264	9·76
Combined:		(P < 1·0E–10)		121			996	5·84
95% confidence interval:								(3·51:9·70)
Heterogeneity: (P > 0·05)								
HLA-Bw38	2	8	(18·2)	44	5	(3·3)	152	6·25
	5	3	(7·0)	43	7	(2·7)	264	2·97
Combined:		(P = 3·2E–04)		87			416	4·52
95% confidence interval:								(1·99:10·27)
Heterogeneity: (P > 0·05)								

References

1. Brewerton, *Sem. in Arthr. & Rheum.* **4**, 191, 1975.
2. Feldmann, *Nouv. Pres. Med.* **5,** 477, 1976.
3. Karvonen, *Ann. Clin. Res.* **7,** 112, 1975.
4. Metzger, *Arthr. & Rheum.* **18,** 111, 1976.
5. Sany, *Rev. Rheum.* **42,** 451, 1975.

HLA	Ref. No.	Pos.	Ptt. (%)	Total	Pos.	Ctr. (%)	Total	Rel. risk X (Haldane)
Disease WHO code: 696.092		**Psoriasis arthropathica—Central**						
HLA-B13	2	5	(19·2)	26	8	(5·3)	152	4·35
	3	7	(36·8)	19	25	(7·7)	326	7·09
	4	2	(8·7)	23	10	(3·9)	254	2·71
	5	3	(16·7)	18	12	(4·5)	264	4·56
Combined:		(P = 7·6E–08)		86			996	4·79
95% confidence interval:								(2·70:8·47)
Heterogeneity: (P > 0·05)								
HLA-B27	1	4	(36·4)	11	3	(4·0)	75	12·43
	2	13	(50·0)	26	6	(3·9)	152	22·54
	3	11	(57·9)	19	46	(14·1)	326	8·16
	4	8	(34·8)	23	15	(5·9)	254	8·47
	5	3	(16·7)	18	23	(8·7)	264	2·32
Combined:		(P < 1·0E–10)		97			1071	8·58
95% confidence interval:								(5·31:13·88)
Heterogeneity: (P > 0·05)								

HLA	Ref. No.	Pos.	Ptt. (%)	Total	Pos.	Ctr. (%)	Total	Rel. risk X (Haldane)
Psoriasis arthropathica—Central (*cont.*):								
HLA-Bw17	2	3	(11·5)	26	9	(5·9)	152	2·25
	3	2	(10·5)	19	12	(3·7)	326	3·59
	4	3	(13·0)	23	23	(9·1)	254	1·68
	5	2	(11·1)	18	11	(4·2)	264	3·34
Combined:		(P = 4·6E–03)		86			996	2·49
95% confidence interval:								(1·32:4·68)
Heterogeneity: (P > 0·05)								
HLA-Bw38	2	7	(26·9)	26	5	(3·3)	152	10·31
	5	3	(16·7)	18	7	(2·7)	264	7·75
Combined:		(P = 5·6E–07)		44			416	9·09
95% confidence interval:								(3·83:21·60)
Heterogeneity: (P > 0·05)								

References

1. Brewerton, *Sem. in Arthr. & Rheum.* **4,** 191, 1975.
2. Feldmann, *Nouv. Pres. Med.* **5,** 477, 1976.
3. Karvonen, *Ann. Clin. Res.* **7,** 112, 1975.
4. Metzger, *Arthr. & Rheum.* **18,** 111, 1976.
5. Sany, *Rev. Rheum.* **42,** 451, 1975.

HLA	Ref. No.	Pos.	Ptt. (%)	Total	Pos.	Ctr. (%)	Total	Rel. risk X (Haldane)
Disease WHO code: 696.093		**Psoriasis arthropathica—Unspecified**						
HLA-B27	1	13	(29·5)	44	172	(8·2)	2103	4·80
	2	10	(90·9)	11	3	(4·0)	75	145·00
Combined:		(P = 2·5E–10)		55			2178	7·06
95% confidence interval:								(3·84:12·98)
Heterogeneity: (P = 5·2E–04)								
HLA-Bw17	1	11	(25·0)	44	170	(8·1)	2103	3·89
Fisher: P = 7·3E–04								

References

1. Zachariae, *Acta Dermatovener* (Stockholm), **54,** 443, 1974.
2. Brewerton, *Sem. in Arthr. & Rheum.* **4,** 191, 1975.

HLA	Ref. No.	Pos.	Ptt. (%)	Total	Pos.	Ctr. (%)	Total	Rel. risk X (Haldane)
Disease WHO code: 712.090		**Juvenile arthritis**						
HLA-A2	1	73	(59·3)	123	53	(42·4)	125	1·97
	2	40	(60·6)	66	143	(47·7)	300	1·68
	4	17	(65·4)	26	125	(46·8)	267	2·09
	5	16	(66·7)	24	285	(47·7)	597	2·12
	7	22	(62·9)	35	491	(49·1)	1000	1·73
Combined:		(P = 1·2E–05)		274			2289	1·87
95% confidence interval:								(1·41:2·48)
Heterogeneity: (P > 0·05)								
HLA-B27	1	18	(14·6)	123	8	(6·4)	125	2·42
	2	16	(24·2)	66	30	(10·0)	300	2·90
	3	8	(17·0)	47	46	(14·1)	326	1·30
	4	11	(42·3)	26	16	(6·0)	267	11·31
	5	7	(29·2)	24	53	(8·9)	597	4·36
	6	19	(35·2)	54	28	(8·9)	314	5·52
	7	20	(57·1)	35	67	(6·7)	1000	18·29
Combined:		(P < 1·0E–10)		375			2929	4·72
95% confidence interval:								(3·54:6·28)
Heterogeneity: (P = 8·9E–06)								

References

1. Gibson, *New Engl. J. Med.* **293,** 636, 1975.
2. Hall, *Ann. Rheum. Dis.* **34** suppl., 36, 1975.
3. Nissilä, *New Engl. J. Med.* **292,** 430, 1975.
4. Rachelefsky, *New Engl. J. Med.* **290,** 892, 1974.
5. Sturrock, *J. Rheum.* **1,** 269, 1974.
6. Buc, *Tissue Antigens*, **4,** 395, 1974.
7. Veys, *Tissue Antigens*, 1976, in press.

HLA	Ref. No.	Pos.	Ptt. (%)	Total	Pos.	Ctr. (%)	Total	Rel. risk X (Haldane)
Disease WHO code: 712.390		**Rheumatoid arthritis**						
HLA-A9	1	12	(11·5)	104	27	(26·5)	102	0·37
	2	11	(17·7)	62	17	(14·8)	115	1·26
	3	8	(15·4)	52	76	(19·1)	398	0·81
	4	10	(25·0)	40	37	(18·5)	200	1·50
	5	24	(20·2)	119	199	(22·0)	906	0·91
	6	17	(17·0)	100	69	(27·2)	254	0·56
	7	12	(26·7)	45	26	(8·0)	326	4·23
Combined:		(P = 6·8E–01)		522			2301	0·95
95% confidence interval:								(0·74:1·22)
Heterogeneity: (P = 1·5E–04)								
HLA-B27	1	10	(9·6)	104	6	(5·9)	102	1·65
	3	2	(3·8)	52	20	(5·0)	398	0·91
	4	7	(17·5)	40	19	(9·5)	200	2·08
	5	10	(8·4)	119	72	(7·9)	906	1·10
	6	12	(12·0)	100	24	(9·4)	254	1·33
	7	22	(48·9)	45	46	(14·1)	326	5·78
Combined:		(P = 6·2E–05)		460			2186	1·94
95% confidence interval:								(1·40:2·68)
Heterogeneity: (P = 6·3E–03)								
HLA-Bw21	3	0	(0·0)	52	60	(15·1)	398	0·05
	5	0	(0·0)	119	45	(5·0)	906	0·08
	6	16	(16·0)	100	17	(6·7)	254	2·65
	7	0	(0·0)	45	0	(0·0)	326	7·18
Combined:		(P = 3·2E–01)		316			1884	1·37
95% confidence interval:								(0·74:2·54)
Heterogeneity: (P = 4·6E–05)								

References

1. Brackertz, *Z. Immun. Forsch.* **146,** 108, 1973.
2. Lies, *Arthr. & Rheum.* **15,** 524, 1972.
3. Marcolongo, *Nouv. Pres. Med.* **3,** 2023, 1974.
4. Nyulassy, *Lancet*, **i,** 450, 1974.
5. Schlossstein, *New Engl. J. Med.* **288,** 704, 1973.
6. Seignalet, *J. Med. Montpellier*, in press.
7. Isomäki, *Ann. Clin. Res.* **7,** 138, 1975.

HLA	Ref. No.	Pos.	Ptt. (%)	Total	Pos.	Ctr. (%)	Total	Rel. risk X (Haldane)
Disease WHO code: 366.000		**Acute anterior uveitis**						
HLA-B27	1	58	(58·0)	100	22	(7·3)	300	17·04
	2	50	(55·6)	90	19	(8·2)	233	13·72
Combined:		(P < 1·0E–10)		190			533	15·39
95% confidence interval:								(10·09:23·46)
Heterogeneity: (P > 0·05)								

References

1. Brewerton, *Lancet*, **ii,** 994, 1973 and *Sem. in Arthr. & Rheum.* **4,** 191, 1975.
2. Mapstone, *Brit. J. Ophthal.* **59,** 270, 1975.

ADDITIONAL NOTES ON RHEUMATOLOGIC DISORDERS

Gout

Was not found associated with HLA in 66 patients (Schlossstein *et al.*, *New Eng. J. Med.* **288,** 704, 1973.

Rheumatic fever and/or rheumatic heart disease

No significant associations (75–222 patients studied).

References

Caughey, D., *Jour. Rheum.* **2,** 319, 1975.
Falk, J. A., *Tissue Antigens*, **3,** 173, 1973.
Copenhagen material (in the Registry).
Ward, C. *et al.*, *Tissue Antigens*, in press.

Chronic uveitis

No significant deviations.

Reference

Ehlers, N. *et al.*, *Lancet*, **i**, 99, 1974.

Paget's disease

No significant deviations (46–140 patients studied).

References

Mercier, P. and Seignalet, J., *Tissue Antigens*, in press.
Cullen, P. *et al.*, *Tissue Antigens*, **7**, 55–6, 1976.

Frozen shoulder

Most likely increase of HLA-B27.

Reference

Bulgen, D. Y. *et al.*, *Lancet*, **i**, 1042, 1976.

NEUROLOGY

HLA	Ref. No.	Pos.	Ptt. (%)	Total	Pos.	Ctr. (%)	Total	Rel. risk X (Haldane)
Disease WHO code: 340.000		**Multiple sclerosis**						
HLA-A2	1	14	(43·8)	32	78	(51·3)	152	0·74
	2	93	(44·5)	209	1054	(53·6)	1067	0·70
	3	34	(36·2)	94	447	(51·3)	871	0·54
	4	23	(41·1)	56	49	(49·0)	100	0·73
	5	33	(44·6)	74	330	(44·1)	749	1·02
	6	432	(43·2)	1000	511	(51·1)	1000	0·73
Combined:		(P = 9·7E–07)		1465			4839	0·72
95% confidence interval:								(0·63:0·82)
Heterogeneity: (P > 0·05)								
HLA-A3	1	13	(40·6)	32	36	(23·7)	152	2·21
	2	76	(36·4)	209	529	(26·9)	1967	1·56
	3	38	(40·4)	94	205	(23·5)	871	2·21
	4	24	(42·9)	56	23	(23·0)	100	2·49
	5	13	(17·6)	74	155	(20·7)	749	0·84
	6	358	(35·8)	1000	288	(28·8)	1000	1·38
Combined:		(P = 9·4E–09)		1465			4839	1·51
95% confidence interval:								(1·31:1·73)
Heterogeneity: (P > 0·05)								
HLA-B7	1	9	(28·1)	32	32	(21·1)	152	1·50
	2	83	(39·7)	209	527	(26·8)	1967	1·80
	3	26	(27·7)	94	205	(23·5)	871	1·25
	4	22	(39·3)	56	21	(21·0)	100	2·41
	5	9	(12·2)	74	75	(14·1)	531	0·88
	6	353	(35·3)	1000	260	(26·0)	1000	1·55
Combined:		(P = 7·6E–10)		1465			4621	1·57
95% confidence interval:								(1·36:1·81)
Heterogeneity: (P > 0·05)								
HLA-B12	1	7	(21·9)	32	55	(36·2)	152	0·52
	2	39	(18·7)	209	496	(25·2)	1967	0·69
	3	18	(19·1)	94	199	(22·8)	871	0·82
	4	8	(14·3)	56	19	(19·0)	100	0·73
	5	16	(21·6)	74	92	(17·3)	531	1·34
	6	158	(15·8)	1000	218	(21·8)	1000	0·67
Combined:		(P = 1·3E–04)		1465			4621	0·72
95% confidence interval:								(0·61:0·85)
Heterogeneity: (P > 0·05)								
HLA-Bw15	1	4	(12·5)	32	18	(11·8)	152	1·15
	2	33	(15·8)	209	352	(17·9)	1967	0·87
	3	3	(3·2)	94	71	(8·2)	871	0·43
	4	1	(1·8)	56	2	(2·0)	100	1·06
	6	93	(9·3)	1000	150	(15·0)	1000	0·58
Combined:		(P = 2·5E–04)		1391			4090	0·67
95% confidence interval:								(0·54:0·83)
Heterogeneity: (P > 0·05)								

References

1. Dausset, J. and Hors, J., *Transpl. Rev.* **22,** 44–74, 1975.
2. Jersild, C. *et al.*, *Transpl. Rev.* **22,** 148–63, 1975.
3. Naito, S. *et al.*, *Tissue Antigens*, **2,** 1–4, 1972.
4. Arnason, B. G. *et al.*, *J. Neurol. Sci.* **22,** 419–28, 1974.
5. Smeraldi, E., *Boll. Inst. Sier. Milan*, **51,** 220–3, 1972.
6. Bertrams, J. and Kuwert, E., Thesis, 1974.

HLA	Ref. No.	Pos.	Ptt. (%)	Total	Pos.	Ctr. (%)	Total	Rel. risk X (Haldane)
Disease WHO code: 733.090	**Myasthenia gravis**							
HLA-A1	1	22	(84·6)	26	184	(30·8)	597	11·21
	2	55	(55·0)	100	158	(29·6)	533	2·89
	3	14	(25·0)	56	22	(24·4)	90	1·04
	4	11	(30·6)	36	55	(16·9)	326	2·21
	5	14	(33·3)	42	76	(22·7)	335	1·73
Combined:		(P = 8·7E–10)		260			1881	2·45
95% confidence interval:								(1·84:3·26)
Heterogeneity: (P = 3·2E–03)								
HLA-B7	2	15	(15·0)	100	158	(29·6)	533	0·43
	3	8	(14·3)	56	20	(22·2)	90	0·60
	5	5	(11·9)	42	92	(27·5)	335	0·39
Combined:		(P = 2·1E–04)		198			958	0·45
95% confidence interval:								(0·30:0·69)
Heterogeneity: (P > 0·05)								
HLA-B8	1	17	(65·4)	26	186	(31·2)	597	4·06
	2	59	(59·0)	100	103	(19·3)	533	5·96
	3	21	(37·5)	56	16	(17·8)	90	2·73
	4	17	(48·6)	35	59	(18·1)	326	4·25
	5	20	(47·6)	42	67	(20·0)	335	3·62
Combined:		(P < 1·0E–10)		259			1881	4·40
95% confidence interval:								(3·33:5·82)
Heterogeneity: (P > 0·05)								

References

1. Behan, P. O. *et al.*, *Lancet*, **ii,** 1033, 1973.
2. Berg-Loonen, E. van den *et al.* Submitted to the Registry, 1973/4.
3. Fritze, D. *et al.*, *Lancet*, **i,** 240, 1974.
4. Pirskanen, R. *et al.*, *Ann. Clin. Res.* **4,** 304, 1972.
5. Säfwenberg, J. *et al.*, *Tissue Antigens*, **3,** 465, 1973.

HLA	Ref. No.	Pos.	Ptt. (%)	Total	Pos.	Ctr. (%)	Total	Rel. risk X (Haldane)
Disease WHO code: 41.990	**Paralytic poliomyelitis**							
HLA-B7	1	14	(20·6)	68	32	(21·1)	152	0·99
	2	42	(37·8)	111	75	(19·0)	395	2·60
Combined:		(P = 6·5E–04)		179			547	1·94
95% confidence interval:								(1·32:2·83)
Heterogeneity: (P = 2·2E–02)								

References

1. Dausset, J., *Transpl. Rev.* **22,** 44, 1975.
2. Pietsch, M. C. and Morris, P. J., *Tissue Antigens*, **4,** 50, 1974.

HLA	Ref. No.	Pos.	Ptt. (%)	Total	Pos.	Ctr. (%)	Total	Rel. risk X (Haldane)
Disease WHO code: 295.000	**Schizophrenia**							
HLA-A28	1	28	(18·9)	148	76	(6·3)	1200	3·48
	3	2	(4·3)	47	88	(7·0)	1263	0·73
Combined:		(P = 2·8E–06)		195			2463	2·82
95% confidence interval:								(1·83:4·36)
Heterogeneity: (P = 1·6E–02)								

References

1. Ivanyi, D. *et al.*, *Tissue Antigens*, in press.
2. Smeraldi, E. *et al.*, *Tissue Antigens*, in press.
3. Eberhard, G. *et al.*, *Neuropsychobiol.* **1,** 211, 1975.

HLA	Ref. No.	Pos.	Ptt. (%)	Total	Pos.	Ctr. (%)	Total	Rel. risk X (Haldane)
Disease WHO code: 296.000		**Manio-depression**						
HLA-Bw16	1	6	(11·8)	51	26	(4·6)	562	2·89
	2	12	(13·0)	92	106	(5·4)	1967	2·71
Combined:		(P = 7·9E-05)		143			2529	2·77
95% confidence interval:								(1·67:4·60)
Heterogeneity: (P < 0·05)								

References

1. Berthelsen and Kissmeyer-Nielsen, F. (Århus). Submitted to the Registry.

2. Shapiro, R. *et al.* (Copenhagen). Submitted to the Registry.

ADDITIONAL NOTES ON NEUROLOGIC DISORDERS

Optic neuritis

No significant deviations with HLA-A and B antigens, but HLA-Dw2 is most probably increased as in multiple sclerosis.

Reference

Sandberg-Wolheim, M. *et al.*, *Acta Neurol. Scand.* **52,** 161, 1975.

Multiple sclerosis

The HLA-Dw2 antigen is definitely more strongly associated than HLA-B7 in several investigations.

DERMATOLOGY

HLA	Ref. No.	Pos.	Ptt. (%)	Total	Pos.	Ctr. (%)	Total	Rel. risk X (Haldane)
Disease WHO code: 696.000		**Psoriasis vulgaris**						
HLA-B7	1	23	(18·4)	125	95	(29·1)	326	0·56
	2	4	(8·0)	50	29	(29·0)	100	0·23
	4	8	(10·5)	76	194	(34·5)	562	0·24
	5	12	(15·0)	80	408	(26·5)	1541	0·51
	6	9	(10·0)	90	82	(23·2)	353	0·38
Combined:		(P = 2·6E-09)		421			2882	0·41
95% confidence interval:								(0·31:0·55)
Heterogeneity: (P > 0·05)								
HLA-B8	1	9	(7·2)	125	59	(18·1)	326	0·37
	2	5	(10·0)	50	16	(16·0)	100	0·62
	4	13	(17·1)	76	130	(23·1)	562	0·70
	5	8	(10·0)	80	367	(23·8)	1541	0·37
	6	9	(10·0)	90	82	(23·2)	353	0·38
Combined:		(P = 3·6E-06)		421			2882	0·47
95% confidence interval:								(0·34:0·65)
Heterogeneity: (P > 0·05)								
HLA-B13	1	30	(24·0)	125	26	(8·0)	326	3·62
	2	1	(2·0)	50	2	(2·0)	100	1·19
	3	3	(6·7)	45	85	(4·3)	1967	1·81
	4	16	(21·1)	76	16	(2·8)	562	9·03
	5	12	(15·0)	80	65	(4·2)	1541	4·11
	6	30	(33·3)	90	24	(6·8)	353	6·78
Combined:		(P < 1·0E-10)		466			4849	4·65
95% confidence interval:								(3·46:6·24)
Heterogeneity: (P > 0·05)								

HLA	Ref. No.	Pos.	Ptt. (%)	Total	Pos.	Ctr. (%)	Total	Rel. risk X (Haldane)
HLA-Bw17	1	23	(18·4)	125	13	(4·0)	326	5·32
	2	6	(12·0)	50	5	(5·0)	100	2·54
	3	13	(28·9)	45	151	(7·7)	1967	4·98
	4	21	(27·6)	76	46	(8·2)	562	4·30
	5	29	(36·3)	80	123	(8·0)	1541	6·58
	6	30	(33·3)	90	38	(10·8)	353	4·13
Combined:		(P < 1·0E–10)		466			4849	4·90
95% confidence interval:								(3·81:6·30)
Heterogeneity: (P > 0·05)								
HLA-Bw37	1	8	(6·4)	125	5	(1·0)	505	6·58
	2	2	(4·0)	50	3	(3·0)	100	1·44
	3	7	(15·6)	45	6	(1·4)	424	12·54
Combined:		(P = 7·3E–08)		220			1029	6·35
95% confidence interval:								(3·24:12·45)
Heterogeneity: (P > 0·05)								
Disease WHO code: 696.000	**Psoriasis nonspecificata**							
HLA-A2	7	61	(70·1)	87	121	(61·1)	198	1·48
	8	84	(67·7)	124	511	(51·1)	1000	2·00
	9	56	(55·4)	101	62	(54·9)	113	1·02
	10	25	(56·8)	44	43	(48·3)	89	1·40
	11	67	(64·4)	104	199	(45·0)	442	2·20
	12	69	(62·7)	110	106	(45·9)	231	1·97
	13	76	(48·7)	156	185	(47·9)	386	1·03
	14	69	(55·2)	125	109	(46·8)	233	1·40
Combined:		(P = 4·3E–07)		851			2692	1·52
95% confidence interval:								(1·29:1·79)
Heterogeneity: (P > 0·05)								
HLA-B7	7	21	(24·1)	87	82	(41·4)	198	0·46
	8	17	(13·7)	124	260	(26·0)	1000	0·46
	9	14	(13·9)	101	36	(31·9)	113	0·35
	10	8	(18·2)	44	18	(20·2)	89	0·90
	11	17	(16·3)	104	124	(28·1)	442	0·51
	12	7	(6·4)	110	41	(17·7)	231	0·33
	13	20	(12·8)	156	85	(22·0)	386	0·53
	14	17	(13·6)	125	75	(32·2)	233	0·34
Combined:		(P < 1·0E–10)		851			2692	0·45
95% confidence interval:								(0·37:0·56)
Heterogeneity: (P > 0·05)								
HLA-B13	7	6	(6·9)	87	2	(1·0)	198	6·27
	8	32	(25·8)	124	43	(4·3)	1000	7·73
	9	9	(8·9)	101	8	(7·1)	113	1·27
	10	12	(27·3)	44	3	(3·4)	89	9·51
	11	24	(23·1)	104	35	(7·9)	442	3·49
	12	14	(12·7)	110	10	(4·3)	231	3·17
	13	23	(14·7)	156	19	(4·9)	386	3·32
	14	9	(7·2)	125	12	(5·2)	233	1·44
Combined:		(P < 1·0E–10)		851			2692	3·88
95% confidence interval:								(3·00:5·03)
Heterogeneity: (P = 3·6E–03)								
HLA-Bw16	9	22	(21·8)	101	6	(5·3)	113	4·68
	11	11	(10·6)	104	13	(2·9)	442	3·91
Combined:		(P = 2·1E–06)		205			555	4·24
95% confidence interval:								(2·33:7·70)
Heterogeneity: (P > 0·05)								

HLA	Ref. No.	Pos.	Ptt. (%)	Total	Pos.	Ctr. (%)	Total	Rel. risk X (Haldane)
Psoriasis nonspecificata (*cont.*):								
HLA-Bw17	7	9	(10·3)	87	1	(0·5)	198	15·93
	8	38	(30·6)	124	80	(8·0)	1000	5·09
	9	31	(30·7)	101	7	(6·2)	113	6·34
	10	10	(22·7)	44	8	(9·0)	89	2·92
	11	22	(21·2)	104	35	(7·9)	442	3·13
	12	24	(21·8)	110	9	(3·9)	231	6·63
	13	41	(26·3)	156	31	(8·0)	386	4·06
	14	63	(50·4)	125	14	(6·0)	233	15·38
Combined:		(P < 1·0E-10)		851			2692	5·38
95% confidence interval:								(4·29:6·76)
Heterogeneity: (P = 7·3E-03)								

Psoriasis vulgaris

References

1. Karvonen, *Ann. Clin. Res.* **7,** 301, 1975.
2. Marcusson, *Acta Dermatovener* (Stockholm), **55,** 297, 1975.
3. Nyfors, *Acta Dermatovener* (Stockholm), 1977, in press.
4. Århus material (quoted in Svejgaard *et al.*, *Brit. J. Derm.* **91,** 145, 1974).
5. Copenhagen material (quoted in Svejgaard *et al.*, *Brit. J. Derm.* **91,** 145, 1974.
6. Schunter, *Der Hautarzt*, **25,** 82, 1974.

Psoriasis nonspecificata

References

7. Beckman, *Human Heredity*, **24,** 496, 1974.
8. Bertrams, 5. internationale Tagung der Gesellschaft für forensische Blutgruppenkunde e.v. 1973.
9. Krulig, *Arch. Dermatol.* **111,** 857, 1975.
10. Russell, *New Engl. J. Med.* **287,** 738, 1972.
11. Schoefinius, *Dtsch. med. Wschr.* **99,** 440, 1974.
12. Seignalet, *Tissue Antigens*, **4,** 59, 1974.
13. White, *New Engl. J. Med.* **287,** 740, 1972.
14. Woodrow, *Brit. J. Dermatol.* **92,** 427, 1975.

HLA	Ref. No.	Pos.	Ptt. (%)	Total	Pos.	Ctr. (%)	Total	Rel. risk X (Haldane)
Disease WHO code: 696.100		**Psoriasis pustulosa**						
HLA-B27	15	9	(56·3)	16	46	(14·1)	326	7·64
	16	4	(12·9)	31	125	(8·1)	1541	1·85
Combined:		(P = 1·8E-04)		47			1867	3·73
95% confidence interval:								(1·87:7·42)
Heterogeneity: (P = 4·3E-02)								

References

15. Karvonen, *Ann. Clin. Res.* **7,** 301, 1975.
16. Svejgaard, *Brit. J. Derm.* **91,** 145, 1974.

HLA	Ref. No.	Pos.	Ptt. (%)	Total	Pos.	Ctr. (%)	Total	Rel. risk X (Haldane)
Disease WHO code: 693.990		**Dermatitis herpetiformis**						
HLA-A1	1	16	(61·5)	26	72	(28·7)	251	3·89
	3	19	(54·3)	35	61	(34·9)	175	2·20
	4	29	(72·5)	40	348	(33·6)	1036	5·07
	5	39	(63·9)	61	55	(16·9)	326	8·59
	6	23	(60·5)	38	57	(31·7)	180	3·26
Combined:		(P < 1·0E-10)		200			1968	4·44
95% confidence interval:								(3·26:6·04)
Heterogeneity: (P = 4·9E-02)								
HLA-B8	1	15	(57·7)	26	60	(23·9)	251	4·27
	2	35	(79·5)	44	405	(24·9)	1628	11·28
	3	21	(60·0)	35	58	(33·1)	175	2·98
	4	34	(85·0)	40	260	(25·1)	1036	15·82
	5	53	(86·9)	61	57	(17·5)	326	29·50
	6	30	(78·9)	38	47	(26·1)	180	10·08
Combined:		(P < 1·0E-10)		244			3596	9·23
95% confidence interval:								(6·74:12·63)
Heterogeneity: (P = 2·3E-04)								

References

1. Katz, *J. Clin. Invest.* **51,** 2977, 1972.
2. Solheim, *Tissue Antigens*, **7,** 57, 1976.
3. White, *Brit. J. Dermatol.* **89,** 133, 1973.
4. Material submitted from Newcastle upon Tyne.
5. Reunala, *Brit. J. Dermat.* **94,** 139, 1976.
6. Seah, *Brit. J. Dermat.* **94,** 131, 1976.

HLA	Ref. No.	Pos.	Ptt. (%)	Total	Pos.	Ctr. (%)	Total	Rel. risk X (Haldane)
Disease WHO code: 694.000	**Pemphigus**							
	1	4	(22·2)	18	39	(15·5)	251	1·67
	2	17	(60·7)	28	19	(20·2)	94	5·89
	3	3	(20·0)	15	96	(11·0)	870	2·25
Combined:		(P < 1·2E–04)		61			1215	3·14
Heterogeneity: (P > 0·05)								

References

1. Katz, *Arch. Dermatol.* **108,** 53, 1973.
2. Krain, *Arch. Dermatol.* **108,** 803, 1973 (Jewish).
3. Krain, *Arch. Dermatol.* **108,** 803, 1973 (non-Jewish).

HLA	Ref. No.	Pos.	Ptt. (%)	Total	Pos.	Ctr. (%)	Total	Rel. risk X (Haldane)
Disease WHO code: 136.020	**Behcet's Disease**							
HLA–B5	1	6	(85·7)	7	13	(8·6)	152	44·78
	2	4	(18·2)	22	71	(10·1)	700	2·14
	3	3	(37·5)	8	33	(16·5)	200	3·18
Combined:		(P = 8·1E–05)		37			1052	4·29
95% confidence interval:								(2·08:8·85)
Heterogeneity: (P = 8·1E–03)								
BEHCET'S DISEASE (JAPANESE)								
HLA–B5	4	33	(75·0)	44	24	(30·8)	78	6·48
Fisher: P = 2·4E–06								

References

1. Dausset, *Transpl. Rev.* **22,** 44, 1975.
2. Chamberlain, *Ann. Rheum. Dis.* **34,** suppl. 53, 1975.
3. Rosselet, *Ophthalmologica*, **172,** 116, 1976.
4. Ohno, *Amer. J. Ophthalmol.* **80,** 636, 1975.

HLA	Ref. No.	Pos.	Ptt. (%)	Total	Pos.	Ctr. (%)	Total	Rel. risk X (Haldane)
Disease WHO code: 54.00	**Recrudescent herpes labialis**							
HLA–A1	1	50	(55·6)	90	152	(25·1)	606	3·72
Fisher: P = 1·3E–08								
HLA–B8	1	30	(33·3)	90	102	(16·8)	606	2·48
Fisher: P = 3·5E–04								

Reference

1. Russell, *Tissue Antigens*, **6,** 257, 1975.

ADDITIONAL NOTES ON DERMATOLOGIC DISORDERS

PSORIASIS VULGARIS

The primary association may involve the C-series antigen, T7 (Ryder and Svejgaard in *T and B Lymphocytes in Immune Responses*, eds. F. Loor and G. E. Roelants. J. Wiley & Sons Ltd., Chichester).

LEPROSY

Combined calculations not performed. The situation unclear. Several different ethnic groups have been studied. The following references exist:

1. Dasgupta, A. *et al., Tissue Antigens*, **5,** 85, 1975.
2. Escobar-Gutierrez *et al., Vox Sang.* **25,** 151, 1973.
3. Kreisler, M. *et al., Tissue Antigens*, **4,** 197, 1974.
4. Reis, A. P. *et al., Lancet*, **ii,** 1384, 1974.
5. Smith, G. S. *et al., Vox Sang.* **28,** 42, 1975.
6. Thorsby, E. *et al., Tissue Antigens*, **3,** 373, 1973.

SCLERODERMA

No significant deviations.

Reference

Crouzet, J. *et al., Nouv. Presse Med.* **4,** 2489, 1975.

ACNE CONGLOBATA

No significant deviations.

Reference

Schackert, K. *et al., Arch. Dermatol.* **110,** 468, 1974.

RECURRENT APHTHOUS STOMATITIS

No significant deviations (104 patients).

References

Dolby, A. E. Data submitted to the Registry.
Platz, P. *et al., Tissue Antigens*, in press.

ENDOCRINOLOGY

HLA	Ref. No.	Pos.	Ptt. (%)	Total	Pos.	Ctr. (%)	Total	Rel. risk X (Haldane)
Disease WHO code: 250.001	**Diabetes, juvenile/insulin-dependent**							
HLA-B7	1	8	(28·6)	28	32	(32·0)	100	0·87
	2	8	(16·0)	50	75	(32·2)	233	0·42
	3	9	(10·6)	85	527	(26·8)	1967	0·34
	4	10	(20·0)	50	21	(21·0)	100	0·96
	5	7	(11·9)	59	42	(15·6)	270	0·77
	6	6	(12·0)	50	117	(26·0)	450	0·41
	7	15	(13·4)	112	260	(26·0)	1000	0·45
Combined:		(P = 4·1E-06)		434			4120	0·52
95% confidence interval:								(0·40:0·69)
Heterogeneity: (P > 0·05)								
HLA-B8	1	10	(35·7)	28	25	(25·0)	100	1·68
	2	74	(49·3)	150	74	(31·8)	233	2·08
	3	38	(44·7)	85	466	(23·7)	1967	2·61
	4	12	(24·0)	50	20	(20·0)	100	1·27
	5	12	(20·3)	59	44	(16·3)	270	1·34
	6	21	(42·0)	50	81	(18·0)	450	3·30
	7	34	(30·4)	112	205	(20·5)	1000	1·70
	8	28	(31·1)	90	17	(11·2)	152	3·53
Combined:		(P < 1·0E-10)		624			4272	2·13
95% confidence interval:								(1·75:2·58)
Heterogeneity: (P > 0·05)								
HLA-B18	1	9	(32·1)	28	23	(23·0)	100	1·61
	2	4	(8·0)	50	10	(4·3)	233	2·06
	3	8	(9·4)	85	140	(7·1)	1967	1·43
	4	5	(10·0)	50	12	(12·0)	100	0·86
	5	14	(23·7)	59	33	(12·2)	270	2·26
	6	6	(12·0)	50	59	(13·1)	450	0·96
	8	28	(31·1)	90	21	(13·8)	152	2·79
Combined:		(P = 3·9E-04)		412			3272	1·72
95% confidence interval:								(1·27:2·33)
Heterogeneity: (P > 0·05)								
HLA-Bw15	1	5	(17·9)	28	7	(7·0)	100	2·92
	2	31	(20·7)	150	28	(12·0)	233	1·90
	3	28	(32·9)	85	352	(17·9)	1967	2·27
	4	18	(36·0)	50	10	(10·0)	100	4·91
	5	9	(15·3)	59	27	(10·0)	270	1·67
	6	13	(26·0)	50	43	(9·6)	450	3·37
	7	28	(25·0)	112	150	(15·0)	1000	1·91
	8	10	(11·1)	90	20	(13·2)	152	0·84
Combined:		(P < 1·0E-10)		624			4272	2·11
95% confidence interval:								(1·69:2·64)
Heterogeneity: (P > 0·05)								

References

1. Finkelstein, S. *et al.*, *Tissue Antigens*, **2,** 74, 1972.
2. Cudworth, A. G. and Woodrow, J. C., *Diabetes*, **24,** 345, 1975.
3. Thomsen, M. *et al.*, *Transpl. Rev.* **22,** 125, 1975.
4. Singal, D. P. and Blajchman, M. A., *Diabetes*, **22,** 429, 1973.
5. Seignalet, J. *et al.*, *Tissue Antigens*, **6,** 272, 1976.
6. Mayr, W. *et al.* (Vienna). Submitted to the Registry.
7. Bertrams, J. *et al.*, *Tissue Antigens*, 1976, in press.
8. Cathelineau, G. *et al.*, *Nouv. Presse Med.* **5,** 586, 1976.

DIABETES, MATURITY ONSET

No significant deviations (61–132 patients).

References

1. Cudworth, A. G. and Woodrow, J. C., *Diabetes*, **24,** 345, 1975.
2. Thomsen, M. *et al.*, *Transpl. Rev.* **22,** 125, 1975.
3. Singal, D. P. *et al.*, *Diabetes*, **22,** 429, 1973.

HLA	Ref. No.	Pos.	Ptt. (%)	Total	Pos.	Ctr. (%)	Total	Rel. risk X (Haldane)
Disease WHO code: 242.090		**Thyrotoxicosis**						
HLA-B8	1	35	(35·0)	100	44	(16·3)	270	2·76
	2	21	(35·0)	60	16	(26·7)	60	1·47
	3	36	(44·4)	81	405	(24·9)	1628	2·42
	4	27	(42·2)	64	168	(24·0)	700	2·32
	6	29	(46·8)	62	24	(21·2)	113	3·22
	5	40	(46·5)	86	467	(23·7)	1967	2·80
Combined:		(P < 1·0E–10)		453			4738	2·52
95% confidence interval:								(2·04:3·12)
Heterogeneity: (P > 0·05)								
				Newfoundland population				
HLA-B8	51	27	(57·4)	47	33	(25·8)	128	3·82
Fisher P = 1·2E–04								
				Japanese population				
HLA-Bw35	52	25	(56·8)	44	17	(20·5)	83	4·97
Fisher P = 4·6E–05								

References

1. Seignalet, J. *et al.*, *Rev. Franc. Transf.* **17,** 305, 1975.
2. Nelson, S. D. and Pollett, J. E., *Tissue Antigens*, **5,** 38, 1975.
3. Thorsby, E. *et al.*, *Tissue Antigens*, **6,** 54, 1975.
4. Whittingham, S. *et al.*, *Tissue Antigens*, **6,** 23, 1975.
5. Bech, K. *et al.* (Copenhagen). Submitted to the Registry.
6. Grumet, F. C. *et al.*, 1974. Data in the Registry.
51. Farid, N. R. *et al.*, *Tissue Antigens*, in press.
52. Grumet, F. C. et *al.*, *Tissue Antigens*, **6,** 347, 1975.

HLA	Ref. No.	Pos.	Ptt. (%)	Total	Pos.	Ctr. (%)	Total	Rel. risk X (Haldane)
Disease WHO code: 255.100		**Idiopathic Addison's Disease**						
HLA-B8	1	4	(20·0)	20	81	(18·0)	450	1·24
	2	22	(68·8)	32	467	(23·7)	1967	6·88
Combined:		(P = 7·3E–06)		52			2417	3·88
95% confidence interval:								(2·14:7·01)
Heterogeneity: (P = 7·4E–03)								

References

1. Ludwig, H. *et al.*, *Z. ImmunForsch.* **149,** 423, 1975.
2. Thomsen, M. *et al.*, *Transpl. Rev.* **22,** 125, 1975.

HLA	Ref. No.	Pos.	Ptt. (%)	Total	Pos.	Ctr. (%)	Total	Rel. risk X (Haldane)
Disease WHO code: 254.020		**Subacute thyroiditis type De Quervain**						
HLA-Bw35	1	13	(86·7)	15	29	(9·2)	314	52·26
	2	17	(70·8)	24	257	(13·1)	1967	15·50
Combined:		(P < 1·0E–10)		39			2281	22·19
95% confidence interval:								(10·93:45·03)
Heterogeneity: (P > 0·05)								

References

1. Nyulassy, S. *et al.*, *Tissue Antigens*, **6,** 105, 1975.
2. Bech, K. *et al.* (Copenhagen). Data in the Registry.

ADDITIONAL NOTES ON ENDOCRINOLOGIC DISORDERS

Thyrotoxicosis

The association with HLA-B8 seems primarily to concern patients with ophthalmopathy (Mayr *et al.* (Vienna). Data submitted to the Registry). The association is apparently strongest with Graves' disease (which term is not always used in the same sense).

Hashimoto's disease

No significant deviations (109 patients).

References

Mayr, W. (Vienna). Data submitted to the Registry.
Whittingham, S. *et al.*, *Clin. Exp. Immunol.* **19,** 289, 1975.

Newfoundland inbred population:

Farid, N. R. *et al.*, *Tissue Antigens*, in press.

HLA-D typing

Has been performed in juvenile diabetes, Graves' disease, and idiopathic Addison's disease, and the association with HLA-Dw3 is stronger than with HLA-B8.

GASTROENTEROLOGY

HLA	Ref. No.	Pos.	Ptt. (%)	Total	Pos.	Ctr. (%)	Total	Rel. risk X (Haldane)
Disease WHO code: 571.931		**Chronic aggressive hepatitis**						
HLA-A1	1	24	(31·2)	77	290	(29·0)	1000	1·12
	2	30	(53·6)	56	15	(18·1)	83	5·09
	3	16	(39·0)	41	188	(27·2)	690	1·72
	4	22	(59·5)	37	109	(31·1)	350	3·20
	5	5	(22·7)	22	130	(28·9)	450	0·77
Combined:		(P = 6·4E–05)		233			2573	1·82
95% confidence interval:								(1·36:2·43)
Heterogeneity: (P = 2·1E–03)								
HLA-B8	1	23	(29·9)	77	205	(20·5)	1000	1·67
	2	34	(60·7)	56	14	(16·9)	83	7·35
	3	19	(46·3)	41	160	(23·2)	690	2·86
	4	25	(67·6)	37	63	(18·0)	350	9·24
	5	2	(9·1)	22	81	(18·0)	450	0·55
Combined:		(P < 1·0E–10)		233			2573	3·04
95% confidence interval:								(2·25:4·13)
Heterogeneity: (P = 1·9E –05)								

References

1. Bertrams, J. *et al.*, *Z. ImmunForsch.* **146,** 300, 1974.
2. Freudenberg, J. *et al.*, *Klin. Wschr.* **51,** 1075, 1973.
3. Lindenberg, J. *et al.*, *Brit. Med. J.* **4,** 77, 1975.
4. Mackay, I. R. and Morris, P. J., *Lancet*, **ii,** 793, 1972.
5. Mayr, W. Submitted to the Registry.

HLA	Ref. No.	Pos.	Ptt. (%)	Total	Pos.	Ctr. (%)	Total	Rel. risk X (Haldane)
Disease WHO code: 273.290		**Idiopathic haemochromatosis**						
HLA-A3	1	40	(78·4)	51	55	(27·0)	204	9·49
Fisher P = 2·1E–11								
HLA-B14	2	13	(25·5)	51	7	(3·4)	204	9·23
Fisher P = 5·3E–06								

References

1. Simon, M. *et al.*, *Gut*, 1976, in press.
2. Shewan *et al.*, *Brit. Med. J.* **1,** 281, 1976. Definitely confirms the increase of HLA-A3.

HLA	Ref. No.	Pos.	Ptt. (%)	Total	Pos.	Ctr. (%)	Total	Rel. risk X (Haldane)
Disease WHO code: 269.000		**Coeliac disease, childhood and adult**						
HLA-A1	1	22	(41·5)	53	32	(21·1)	152	2·65
	2	31	(57·4)	54	71	(29·6)	240	3·18
	4	82	(70·1)	117	89	(33·2)	268	4·66
	5	28	(70·0)	40	117	(29·3)	400	5·50
	6	34	(64·2)	53	125	(27·1)	462	4·76
	8	16	(66·7)	24	70	(35·0)	200	3·59
	9	27	(75·0)	36	57	(31·7)	180	6·22
Combined:		(P < 1·0E–10)		377			1902	4·20
95% confidence interval:								(3·31:5·32)
Heterogeneity: (P > 0·05)								
HLA-B7	1	5	(9·4)	53	32	(21·1)	152	0·42
	2	3	(5·6)	54	70	(29·2)	240	0·16
	5	7	(17·5)	40	109	(27·3)	400	0·60
	8	2	(8·3)	24	40	(20·0)	200	0·44
	9	4	(11·1)	36	39	(21·7)	180	0·50
Combined:		(P = 6·9E–05)		207			1172	0·41
95% confidence interval:								(0·27:0·64)
Heterogeneity: (P > 0·05)								

HLA	Ref. No.	Pos.	Ptt. (%)	Total	Pos.	Ctr. (%)	Total	Rel. risk X (Haldane)
HLA-B8	1	24	(45·3)	53	17	(11·2)	152	6·43
	2	30	(55·6)	54	39	(16·3)	240	6·35
	3	31	(67·4)	46	405	(24·9)	1628	6·13
	4	94	(80·3)	117	79	(29·5)	268	9·59
	5	33	(82·5)	40	88	(22·0)	400	15·77
	6	35	(66·0)	53	88	(19·0)	462	8·12
	7	16	(76·2)	21	69	(27·3)	253	7·96
	8	21	(87·5)	24	43	(21·5)	200	22·24
	9	32	(88·9)	36	47	(26·1)	180	20·30
Combined:		($P < 1{\cdot}0E{-}10$)		444			3783	8·84
95% confidence interval:								(6·98:11·18)
Heterogeneity: ($P > 0{\cdot}05$)								
HLA-Bw35	1	4	(7·5)	53	29	(19·1)	152	0·38
	2	5	(9·3)	54	31	(12·9)	240	0·74
	4	12	(10·3)	117	39	(14·6)	268	0·69
	5	2	(5·0)	40	75	(18·8)	400	0·28
	8	0	(0·0)	24	41	(20·5)	200	0·08
	9	0	(0·0)	36	27	(15·0)	180	0·08
Combined:		($P = 3{\cdot}9E{-}04$)		324			1440	0·47
95% confidence interval:								(0·30:0·71)
Heterogeneity: ($P > 0{\cdot}05$)								

References

1. Dausset, J. and Hors, J., *Transpl. Rev.* **22,** 44, 1975.
2. Ludwig, H. *et al., J. Immunogenet.* **1,** 91, 1974.
3. Solheim, B. *et al., Tissue Antigens,* **7,** 57, 1976.
4. Stokes, P. L. *et al., Gut,* **14,** 627, 1973.
5. Rood, J. J. van, *et al., Transpl. Rev.* **22,** 75, 1975.
6. Albert, E. D. *et al., Transpl. Proc.* **5,** 1785, 1973.
7. Evans, D. A. P., *Lancet,* **ii,** 1096, 1973.
8. Falchuk, M. *et al., J. Clin. Invest.* **51,** 1602, 1972.
9. Seah, P. P. *et al., Brit. J. Derm.* **94,** 131, 1976.

HLA	Ref. No.	Pos.	Ptt. (%)	Total	Pos.	Ctr. (%)	Total	Rel. risk X (Haldane)
Disease WHO code: 70.001	**Healthy carriers of hepatitis associated antigen**							
HLA-Bw41	3	5	(11·9)	42	6	(1·2)	500	11·16
Fisher $P = 7{\cdot}2E{-}04$								

References

1. Bertrams, J. Submitted for the Registry.
2. Gyodi, E. *et al., Haematol.* **7,** 199, 1973.
3. Jeannet, M. and Farquet, J. J., *Lancet,* **ii,** 1383, 1974.
4. Seignalet, J. *et al., Nouv. Rev. Franc. Hematol.* **14,** 89, 1974.

AUSTRALIAN ABORIGINES

Two consecutive studies of asymptomatic Australian antigen (Au) carriers among Australian aborigines showed both a decreased frequency of HLA-Bw15.

Reference

Boettcher, B. *et al., J. Immunogenet.* in press.

HLA	Ref. No.	Pos.	Ptt. (%)	Total	Pos.	Ctr. (%)	Total	Rel. risk X (Haldane)
Disease WHO code: 281.000	**Pernicious anaemia**							
HLA-B7	1	15	(51·7)	29	107	(26·8)	400	2·92
	2	16	(38·1)	42	112	(19·0)	591	2·65
	3	18	(27·3)	66	19	(22·1)	86	1·32
Combined:		($P = 1{\cdot}2E{-}04$)		137			1077	2·20
95% confidence interval:								(1·47:3·30)
Heterogeneity: ($P > 0{\cdot}05$)								

References

1. Mawhinney, H. *et al., Clin. Exp. Immunol.* **22,** 47, 1975.
2. Zittou, R., *New Engl. J. Med.* **293,** 1324, 1975.
3. Horton, M. A. and Oliver, R. T. D., *Tissue Antigens,* 1976, in press.

ADDITIONAL NOTES ON GASTROENTEROLOGIC DISORDERS

Persistent chronic hepatitis

No significant deviations (19–70 patients studied).

References

1. Bertrams, J. *et al.*, *Z. ImmunForsch.* **146,** 300, 1974.
2. Freudenberg, J. *et al.*, *Klin. Wschr.* **51,** 1075, 1973.

Ulcerative colitis

No significant deviations (51–152 patients).

References

1. Asquith, P. *et al.*, *Lancet*, **i,** 113, 1976.
2. Bergman, L. *et al.*, *Tissue Antigens*, **7,** 145, 1976.
3. Gleeson, M. H. *et al.*, *Gut*, **13,** 438, 1972.
4. Lewkonia, R. M. *et al.*, *Lancet*, **i,** 574, 1974.

Crohn's disease

No significant deviations (62–262 patients).

References

1. Asquith, P. *et al.*, *Lancet*, **i,** 113, 1974.
2. Bergman, L. *et al.*, *Tissue Antigens*, **7,** 145, 1976.
3. Gleeson, M. H. *et al.*, *Gut*, **13,** 438, 1972.
4. Lewkonia, R. M. *et al.*, *Lancet*, **i,** 574, 1974.
5. Russell, A. S. *et al.*, *Amer. J. Digest. Dis.* **20,** 359, 1975.

ALLERGOLOGY

A variety of allergic disorders have been studied in terms of HLA, both in unrelated patients and in families. Some trends have emerged, but the situation is far from clear. The heterogeneity of the allergies (in terms of specificity) have not allowed us to do any combined calculations. The following list of references is not complete, but we have a feeling (and hope) that some of the new data which are to be presented in Paris will bring more clarity. Nevertheless, we know we have not worked enough on these data and wish to apologize for this, the poorest part of the report.

References

1. Blumenthal, M. N., Genetic mapping of Ir locus in man: linkage to second locus of HLA. *Science*, **184,** 1301, 1974.
2. Geerts, S. J. *et al.*, Predisposition for atopy or allergy linked to HLA. *Lancet*, **i,** 461, 1975.
3. Krain, L. S. and Terasaki, P. I., HLA types in atopic dermatitis. *Lancet*, **i,** 1059, 1973.
4. Krain, L. S., Histocompatibility antigens: a laboratory and epidemiologic tool. *J. Invest. Dermatol.* **62,** 67, 1974.
5. Levine, B. B. *et al.*, Ragweed hay fever: genetic control and linkage to HLA haplotypes. *Science*, **178,** 1201, 1972.
6. Marsh, D. G. *et al.*, Association of the HL-A7 cross-reacting group with a specific reaginic antibody response in allergic man. *Science*, **179,** 693, 1973.
7. McDevitt, H. O. and Bodmer, W. F., HL-A, immune response genes, and disease. *Lancet*, **i,** 1269, 1974.
8. Pillier-Loriette, C. *et al.*, Search for a correlation between familial allergy to dactyl (pollen-hypersensitivity) and HLA antigens. *Tissue Antigens*, in press.
9. Schunter, F. *et al.*, Histocompatibility antigens in hay fever. *Z. ImmunForsch.* **150,** 105, 1975.
10. Terasaki, P. I. and Mickey, M. R., HL-A haplotypes of 32 diseases. *Transpl. Rev.* **22,** 105, 1975.
11. Thorsby, E. *et al.*, HL-A antigens and susceptibility to diseases. *Tissue Antigens*, **1,** 147, 1971.
12. Yoo, T.-J. *et al.*, The relationship between HLA antigens and lymphocyte response in ragweed allergy. *J. Allergy Clin. Immunol.* **57,** 25, 1976.

IMMUNOPATHOLOGY

HLA	Ref. No.	Pos.	Ptt. (%)	Total	Pos.	Ctr. (%)	Total	Rel. risk X (Haldane)
Disease WHO code: 734.900	**Sicca syndrome**							
HLA-B8	1	14	(58·3)	24	253	(21·0)	1205	5·19
	2	19	(52·8)	36	77	(22·0)	350	3·93
	3	8	(38·1)	21	186	(31·2)	597	1·39
Combined:		(P = 1·9E–07)		81			2152	3·25
95% confidence interval:								(2·08:5·05)
Heterogeneity: (P > 0·05)								

References

1. Gershwin, M. E. *et al.*, *Tissue Antigens*, **6,** 342, 1975.
2. Ivanyi, D. *et al.*, *Tissue Antigens*, **7,** 45, 1976.
3. Sturrock, R. D. *et al.*, *Ann. Rheum. Dis.*, **33,** 165, 1974.

ADDITIONAL NOTES ON IMMUNOPATHIC DISORDERS

Systemic lupus erythematosus

No significant associations, but a slight increase of HLA-B8 (rel. risk = 1·66, 226 patients studied).

References

1. Dostal, C. *et al.*, *Ann. Rheum. Dis.*, in press.
2. Grumet, F. C. *et al.*, *New Engl. J. Med.* **285,** 193, 1971.
3. Kissmeyer-Nielsen, F. *et al.*, *Transpl. Rev.* **22,** 164, 1975.
4. Nies, K. M. *et al.*, *Arthr. Rheum.* **17,** 397, 1974.
5. Goldberg, M. A. *et al.*, *Arthr. Rheum.* **19,** 129, 1976,

Sarcoidosis

No significant associations (130–262 patients, HLA-B7: rel. risk = 1·37, P = 3·1E–02).

References

1. Hedfors, E. and Möller, E., *Tissue Antigens*, **3,** 95, 1973.
2. Kueppers, F. *et al.*, *Tissue Antigens*, **4,** 56, 1974.
3. Persson, I. *et al.*, *Tissue Antigens*, **6,** 50, 1975.

Chronic glomerulonephritis

No significant associations (183–890 patients, HLA-A2: rel. risk = 1·31, P = 2·2E–03).

References

1. Mickey, M. R. *et al.*, *Histocompatibility Testing 1970*, p. 237, Munksgaard, Copenhagen.
2. Jensen, H. *et al.*, *Tissue Antigens*, **6,** 368, 1975.

Polycystic kidney disease

No significant deviations (75 patients).

Reference

Dausset, J. *et al.*, *Transpl. Rev.* **22,** 44, 1975.

Acquired haemolytic anaemia

No significant deviations. For references see Dausset and Hors, *Transpl. Rev.* **22,** 44, 1975.

Idiopathic thrombocytopenic purpura

No significant deviations.

Reference

Dausset and Hors, *Transpl. Rev.* **22,** 44, 1975.

Complement deficiencies

It is well known that complement factor 2 (C2) deficiency is strongly associated with HLA-Dw2, Bw18, and Aw25 (in the order mentioned), but unbiased association studies of disease, C2-deficiency, and HLA have to our knowledge not been done.

References

1. Fu, S. M. *et al.*, *J. Exp. Med.* **142,** 495, 1975.
2. Gibson, D. J. *et al.*, *J. Immunol.* **116,** 1065, 1976.

MALIGNANT DISEASES

HLA	Ref. No.	Pos.	Ptt. (%)	Total	Pos.	Ctr. (%)	Total	Rel. risk X (Haldane)
Disease WHO code: 190.030	**Retinoblastoma**							
HLA-B12	1	12	(9·8)	122	64	(25·1)	255	0·34
Fisher P = 2·7E–04								
HLA-Bw35	1	31	(25·4)	122	28	(11·0)	255	2·75
Fisher P = 3·8E–04								

Reference

1. Schildberg, P. *et al.*, *Arch. Klin. Exp. Ophthal.* **186,** 33, 1973.

TABLE II

Combined risks of Hodgkin's disease

Antigens	No. of patients	No. of controls	Combined risk	χ_1^2 for significance	χ^2 for heterogeneity	d.f. for heterogeneity	References
HL-A1	1509	5464	1·42	29·69***	22·13	16	1–17
HL-A9	1459	5375	1·22	7·47**	17·57	15	do., excl. 9
HL-A10	1424	4973	1·35	9·75**	13·47	14	do., excl. 9, 14
HL-A11	1475	5288	0·77	6·49*	13·17	15	do., excl. 14
Total LA:				$\chi_7^2 = 58{\cdot}64$*** P = 10^{-10}		$\chi_{107}^2 = 113{\cdot}44$ P = 0·32	
HL-A5	1508	5474	1·59	25·82***	27·15*	16	1–17
HL-A7	1510	5475	0·92	1·45	29·98*	16	do.
HL-A8	1510	5475	1·33	16·33***	17·81	16	do.
W10	1474	5042	0·80	6·21*	15·12	15	do., excl. 14
W18	1165	3677	1·85	29·08***	8·28	11	do., excl. 2, 4, 5, 6, 14
Total FOUR:				$\chi_{15}^2 = 91{\cdot}14$*** P = 10^{-44}		$\chi_{187}^2 = 223{\cdot}3$* P = 0·04	

Only antigens showing probably significant ($P < 0{\cdot}05$) deviation or heterogeneity are shown. One, two, and three asterisks indicate significance at the 5, 1, and 0·1 per cent probability levels, respectively. References: 1, Bertrams *et al.* (1972); 2, Dick *et al.* (1972); 3, van der Does *et al.* (1972); 4, Engelfriet *et al.* (1972); 5, Falk *et al.* (1971); 6, Falk *et al.* (1974); 7, Festenstein *et al.* (1972); 8, Graff *et al.* (1974); 9, Harris *et al.* (1972); 10, Henderson *et al.* (1973); 11, Kissmeyer-Nielsen *et al.* (1972); 12, Morris *et al.* (1972); 13, Singal *et al.* (1972); 14, Sybesma *et al.* (1972); 15, Takasugi *et al.* (1973); 16, Thorsby *et al.* (1972); 17, Tittor *et al.* (1972).

From: Svejgaard *et al.*, *Transpl. Rev.* **22,** 3, 1975.

TABLE III

Combined risks of acute lymphatic leukaemia

Antigen	No. of patients	No. of controls	Combined risk	χ_1^2 for significance	χ^2 for heterogeneity	d.f. for heterogeneity	References
HL-A2	527	3215	1·34	8·81**	25·65**	9	1–10
HL-A9	425	2981	0·87	0·90	16·92*	8	1–9, excl. 5
Total LA:				$\chi_8^2 = 18{\cdot}23$ P = 0·02		$\chi_{57}^2 = 91{\cdot}41$ P = 0·003	
HL-A8	527	3215	1·28	4·52*	15·62	9	1–10
HL-A12	527	3215	1·24	3·98*	30·88***	9	do.
W18	135	1064	1·08	0·04	7·44*	2	3, 4, 7
Total FOUR:				$\chi_{13}^2 = 27{\cdot}50$ P = 0·01		$\chi_{81}^2 = 112{\cdot}31$ P = 0·01	

See Table II for explanations. References: 1, Davey *et al.* (1974); 2, Dick *et al.* (1972); 3, Jeannet *et al.* (1971); 4, Klouda *et al.* (1974); 5, Kourilsky *et al.* (1967); 6, Lawler *et al.* (1971); 7, Rogentine *et al.* (1973); 8, Sanderson *et al.* (1973); 9, Thorsby *et al.* (1971); 10, Walford *et al.* (1971).

From: Svejgaard, A. *et al.*, *Transpl. Rev.* **22,** 3, 1975.

Leukaemias

Apart from acute lymphatic leukaemia (cf. above) we have not had time to make combined calculations on these disorders. Reviews on AML, CML, and CLL have been given by:

1. Morris, P. J., *Contemporary topics in immunobiology*, vol. 3, Plenum Press, N.Y./London, 1974.
2. Dausset, J. *et al.*, *Clin. Immunol. Immunopath.* **3,** 127, 1974.
3. Dausset, J. and Hors, J., *Transpl. Rev.* **22,** 44, 1975.

The suggestion of Falk and co-workers and Rogentine and co-workers that some HLA antigens confer survival value once Hodgkin's disease or ALL have developed is gaining increasing support. Most of the reports on both of these diseases have treated both retrospective and prospective studies.

Multiple myeloma

No significant deviations (32–149 patients).

References

1. Bertrams, J. *et al.*, *Tissue Antigens*, **2,** 41, 1972.
2. Smith, G. *et al.*, *Tissue Antigens*, **4,** 374, 1974.
3. Mason, D. Y. and Cullen, P., *Tissue Antigens*, **5,** 238, 1975.
4. Jeannet, M. and Magnin, C., *Eur. J. Clin. Invest.* **2,** 39, 1976.

Burkitt's lymphoma

No significant deviations in African Blacks (106 patients) in three independent studies.

Reviewed by:

Bodmer *et al.*, *Tissue Antigens*, **5,** 63, 1975.

Malignant melanoma

No significant deviations (104–349 patients).

References

1. Cordon, A. L., *Lancet*, **i,** 938, 1973.
2. Lamm, L. U. *et al.*, *Cancer*, **33,** 1458, 1974.
3. Takasugi, M. *et al.*, *Cancer Res.* **33,** 648, 1973.
4. Clark, D. A. *et al.*, *Israel J. Med. Sci.* **10,** 836, 1974.
5. Singal, D. P. *et al.*, *Transpl.* **18,** 186, 1974.

Mammary carcinoma

No significant deviations (200–966 patients).

References

1. Bertrams, J. *et al.*, *Cancer Res. Clin. Oncol.* **83,** 219, 1975.
2. Jong-Bakker, M. *et al.*, *Eur. J. Cancer*, **10,** 555, 1974.
3. Cordon, A. L. and James, D. C. O., *Lancet*, **ii,** 565, 1973.
4. Patel, R. *et al.*, *Amer. J. Surg.* **124,** 31, 1972.
5. Takasugi, M. *et al.*, *Cancer Res.* **33,** 648, 1973.
6. Martz, E. and Benacerraf, B., *Tissue Antigens*, **3,** 30, 1973.
7. Darke, C. (Cardiff). Submitted to the Registry.

Trophoblastic neoplasia

No significant deviations (98–151 patients).

References

1. Lawler, S. D. *et al.*, *Lancet*, **ii,** 834, 1971.
2. Mittal, K. K. *et al.*, *Tissue Antigens*, **6,** 57, 1975.

Nasopharyngeal carcinoma

Studies of Chinese have given evidence of an association with an HLA antigen specific for Chinese.

References

Simons, M. J. *et al.*, *Int. J. Cancer*, **13,** 122, 1974.
Simons, M. J. *et al.*, *Lancet*, **i,** 142, 1975.
Simons, M. J. *et al.*, *Histocompatibility Testing 1975*, p. 809, Munksgaard, Copenhagen.

OTHER DISEASES

Haemophilus influenza type B

No clearly significant deviations, but rather many low P-values; highest risk for HLA-Bw17 (4·5 with P = 3·1E–03; 65 patients).

Reference

Robbins, J. B. *et al.*, *Ann. Int. Med.* **78,** 259, 1973.

Mononucleosis

No significant deviations (40–159 patients).

References

Schiller, J. and Davey, F. R., *A.J.C.P.* **62,** 325, 1974.
Ting, A. *et al.*, *Symp. Series Immunobiol. Standard*, **18,** 276, 1973.

Congenital rubella

No significant deviations (58 patients, rel. risk for HLA-A1: = 2·3, P = 2·0E–03).

Reference

Honeyman, M. C. *et al.*, *Tissue Antigens*, **5,** 12, 1975.

Essential hypertension

Gelsthorpe, K. *et al.*, *Lancet*, **i,** 1039, 1975.

Spina bifida

Family studies.

References

Bobrow, M. *et al.*, *Tissue Antigens*, **5,** 234, 1975.
Amos, D. B. *et al.*, *Transpl. Proc.* **7,** 93, 1975.

Brachymetacarpia

Saint-Hillier, Y. *et al.*, *Nouv. Presse Med.* **5,** 1003, 1976.

HLA	Ref. No.	Pos.	Ptt. (%)	Total	Pos.	Ctr. (%)	Total	Rel. risk X (Haldane)
Disease WHO code: 746.000	**Congenital heart malformation**							
HLA-A2	1	40	(80·0)	50	138	(43·9)	314	4·92
Fisher P = 1·3E-06								

Reference

1. Buc, M. *et al.*, *Tissue Antigens*, **5**, 128, 1975.

HARE-LIP CLEFT PALATE

Family studies.

References

Rapaport, F. T. *et al.*, *Transpl. Proc.* **5,** 1823, 1973.
Rapaport, F. T. *et al.*, *Transpl. Proc.* **5,** 1817, 1973.

CYSTIC FIBROSIS

Reference

Polymenidis, Z. *et al.*, *Lancet*, **ii,** 1452, 1973.

DOWN'S SYNDROME

No significant deviations (76 patients).

Reference

Segal, D. J. *et al.*, *Humangenetik*, **27,** 45, 1975.

ASBESTOSIS

No significant deviations (56 patients, HLA-B27: rel. risk = 3·9, P = 6·6E-03).

Reference

Merchant, J. A. *et al.*, *Brit. Med. J.* **1,** 189, 1975.

FARMER'S LUNG

References

Evans, C. C. and Evans, J. M., *Lancet*, **ii,** 975, 1975.
Flaherty, D. K. *et al.*, *Lancet*, **ii,** 507, 1975.

Post scriptum

We are well aware that the above tables and notes lack a number of references and some diseases in which HLA typing has been performed and even published—this has become particularly clear during the preparation of the tables and it is due to the shortage of time inherent in the necessity of finishing the report before the first international symposium on HLA and disease. Nevertheless, we hope that the diseases included cover the over-all field in general.

A summary of the above tables will be given in a chapter of the book *HLA and Disease* (Dausset and Svejgaard, eds.) to be published by Munksgaard, Copenhagen, after the symposium. However, this chapter will only contain the *combined* estimates of relative risks, etc., while there will not be space for the data of the individual studies as represented here (and perhaps not all the references). There are still a number of extra copies available which can be obtained from the Registry on request; unfortunately we have to charge for such extra copies to cover manifolding and postage.

L. P. Ryder and A. Svejgaard
Copenhagen, 11 June 1976
at the very last minute.

BIBLIOGRAPHY

Adamo, F. (1961*a*). Gruppi sanguigni e sottogruppi in alcune emopatie sistemiche. *Rass. med. sarda* **63**, 305–11.

Adamo, F. (1961*b*). Gruppi sanguigni e sottogruppi nell'asma bronchiale. *Rass. med. sarda* **63**, 603–8.

Adamo, F. (1961*c*). Rapporti tra gruppi sanguigni e sottogruppi in alcune emopatie sistemiche. *Rass. med. sarda* **63**, 635–40.

Addis, G. J. (1959). Blood groups in acute rheumatism. *Scot. med. J.* **4**, 547–8.

Addis, S. & D'Ovidio, N. (1977). Glucose-6-phosphate dehydrogenase deficiency and duodenal ulcer. *Brit. med. J.* **i**, 1533–4.

Aird, I., Bentall, H. H., & Roberts, J. A. Fraser (1953). A relationship between cancer of stomach and the ABO blood groups. *Brit. med. J.* **i**, 799–801.

Aird, I., Bentall, H. H., Mehigan, J. A., & Roberts, J. A. Fraser (1954). The blood groups in relation to peptic ulceration and carcinoma of colon, rectum, breast, and bronchus: an association between the ABO groups and peptic ulceration. *Brit. med. J.* **ii**, 315–21.

Aird, I., *et al.* (1956). An association between blood group A and pernicious anaemia. A collective series from a number of centres. *Brit. med. J.* **ii**, 723–4.

Aird, I., Lee, D. R., & Roberts, J. A. Fraser (1960). ABO blood groups and cancer of oesophagus, cancer of pancreas, and pituitary adenoma. *Brit. med. J.* **i**, 1163–6.

Åkesson, H. O. (1959). Taste sensitivity to phenyl-thio-urea in tuberculosis and diabetes mellitus. *Ann. hum. Genet.* **23**, 262–5.

Alcober Coloma, T. (1944). Distribución de los grupos sanguíneos entre los enfermos mentales. *Med. esp.* **11**, 204.

Alexander, L., Loman, J., Lesses, M. F., & Green, I. (1950). Blood and plasma transfusions in multiple sclerosis. *Res. Publ. Ass. nerv. ment. Dis.* **28**, 179–200.

Alexander, W. (1921). An inquiry into the distribution of the blood groups in patients suffering from 'malignant disease'. *Brit. J. exp. Path.* **2**, 66–9.

Ali, M. (1931). Blood-groups among lepers. *J. Egypt. med. Ass.* **14**, 119–22.

Allan, T. M. (1958). Rh blood groups and sex ratio at birth. *Brit. med. J.* **ii**, 248.

Allan, T. M. (1959). ABO blood groups and sex ratio at birth. *Brit. med. J.* **i**, 553–4.

Allan, T. M. & Dawson, A. A. (1968). ABO blood groups and ischaemic heart disease in men. *Brit. Heart J.* **30**, 377–82.

Allan, T. M. (1970). ABO blood groups and myelomatosis. *Brit. med. J.* **ii**, 178.

Allan, T. M. & Stewart, K. S. (1971). ABO blood-groups and superficial puerperal thrombophlebitis. *Lancet* **i**, 1125.

Allan, T. M. (1972). ABO and Rh blood groups in relation to sex ratio of sibs. *Hum. Hered.* **22**, 578–83.

Allan, T. M. (1973). ABO blood groups and sex ratio at birth. *Brit. med. J.* **i**, 236–7.

Allen, C. M. (1964). Blood groups and abortions. *J. chron. Dis.* **17**, 619–26.

Allen, J. G. & Sayman, W. A. (1962). Serum hepatitis from transfusions of blood. *J. Amer. med. Ass.* **180**, 1079–85.

Allison, A. C. (1954*a*). The distribution of the sickle-cell trait in East Africa and elsewhere, and its apparent relationship to subtertian malaria. *Trans. R. Soc. trop. Med. Hyg.* **48**, 312–18.

Allison, A. C. (1954*b*). Protection afforded by sickle-cell trait against subtertian malarial infection. *Brit. med. J.* **ii**, 290–4.

Allison, A. C. & Clyde, D. F. (1961). Malaria in African children with deficient erythrocyte glucose-6-phosphate dehydrogenase. *Brit. med. J.* **i**, 1346–9.

Allison, A. C. (1973). Polymorphism and natural selection in human populations. In *Heredity and society* (ed. A. S. Baer), pp. 255–76. N. York, Macmillan Co.

Aloigi, S. (1929). Gruppi sanguigni e tubercolosi polmonare. *Riv. Clin. med.* **30**, 1119–23.

Alperin, M. M. (1926). Über die Beziehungen zwischen Blutgruppen und Tuberkulose. *Beitr. Klin. Tuberk.* **64**, 500.

Alsbirk, P. H. (1975). Anterior chamber of the eye. A genetical and anthropological study in Greenland Eskimos. *Hum. Hered.* **25**, 418–27.

Altobella, L. (1967–8). Osservazioni sul rapporto fra gruppi sanguigni e dermatosi varie. *Arch. ital. Derm.* **35**, 319–26.

Ammerman, A. J. & Cavalli-Sforza, L. L. (1971). Measuring the rate of spread of early farming in Europe. *Man* n.s. **6**, 674–88.

Amzel, R. & Halber, W. (1924). Sur la réaction de Wassermann chez les individus appartenant aux différents groupes sérologiques. *C. R. Soc. Biol., Paris* **91**, 1479–80.

Amzel, R. & Halber, W. (1925). Ueber das Ergebnis der Wassermannschen Reaktion innerhalb verschiedener Blutgruppen. *Z. ImmunForsch.* **42**, 89–98.

Anand, S. (1961). ABO blood group in relation to eosinophilia. *Anthropologist* **8**, 33–9.

Anand, S. (1964*a*). Association of ABO blood groups with incidence of renal lithiasis. *Acta Genet. med. Gemell.* **13**, 167–72.

Anand, S. (1964*b*). The relationship of ABO, MN and Rhesus blood groups to asthma. *Indian J. Chest Dis.* **6**, 74–9.

Anand, S. (1965). Filariasis in its relation to A_1A_2BO, MN, Kell, Duffy and Rhesus blood groups and secretor factor. *Acta Genet. med. Gemell.* **14**, 326–35.

Ananthakrishnan, R. & Walter, H. (1972). Some notes on the geographical distribution of the human red cell acid phosphatase phenotypes. *Humangenetik* **15**, 177–81.

Ananthakrishnan, R., Beck, W., Walter, H., Arndt Hauser, A., Gumbel, W., Leithoff, H., Wigand, R., Zimmermann, W., & Boros, B. (1973). A mother-child combination analysis for ABO-Hp interaction. *Humangenetik* **18**, 203–6.

Anders, W. (1956). Poliomyelitis und Blutgruppen. *Zbl. Bakt.* Abt. i, Orig. **165**, 221–5.

Andersen, J. & Lauritzen, E. (1960). Blood groups and diabetes mellitus. *Diabetes* **9**, 20–4.

Andersen, S. B. (1955). Blodtypefordelingen i København. *Ugeskr. Laeg.* **21**, 932–3.

André, F., André, C., Lambert, R., & Descos, F. (1974). Prevalence of alpha$_1$-antitrypsin deficiency in patients with gastric or duodenal ulcer. *Biomedicine 'Express'* **21**, 222–4.

Andreani (1954). Quoted by Asaro (1955).

Andrews, G. S. (1959). Blood groups and toxaemia of pregnancy. *Brit. med. J.* **ii**, 806–7.

Araújo, H. M. Mendez de, Salzano, F. M., & Wolff, H. (1972). New data on the association between PTC and thyroid diseases. *Humangenetik* **15**, 136–44.

Arfors, K. E., Beckman, L., & Lundin, L. G. (1963). Genetic variations of human serum phosphatases. *Acta genet. Stat. med.* **13**, 89–94.

Arias, S. & Bermúdez, C. (1963). Ulcera péptica y grupos sanguíneos. Estudio de la distribución de los grupos ABO y caracter secretor en 102 ulcerosos. *Rev. clin. esp.* **91**, 227–35.

Asaro, F. (1955). Gruppi sanguigni e malattie mentali. I. Gruppi O–A–B–AB. *Rass. Neuropsich.* **9**, 579–95.

Aschner, B. M. & Post, R. H. (1956–7). Modern therapy and hereditary diseases. *Acta genet. Stat. med.* **6**, 362–9.

Ashley, D. J. B. (1969). Blood groups and lung cancer. *J. med. Genet.* **6**, 183–6.

Ashton, G. C. (1965). Cattle serum transferrins: a balanced polymorphism. *Genetics* **52**, 983–97.

Astwood, E. B., Sullivan, J., Bissell, A., & Tyslowitz, R. (1943). Action of certain sulfamides and of thiourea upon the function of the thyroid gland of the rat. *Endocrinology* **32**, 210–25.

Astwood, E. B., Nissel, A., & Hughes, A. M. (1945). Further studies on the chemical nature of compounds which inhibit the function of the thyroid gland. *Endocrinology* **37**, 456–81.

Athreya, B. H. & Coriell, L. L. (1967). Relation of blood groups to infection. i. A survey and review of data suggesting possible relationship between malaria and blood groups. *Amer. J. Epidemiol.* **86,** 292–304.

Atwell, J. D. (1962). Distribution of ABO blood groups in children with embryonic tumours. *Brit. med. J.* **i,** 89–90.

Auteri-Madia. Quoted by Asaro (1955).

Awdiejewa & Grycewicz (1924). Quoted by Poppoff (1927).

Awny, A. Y. & Kamel, K. (1959). The relation between ABO system of blood groups and the incidence of certain diseases. *Bull. clin. sci. Soc. Abbassiah* **10,** nos. 1–2, 61–4.

Ayres, M., Salzano, F. M., & Ludwig, O. K. (1966). Blood group changes in leukaemia. *J. med. Genet.* **3,** 180–5.

Ayres, M., Salzano, F. M., Helena, M., Franco, L. P., & Souza Barros, M. de (1976). The association of blood groups, ABH secretion, haptoglobins and hemoglobins with filariasis. *Hum. Hered.* **26,** 105–9.

Azevêdo, E., Krieger, H., Mi, M. P., & Morton, N. E. (1965). PTC taste sensitivity and endemic goiter in Brazil. *Amer. J. hum. Genet.* **17,** 87–90.

Baer, A., Lie-Injo, L. E., Welch, Q. B., & Lewis, A. N. (1976). Genetic factors and malaria in the Temuan. *Amer. J. hum. Genet.* **28,** 179–88.

Bagshawe, K. D., Rawlins, G., Pike, M. C., & Lawler, S. D. (1971). ABO blood-groups in trophoblastic neoplasia. *Lancet* **i,** 553–7.

Bagshawe, K. D. (1976). Risk and prognostic factors in trophoblastic neoplasia. *Cancer* **38,** 112–18.

Baisi, F. (1959). Cancro del collo dell'utero e gruppi sanguigni. *Boll. Soc. med.-chir. Pisa* **27,** 423–7.

Bajusz, G. & Hoffman, J. (1965). Gastric cancer and the A blood group. (In Hungarian.) *Orv. Hétil.* **106,** 2091.

Balestra, V. & Mattioli, F. (1958). Les groupes sanguins et l'ulcère gastroduodénal. *Schweiz. Z. allg. Path.* **21,** 331–3.

Balgairies, E. (1934). Réaction de Schick et groupes sanguins. *Ann. Mèd. lég.* **14,** 575–7.

Ball, P. A. J. (1962). Influence of the secretor and Lewis genes on susceptibility to duodenal ulcer. *Brit. med. J.* **ii,** 948–50.

Balme, R. H. & Jennings, D. (1957). Gastric ulcer and the ABO blood groups. *Lancet* **i,** 1219–20.

Barber, M. & Dunsford, I. (1959). Excess blood-group substance A in serum of patient dying with carcinoma of stomach. *Brit. med. J.* **i,** 607–9.

Bárdosi, Z., Dubecz, S., & Adám, M. (1965). Über die Blutgruppen unserer Magenkrebskranken. *Zbl. Chir.* **90,** 481–4.

Bartlett, A., Dormandy, K. M., Hawkey, C. M., Stableforth, P., & Voller, A. (1976). Factor-VIII-related antigen: measurement by enzyme immunoassay. *Brit. med. J.* **i,** 994–6.

Barura, D. & Paguio, A. S. (1976). ABO blood groups and cholera. MS. Pers. comm. to A. E. Mourant.

Bast, R. C., Whitlock, J. P., Miller, H., Rapp, H. J., & Gelboin, H. V. (1974). Aryl hydrocarbon (benzo(a)pyrene) hydroxylase in human peripheral blood monocytes. *Nature, Lond.* **250,** 664–5.

Batchelor, J. R. (1977) Histocompatibility antigens and their relevance to multiple sclerosis. *Brit. med. Bull.* **33,** 72–7.

Baum, G. L., Racz, I., Bubis, J. J., Molho, M., & Shapiro, B. L. (1966). Cystic disease of the lung. Report of eighty-eight cases, with an ethnologic relationship. *Amer. J. Med.* **40,** 578–602.

Beasley, W. H. (1960*a*). Blood groups of gastric ulcer and carcinoma. *Brit. med. J.* **i,** 1167–72.

Beasley, W. H. (1960*b*). The blood groups of gastric ulcer-cancer. *J. clin. Path.* **13,** 315–24.

Beasley, W. H. (1964). The ABO blood groups of carcinoma of the oesophagus and of benign prostatic hyperplasia. *J. clin. Path.* **17,** 42–4.

Beaven, G. H. (1973). Biological studies of Yemenite and Kurdish Jews in Israel and other groups in south-west Asia. X. Haemoglobin studies of Yemenite and Kurdish Jews in Israel. *Phil. Trans.* ser. B **266,** 185–93.

Becker, B. & Morton, W. R. (1964*a*). Phenylthiourea taste testing and glaucoma. *Arch. Ophthal., Chicago* **72,** 323–7.

Becker, B. & Morton, W. R. (1964*b*). Taste sensitivity to phenylthiourea in glaucoma. *Science* **144,** 1347–8.

Becker, B., Kolker, A. E., & Ballin, N. (1966). Thyroid function and glaucoma. *Amer. J. Ophthal.* **61,** 997–9.

Beckman, L. & Eklund, A. E. (1961). ABO blood groups and gastric carcinoma. *Acta genet. Stat. med.* **11,** 363–9.

Beckman, L. (1968). Blood groups and serum alkaline phosphatase. *Ser. haemat.* **1,** no. 1, 137–52.

Beckman, L., Brönnestam, R., Cedergren, B., & Lidén, S. (1974). HL–A antigens, blood groups, serum groups and red cell enzyme types in psoriasis. *Hum. Hered.* **24,** 496–506.

Beet, E. A. (1946). Sickle-cell disease in the Balovale District of Northern Rhodesia. *E. Afr. med. J.* **23,** 75–86.

Beet, E. A. (1947). Sickle-cell disease in Northern Rhodesia. *E. Afr. med. J.* **24,** 212–22.

Beet, E. A. (1949). The genetics of the sickle-cell trait in a Bantu tribe. *Ann. Eugen., Lond.* **14,** 279–84.

Beffa, A. della, Mortara, A., & Serra, A. (1960). Gozzismo, cretinismo endemico, sordomutismo e gruppi sanguigni del sistema ABO. *Folia endocrin., Pisa* **13,** 670–80.

Behrman, S. J., Buettner-Janusch, J., Heglar, R., Gershowitz, H., & Tew, W. L. (1960). ABO(H) blood incompatibility as a cause of infertility: a new concept. *Amer. J. Obstet. Gynec.* **79,** 847–55.

Behzad, O., Lee, C. L., Gavin, J., & Marsh, W. L. (1973). A new anti-erythrocyte antibody in the Duffy system: anti-Fy4. *Vox Sang.* **24,** 337–42.

Beiguelman, B. (1962). Reação gustativa à fenil-tio-carbamida (PTC) e lepra. *Rev. bras. Leprol.* **30,** 111–24.

Beiguelman, B. (1963). Grupos sangüíneos e lepra. *Rev. bras. Leprol.* **31,** 34–44.

Beiguelman, B. (1964*a*). Sistema ABO e epidemiologia de lepra. *Rev. paulist. Med.* **65,** 80–6.

Beiguelman, B. (1964*b*). Taste sensitivity to phenylthiourea and leprosy. *Acta Genet. med. Gemell.* **13,** 193–6.

Belec, C., Chojnowski, J. R., Tkaczyk, F., & Żydowicz, L. (1971). Distribution of ABO blood groups and presence of group substances in the saliva of patients with gastric and duodenal ulcer. (In Polish.) *Pol. Arch. Med. wewnęt.* **46,** 557–62.

Benassi, G. & Atzeni, V. (1934). Contributo allo studio dei gruppi sanguigni e dei principali caratteri etno-antropologici nella popolazione sarda. II. I gruppi sanguigni negli alienati del Manicomio di Cagliari. *Atti Soc. Sci. med. nat. Cagliari* **36,** 3–18 in reprint.

Benda, C. E. & Bixby, E. M. (1939). Function of the thyroid and the pituitary in mongolism. *Amer. J. Dis. Child.* **58,** 1240–55.

Benda, N. & Menghini, G. (1957). Correliazioni tra gruppi sanguigni ed incidenza di alcune forme morbose. *Rif. med.* **71,** 169–72.

Benda, N. & Gambelunghe, C. (1962). Gruppi sanguigni e tumori. *Rif. med.* **76,** 266–8.

Bendien, S. G. T. (1926). Haemagglutinegehalte van het bloedserum bij carcinoompatiënten. *Ned. Tijdschr. Geneesk.* **1,** 2856–8.

Bennett, J. H. & Walker, C. B. V. (1955–6). Fertility and blood groups of some East Anglian blood donors. *Ann. hum. Genet.* **20,** 299–308.

Beolchini, P. E., Cresseri, A., Maria, B. de, Morganti, G., Peruzzotti, R., & Serra, A. (1958*a*). Rapporti tra neoplasie del collo dell'utero e gruppi sanguigni del sistema ABO (dati preliminari). *Analecta genet.* **6,** 109–11.

Beolchini, P. E., Cresseri, A., Maria, B. de, Morganti, G., Peruzzotti, R., & Serra, A. (1958*b*). Carcinoma gastrico e gruppi sanguigni del sistema ABO. *Analecta genet.* **6,** 112–17.

Berg, G., Wicke, D., & Schricker, T. (1967). Über die Beziehungen zwischen Blutgruppenfaktoren und Erkrankungen des Verdauungstraktes. *Med. Welt* **1,** 136–41.

Berg, K., Aarseth, S., Lundevall, J., & Reinskou, T. (1967). Blood groups and genetic serum types in diabetes mellitus. *Diabetologia, Berl.* **3,** 30–4.

Bergsjö, P. & Kolstad, P. (1962*a*). The ABO blood groups and cancer of the female genital tract. *Acta obstet. gynec. scand.* **41,** 397–404.

Bergsjö, P. & Kolstad, P. (1962*b*). The Rhesus factor and cancer of the female genital tract. *Acta obstet. gynec. scand.* **41,** 310–12.

BERNDT, H. (1966). Blutgruppe und Magenkrebs. *Folia haemat., Lpz.* **85,** 138-43.

BERNDT, H. & PIETSCHKER, H. (1966). Magenkrebs und Blutgruppe. *Dtsch Gesundheitswes.* **21,** 1864-9.

BERNECKER, L. (1936). Die Blutgruppenverteilung bei Scharlachkranken. *Mschr. Kinderheilk.* **66,** 391-6.

BERTRAMS, J. & KUWERT, E. (1976). Pers. comm. to A. E. Mourant.

BEST, W. R., LIMARZI, L. R., & PONCHER, H. G. (1949). Distribution of blood type in the leukemics. *J. Lab. clin. Med.* **34,** 1587.

BHATTACHARYYA, L. M., SENGUPTA, D. N., PAIN, G. C., BOSE, D. K., MUKHERJEE, S., & MONDAL, A. (1965). ABO blood group and smallpox. *J. Indian med. Ass.* **45,** 234-6.

BHENDE, Y. M., DESHPANDE, C. K., BHATIA, H. M., SANGER, R., RACE, R. R., MORGAN, W. T. J., & WATKINS, W. M. (1952). A 'new' blood-group character related to the ABO system. *Lancet* **i,** 903.

BIANCHI, C. M. (1960). Sull'associazione emogruppo A e carcinoma gastrico in Provincia di Cremona. *Boll. Soc. med.-chir. Cremona* **14,** 171-9.

BIANCHINI, F. (1937). Quoted by Marzi & Turchini (1952) and Asaro (1955).

BIBAWI, E. & KHATWA, H. A. (1961). The blood groups in relation to diabetes. *J. Egypt. med. Ass.* **44,** 655-9.

BIENZLE, U., AYENI, O., LUCAS, A. O., & LUZZATTO, L. (1972). Glucose-6-phosphate dehydrogenase and malaria. Greater resistance of females heterozygous for enzyme deficiency and of males with non-deficient variant. *Lancet* **i,** 107-10.

BILLINGTON, B. P. (1956*a*). ABO blood groups and gastro-duodenal diseases. *Australas. Ann. Med.* **5,** 141-8.

BILLINGTON, B. P. (1956*b*). Gastric cancer; relationships between ABO blood-groups, site, and epidemiology. *Lancet* **ii,** 859-62.

BILLINGTON, B. P. (1956*c*). A note on the distribution of ABO blood groups in bronchiectasis and portal cirrhosis. *Australas. Ann. Med.* **5,** 20-2.

BILLINGTON, B. P. (1957). A note on ABO blood group distribution in carcinoma of the oesophagus and cardia. *Australas. Ann. Med.* **6,** 56-7.

BIRNBAUM, D. & MENCZEL, J. (1959). ABO blood group distribution in ulcerative and malignant diseases of the gastrointestinal tract; incidence in three communal groups in Israel. *Gastroenterology* **37,** 210-13.

BJARNASON, O., BJARNASON, V., EDWARDS, J. H., FRIDRIKSSON, S., MAGNUSSON, M., MOURANT, A. E., & TILLS, D. (1973). The blood groups of Icelanders. *Ann. hum. Genet., Lond.* **36,** 425-58.

BLAKESLEE, A. F. & SALMON, M. R. (1931). Odour and taste blindness. *Eugen. News* **16,** 105-8.

BLAKESLEE, A. F. (1932). Genetics of sensory thresholds: taste for phenyl thio carbamide. *Proc. nat. Acad. Sci., Wash.* **18,** 120-30.

BLEGVAD, B. (1960*a*). ABO blood groups and stomal ulcer. *Dan. med. Bull.* **7,** 72-3.

BLEGVAD, B. (1960*b*). ABO blood groups and gastric acidity. *Dan. med. Bull.* **7,** 73-5.

BLOTEVOGEL, H. & BLOTEVOGEL, W. (1934). Blutgruppe und Daktylogram als Konstitutions-merkmale der Poliomyelitiskranken. *Z. Kinderheilk.* **56,** 143-69.

BLUMBERG, B. S. & HESSER, J. E. (1975). Anthropology and infectious disease. In *Physiological anthropology*, pp. 260-94. London, Oxford University Press.

BODMER, W. F., CANN, H., & PIAZZA, A. (1973). Differential genetic variability among polymorphisms as an indicator of natural selection. In *Histocompatibility testing 1972* (ed. J. Dausset & J. Colombani), pp. 753-67. Copenhagen, Munksgaard.

BODVALL, B. & ÖVERGAARD, B. (1966). The association between ABO blood groups and cholelithiasis with special reference to biliary distress following cholecystectomy. *Acta chir. scand.* **131,** 334-42.

BOERO, G. & CORADDU, M. (1965). Rapporti tra gruppi sanguigni e tumori delle ghiandole salivari nella provincia di Cagliari. *Rass. med. sarda* **68,** 117-21.

BONVINI, E. (1961). Rapporti tra gruppi sanguigni e leucemia acuta nell' infanza. *Minerva pediat.* **13,** 757-76.

BONVINI, E. & ZANETTI, P. (1961). Distribuzione dei gruppi sanguigni ABO negli immaturi. *Minerva pediat.* **13,** 1760-2.

BONZANINI, C. (1961). Gruppi sanguigni e malatie. *Fracastoro* **54,** 280-92.

BORSCHELL (1961). Quoted by Vogel & Helmbold (1972).

BOSTON COLLABORATIVE DRUG SURVEILLANCE PROGRAMME (1971). Relation between breast cancer and S blood-antigen system. *Lancet* **i,** 301-5.

BOTSZTEJN, C. (1942). Malignome und Blutgruppen. *Arch. Klaus-Stift. VererbForsch.* **17,** 413-20.

BOTTINI, E., LUCARELLI, P., AGOSTINO, R., PALMARINO, R., BUSINCO, L., & ANTOGNONI, G. (1971). Favism: association with erythrocyte acid phosphatase phenotype. *Science* **171,** 409-11.

BOTTINI, E., LUCARELLI, P., ORZALESI, M., PALMARINO, R., DI MINO, M., GLORIA, M., TERRENATO, L., & SPENNATI, G. F. (1972). Interaction between placental alkaline phosphatase and ABO system polymorphisms. (Effects on the clinical manifestations of feto-maternal ABO incompatibility.) *Vox Sang.* **23,** 413-19.

BOURKE, G. J., CLARKE, N., & THORNTON, E. H. (1965). Smallpox vaccination: ABO and Rhesus blood groups. *J. med. Genet.* **2,** 122-5.

BOURKE, J. B. & GRIFFIN, J. P. (1962). Blood-groups in benign and malignant prostatic hypertrophy. *Lancet* **ii,** 1279-80.

BRADBURY, F. C. S. (1934-5). Tuberculosis in relation to blood groups. *Tubercle* **16,** 113-19.

BRADLEY, M. A. & WALSH, R. J. (1965). Blood group distribution in patients with haemochromatosis. *Vox Sang.* **10,** 107-8.

BRAIN, P. (1952*a*). Sickle-cell anaemia in Africa. *Brit. med. J.* **ii,** 880.

BRAIN, P. (1952*b*). The sickle-cell trait: its clinical significance. *S. Afr. med. J.* **26,** 925-8.

BRAIN, P. (1953). The sickle-cell trait. A study of its distribution and effects in some Bantu tribes of South Central Africa. Thesis, Univ. of Capetown. Unpubl.

BRAND, N. (1963). Taste sensitivity and endemic goitre in Israel. *Ann. hum. Genet.* **26,** 321-4.

BRANDT, E. N. & WELSH, J. D. (1962). The ABO blood groups and muscular dystrophy. *Arch. Neurol., Chicago* n.s. **6,** 387-9.

BRAVETTA, G. (1930). Quoted by Marzi & Turchini (1952) and Asaro (1955).

BREITFELD (1963). Quoted by Vogel & Helmbold (1972).

BREMNER, C. G. (1961). Secretor status in carcinoma of the breast. *Lancet* **ii,** 1338.

BRENDEMOEN, O. J. (1960). The ABO groups in kryptogenetic epilepsy. *Acta path. microbiol. scand.* **48,** 176.

BRENDEMOEN, O. J. (1969). ABO blood-groups in patients with septal defects. *Lancet* **ii,** 1140.

BRITISH MEDICAL JOURNAL (1972). ABO blood groups and abortion. (Leading article.) **iv,** 314-15.

BROCKMÜLLER (1962). Quoted by Vogel & Helmbold (1972).

BRODY, H., SMITH, L. W., & WOLFF, W. I. (1936). Blood grouping in the infectious diseases. *J. Lab. clin. Med.* **21,** 705-10.

BRONTE-STEWART, B., BOTHA, M. C., & KRUT, L. H. (1962). ABO blood groups in relation to ischaemic heart disease. *Brit. med. J.* **i,** 1646-50.

BUBNOV, YU. I. & KIRDAN, G. V. (1972). ABO blood groups and their correlation with malignant tumours in children. (In Russian.) *Genetika* **8,** no. 11, 144-6.

BUCHANAN, J. A. & HIGLEY, E. T. (1921). The relationship of blood-groups to disease. *Brit. J. exp. Path.* **2,** 247-55.

BUCKWALTER, J. A., TURNER, J. H., RATERMAN, L., & TIDRICK, R. T. (1957). On the etiological role of heredity in fractures. *Surg. Forum* **7,** 610-14.

BUCKWALTER, J. A. & KNOWLER, L. A. (1958). Blood donor controls for blood group disease researches. *Amer. J. hum. Genet.* **10,** 164-74.

BUCKWALTER, J. A., TIDRICK, R. T., KNOWLER, L. A., WOHLWEND, E. B., COLTER, D. C., TURNER, J. H., RATERMAN, L., GAMBER, H. H., ROLLER, G. J., POLLOCK, C. B., & NAIFEH, V. K. (1958). The Iowa blood type disease research project. *J. Iowa med. Soc.* **48,** 78-81.

BUCKWALTER, J. A., TURNER, J. H., GAMBER, H. H., RATERMAN, L., SOPER, R. T., & KNOWLER, L. A. (1959). Psychoses, intracranial neoplasms, and genetics. *Arch. Neurol. Psychiat.* **81,** 480–5.

BUCKWALTER, J. A., SCOY, R. E. VAN, & KNOWLER, L. E. (1960). ABO blood groups of siblings of duodenal ulcer patients. *Brit. med. J.* **ii,** 1643–4.

BUCKWALTER, J. A., KARK, A. E., & KNOWLER, L. A. (1961). A study in human genetics. The ABO blood groups and disease in South Africa. *Arch. inter. Med.* **107,** 558–67.

BUCKWALTER, J. A. (1962). Peptic ulcer and the blood groups. *Ann. N. Y. Acad. Sci.* **99,** 81–8.

BUCKWALTER, J. A., NAIFEH, G. S., & AUER, J. E. (1962). Rheumatic fever and the blood groups. *Brit. med. J.* **ii,** 1023–7.

BUCKWALTER, J. A. & TWEED, G. V. (1962). The Rhesus and MN blood groups and disease. *J. Amer. med. Ass.* **179,** 479–85.

BUCKWALTER, J. A. (1964). Diabetes mellitus and the blood groups. *Diabetes* **13,** 164–8.

BUCKWALTER, J. A., POLLOCK, C. B., HASELTON, G., KROHN, J. A., NANCE, M. J., FERGUSON, J. L., BONDI, R. L., JACOBSEN, J. J., & LUBIN, A. H. (1964). The Iowa blood type disease research project: II. *J. Iowa med. Soc.* **54,** 58–66.

BUNKER, H. A. & MEYERS, S. (1927). Blood groups in general paralysis. *J. Lab. clin. Med.* **12,** 415–26.

BURNETT, D., WOOD, S. M., & BRADWELL, A. R. (1975). Plasma protein profiles of serum and amniotic fluid in normal pregnancy and pre-eclampsia. *Protides of the biological fluids*, 23rd Coll., Brugge, 349–52.

BUSI, B. R. (1972). Taste sensitivity to phenylthiourea among leprosy and filarial patients in coastal Andhra Pradesh. *Acta Genet. med. Gemellol.* **21,** 332–6.

BUTTS, D. C. A. (1950). A heretofore unreported agglutinable human blood factor and its possible relationship to blackwater fever. *Amer. J. trop. Med.* **30,** 663–7.

CAGLIERO, L. (1961). Rapporti fra gruppi sanguigni, carcinoma e fibromioma dell'utero. *Trasfus. Sangue* **6,** 58–64.

CALLENDER, S. T., DENBOROUGH, M. A., & SNEATH, J. (1957). Blood groups and other inherited characters in pernicious anaemia. *Brit. J. Haemat.* **3,** 107–14.

CAMERINI RIVIERA, L. (1960). Distribuzione dei gruppi sanguigni nei portatori di carcinoma gastrico e ulcere peptiche. *Folia hered. path.* **9,** 179–84.

CAMERON, G. L. & STAVELEY, J. M. (1957). Blood group P substance in hydatid cyst fluids. *Nature, Lond.* **179,** 147–8.

CAMERON, J. M. (1958). Blood-groups in tumours of salivary tissue. *Lancet* **i,** 239–40.

CAMERON, J. M. & IZATT, M. M. (1962). The ABO and rhesus blood groups in Perthes' disease. *J. clin. Path.* **15,** 163–8.

CAMPBELL, A. C. P., GAISFORD, W., PATERSON, E., & STEWARD, J. K. (1961). Tumours in children. A survey carried out in the Manchester region. *Brit. med. J.* **i,** 448–60.

CAMPBELL, A. E. R. (1956). Blood groups in tuberculosis. *Tubercle* **37,** 89–92.

CAMPS, F. E., DODD, B. E., & LINCOLN, P. J. (1969). Frequencies of secretors and non-secretors of ABH group substances among 1,000 alcoholic patients. *Brit. med. J.* **iv,** 457–9.

CANESTRI, G. (1963). I gruppi sanguigni A-B-O in relazione alla prematuranza e alla postmaturanza. *Minerva pediat.* **15,** 239–42.

CANÓNICO, A. N. & STAGNARA, R. F. (1955). Quoted by Hogg & Pack (1957).

CAPITOLO, G., GUALANDRI, V., & SERRA, A. (1965). Nota sull'associazione tra varici agli arti inferiori e gruppi sanguigni. *Minerva med.* **56,** 2514–15.

CAPPELLINI, E. & GUFFANTI, A. (1956). Gruppi sanguigni e neoplasie. Inchiesta su 449 casi di tumori gastrici e 248 casi di tumori broncopolmonari. *Rass. ital. Chir. Med.* **5,** 555–65.

CARCASSI, U., CEPPELLINI, R., & PITZUS, F. (1957). Frequenza della talassemia in quattro popolazioni sarde e suoi rapporti con la distribuzione dei gruppi sanguigni e della malaria. *Boll. Ist. sieroter. milan.* **36,** 206–18.

CARLO, G. DI & RIDULFO, S. (1958). Gruppi sanguigni, carcinoma dello stomaco ed ulcera gastro-duodenale. *Sintesi* **2,** 1–10.

CARRERA, F. (1963). Rapporti fra i gruppi sanguigni e malattie: fibroma e carcinoma dell'utero. *Minerva ginec.* **15,** 39–41.

CARRESCIA. Quoted by Asaro (1955).

CARTER, C. O. & HESLOP, B. (1957). ABO blood groups and broncho-pneumonia in children. *Brit. J. prev. & soc. Med.* **11,** 214–16.

CARTER, C. O. (1976). The global incidence of genetic illnesses. In *Equalities and inequalities in health* (eds. C. O. Carter & J. Peel), pp. 1–12.

CARTER, C. O. & PEEL, J. eds. (1976). *Equalities and inequalities in health. Proceedings of the twelfth annual symposium of the Eugenics Society, London 1975.* London, Academic Press.

CARTER, R. L., HITCHCOCK, E. R., & SATO, F. (1964). Malignant glioma and ABO blood group. *Brit. med. J.* **i,** 122.

CARTWRIGHT, R. A. & SUNDERLAND, E. (1967). Phenylthiocarbamide (PTC) tasting ability in populations in the North of England: with a note on endemic goitre. *Acta genet. Stat. med.* **17,** 211–21.

CASELLI, G. (1955). Ricerche sulla distribuzione del fattore Rh e dei gruppi sanguigni nella frenastenia. *G. Psichiat. Neuropat.* **83,** 281–5.

CAVALLI, A., CORRADI, C., & CALDERINI, P. (1964). Indagine statistica nei rapporti fra emogruppi del sistema ABO ed affezioni cancerose. *Minerva med. parte sci.* **55,** 326–9.

CAVALLI-SFORZA, L. L. & BODMER, W. F. (1971). *The genetics of human populations.* San Francisco, W. H. Freeman.

CELAYA, M. (1939). Los grupos sanguíneos en relación con la tuberculosis pulmonar y los habitos constitucionales. *Rev. argent. Tuberc.* **5,** 49–74.

CELESTINO, D. & SILVAGNI, C. (1964). Sulla distribuzione dei gruppi sanguigni del sistema ABO negli individui affetti da carcinoma laringeo. *Valsalva* **40,** 211–16.

CERRATO, O. & GHIBAUDI, D. (1968). Gruppi sanguigni e artrite reumatoide. *Arch. Ist. Osped. S. Corona* **33,** 468–73.

CERRI, B. (1938). I gruppi sanguigni nella lebbra come eventuale elemento di resistenza. *G. ital. Derm. Sif.* **79,** 791–809.

CESARINO-NETTO, J. B. (1952). Grupos sanguíneos na lepra. *Arch. min. Leprol.* **12,** 271–81.

CHAKRAVARTTI, M. R., VERMA, B. K., HANURAV, T. V., & VOGEL, F. (1966). Relation between smallpox and the ABO blood groups in a rural population of West Bengal. *Humangenetik* **2,** 78–80.

CHAKRAVARTTI, M. R. & VOGEL, F. (1966). Relation between incidence of small-pox and the OAB system of blood groups. *J. Indian anthrop. Soc.* **1,** 119–28.

CHALMERS, J. N. M., IKIN, E. W., & MOURANT, A. E. (1948). Basque blood groups. *Nature, Lond.* **162,** 27.

CHALMERS, J. N. M., IKIN, E. W., & MOURANT, A. E. (1949). The ABO Mn and Rh blood groups of the Basque people. *Amer. J. phys. Anthrop.* n.s. **7,** 529–44.

CHARNEY, M. (1969). *ABO blood groups and asthma—a suspected correlation.* Ph.D. thesis, Univ. of Colorado.

CHESNEY, A. M., CLAWSON, T. A., & WEBSTER, B. (1928). Endemic goitre in rabbits. i. Incidence and characteristics. *Bull. Johns Hopkins Hosp.* **43,** 261–77.

CHEW, B. K., SEAH, C. S., ONG, Y. W., & TAN, L. (1973). ABO blood groups in primary carcinoma of the liver. *Aust. N. Z. J. Med.* **3,** 129–30.

CHISALE, E. (1963). Il gruppo sanguigno delle pazienti con carcinoma uterino. *Pathologica* **55,** 133–5.

CHOMINSKIJ, B. & SCHUSTOVA, L. (1928). Zur Frage des Zusammenhangs zwischen Blutgruppe und psychischer Erkrankung. *Z. ges. Neurol. Psychiat.* **115,** 303–8.

CHOWN, B. & LEWIS, M. (1963). ABO blood groups of mongols. *Canad. med. Ass. J.* **89,** 906.

CHUDINA, A. P. (1963). On blood groups in stomach carcinoma. (In Russian.) *Vopr. Onkol.* **8,** 18–23.

CHUNG, C. S. & MORTON, N. E. (1961). Selection at the ABO locus. *Amer. J. hum. Genet.* **13,** 9–27.

CHUNG, C. S., WITKOP, C. J., & HENRY, J. L. (1964). A genetic study of dental caries with special reference to PTC taste sensitivity. *Amer. J. hum. Genet.* **16,** 231–45.

CICHECKA, K. (1965). Distribution of the blood groups of the ABO and Rh systems in diseases of the blood-forming organs. (In Polish.) *Folia med. cracov.* **7,** 401–27.

CISWICKA-SZNAJDERMAN, M., SZNAJDERMAN, M., JANUSZEWICZ, W., DZIERZYKRAY-ROGALSKI, T., PROMINSKA, E., & CHARZEWSKI, J. (1973). Studi clinici e metabolici in soggetti giovani con infarto miocardico. *Minerva med.* **64,** 399–404.

CITRON, K. M. (1956). Rhesus (D) factor in sarcoidosis. *Lancet* **i,** 969.

CLARKE, C. A., EDWARDS, J. Wyn, HADDOCK, D. R. W., HOWEL-EVANS, A. W., MCCONNELL, R. B., & SHEPPARD, P. M. (1956). ABO blood groups and secretor character in duodenal ulcer. *Brit. med. J.* **ii,** 725–31.

CLARKE, C. A., EVANS, D. A. Price, MCCONNELL, R. B., & SHEPPARD, P. M. (1959). Secretion of blood group antigens and peptic ulcer. *Brit. med. J.* **i,** 603–7.

CLARKE, C. A., MCCONNELL, R. B., & SHEPPARD, P. M. (1960). ABO blood groups and secretor character in rheumatic carditis. *Brit. med. J.* **i,** 21–3.

CLARKE, C. A. (1961). Blood groups and disease. In *Progress in medical genetics.* Vol. 1, pp. 81–119. Grune and Stratton, New York.

CLARKE, C. A., HOBSON, D., MCKENDRICK, O. M., ROGERS, S. C., & SHEPPARD, P. M. (1975). Spina bifida and anencephaly: miscarriage as possible cause. *Brit. med. J.* **iv,** 743–6.

CLEMENS, K. & WALSH, R. J. (1955). Blood groups and acquired haemolytic anaemia. *Aust. J. Sci.* **17,** 136–7.

CLEMENTS, F. W. (1955). A thyroid blocking agent as a cause of endemic goitre in Tasmania: preliminary communication. *Med. J. Austr.* **ii,** 369–70.

CLEVE, H. (1966). Die Verteilung der Gc-Typen und Gc-Allele bei Kranken mit Diabetes mellitus und chronischer Polyarthritis. *Humangenetik* **2,** 355–62.

CLEVE, H. (1973). The variants of the group-specific component. A review of their distribution in human populations. *Israel J. med. Sci.* **9,** 1133–46.

CLIFFORD, P. (1970). Blood-groups and nasopharyngeal carcinoma. *Lancet* **ii,** 48–9.

COCCHIA, N., MESSINA, N., & PISCICELLI, I. (1963). Gruppi sanguigni e malattie chirurgiche. *Rass. int. Clin. Terap.* **43,** 129–36.

COFFEY, V. P. (1974). Twenty-one years' study of anencephaly in Dublin. *Irish med. J.* **67,** 553–8.

COHEN, A. S., BOYD, W. C., GOLDWASSER, S., CATHCART, E. S., & HEISLER, M. (1963). Correlation between rheumatic diseases and Rh blood groups. *Nature, Lond.* **200,** 1215.

COHEN, B. H. & SAYRE, J. E. (1968). Further observations on the relationship of maternal ABO and Rh types to fetal death. *Amer. J. hum. Genet.* **20,** 310–44.

COHEN, B. H. (1970). ABO and Rh incompatibility. *Amer. J. hum. Genet.* **22,** 412–52.

COMPSTON, D. A. S., BATCHELOR, J. R., & MCDONALD, W. I. (1976). B-lymphocyte alloantigens associated with multiple sclerosis. *Lancet* **ii,** 1261–5.

CONNERTH, O. (1927). Über Blutgruppen bei Tuberkulose. *Z. Tuberk.* **48,** 140–2.

CONSTANS, J. & VIAU, M. (1975). Hématologie géographique.—Une nouvelle mutation Pi^N au locus Pi dans les populations humaines. *C. R. Acad. Sci. Paris* **281,** 1361–4.

CORDONE, G. & TAVELLA, F. (1963). Gruppi sanguigni e leucemia nell'età pediatrica. *Minerva pediat.* **15,** 631–3.

CORDONE, G. & MARCHI, A. G. (1964). Gruppi sanguigni e immaturità. *Minerva pediat.* **16,** 899–901.

CORNIL, A. & PIRART, J. (1961). Diabète, hémachromatose et groupes sanguins. *Path. Biol.* **9,** 1911–15.

CORCIANU, V., OPREANU, O., & BRATU, I. (1958). Blutgruppe und Magen-Zwölffingerdarmgeschwür bzw. Magenkrebs. *Zbl. Chir.* **83,** 2201–5.

COTTER, C. A., STAVELEY, J. M., & THOMPSON, H. R. (1961). ABO and Rh(D) blood groups and cancer of the stomach in Auckland. *N. Z. med. J.* **60,** 372–4.

COTTER, C. A., STAVELEY, J. M., & THOMPSON, H. R. (1962). ABO and Rh(D) blood groups in cancer of the female genital tract and cancer of the lung in Auckland. *N. Z. med. J.* **61,** 147–8.

COULTER, J. R. (1962). Staphylococcal infection and blood groups. *Nature, Lond.* **195,** 301.

COVARRUBIAS, E., BARZELATTO, J., STEVENSON, C., BOBADILLA, E., PARDO, A., & BECKERS, C. (1965). Taste sensitivity to phenylthio-carbamide and endemic goitre among Pewenche Indians. *Nature, Lond.* **205,** 1036.

COX, D. Wilson & HUBER, O. (1976). Rheumatoid arthritis and alpha-l-antitrypsin. *Lancet* **i,** 1216–17.

CRAIG, J. & WANG, I. (1955). Blood groups in diabetes mellitus. *Glasg. med. J.* **36,** 261–6.

CRAWFORD, H., CUTBUSH, M., & MOLLISON, P. L. (1953). Hemolytic disease of the newborn due to anti-A. *Blood* **8,** 620–39.

CREGER, W. P. & SORTOR, A. T. (1956). The incidence of blood group A in pernicious anemia. *Arch. int. Med.* **98,** 136–41.

CUADRADO, R. R. & DAVENPORT, F. M. (1970). Antibodies to influenza viruses in military recruits from Argentina, Brazil and Colombia. *Bull. World Hlth Org.* **42,** 873–84.

CUDKOWICZ, L. (1956). Rhesus (D) factor in sarcoidosis. *Lancet* **i,** 480.

CUDWORTH, A. G. & WOODROW, J. C. (1975). Evidence for HL-A-linked genes in 'juvenile' diabetes mellitus. *Brit. med. J.* **iii,** 133–5.

CURTAIN, C. C., GAJDUSEK, D. C., & ZIGAS, V. (1961). Studies on kuru. ii. Serum proteins in natives from the kuru region of New Guinea. *Amer. J. trop. Med. Hyg.* **10,** 92–109.

CURTONI, E. & MORGANTE, F. (1964). Rapporti fra gruppi sanguigni e malattie in Abruzzo. *Trasfus. Sangue.* **9,** 350–7.

CUTBUSH, M., MOLLISON, P. L., & PARKIN, D. M. (1950). A new human blood group. *Nature, Lond.* **165,** 188.

CUTRERA, A. & LEONI, R. (1959). L'incidenza di gruppo (sistema ABO) nelle portatrici di neoplasia mammaria, ovarica ed uterina. *Riv. Ostet. Ginec.* **14,** 737–44.

CZAPLICKI, S., STANOWSKI, E., & SZEPIETOWSKI, J. (1964). Blood groups in cholelithiasis, gastric cancer and ulcer. (In Polish.) *Pol. Tyg. lek.* **19,** 630–2.

DAMBROSIO, F. (1965). Gruppi sanguigni e predisposizione alle malatie. Nota I. Rapporti tra emogruppi del sistema ABO e neoplasie maligne dell'apparato genitale femminile. *Ann. Ostet. Ginec.* **5,** 343–63.

DAMIAN, R. T. (1964). Molecular mimicry: antigen sharing by parasite and host and its consequences. *Amer. Naturalist* **98,** 129–49.

DAMON, A. (1957). Blood groups in pituitary adenoma—'suspected correlation' reexamined. *Science* **126,** 452–3.

DAO, C., T'ANG, Y., CH'I, W. L., & TS'AI, Y. H. (1958). The ABO blood groups and peptic ulceration in Shanghai. *Chin. med. J.* **77,** 76–8.

DAS GUPTA, C. R., CHATTERJEA, J. B., & RAY, R. N. (1955). Incidence of Rh(D) in Cooley's anaemia. *Bull. Calcutta Sch. trop. Med.* **3/4,** 148.

DAUSSET, J. (1954). Leuco-agglutinins. iv. Leuco-agglutinins and blood transfusion. *Vox. Sang.* **4,** 190–8.

DAUSSET, J. & BRECY, H. (1957). Identical nature of leucocyte antigens detectable in monozygotic twins by means of immune iso-leuco-agglutinins. *Nature, Lond.* **180,** 1430.

DAUSSET, J. (1958). Iso-leuco-anticorps. *Acta haemat.* **20,** 156–66.

DAUSSET, J. & COLOMBANI, J. (ed.) (1973). *Histocompatibility testing 1972.* Copenhagen, Munksgaard.

DAUSSET, J. & SVEJGAARD, A. (presidents) (1977). *HLA and disease. Predisposition to disease and clinical implications.* Abstracts of the 1st International Symposium on HLA and diseases. Paris. INSERM.

DAVEY, W. W. & ELEBUTE, E. A. (1963). ABO blood groups in relation to duodenal ulceration among the Yorubas of Western Nigeria. *Gut* **4,** 367.

DAVID, T. J. (1970). Blood-groups and heart-disease in Bristol. *Lancet* **i,** 570.

DAWSON, T. A. J., WELSHMAN, S. G., & KOPEĆ, A. C. (1966). Serum protein bound iodine and the ABO blood groups. *Vox Sang.* **11,** 230–1.

DE GEORGE, F. V. (1970). Differences in Rh type between age groups of leukaemia patients. *Nature, Lond.* **228,** 168–9.

DENBOROUGH, M. A. (1962). Blood groups and ischaemic heart disease. *Brit. med. J.* **ii,** 927.

DENBOROUGH, M. A. & DOWNING, H. J. (1968). Secretor status in asthma and hay fever. *J. med. Genet.* **5,** 302–5.

DEROM, R. & THIERY, M. (1964). ABO blood-groups and cancer. *Lancet* **ii,** 822.

DESAI, R. G. & CREGER, W. P. (1964*a*). Present knowledge of the association of blood groups and diseases with special reference to the studies on gastric cancer in U.S.A. and Japan. 9th *Congr. int. Soc. Blood Transfus.*, Mexico, 1962. *Bibl. haemat.* **19,** 709–18.

DESAI, R. G. & CREGER, W. P. (1964*b*). Salivary secretion of A, B and H substances in gastric cancer in Japan and the U.S.A. *Transfusion, Philad.* **4,** 188–94.

DIAMANTOPOULOS, J. (1928). Die Blutgruppen bei verschiedenen Krankheiten, *Dtsch. med. Wschr.* **54,** 1839–40.

DICK, W., SCHNEIDER, W., & BROCKMÜLLER, K. (1962). Über das gegensätzliche Verhalten der Blutgruppen A_1 und A_2. Ein weiterer Beitrag zur Frage: Blutgruppen und Krankheiten. *Dtsch. med. Wschr.* **87,** 2567–73.

DICK, W., SCHNEIDER, W., BROCKMÜLLER, K., & MAYER, W. (1963). Thromboembolische Erkrankungen und Blutgruppenzugehörigkeit. *Med. Welt* **24,** 1296–8.

DICKINS, A. M., RICHARDSON, J. R. E., PIKE, L. A., & ROBERTS, J. A. Fraser (1956). Further observations on ABO blood-group frequencies and toxaemia of pregnancy. *Brit. med. J.* **i,** 776–7.

DIENST, A. (1905). Das Eklampsiegift. *Zbl. Gynäk.* **29,** 353–64.

DIMITRI, V., PALAZZO, R., TENCONI, J., & MENZANI, A. C. (1939). Los grupos sanguíneos en algunas affecciones del sistema nervioso y en particular en las heredofamiliares. *Sem. Méd., B. Aires* **46,** 1125–35.

DODGE, J. A. (1971). Abnormal distribution of ABO blood groups in infantile pyloric stenosis. *J. med. Genet.* **8,** 468–70.

DOES, J. A. VAN DER, ELKERBOUT, F., D'AMARO, J., STEEN, G. VAN DER, LOGHEM, E. VAN, MEERA KHAN, P., BERNINI, L. F., LEEUWEN, A. VAN, & ROOD, J. J. VAN (1973). HL-A typing in Dutch patients with Hodgkin's disease. In *Histocompatibility testing 1972* (ed. J. Dausset and J. Colombani), pp. 579–86. Copenhagen, Munksgaard.

DOLL, R., SWYNNERTON, B. F., & NEWELL, A. C. (1960). Observations on blood group distribution in peptic ulcer and gastric cancer. *Gut* **1,** 31–5.

DOLL, R., DRANE, H., & NEWELL, A. C. (1961). Secretion of blood group substances in duodenal, gastric and stomal ulcer, gastric carcinoma, and diabetes mellitus. *Gut* **2,** 352–9.

DOMARADZKA-WOŹNIAK, A. (1964). Correlation between blood-group and occurrence of cervix uteri and breast cancer. (In Polish.) *Pol. Tyg. lek.* **19,** 1726–9.

DOMINICI, L. M. (1965). Rapporti fra diabete mellito e gruppi sanguigni ABO ed Rh nella Repubblica di San Marino. *Ann. Sclavo* **7,** 318–23.

DOONER, H. & AGUAYO, E. (1960). Cancer gástrico y grupos sanguíneos. *Rev. méd. Chile* **88,** 287–9.

D'ORMEA & CENTINI (1942). Quoted by Marzi & Turchini (1952) and Asaro (1955).

DORN, H. (1959). Blutgruppen und endogenes Ekzem. *Acta Allergol.* **13,** 442–53.

DOSSENA, G. & LANZARA, V. (1925). L'isoagglutinazione studiata nei riguardi dell'abito morfologico e delle neoplasie della sfera genitale mulierre. *Ann. Ostet. Ginec.* **47,** 163–79.

DOWNIE, A. W., MEIKLEJOHN, G., VINCENT, L. S., RAO, A. R., BABU, B. V. S., & KEMPE, C. H. (1965). Smallpox frequency and severity in relation to A, B and O blood groups. *Bull. World Hlth Org.* **33,** 623–5.

DUBLIN, T. D., BERNANKE, A. D., PITT, E. L., MASSELL, B. F., ALLEN, F. H., & AMEZCUA, F. (1964). Red blood cell groups and ABH secretor system as genetic indicators of susceptibility to rheumatic fever and rheumatic heart disease. *Brit. med. J.* **ii,** 775–9.

DUFOURT, A., ETIENNE-MARTIN, P., & MARTIN, Q. (1933). Tuberculose pulmonaire et groupes sanguins. *C. R. Soc. Biol., Paris* **112,** 1407–8.

DUJARRIC DE LA RIVIÈRE, R., & KOSSOVITCH, N. (1928). Recherches sur les groupes sanguins dans quelques états pathologiques. *Ukr. Zbl. Blutgr.* **3,** 44–7.

DUNGERN, E. VON & HIRSZFELD, L. (1910). Über Vererbung gruppenspezifischer Strukturen des Blutes. ii. *Z. ImmunForsch. i.* Originale **6,** 284–92.

DUNSFORD, I. & OWEN, G. (1960). Distribution of the ABO blood groups in cases of acquired haemolytic anaemia. *Brit. med. J.* **i,** 1172–3.

DUTTA, A. K., MONDAL, S. B., & DUTTA, S. B. (1969). ABO blood group and secretory status in vitiligo. *J. Indian med. Ass.* **53,** 186–9.

EDWARDS, J. H. (1976). Single factor predisposition to disease. In *Equalities and inequalities in health* (eds. C. O. Carter & J. Peel), pp. 35–44.

EHRLICH, P. & MORGENROTH, J. (1900). Ueber Haemolysine. iii. Mitteilung. *Berl. klin. Wschr.* **37,** 453–8.

EISENBERG, H., GREENBERG, R. A., & YESNER, R. (1958). ABO blood groups and gastric cancer. *J. chronic Dis.* **8,** 342–8.

EKLUND, A. E. (1965). Studies on the relation between ABO blood groups and gastric carcinoma. *Acta chir. scand.* **129,** 211–26.

ERB, I. H., DOYLE, H. S., & HEAL, F. C. (1938). Blood groups in poliomyelitis. *Canad. pub. Hlth J.* **29,** 441–2.

ERIKSSON, S. (1964). Pulmonary emphysema and alpha$_1$-antitrypsin deficiency. *Acta med. scand.* **175,** 197–205.

ERIKSSON, S. (1965). *Studies in α_1-antitrypsin deficiency*. Lund, Carl Bloms. Also published as supplement to *Acta med. scand.* **177.**

ERNST, F. (1928). Blutgruppen und Tuberkulose. *Klin. Wschr.* **7,** 1036–7.

ESPEJO SOLÁ, J. (1931). Los grupos sanguíneos en las diferentes formas de alienación mental. *Sem. méd., B. Aires* **38,** 699–706.

ESQUIVEL, E. L. (1960). The ABO blood group and breast carcinoma in Filipinos. *Philipp. J. Surg.* **15,** 284–5.

ESTEVEZ, R. A. (1963). Grupos sanguíneos y cancer. *Sem. méd., B. Aires* **122,** 1121–8.

ETCHEVERRY, M. A. (1945). El factor rhesus; su genética e importancia clínica. *Día méd.* **17,** 1237–59.

EVANS, C. C., LEWINSÖHN, H. C., & EVANS, J. M. (1977). Frequency of HLA antigens in asbestos workers with and without pulmonary fibrosis. *Brit. med. J.* **i,** 603–5.

EVANS, D. A. Price, KITCHIN, F. D., & RIDING, J. E. (1962). The metabolism of methylthiouracil and thiopentone in tasters and non-tasters of P.T.C. *Ann. hum. Genet.* **26,** 123–33.

EVANS, D. A. Price, DONOHOE, W. T. A., BANNERMAN, R. M., MOHN, J. F., & LAMBERT, R. M. (1966). Blood-group gene localization through a study of mongolism. *Ann. hum. Genet.* **30,** 49–67.

EVANS, D. A. Price, HORWICH, L., MCCONNELL, R. B., & BULLEN, M. F. (1968). Influence of the ABO blood groups and secretor status on bleeding and on perforation of duodenal ulcer. *Gut* **9,** 319–22.

FAGERHOL, M. K. & BRAEND, M. (1965). Serum prealbumin: polymorphism in man. *Science* **149,** 986–7.

FANCONI (1945). Quoted by Jungeblut *et al.* (1947).

FARJOT, A. (1933). Réaction de Schick et groupes sanguins. *C. R. Soc. Biol., Paris* **113,** 773.

FARJOT, A. & SPRIET, A. (1934). Les groupes sanguins chez les paralytiques généraux. *Ann. Méd. lég.* **14,** 574.

FARR, A. D. (1960). Blood group frequencies in some allergic conditions and in malaria. *J. Inst. Sci. Tech.* **6,** 32–3.

FATTOVICH, G. (1928). Gruppi sanguigni e malattie mentali. *Riv. Neurol.* **1,** 207–12.

FAVILLI, G. (1959). La ricerca dei gruppi sanguigni negli epilettici. *Riv. Pat. nerv. ment.* **80,** 367–9.

FEDELI, M. (1959). Sensibilità alla PTC, funzione tiroidea e metabolismo basale. *Riv. Antrop.* **46,** 149–58.

FEDRICK, J. (1972). ABO blood-groups and epilepsy. *Lancet* **ii,** 1034.

FERRARI, A. V. (1930). Psoriasi e gruppi sanguigni. *G. ital. Derm.* **71,** 1087–9.

FIORI, E. (1932). Dei rapporti tra gruppi sanguigni e splenomegalie malariche. *Riv. Malariol.* **11,** 487–92.

FISCHER, W. (1928–31). Untersuchungen über die Vererbung der Disposition bei Scharlach. *Arb. Staatsinst. exp. Ther. Frankfurt* **21–5,** 219–29.

FITCH, W. M. & MARGOLIASH, E. (1967). Construction of phylogenetic trees. *Science* **155,** 279–84.

FLAMM, L. & FRIEDRICH, R. (1929). Blutgruppen und chirurgische Erkrankungen. *Dtsch. Z. Chir.* **219,** 289–96.

FLEMING, T. C., CAPLAN, H. W., HYMAN, G. A., & KITCHIN, F. D. (1967). ABO blood groups and polyps of the colon. *Brit. med. J.* **ii,** 526–7.

FOCHI. Quoted by Tagliaferro (1937*b*).

FODOR, O. & URCAN, S. (1966). Hereditary aspects of duodenal ulcer in relation to blood group and secretor status. *Rev. roum. Med. interne* **3,** 301–3.

FORBAT, A., LEHMANN, H., & SILK, E. (1953). Prolonged apnoea following injection of succinyldicholine. *Lancet* **ii,** 1067.

FOSSATI, C. (1968). Studio dei gruppi sanguigni e del fattore Rh- negativo in pazienti arabo-libici della Cirenaica affetti da tuberculosi polmonare. *Rass. clin.-sci. Ist. biochim. ital.* **44,** 113–15.

FOX, A. L. (1931). Six in ten 'tasteblind' to bitter chemical. *Sci. News Lett., Wash.* **19,** 249.

FOX, A. L. (1932). The relationship between chemical constitution and taste. *Proc. nat. Acad. Sci., U.S.A.* **18,** 115–20.

FRANKS, M. B. (1946). Blood agglutinins in filariasis. *Proc. Soc. exp. Biol. Med.* **62,** 17–18.

FRANQUELO RAMOS, E. & ELOY-GARCIA, F. (1966). Grupos sanguíneos y enfermedades del aparato digestivo. *Rev. esp. Enferm. Apar. dig.* **25,** 654–61.

FRASER, G. R. (1963). A genetical study of goitre. *Ann. hum. Genet.* **26,** 335–46.

FRASER, G. R. (1970). Some aetiological aspects of non-endemic childhood hypothyroidism. *J. Génét. hum.* **18,** 169–89.

FREIRE-MAIA, N., KARAM, E., & MEHL, H. (1968). P.T.C. sensitivity among psychiatric patients. *Acta genet. Stat. med.* **18,** 31–7.

FURUHATA, T., TSUGE, K., YOKOYAMA, M., & ISHII, T. (1954). Racial difference of blood groups and blood types. *Proc. Japan Acad.* **30,** 405–8.

GAISFORD, W. & CAMPBELL, A. C. P. (1958). In *British Empire Cancer Campaign 36th annual report 1958*, part ii, 533–8.

GALA, J. & GALA, J. (1966). ABO blood groups and mental diseases. (In Polish.) *Wiad. lek.* **19,** 29–31.

GARCIA, J. H., OKAZAKI, H., & ARONSON, S. A. (1963). Blood-group frequencies and astrocytomata. *J. Neurosurg.* **20,** 397–9.

GARG, M. P. & PAHWA, J. M. (1965). Primary glaucoma and blood groups. *J. All-India Ophthal. Soc.* **13,** 127–9.

GARRETT, J. V., NICHOLSON, A., WHITTAKER, J. S., RIDWAY, J. C., & BOWMAN, C. M. (1971). Blood-groups and secretor status in patients with salivary-gland tumours. *Lancet* **ii,** 1177–9.

GARRIGA, R. & GHOSSEIN, N. A. (1963). The ABO blood groups and their relation to the radiation response in carcinoma of the cervix. *Cancer, Philad.* **16,** 170–2.

GEDICKE, K. H. & WELLHÖNER, H. H. (1961). Beitrag zur Frage der Korrelation zwischen ABO-Blutgruppensystem, Magenkarzinom und Magenulcus. *Zbl. Chir.* **86,** 652–6.

GEISLER, P. & SARAF, I. (1965). Zur Frage der Beziehungen zwischen Blutgruppenzugehörigkeit und Bronchuskarzinom. *Zbl. Chir.* **90,** 2301–6.

GERAGA, W., GDULEWICZ, T., & WILCZYŃSKA, U. (1972). ABO blood-groups and the myocardial infarction. (In Polish.) *Wiad. lek.* **25,** 401–4.

GERSHOWITZ, H. & NEEL, J. V. (1965). The blood groups and secretor types in five potentially fatal diseases of Caucasian children. *Acta genet. Stat. med.* **15,** 261–308.

GERTLER, M. M. & WHITE, P. D. (1954). *Coronary heart disease in young adults. A multidisciplinary study.* Harvard University Press, Cambridge, Massachusetts.

GHOOI, A. M., KAMALPURIA, S. K., JAIN, P. K., & TANDON, P. L. (1970). Distribution of blood groups in cancer. *Indian J. Cancer* **7,** 296–305.

GHOSH, M. N., BISWAS, B. N., & CHATTERJEA, M. L. (1957). ABO blood groups and peptic ulcer in Indians. *Bull. Calcutta Sch. trop. Med.* **5,** 169.

GIANNANTONI, C. (1928). I gruppi sanguigni in relazione ad alcune malatie oculari. *Ann. Oftal. Clin. ocul.* **56,** 673–92.

GIBBS, P. (1974). Three cases of acute ketotic diabetes mellitus with myocarditis: a common viral origin? *Brit. med. J.* **iii,** 781–3.

GIBLETT, E. R. (1969). *Genetic markers in human blood.* Blackwell Scientific Publications, Oxford.

GIBLETT, E. R., KLEBANOFF, S. J., PINCUS, S. H., SWANSON, J., PARK, B. H., & MCCULLOUGH, J. (1971). Kell phenotypes in chronic granulomatous disease: a potential transfusion hazard. *Lancet* **i,** 1235–6.

GIMÉNEZ CAMARASA, J. M. (1968). Algunos aspectos en la genética del psoriasis. *Rev. clín. esp.* **108,** 40–2.

GIULI, P. DE (1959). Les groupes sanguins du système ABO et le facteur Rh dans les maladies mentales, 7th *Congr. int. Soc. Blood Tranfus.*, Rome, 1958. *Bibl. haemat.* **10,** 186–8.

GJØRUP, L. (1963). Blood groups and coronary occlusion. *Acta genet. Stat. med.* **13,** 178–83.

GLASS, G. B. J., ISHIMORI, A., & BUCKWALTER, J. A. (1962). ABO(H) blood group substances of the gastric juice in peptic ulcer, cancer of the stomach, and atrophic lesions of the gastric mucosa. *Gastroenterology* **42,** 443–54.

GLIDŽIĆ, V. & KRAJINOVIĆ, S. (1964). ABO groupes sanguins des malades avec ulcère duodenal. (In Serbo-Croat.) *Srpski Arkh. tselok. Lek.* **94,** 1191–6.

GLOBER, G., PEÑA, A. S., WHITEHEAD, R., GEAR, M. W. L., ROCA, M., KERRIGAN, G., & TRUELOVE, S. C. (1972). ABO blood groups, Rhesus factor and intestinal metaplasia of the stomach. *Brit. J. Cancer* **26,** 420–2.

GLYNN, A. A., GLYNN, L. E., & HOLBOROW, E. J. (1956). The secretor status of rheumatic-fever patients. *Lancet* **ii,** 759–62.

GLYNN, L. E. (1959). Pers. comm. to Clarke *et al.* (1960).

GLYNN, L. E. & HOLBOROW, E. J. (1961). Relation between blood groups, secretor status and susceptibility to rheumatic fever. *Arthr. Rheum.* **4,** 203–7.

GODBOLE, A. S. (1960). Distribution of ABO blood groups in cases of myocardial infarction. *J. postgrad. Med.* (*Bombay*) **6,** 144–6.

GÖHLER, W. & GÖHLER, I. (1963). Haptoglobinbestimmung bei Krankheiten unter besonderer Berücksichtigung von Nerven- und Geisteskrankheiten. *Acta Med. leg. soc.* **16,** 73–8.

GOEMINNE, L. (1962). De ABO-bloedgroepenverdeling bij leukemiepatiënten. *Belg. Tijdschr. Geneesk.* **18,** 386–8.

GOŁĄBEK, A. (1965). Gastric and duodenal ulcer and the ABO blood groups. (In Polish.) *Wiad. lek.* **18,** 731–5.

GOLDENBERG, I. S. & HAYES, M. A. (1958). Breast carcinoma and ABO blood groups. *Cancer, Philad.* **11,** 973–4.

GOLDFEDER, A. & FERSHING, J. L. (1937). Iso-agglutinins in association with malignant growth. *Amer. J. Cancer* **29,** 307–12.

GOLDSTEIN, M. (1929). La répartition des groupes sanguins parmi les cancereux. *Boll. Sez. ital. Soc. int. Microbiol.* **1,** no. 6, 134–5.

GOLOVACHEV, G. D. & BOKARIUS, L. V. (1972). Intrauterine selection and ABO incompatibility in humans. (In Russian.) *Genetika* **8,** 147–54.

GOODMAN, H. O. & THOMAS, J. J. (1966). ABO frequencies in mongolism. *Ann. hum. Genet.* **30,** 43–8.

GÓRECKI, J. & KULESZA, S. (1949). Typhoid fever and blood groups. (In Polish.) *Pol. med. Wkly.* **4,** 1254–7.

GOTI ITURRIAGA, J. L. & VELASCO ALONSO, R. (1965). Grupos sanguíneos y ulcera peptica. Sustancias antigenicas ABH y Le^a en la úlcera péptica. *Rev. clin. esp.* **98,** 119–29.

GRABOWSKA, M. J. (1969). Blood groups and diabetes. (In Polish.) *Pol. Arch. Med. wewnęt.* **42,** 155–9.

GRAHAME, E. W. (1961). The ABO blood groups and peptic ulceration. (A survey of 1,080 cases on south Tees-side.) *Brit. med. J.* **i,** 95–6.

GREEN, H. N. & DUNSFORD, I. (1954). Relationship of blood groups to cancer. *Acta Un. int. Cancr.* **10,** 125–7.

GREEN, P. T. & DUNDEE, J. C. (1952). The association of chronic pulmonary emphysema with chronic peptic ulceration. *Canad. Med. Ass. J.* **67,** 438–9.

GRIKUROV, V. S. (1936). Isoagglutinating properties of blood in healthy and goitrous inhabitants of Dagestan. (In Russian.) *Trud. kubansk. med. Inst.* **16,** no. 3, 165–70.

GRÖNVIK KORNSTAD, A. M., KORNSTAD, L., & GULDBERG, D. (1965). Blood groups in rheumatoid arthritis. *Nature, Lond.* **206,** 836–7.

GRÖNVIK KORNSTAD, A. M., KORNSTAD, L., & GULDBERG, D. (1968). Blood groups in ankylosing spondylitis. *Ann. rheum. Dis.* **27,** 472–3.

GROOTEN, O. & KOSSOVITCH, N. (1930). Sur les groupes sanguins chez les enfants poliomyélitiques. *C. R. Soc. Biol., Paris* **105,** 428–9.

GRUBB, R. & SJØSTEDT, S. (1954–5). Blood groups in abortion and sterility. *Ann. hum. Genet.* **19,** 183–95.

GUALANDRI, V. & BALLABIO, A. (1965). Sui rapporti fra vizi cardiaci acquisiti e gruppi sanguigni del sistema ABO. *Acta Genet. med. Gemell.* **14,** 392–405.

GUARINI, L. & FURLANI, E. (1968). Sui rapporti fra gruppi sanguigni del sistema ABO e colecistopatie litiasiche. *Trasfus. Sangue* **13,** 103–8.

GUNDEL, M. (1928). Weitere Untersuchungen über Lues und Blutgruppenzugehörigkeit. *Münch. med. Wschr.* **75,** 1337–8.

GUNDEL, M. & TORNQUIST, A. (1929). Über Beziehungen zwischen Blutgruppen und Geisteskrankheiten. *Arch. Psychiat. Nervenkr.* **86,** 576–86.

GUNELLA (1936). Quoted by Valentini (1938).

GUNSON, H. H. & LATHAM, V. (1972). An agglutinin in human serum reacting with cells from Le(a–b–) non-secretor individuals. *Vox Sang.* **22,** 344–53.

GUPTA, M. C. & GUPTA, S. R. (1966). Blood groups in relation to pulmonary tuberculosis and leprosy. *Indian J. med. Sci.* **20,** 353–6.

GUPTA, P. (1968). ABO blood groups and their relationship with cancer of the cervix uteri. *J. Indian med. Ass.* **51,** 69–71.

GUPTA, S. R. & GUPTA, M. C. (1965). Relationship between azoospermia and blood groups. *Indian Practit.* **18,** 339–40.

GUPTA, S. R. & GUPTA, M. C. (1966). Blood groups in skin diseases. *Indian J. Derm.* **11,** 49–50.

GUPTA, S. R., MAJUPURIA, K. C., & GUPTA, L. C. (1967). The study of ABO blood groups and relationship with acne vulgaris. (A preliminary report.) *Indian J. Derm.* **12,** 63–4.

GURDA, M. & TUROWSKA, B. (1970). Distribution of ABO and Rh D characters in leukemia patients. (In Polish.) *Przegl. lek.* **26,** 606–7.

GUREVIČ, N. & GELLERMAN-GUREVIČ, F. (1929). Isohämagglutinationseigenschaften des Blutes bei Syphilitikern. *Zbl. Haut-u. GeschlKr.* **30,** 511.

GUTHOF, O. Quoted by Helmbold (1961).

HADDOCK, D. R. & MCCONNELL, R. B. (1956). Carcinoma of stomach and ABO blood-groups. *Lancet* **ii,** 146–7.

HÄGELE, R., EVERS, K. G., LEVEN, B., & KRÜGER, J. (1976). HLA frequencies in primary immunodeficiency diseases (IDD). In *HLA and disease. 1st int. Symp.*, p. 200. Abstracts, Paris. INSERM.

HÄKKINEN, I. P. T. & VIRTANEN, S. (1967). The blood group activity of gastric sulphoglycoproteins in patients with gastric cancer and normal controls. *Clin. exp. Immunol.* **2,** 669–75.

HAEMMERLI, U. P., KISTLER, H., AMMANN, R., MARTHALER, T., SEMENZA, G., AURICCHIO, S., & PRADER, A. (1965). Acquired milk intolerance in the adult caused by lactose malabsorption due to a selective deficiency of intestinal lactase activity. *Amer. J. med.* **38,** 7–30.

HAKOMORI, S., KOŚCIELAK, J., BLOCH, K. J., & JEANLOZ, R. W. (1967). Immunologic relationship between blood group substances and a fucose-containing glycolipid of adenocarcinoma. *J. Immunol.* **98,** 31–8.

HALBRECHT, I. (1944). Role of hemoagglutinins anti-A and anti-B in pathogenesis of jaundice of the newborn (icterus neonatarum precox). *Amer. J. Dis. Child.* **68,** 248–9.

HALDANE, J. B. S. (1942). Selection against heterozygosis in man. *Ann. Eugen., Lond.* **11,** 333–40.

HALDANE, J. B. S. (1949*a*). Disease and evolution. *Ric. sci.* **19,** Suppl., 68–76.

HALDANE, J. B. S. (1949*b*). Mutation in man. *Hereditas, Lund,* Suppl., 267–73.

HALDANE, J. B. S. (1955–6). The estimation and significance of the logarithm of a ratio of frequence. *Ann. hum. Genet.* **20,** 309–11.

HALL, R., BUNCH, G. A., & HUMPHREY, C. S. (1971). Arteriosclerosis, duodenal ulcer, blood group, and secretor status. *Brit. med. J.* **iii,** 767.

HANDZEL, L. & NOWAKOWSKI, T. K. (1961). An attempt to find a relationship between cleft palate, blood groups and Rh factor. (In Polish.) *Otolaryng. pol.* **15,** 469–73.

HANINGTON, E. (1961). The relationship of the ABO blood groups to pregnancy, and toxaemia. *Path. Microbiol.* **24,** 687–9.

HARGREAVES, G. K. & HELLIER, F. F. (1958). The association of psoriasis with blood groups. *Arch. Derm.* **78,** 438–9.

HARLAP, S. & DAVIES, A. M. (1974). Maternal blood group A and pre-eclampsia. *Brit. med. J.* **iii,** 171–2.

HARPER, R. M. J. (1975). *Evolutionary origins of disease.* G. Mosdell, Barnstaple (England).

HARRIS, H. & KALMUS, H. (1949). Genetical differences in taste sensitivity to phenylthiourea and to anti-thyroid substances. *Nature, Lond.* **163,** 878.

HARRIS, H., KALMUS, H., & TROTTER, W. R. (1949). Taste sensitivity to phenylthiourea in goitre and diabetes. *Lancet* **ii,** 1038–9.

HARRIS, H. & KALMUS, H. (1950). The measurement of taste sensitivity to phenylthiourea (P.T.C.). *Ann. Eugen., Lond.* **15,** 24–31.

HARRIS, R. & GILLES, H. M. (1961). Glucose-6-phosphate dehydrogenase deficiency in the peoples of the Niger Delta. *Ann. hum. Genet.* **25,** 199–206.

HARRIS, R., WENTZEL, J., CARROLL, C. A., GARRETT, J. V., JACKSON, S. M., & DODGE, O. G. (1973). A study of HL-A in patients with Hodgkin's disease. In *Histocompatibility testing 1972* (ed. J. Dausset and J. Colombani), pp. 603–9. Copenhagen, Munksgaard.

HARRISON, G. A., BOYCE, A. J., HORNABROOK, R. W., & CRAIG, W. J. (1976). Associations between polymorphic variety and disease susceptibility in two New Guinea populations. *Ann. hum. Biol.* **3,** 253–67.

HARTMANN, G. (1941). *Group antigens in human organs.* Kopenhagen, Munksgaard. Reprinted in: US Army Med. Res. Lab. *Selected contributions to the literature of blood groups and immunology.* Fort Knox, Kentucky, 1970.

HARTMANN, O. & STAVEM, P. (1964). ABO blood-groups and cancer. *Lancet* **i,** 1305–6.

HASEGAWA (1937). Quoted by Vogel & Helmbold (1972).

HATZESOTERIOS, G. D. (1959). Frequencies of blood groups ABO and Rh factors in malignant neoplasms. (In Greek.) *Acta microbiol. hellen.* **4,** 200–5.

HATZKY, K. (1933). Untersuchungen über die Blutgruppenverteilung bei Poliomyelitikern. *Münch. med. Wschr.* **80,** 1973–4.

HAUCH, E. W. & MOORE, F. J. (1963). Is cholelithiasis associated with a specific blood group? *Gastroenterology* **44,** 125–6.

HAVERKORN, M. J. & GOSLINGS, W. R. O. (1969). Streptococci, ABO blood groups and secretor status. *Amer. J. hum. Genet.* **21,** 360–75.

HAVLIK, R. J., FEINLEIB, M., GARRISON, R. J., & KANNEL, W. B. (1969). Blood-groups and coronary heart-disease. *Lancet* **ii,** 269–70.

HEDENSTEDT, S. (1961). ABO-blodgruppsfördelning vid ulcus. *Nord. Med.* **65,** 697–9.

EL-HEFNAWI, H., MOHIEDDIN, O., & RASHEED, A. (1963). ABO system of blood groups and its incidence in selected dermatoses in U.A.R. i. Allergic skin diseases. ii. Photosensitivity skin diseases. iii. Miscellaneous skin diseases. *J. Egypt med. Ass.* **46,** 1097–106.

HEGETSCHWEILER, W., HUNZIKER, A., & MARANTA, E. (1960). Zur Ulcushaüfung beim Emphysem. *Schweiz. med. Wschr.* **90,** 1012–16.

HEISTØ, H. (1956). Relasjonen mellom blodtype og ulcus-sykdom. *Tidsskr. norske Laegeforen* **1,** 10–12.

HELMBOLD, W., KRAH, E., & BITZ, H. (1958). Über den Zusammenhang zwischen ABO-Blutgruppen und weiblichem Genital-Carcinom. *Acta genet. Stat. med.* **8,** 207–18.

HELMBOLD, W. (1961). Sammelstatistik zur Prüfung auf Korrelationen zwischen dem weiblichen Genitalcarcinom und dem ABO- und Rhesus-System. *Acta genet. Stat. med.* **11,** 29–51.

HELMBOLD, W. (1963). Quoted by Vogel (1963).

HENLEY, W. L., LEOPOLD, I. H., & AVINER, Z. (1974). Glaucoma and HL-A antigens. *Lancet* **ii,** 1273.

HENRY, M. U. & POON-KING, T. (1961). Blood groups in diabetes. A preliminary survey in Trinidad. *W. Indian med. J.* **10,** 156-60.

HEPP, R., KRÜGER, J., KURZEN, S., RUPP, H., & VOGEL, F. (1975). ABO blood groups and chicken pox. *Humangenetik* **27,** 329-32.

HERCUS, C. E. & PURVES, H. D. (1936). Studies on endemic and experimental goitre. *J. Hyg.* **36,** 182-203.

HÉRIVAUX, A. (1931). Les groupes sanguins dans la lèpre. *Bull. Soc. Path. exot.* **24,** 618-19.

HERMAN, M. & DERBY, I. M. (1937). The blood groups and M-N types in mental diseases. *J. Immunol.* **33,** 87-99.

HERMANNS, L. & KRONBERG, J. (1927). Blutgruppe und Krankheitsdisposition. *Münch. med. Wschr.* **74,** 967-9.

HERRMAN, J. B. (1971). Lymphoproliferative disease secondary to breast cancer, *N.Y. State J. Med.* **71,** 1108-11.

HEVÉR, Ö. (1966). Die Verteilung der genetisch bedingten Haptoglobintypen bei Geschwulstkrankheiten. *Experientia* **22,** 41.

HEVÉR, Ö. (1969). Relations entre les phénotypes d'haptoglobine dans diverses maladies. *Presse méd.* **77,** 1081-2.

HEWITT, D. & SPIERS, P. S. (1964). Low prevalence of A-antigen in children with acute myeloid leukaemia. *Lancet* **ii,** 93-4.

HILL, Z., MAKEŠOVÁ, D., & KREJČOVÁ, O. (1968). The factors Gm(1), Gm(2), Gm(4), Gm(5) and Inv(1) in the sera of patients with allergic diseases. *Acta allerg., Kbh.* **23,** 124-9.

HIRAIZUMI, Y., SPRADLIN, C. T., ITO, R., & ANDERSON, S. A. (1973). Birth-order dependent segregation frequency in the ABO blood groups of man. *Amer. J. hum. Genet.* **25,** 277-86.

HIROSE, Y. & HONMA, R. (1962). ABO blood groups and surgical diseases. 8th *Congr. int. Soc. Blood Transfus.*, Tokyo, 1960. *Bibl. haemat.* **13,** 270-5.

HIRSCHFELD, H. & HITTMAIR, A. (1926). Über Blutgruppenbestimmungen bei Krebskranken. *Med. Klin.* **22,** 1494-6.

HIRSZFELD, H., HIRSZFELD, L., & BROKMAN, H. (1924). On the susceptibility to diphtheria (Schick test positive) with reference to the inheritance of blood groups. *J. Immunol.* **9,** 571-91.

HIRSZFELD, L. & HIRSZFELD, H. (1918-19). Essai d'application des méthodes sérologiques au problème des races. *Anthropologie, Paris,* **29,** 505-37.

HIRSZFELD, L. & HIRSZFELD, H. (1919). Serological differences between the blood of different races. The result of researches on the Macedonian front. *Lancet* **ii,** 675-9.

HIRSZFELD, L. & HIRSZFELD, H. (1919). Serološka diferenciacija krvi kod raznich naroda i rasa. *Srpski Arh.* **21,** 105-11.

HIRSZFELD, L. & ZBOROWSKI, H. (1925). Gruppenspezifische Beziehungen zwischen Mutter und Frucht und elektive Durchlässigkeit der Placenta. *Klin. Wschr.* **4,** 1152-7.

HIRSZFELD, L. (1928). *Konstitutionsserologie und Blutgruppenforschung.* Translation in: US Army Med. Res. Lab. *Selected contributions to the literature of blood groups and immunology.* Fort Knox, Kentucky, 1969, **3,** pt. 1.

HOBBS, M. S. T. (1968). Blood groups and pyloric stenosis. *Brit. med. J.* **ii,** 51-2.

HOCHE, O. & MORITSCH, P. (1926). Zur Frage der Blutgruppenspezifität der malignen Tumoren und deren gruppenspezifische Bekämpfung. *Mitt. Grenzgeb. Med. Chir.* **39,** 409-14.

HOFFBAUER, H. Quoted by Helmbold (1961).

HOGG, L. & PACK, G. T. (1957). The controversial relationship between blood group A and gastric cancer. *Gastroenterology* **32,** 797-806.

HOLLÄNDER, L. *et al.* Quoted by Aird *et al.* (1953).

HOLLINGSWORTH, D. R. (1963). Phenylthiourea taste testing in Hiroshima subjects with thyroid disease. *J. clin. Endocrin.* **23,** 961-3.

HOLLÓ, J. & LÉNARD, W. (1926). Gibt es einen Unterschied in der Häufigkeit der einzelnen Blutgruppen bei Lungentuberkulösen und bei gesunden Menschen? *Beitr. Klin. Tuberk.* **64,** 513-14.

HOOPER, W. L. (1960). Blood groups in rheumatic carditis. *Brit. med. J.* **i,** 565-6.

HOPKINSON, D. A., SPENCER, N., & HARRIS, H. (1963). Red cell acid phosphatase variants: a new human polymorphism. *Nature, Lond.* **199,** 969-71.

HORTON, M. A. & OLIVER, R. T. D. (1976). HLA antigen (A & B loci) frequency in Addisonian pernicious anaemia. *Tissue Antigens* **7,** 239-42.

HORTON, R. J. & POVEY, M. S. (1966). *Cambridge medico-sociological expedition to India 1964.* Report on project. (Stencilled.)

HORWICH, L., EVANS, D. A. P., MCCONNELL, R. B., & DONOHOE, W. T. A. (1966). ABO blood groups in gastric bleeding. *Gut* **7,** 680-5.

HOSKINS, L. C., LOUX, H. A., BRITTEN, A., & ZAMCHECK, N. (1965). Distribution of ABO blood groups in patients with pernicious anaemia, gastric carcinoma and gastric carcinoma associated with pernicious anaemia. *New Engl. J. Med.* **273,** 633-7.

HOUTE, O. VAN & KESTELOOT, H. (1972). An epidemiological survey of risk factors for ischemic heart disease in 42,804 men. *Acta cardiol., Brux.* **27,** 527-64.

HOVE, G. M. (1976). The geography of disease. In *Equalities and inequalities in health* (eds. C. O. Carter & J. Peel), pp. 45-64.

HSIA, D. Y.-Y., SHIH, L.-Y., EASTERBERG, S., FARQUHAR, J., KIM, C.-B., YEH, S., & YOUNG, A. (1969). The distribution of genetic polymorphisms among patients with Down's syndrome, phenylketonuria and cystic fibrosis of the pancreas. *Amer. J. hum. Genet.* **21,** 285-9.

HSUEN, J., THOMAS, E., & JESUDIAN, G. (1963). A, B, O blood groups and leprosy. *Leprosy Rev.* **34,** 143-7.

HUGUENIN, R. & DELAGE, J. (1933). Groupes sanguins et cancer. *C. R. Soc. Biol., Paris* **112,** 152-4.

HUNT, M. L. & LUCIA, S. P. (1953). The occurrence of acquired hemolytic anemia in subjects of blood group O. *Science* **118,** 183-4.

HUTTON, A. C. & SMITH, G. F. (1964). Haptoglobins and transferrins in patients with Down's syndrome. *Ann. hum. Genet.* **27,** 413-15.

IHM, P. & WENDT, G. G. (1966). Statistische Betrachtung über die Häufigkeit der Haptoglobin-Typen bei verschiedenen Krankheiten. *Humangenetik* **2,** 186-91.

IKIN, E. W., MOURANT, A. E., PETTENKOFER, H. J., & BLUMENTHAL, G. (1951). Discovery of the expected haemagglutinin anti-Fy^b. *Nature, Lond.* **168,** 1077.

INADA, R. (1934). Quoted by Desai & Creger (1964).

ING, R., PETRAKIS, N. L., & HO, H. C. (1973). Evidence against association between wet cerumen and breast cancer. *Lancet* **i,** 41.

IONESCU, D. A., MARCU, I., & BICESCU, E. (1976). Cerebral thrombosis, cerebral haemorrhage, and ABO blood-groups. *Lancet* **i,** 278-80.

IRACI, G. & CARTERI, A. (1964). Frequenza dei gruppi ABO nei tumori intracranici di origine neuroectodermica. *Tumori* **50,** 187-200.

IRACI, G. & TOFFOLO, G. G. (1964*a*). Frequenza dei gruppi ABO negli adenomi ipofisari. *Tumori* **50,** 469-72.

IRACI, G. & TOFFOLO, G. G. (1964*b*). Frequenza dei gruppi ABO nei meningiomi. *Tumori* **50,** 473-5.

ISTVÁN, L. & SZÉLL, K. (1961). Distribution of blood groups between patients with gastric cancer and ulcer. (In Hungarian.) *Orv. Hétil.* **102,** 986-90.

JACKSON, —, KENNETH, H., & HERMAN, B. (1959). Los grupos sanguínos ABO en relación a las ulceras gastroduodenales y el cancer gastrico. *Rev. méd. Valparaiso* **12,** 255-7.

JACKSON, I. M. D., BOYLE, J. A., & HARDEN, R. MCG. (1965). Distribution of the ABO blood groups in thyrotoxicosis. *Vox Sang.* **10,** 246-8.

JACOBSOHN, H. (1926). Über die Blutgruppenzugehörigkeit der Paralytiker. *Z. ges. Neurol. Psychiat.* **105,** 810-14.

JAEGERMANN, K. (1964). Coronary atherosclerosis and blood groups. *Pol. med. J.* **3,** 626-33.

JAIN, R. C. (1970). ABO blood groups and pulmonary tuberculosis. *Tubercle* **51,** 322-3.

JAKOUBKOVÁ, J. & MÁJSKÝ, A. (1965). Blood groups and neoplastic disease. *Neoplasma* **12,** 611-16.

JANUS, Z. L., BAILAR, J. C., & EISENBERG, H. (1967). Blood group and uterine cancer. *Amer. J. Epidemiol.* **86,** 569–78.

JAYAKAR, S. D. (1974). Pers. comm. to A. E. Mourant.

JAYANT, K. (1971). Relationship of ABO blood groups to certain types of cancer common in Western India. *Indian J. Cancer* **8,** 185–8.

JENKINS, D. M., NEED, J. A., SCOTT, J. S., & RAJAH, S. M. (1976). HLA and severe pre-eclampsia. In *HLA and disease. 1st int. Symp.*, p. 250. Abstracts, Paris, INSERM.

JENKINS, T., LEHMANN, H., & NURSE, G. T. (1974). Public health and genetic constitution of the San ('Bushmen'): carbohydrate metabolism and acetylator status of the !Kung of Tsumkwe in the North-western Kalahari. *Brit. med. J.* **ii,** 23–6.

JERSILD, C., FOG, T., HANSEN, G. S., THOMSEN, M., SVEJGAARD, A., & DUPONT, B. (1973). Histocompatibility determinants in multiple sclerosis, with special reference to clinical course. *Lancet* **ii,** 1221–5.

JICK, H., SLONE, D., WESTERHOLM, B., INMAN, W. H. W., VESSEY, M. P., SHAPIRO, S., LEWIS, G. P., & WORCESTER, J. (1969). Venous thromboembolic disease and ABO blood type. *Lancet* **i,** 539–42.

JÖRGENSEN, G. (1965). *Untersuchungen zur Genetik der Sarkoidose.* Heidelberg, Alfred Hüthig (Habilitationsschrift).

JÖRGENSEN, G. (1967). The ABO blood group-polymorphism in the multifactorial genetic system. *Humangenetik* **3,** 264–8.

JÖRGENSEN, G. & HOPFER, A. (1967). Die Verteilung der Gc-Phänotypen und Gc-Allele bei einigen Krankheiten (Diabetes mellitus, Leberparenchymschaden, Psoriasis vulgaris). *Humangenetik* **3,** 273–6.

JÖRGENSEN, G. & HOPFER, U. (1967). Die Verteilung der Haptoglobinphänotypen und Haptoglobinallele bei einigen Krankheiten (Diabetes mellitus, Leberparenchymschaden, Psoriasis vulgaris). *Humangenetik* **3,** 277–81.

JÖRGENSEN, G., BEUREN, A. J., STOERMER, J., & HAHN, H. J. (1968). Untersuchungen über die Verteilung der ABO-Blutgruppen bei angeborenen Herzfehlern. *Humangenetik* **5,** 266–70.

JÖRGENSEN, G. & KALLENBACH, H. H. (1968). Untersuchungen zur Frage der statistischen Beziehungen zwischen Rhesusfaktoren (D-System) und Krankheiten. *Humangenetik* **5,** 261–5.

JÖRGENSEN, G. & RÜBBERDT, V. (1968). Die Verteilung der Haptoglobin-Phänotypen und Haptoglobin-Allele bei der Lungentuberkulose. *Humangenetik* **6,** 340–4.

JÖRGENSEN, G. Quoted by Vogel & Helmbold (1972).

JÖRGENSEN, G. & LAL, V. B. (1972). Serogenetic investigations on malignant melanomas with reference to the incidence of ABO system, Rh system, Gm, Inv, Hp and Gc systems. *Humangenetik* **15,** 227–31.

JOHANNSEN, E. W. (1927). A classification of cancer patients according to their blood groups and some investigations concerning isohemagglutination. *Acta path. microbiol. scand.* **4,** 175–97.

JOHNSON, H. D., LOVE, A. H. G., ROGERS, N. C., & WYATT, A. P. (1964). Gastric ulcers, blood groups, and acid secretion. *Gut* **5,** 402–11.

JOHNSON, H. D. (1965). Gastric ulcer: classification, blood group characteristics, secretion patterns and pathogenesis. *Ann. Surg.* **162,** 996–1004.

JOHNSTON, F. E., HERTZOG, K. P., & MALINA, R. M. (1966). Phenylthiocarbamide taste sensitivity and its relationship to growth variation. *Amer. J. phys. Anthrop.* **24,** 253–5.

JOHNSTON, S. J., JONES, P. F., KYLE, J., & NEEDHAM, C. D. (1973). Epidemiology and course of gastrointestinal haemorrhage in North-east Scotland. *Brit. med. J.* **iii,** 655–64.

JOLLY, J. G., SARUP, B. M., & AIKAT, B. K. (1969). Diabetes mellitus and blood groups. *J. Indian med. Ass.* **52,** 104–7.

JORDAL, K. (1956). Blood groups and disease; ABO, rhesus, and Lewis blood groups in relation to cancer of stomach, rectum, and colon, and to peptic ulceration. *Acta med. leg. soc.* **9,** special no., 195–203.

JOSHI, M. S., NIMBKAR, N. V., & RINDANI, A. B. (1958). Blood groups in relation to peptic ulceration. *Indian J. Surg.* **20,** 169–72.

JOSKE, R. A. & BENSON, J. A. (1958). ABO blood groups and non-tropical sprue. *Gastroenterology* **34,** 408–9.

JOVINO, R. & MUSELLA, S. (1958). Gruppi sanguigni e cancro del polmone. *Chir. torac.* **11,** 186–91.

JUNGEBLUT, C. W. & SMITH, L. W. (1932). Blood grouping in poliomyelitis. *J. Immunol.* **23,** 35–47.

JUNGEBLUT, C. W., KAROWE, H. E., & BRAHAM, S. B. (1947). Further observations on blood grouping in poliomyelitis. *Ann. intern. Med.* **26,** 67–75.

KACZYNSKY, R. (1926). Les groupes sanguins et les réactions de Dick et de Schick. *C. R. Soc. Biol., Paris* **95,** 933.

KAFKAS, M. & GERCEL, R. (1967). Blood groups in patients with prostatic hyperplasia or urinary stones. (In Turkish.) *Tip. Fakült. Mecmuasi* **20,** 238–41.

KAIPANEN, W. J. & VUORINEN, Y. V. (1960). ABO blood groups in pernicious anaemia and pernicious tapeworm anaemia. *Ann. Med. exp. Fenn.* **38,** 212–13.

KAISER-MEINHARDT, I. (1962). ABO-Blutgruppen und Se/se-Eigenschaft bei Karzinomen des Hals-Nasen-Ohren-Gebietes. *Z. Laryng. Rhinol.* **41,** 386–90.

KAK, V. K. & GORDON, D. S. (1970). ABO blood groups and Parkinson's disease. *Ulster med. J.* **39,** 132–4.

KALLABIS, B. (1927). Blutgruppenbestimmung und Tuberkulose. *Beitr. Klin. Tuberk.* **66,** 391–4.

KALLIOMÄKI, J. L. & SAARIMAA, H. A. (1962). The A–B–O–Rh groups and myocardial infarction; association between the blood groups and the patient's age, mortality rate in first month of illness, and the requirement of anticoagulants. *Cardiologia* **41,** 109–12.

KALLIOMÄKI, J. L. & SEPPÄLÄ, P. O. (1971). Observations on serum alpha$_1$-antitrypsin with special reference to peptic ulcer and the combination of peptic ulcer and pulmonary emphysema. *R. C. R. Gastroenterol.* **3,** 159–62.

KALMUS, H. & LEWKONIA, I. (1973). Relation between some forms of glaucoma and phenylthiocarbamide tasting. *Brit. J. Ophthal.* **57,** 503–6.

KAMINSKY (1928). Quoted by Penzik (1930).

KAPLAN, A. R., FISCHER, R., GLANVILLE, E., POWELL, W., KAMIONKOWSKI, M., & FLESHLER, B. (1964). Differential taste sensitivities in duodenal and gastric ulcer patients. *Gastroenterology* **47,** 604–9.

KAPLAN, H. (1961). Quoted by Shirley & Desai (1965).

KAPLAN, S., LI, C. C., WALD, N., & BORGES, W. (1964). ABO frequencies in mongols. *Ann. hum. Genet.* **27,** 405–12.

KARNAUKHOVA, E. I. (1930). Blutgruppen und Epilepsie. *Ukr. Zbl. Blutgr.* **4,** 232–6.

KAY, H. E. M. & SHORTER, R. G. (1956). Blood groups in leukaemia and the reticuloses. *Vox Sang.* n.s. **1,** 255–8.

KELLERMANN, G., LUYTEN-KELLERMANN, M., & SHAW, C. R. (1973*a*). Genetic variation of aryl hydrocarbon hydroxylase in human lymphocytes. *Amer. J. hum. Genet.* **25,** 327–31.

KELLERMANN, G., SHAW, C. R., & LUYTEN-KELLERMANN, M. (1973*b*). Aryl hydrocarbon hydroxylase inducibility and bronchogenic carcinoma. *New Engl. J. Med.* **289,** 934–7.

KENNEDY, T. H. (1942). Thio-ureas as goitrogenic substances. *Nature, Lond.* **150,** 233–4.

KERDE, C., DOMINOK, G. W., & GILLNER, E. (1962). Blutgruppenuntersuchungen anlässlich der Ruhrepidemie. *Dtsch. GesundheitsWes.* **17,** 1469–72.

KHALIL, M. (1960). The ABO blood groups and disease in infants and children. *Acta paediat.* **49,** 76–81.

KHATTAB, M., EL-GENGEHY, M. T., & SHARAF, M. (1968). ABO blood groups in bilharzial hepatic fibrosis. *J. Egypt. med. Ass.* **51,** 245–50.

KHATTAB, T. M. & ISMAIL, A. A. (1960). ABO blood groups in relation to rheumatic heart disease. *J. Egypt. med. Ass.* **43,** 441–5.

KHER, M. & GROVER, S. (1969). Glucose-6-phosphate-dehydrogenase deficiency in leprosy. *Lancet* **i,** 1318–19.

KHÉRUMIAN, R. & MOULLEC, J. (1959). Les groupes sanguins ABO dans les cancers et les ulcères de l'estomac et du duodénum. *Rev. Hémat.* **14,** 144–55.

KHOMINSKY, B. & SHUSTOVA, L. (1927). Über die Verteilung der Blutgruppen unter Geisteskranken. (In Russian.) *Sovr. Psikhonevrol.* **4,** 495–8.

KINGSBURY, K. J. (1971). Relation of ABO blood-groups to atherosclerosis. *Lancet* **i**, 199–203.

KIRCHER, W. (1964). Weitere Untersuchungen über den Zusammenhang zwischen Verlauf und Häufigkeit der Säuglingsenteritis und ABO-Blutgruppenzugehörigkeit. *Mschr. Kinderheilk.* **112**, 415–18.

KIRCHER, W. (1965). Zur Frage der Selektion von Kindern in ABO-Blutgruppenunverträglichen Ehen. *Humangenetik* **1**, 668–75.

KIRCHER, W. (1968). Untersuchungen über die Verteilung der ABO-Blutgruppen bei verschiedenen Erkrankungen im Säuglingsalter. *Humangenetik* **6**, 171–80.

KIRCHER, W. (1969). Zur Frage der Verteilung der ABO-Blutgruppen bei an Scharlach erkrankten Kindern. *Humangenetik* **8**, 249–52.

KIRCHMAIR, H. & BLIXENKRONE MØLLER, N. (1935–6). Blutgruppe und Daktylogramm von Poliomyelitiskranken in Hadersleben (Dänemark) 1934. *Z. Kinderheilk.* **57**, 595–601.

KIRK, R. L., KINNS, H., & MORTON, N. E. (1970). Interaction between the ABO blood group and haptoglobin systems. *Amer. J. hum. Genet.* **22**, 384–9.

KIRK, R. L. (1971). A haptoglobin mating frequency, segregation and ABO blood-group interaction analysis for additional series of families. *Ann. hum. Genet.* **34**, 329–37.

KISS, P. VON & TEVELI, Z. (1930). Blutgruppe und Scharlach. *Jb. Kinderheilk.* **127**, 110–13.

KITCHIN, F. D., HOWEL-EVANS, W., CLARKE, C. A., MCCONNELL, R. B., & SHEPPARD, P. M. (1959). P.T.C. taste response and thyroid disease. *Brit. med. J.* **i**, 1069–74.

KITCHIN, F. D., BEARN, A. G., ALPERS, M., & GAJDUSEK, D. C. (1972). Genetic studies in relation to kuru. iii. Distribution of the inherited serum group-specific protein (Gc) phenotypes in New Guineans: an association of kuru and the Gc Ab phenotype. *Amer. J. hum. Genet.* **24** Suppl., S72–S85.

KJAERSGAARD, A. R. (1959). A preliminary report on the association between blood groups and disease in patients admitted to a hospital for functional nervous disorders. *Acta psychiat. scand.* **34** (Suppl. 136), 170–1.

KJØLBYE, J. E. & LYKKEGAARD NIELSEN, E. (1959). ABO blood groups in cholelithiasis. *Acta genet. Stat. med.* **9**, 213–20.

KLAUS (1963). Quoted by Vogel & Helmbold (1972).

KLEBANOFF, S. J. & WHITE, L. R. (1969). Iodination defect in the leucocytes of a patient with chronic granulomatous disease of childhood. *N. England J. Med.* **280**, 460–6.

KLEBE, J. G. & NIELSEN, J. C. (1972). The ABO and Rhesus blood groups of diabetic mothers and their newborn babies. *Hum. Hered.* **22**, 294–300.

KLEINSCHMIDT (1939). Quoted by Jungeblut *et al.* (1947).

KLÖVEKORN, G. H. & SIMON, A. (1927). Die Bedeutung der Blutgruppenuntersuchungen bei Haut- und Geschlechtskrankheiten. *Derm. Z.* **50**, 294–7.

KNOX, E. G. (1974). Twins and neural tube defects. *Brit. J. prev. soc. Med.* **28**, 73–80.

KOBIELOWA, Z., KOBIELA, J., GROCHOWSKI, J., & SLATNIK, J. (1962). The haptoglobin (Hp) group system in some diseases of children. (In Polish.) *Pol. Tyg. lek.* **17**, 1497–9.

KOCHS, K. & WILCKENS, H. (1928). Blutgruppen und Tuberkulosedisposition. *Med. Welt* **2**, 439–40.

KÖRWER, H. (1932). Blutgruppe und Scharlach. *Jb. Kinderheilk.* **136**, 59–70.

KØSTER, K. H., SINDRUP, E., & SEELE, V. (1955). ABO blood groups and gastric acidity. *Lancet* **ii**, 52–5.

KOÏDAKIS, A., GEORGIOU, V., ANTONAKIS, E., & MICHAELIDIS, G. (1970). ABO blood groups and myocardial infarction. (In Greek.) *Hellen. armed Forces med. Rev.* **4**, 759–68.

KOLPAKOV & ANDRUSSON (1928). Quoted by Vogel & Helmbold (1972).

KOMAROVICH, N. I. & RYCHKOV, YU. G. (1966). Blood-group system ABO (H) and immunity against the smallpox. (In Russian.) *Vop. Antrop.* **23**, 39–48.

KOOPTZOFF, O. & WALSH, R. J. (1957). Blood groups and disease: pulmonary tuberculosis. *Aust. Ann. Med.* **6**, 53–5.

KOPEĆ, A. C. (1970). *The distribution of the blood groups in the United Kingdom.* London, Oxford University Press.

KORDAČ, V. I. (1965). Die Blutgruppen des ABO-systems und Rh_0(D)-Faktor bei Leberzirrhose. *Z. ges. inn. Med.* **20**, 290–2.

KORFEL, A. (1966). Morphological and serological investigations of women suffering from the cancer of the uterus. (In Polish.) *Mater. Prace antrop.* **73**, 259–80.

KORFEL, Z., PODSIADŁY, P., & OSTROWSKI, L. (1967). Rh factor and ABO blood groups in patients with cholecystitis. (In Polish.) *Pol. Tyg. lek.* **22**, 339–41.

KOŚCIELAK, J., GROCHOWSKA, E., SEYFRIED, H., RUDOWSKI, W., & SCHARF, R. (1971). A cold agglutinin with anti-blood group A and anti-cancer specificity. 12th *Congr. int. Soc. Blood Transfus.*, Moscow 1969. *Bibl. haemat.* **38**, 424–9.

KOSIŃSKI, W., MŁODZKI, M., & SZKLARSKA, Z. (1959). Blood groups in certain internal diseases. *Pol. med. Wkly.* **14**, 149–54.

KOSSOVITCH, N., BROUSSEAU, A., & BUISSON, M. (1940). Sur quelques particularités de la répartition des groupes sanguins chez les aliénés médico-légaux. *C. R. Soc. Biol., Paris* **134**, 82–3.

KOSSOVITCH, N. & SÉRANE, F. (1941). Séro-agglutination de Hollande dans la démence précoce. Groupes sanguins chez les déments précoces. *C. R. Soc. Biol., Paris* **135**, 172–4.

KOTHARE, S. N. (1959). ABO blood groups in relation to pulmonary tuberculosis. A preliminary report. *J. postgrad. Med.* **5**, 94–8.

KOZACZENKO, J. (1966). Neoplasms of the female genital organs and blood groups. *Pol. med. J.* **5**, 1442–6.

KRAH, E., BITZ, H., & LAU, H. Quoted by Helmbold (1961).

KRANT, M. J., MARTIN, M. S., & BRANDRUP, C. S. (1968). Salivary secretion of blood-group factors in cancer. *J. Amer. med. Ass.* **204**, 153–4.

KRANZ, J. (1942). Die Bedeutung der Blutgruppen bei der Impfmalaria. *Nervenarzt* **15**, 166–70.

KREIL, R. (1966). Besteht eine Abhängigkeit viröser Erkrankungen (Poliomyelitis) vom ABO- und Rh-System? *Folia haemat., Lpz.* **85**, 132–7.

KRIEG, H. & KASPER, K. (1968). ABO incompatibility as a cause of abortion. *Germ. med. Mon.* **13**, 171–5.

KROKFORS, E. & KINNUNEN, O. (1954). Blood groups and gynaecological cancer. *Brit. med. J.* **i**, 1305–6.

KRÓLIKOWSKA, I. & ŻUPAŃSKA, B. (1964). Distribution of the ABO groups in some hematologic diseases. (In Polish.) *Pol. Tyg. lek.* **19**, 168–71.

KRUSZEWSKI, K. (1966). The ABO and Gm(a) blood group systems in rheumatic diseases. (In Polish.) *Przegl. lek.* **22**, 608–10.

KUBÍČKOVÁ, Z. & VESELÝ, K. T. (1966). Die Blutgruppen A_1A_2BO, Rh_0 (D), die Ausscheidungsfähigkeit der ABH-Substanzen und die Ulcuskrankheit. *Gastroenterologia, Basel* **105**, 1–11.

KUBÍČKOVÁ, Z. & VEŠELÝ, K. T. (1972). The value of investigations of the incidence of peptic ulcer in the families of patients with duodenal ulcer. *J. med. Genet.* **9**, 38–42.

KUKOWKA, A. (1935). Die Blutgruppenverteilung bei Krebskranken. *Z. Krebsforsch.* **42**, 510–11.

KURDI, A., AYESH, I., ABDALLAT, A., MAAYTA, U., MCDONALD, W. I., COMPSTON, D. A. S., & BATCHELOR, J. R. (1977). Different B lymphocyte alloantigens associated with multiple sclerosis in Arabs and north Europeans. *Lancet* **i**, 1133–5.

KUROKAWA, T. & MASUDA, H. (1958). Geographic pathology of gastro-duodenal ulcer in Japan. *Acta path. jap.* **8**, 343–86.

KYANK, H. & KULISCH, B. (1958). Blutgruppen, Rh-Faktor und Schwangerschaftstoxikose. *Geburtsh. u. Frauenheilk.* **18**, 946–50.

LADENSON, R. P., SCHWARTZ, S. O., & IVY, A. C. (1949). Incidence of the blood groups and the secretor factor in patients with pernicious anemia and stomach carcinoma. *Amer. J. med. Sci.* **217**, 194–7.

LAFFERTY, C. R., KNOX, W. J., & BURKETT, M. L. (1960). Relationship of secretors and non-secretors of blood group substances in schizophrenics and non-schizophrenics. *Dis. nerv. Syst.* **21**, 620–1.

LAHA, P. N. & DUTTA, M. (1963). Association between blood groups and pulmonary tuberculosis. *J. Ass. Physicians India* **11**, 287–91.

LAL, V. B. & SPEISER, P. (1957). Untersuchungen über Zusammenhänge zwischen erworbenen hämolytischen Anämie, klassischen Blutgruppen, Rhesusfaktor, Geschlecht und Alter. *Blut.* **3**, 15–19.

Lamba, D. L., Singha, P., & Chandra, S. (1974). A study of diabetes in relation to blood groups and cholesterol levels. *Humangenetik* **23,** 51–8.

Lambotte, C. & Israel, E. (1967). Variole et groupes sanguins ABO au Congo. *Ann. Soc. belge Méd. trop.* **47,** 405–12.

Lamp, C. A. (1963). The agricultural significance of goitrogenic activity in *Brassicae*. *J. Austr. Inst. agr. Sci.* **29,** 8–14.

Lancet (1974). Aryl hydrocarbon hydroxylase inducibility and lung cancer (Leading article). **i,** 910–12.

Landsteiner, K. (1900). Zur Kenntnis der antifermentativen, lytischen und agglutinierenden Wirkungen des Blutserums und der Lymphe. *Zbl. Bakt.* Abt. i, **27,** 357–62. Translation in: US Army Med. Res. Lab. *Selected contributions to the literature of blood groups and immunology*. Fort Knox, Kentucky, 1970, **1.**

Landsteiner, K. & Levine, P. (1927*a*). A new agglutinable factor differentiating individual human bloods. *Proc. Soc. exp. Biol., N. Y.* **24,** 600–2.

Landsteiner, K. & Levine, P. (1927*b*). Further observations on individual differences of human blood. *Proc. Soc. exp. Biol., N. Y.* **24,** 941–2.

Landsteiner, K. & Levine, P. (1928). On individual differences in human blood. *J. exp. Med.* **47,** 757–75.

Landsteiner, K. & Wiener, A. S. (1940). An agglutinable factor in human blood recognized by immune sera for rhesus blood. *Proc. Soc. exp. Biol., N. Y.* **43,** 223.

Lang, C. A. (1959). Rilievi statistici iniziali sul rapporto tra gruppi sanguigni e malattie nelle popolazioni italiane. 7th *Congr. int. Soc. Blood Transfus.*, Rome, 1958. *Bibl. haemat.* **10,** 163–6.

Lang-Brown, H., Lawler, S. D., & Penrose, L. S. (1952–3). The blood typing of cases of mongolism, their parents and sibs. *Ann. Eugen., Lond.* **17,** 307–36.

Langman, M. J. S. & Doll, R. (1965). ABO blood group and secretor status in relation to clinical characteristics of peptic ulcers. *Gut* **6,** 270–3.

Langman, M. J. S., Doll, R., & Saracci, R. (1967). ABO blood group and secretor status in stomal ulcer. *Gut* **8,** 128–32.

Langman, M. J. S., Banwell, J. G., Stewart, J. S., & Robson, E. B. (1969). ABO blood groups, secretor status, and intestinal alkaline phosphatase concentrations in patients with celiac disease. *Gastroenterology* **57,** 19–23.

Languillon, J., Linhard, J., Diebolt, G., & Peyrot, N. (1973). Maladie de Hansen et génétique recherche sur l'association entre differents facteurs génétiques et la lèpre chez l'africain. *Méd. trop.* **33,** 9–18.

Larkin, M. F. (1967). Serum haptoglobin type and cancer. *J. nat. Cancer Inst.* **39,** 630–8.

Larrouy, G. (1960). *La répartition des groupes sanguins chez les sujets porteurs de tumeurs malignes.* Toulouse, Cléder. Thèse—Univ. de Toulouse.

Latner, A. L. & Zaki, A. H. (1960). Clinical uses of starch gel electrophoresis with special reference to leukaemia. *Clin. chim. Acta.* **5,** 22–5.

Latts, E. M., Cummins, J. F., & Zieve, L. (1956). Peptic ulcer and pulmonary emphysema. *Arch. int. Med.* **97,** 576–84.

Lauer, V. V. (1929). Studium der Isoagglütinationseigenschaften des Blutes bei der gesunden und an Kropf leidenden Bevölkerung des Karatschaj Autonomgebietes. (In Russian.) *Proc. N. Cauc. Ass. sci. Res. Inst.* **3,** 121–33.

Laurà (1938). Quoted by Asaro (1955).

Laurell, C. B. & Eriksson, S. (1963). The electrophoretic α_1-globulin pattern of serum in α_1-antitrypsin deficiency. *Scand. J. clin. Lab. Invest.* **15,** 132–40.

Lauritsen, J. G., Grunnet, N., & Jensen, O. M. (1975). Materno-fetal ABO incompatibility as a cause of spontaneous abortion. *Clin. Genet.* **7,** 308–16.

Lawler, S. D. (1976). Immunogenetics of trophoblastic tumours. *In press.*

Lechat, M. F., Bile, T., & Rasi, E. (1967). A study of blood groups and leprosy in the population of Colonia Tovar, Venezuela. *Int. J. Leprosy* **35,** 488–93.

Lechat, M. F., Bias, W. B., Guinto, R. S., Cohen, B. H., Tolentino, J. G., & Abalos, R. M. (1968). A study of various blood group systems in leprosy patients and controls in Cebu, Philippines. *Int. J. Leprosy* **36,** 17–31.

Lehmann, H. (1959). The maintenance of the haemoglobinopathies at high frequency. A consideration of the relation between sickling and malaria and of allied problems. In *Abnormal haemoglobins* (ed. J. H. P. Jonxis & J. F. Delafresnaye), pp. 307–21. Blackwell Scientific Publications, Oxford.

Lehmann, H. & Huntsman, R. G. (1974). *Man's haemoglobins*, 2nd ed. Amsterdam and Oxford, North-Holland.

Lehrs, H. (1930). Ueber gruppenspezifische Eigenschaften des menschlichen Speichels. *Z. ImmunForsch.* **66,** 175–92.

Leischner, A. (1936) Über die Blutgruppenverteilung bei Geisteskrankheiten. *Mschr. Psychiat. Neurol.* **93,** 259–77.

Leite, G. Moreira & Goffi, F. Schmidt (1958). A distribuição dos grupos sangüíneos A–B–O em doentes de úlcera gastroduedenal e de carcinoma gástrico. *Rev. paulist. Med.* **52,** 31–6.

Lessa, A. & Alarcão, J. (1947). Contribuição para o estudo das incidências dos tipos do sistema clássico ABO, sobre os estados mórbidos. *J. Soc. Ciên. méd. Lisboa* **111,** no. 7, 1–48 in reprint.

Lessa, A. & Ruffié, J. (1960). Sur la fréquence des groupes sanguins et de certaines maladies. *C. R. Soc. Biol., Paris* **154,** 211–13.

Lev, M., Okada, R., Kerstein, M. D., Paiva, R., & Rimoldi, H. J. A. (1967). Blood groups and congenital heart disease. *Dis. Chest* **52,** 616–20.

Levene, H. & Rosenfield, R. E. (1961). ABO incompatibility. *Progress in medical genetics* **1,** 120–57.

Levine, P. & Stetson, R. E. (1939). An unusual case of intragroup agglutination. *J. Amer. med. Ass.* **113,** 126–7.

Levine, P., Burnham, L., Katzin, E. M., & Vogel, P. (1941*a*). The role of iso-immunization in the pathogenesis of erythroblastosis fetalis. *Amer. J. Obstet. Gynec.* **42,** 925–37.

Levine, P., Katzin, E. M., & Burnham, L. (1941*b*). Isoimmunisation in pregnancy. Its possible bearing on the etiology of erythroblastosis foetalis. *J. Amer. med. Ass.* **116,** 825–7.

Levine, P., Katzin, E. M., Vogel, P., & Burnham, L. (1941*c*). Pathogenesis of erythroblastosis fetalis: statistical evidence. *Science* **94,** 371–2.

Levine, P. (1943). Serological factors as possible causes in spontaneous abortions. *J. Hered.* **34,** 71–80.

Levine, P., Bobbitt, O. B., Waller, R. K., & Kuhmichel, A. (1951*a*). Isoimmunization by a new blood factor in tumour cells. *Proc. Soc. exp. Biol., N. Y.* **77,** 403–5.

Levine, P., Kuhmichel, A. B., Wigod, M., & Koch, E. (1951*b*). A new blood factor, s, allelic to S. *Proc. Soc. exp. Biol., N. Y.* **78,** 218–24.

Levine, P., Celano, M. J., & Falkowski, F. (1963). The specificity of the antibody in paroxysmal cold hemoglobinuria (P.C.H.). *Transfusion, Philad.* **3,** 278–80.

Levitan, R., Razis, D. V., Diamond, H. D., & Craver, L. F. (1959). ABO blood groups in Hodgkin's disease. *Acta haemat.* **22,** 12–19.

Lewin, E. (1960). Gastric cancer. *Acta chir. scand.* **262,** 1–89.

Lewis, J. G. & Woods, A. C. (1961). The ABO and Rhesus blood groups in patients with respiratory disease. *Tubercle* **42,** 362–5.

Lewis, M., Kaita, H., & Chown, B. (1972). The Duffy blood group system in Caucasians. *Vox Sang.* **23,** 523–7.

Lewkonia, R. M. & Finn, R. (1969). ABO blood group distribution in serum hepatitis. *Brit. med. J.* **iii,** 268–9.

Li, C. C. (1953). Is Rh facing a crossroad?—A critique of the compensation effect. *Amer. Naturalist* **87,** 257–61.

Lickint, F. & Tröltzsch, J. (1929). Ist die Blutgruppenbestimmung als differentialdiagnostisches Hilfsmittel verwendbar? *Dtsch. med. Wschr.* **55,** 1339–40.

Lingren, J. (1934). Quoted by Mustakallio (1937).

Liotta, I., Frattaroli, W., & Herzel, A. (1957). Rapporti tra carcinoma dell'utero e gruppi sanguigni. *Riv. Emoter. Immunoemat.* **4,** 205–9.

Lisker, R., Taboada, C., & Reyes, J. L. (1964). Distribution of the ABO blood groups in peptic ulcer, gastric carcinoma and liver cirrhosis in a Mexican population. *Vox Sang.* **9,** 202–3.

Livingstone, F. B. (1967). *Abnormal hemoglobins in human populations.* Chicago, Aldine Publishing Company.

LIZUNOVA, —. (1925). Blood group agglutination and malaria. (In Russian.) *Trud. 3-go vseross. Syezd. Malyarii*, Moskva, 173–5.

LOBECK, E. (1932). Blutgruppen und Glaukom. *Arch. Ophthal.* **128,** 620–47.

LOBSTEIN, J. J. (1958). *Relations des groupes sanguins et de certains états pathologiques.* Thèse de médecine, no. 59, Strasbourg.

LOBSTEIN, J. J. & VOEGTLIN, R. (1959). Répartition de groupes sanguins dans les populations de malades atteints d'ulcères gastroduodénaux, de cancers gastriques ou de lithiase biliaire. *Strasbourg méd.* **10,** 426–40.

LOVEGROVE, T. D. & NICHOLLS, D. M. (1965). Haptoglobin subtypes in a schizophrenic and control population. *J. nerv. ment. Dis.* **141,** 195–6.

LOWE, J. (1942). Leprosy and blood groups. *Leprosy in India* **14,** 23–5.

LUBS, M. L., NORA, J. J., & LUBS, H. A. (1972). Blood-groups and congenital heart-disease. *Lancet* **ii,** 825–6.

LUCA, F. DE & CRAMAROSSA, L. (1965). Phenylthiourea and endemic goitre. *Lancet* **i,** 1399–400.

LUCARELLI, P., AGOSTINO, R., PALMARINO, R., & BOTTINI, E. (1971). Adenosine deaminase polymorphism in Sardinia. *Humangenetik* **14,** 1–5.

LUCIA, S. P., HUNT, M. L., & PETRAKIS, N. L. (1958). The leukemias in relation to age, sex, and blood group. *Vox Sang.* n.s. **3,** 354–62.

LUDWIG (1964). Quoted by Vogel & Helmbold (1972).

LÜTZELER, H. & DORMANNS, E. A. (1929). Blutgruppenstudien an der Leiche. ii. Mitteilung. *Krankheitsforschung* **7,** 144–62.

LUKETIĆ, G., ČERLEK, N., & KULČAR, Ž. (1959). Blood groups and gastrointestinal diseases. (In Serbo-Croat.) *Liječn. Vijesn.* **81,** 827–30.

MACAFEE, A. L. (1962). *A study of blood groups and disease.* D.M. thesis, Queen's Univ. of Belfast.

MACAFEE, A. L. (1964*a*). ABO blood groups and carcinoma of pancreas. *Ulster med. J.* **33,** 129–31.

MACAFEE, A. L. (1964*b*). Blood groups and diabetes mellitus. *J. clin. Path.* **17,** 39–41.

MACAFEE, A. L. (1965*a*). ABO blood groups and gastric ulcer. *J. med. Genet.* **2,** 24–5.

MACAFEE, A. L. (1965*b*). ABO blood groups and rheumatic heart disease. *Ann. rheum. Dis.* **24,** 392–3.

MACAFEE, A. L. (1967*a*). ABO blood group and thyrotoxicosis. *Vox Sang.* **12,** 143–4.

MACAFEE, A. L. (1967*b*). Blood groups and gastrointestinal cancer. A comparison of the ABO distribution by site of lesion. *Ulster med. J.* **36,** 51–2.

MACAFEE, A. L. (1973). Pers. comm. to A. E. Mourant.

MCALPINE, D., LUMSDEN, C. E., & ACHESON, E. D. (1965). *Multiple sclerosis: a reappraisal.* Edinburgh and London, E. & S. Livingstone.

MACANDREW, R. (1969). Venous thromboembolism and blood-group. *Lancet* **i,** 1263.

MCCONNELL, R. B., CLARKE, C. A., & DOWNTON, F. (1954). Blood groups in carcinoma of the lung. *Brit. med. J.* **ii,** 323–5.

MCCONNELL, R. B., CLARKE, C. A., & DOWNTON, F. (1955). Blood groups in carcinoma of lung. *Brit. med. J.* **ii,** 674.

MCCONNELL, R. B., PYKE, D. A., & ROBERTS, J. A. Fraser (1956). Blood groups in diabetes mellitus. *Brit. med. J.* **i,** 772–6.

MCCONNELL, R. B. (1959). Secretion of blood group antigens in gastro-intestinal diseases. *Gastroenterologia, Basel* **92,** 103–13.

MCCONNELL, R. B. (1961). Blood groups and peptic ulcer. *Practitioner* **186,** 350–4.

MCCONNELL, R. B. (1966). *The genetics of gastro-intestinal disorders.* Oxford University Press, London.

MCDEVITT, H. O. & BODMER, W. F. (1974). HL-A immune-response genes, and disease. *Lancet* **i,** 1269–75.

MCDONALD, J. C. & ZUCKERMAN, A. J. (1962). ABO blood groups and acute respiratory virus disease. *Brit. med. J.* **ii,** 89–90.

MACDONALD, J. L., ROBERTS, D. F., SHAW, D. A., & SAUNDERS, M. (1976). Blood groups and other polymorphisms in multiple sclerosis. *J. med. Genet.* **13,** 30–3.

MACHALSKI, M. & WANTOŁA, J. (1967). Blood groups and Rh factor in liver cirrhosis. (In Polish.) *Pol. Tyg. lek.* **22,** 1765–6.

MACHALSKI, M., KALINA, Z., & WODNIEWSKI, J. (1968). Blood groups in some diseases of the alimentary tract, sclerosis and rheumatic disease. (In Polish.) *Pol. Arch. Med. wewn.* **40,** 613–19.

MACKENZIE, C. G. & MACKENZIE, J. B. (1943). Effect of sulfonamides and thioureas on the thyroid gland and basal metabolism. *Endocrinology* **32,** 185.

MCLAREN, E. H., BURDEN, A. C., & MOORHEAD, P. J. (1977). Acetylator phenotype in diabetic neuropathy. *Brit. med. J.* **ii,** 291–3.

MACLEOD, K. I. E. (1937). The relation of the blood group of the individual to blood diseases and neoplasms. *Brit. med. J.* **ii,** 745–7.

MACLEOD, K. I. E. (1954). Blood groups in relation to certain diseases. *Brit. med. J.* **ii,** 754.

MACMAHON, B. & FOLUSIAK, J. C. (1958). Leukemia and ABO blood groups. *Amer. J. hum. Genet.* **10,** 287–93.

MCNEIL, C., WARENSKI, L. C., FULLMER, C. D., & TRENTELMAN, E. F. (1954). A study of the blood groups in habitual abortion. *Amer. J. clin. Path.* **24,** 767–73.

MCNEIL, C., TRENTELMAN, E. F., LADLE, J. N., HELMICK, W. M., & PLENK, H. P. (1965). Blood group secretion factors in bronchogenic carcinoma. *Nature, Lond.* **208,** 299.

MACSWEEN, M. P. & SYME, U. A. (1965). ABO blood groups and skin diseases. *Brit. J. Derm.* **77,** 30–4.

MADSEN, T., ENGLE, E. T., JENSEN, C., & FREUCHEN, I. B. (1936). Blood grouping and poliomyelitis. Report based on 1118 cases in the 1934 epidemic in Denmark. *J. Immunol.* **30,** 213–19.

MÄHR, G. (1959). Die Verteilung der ABO-Blutgruppen beim Diabetes mellitus. *Wien. klin. Wschr.* **71,** 536–8.

MAJOR, L. (1960). Die Relation der Karzinome und Ulcera des Verdauungstraktes zum ABO Blutgruppensystem. *Wien. klin. Wschr.* **72,** 322–33.

MÁJSKÝ, A. (1964). Incidence of disease in the relation to the ABO blood groups and to the Rh_o(D) system. Some remarks based on personal experience with blood diseases. (In Czech.) *Vnitř. Lék.* **10,** 253–8.

MAJUPURIA, K. C. & GUPTA, L. C. (1966). The study of ABO blood groups and relationship with cancer cervix. *J. Obstet. Gynaec., Lahore* **16,** 64–5.

MAJUPURIA, K. C., GUPTA, S. R., & GUPTA, L. C. (1966). The study of ABO blood groups and relationship with cancer breast (a preliminary report). *Indian J. Cancer* **3,** 182–3.

MALAIHOLLO, J. F. (1940). Lepra in de desa Wates (Res. Batavia) en het resultaat van een bloedgroeponderzoek onder leprozen en gezonden in Wates en Blora. *Geneesk. Tijdschr. Ned.-Ind.* **80,** 2296–312.

MALAMOS, B., KOUTRAS, D. A., KOSTAMIS, P., KRALIOS, A. C., RIGOPOULOS, G., & ZEREFOS, N. (1966). Endemic goiter in Greece: epidemiologic and genetic studies. *J. clin. Endocrin.* **26,** 688–95.

MALTONI, G. & CANALI, E. (1956). I gruppi sanguigni in relazione al cancro gastrico e all'ulcera gastro-duodenale. *Ann. ital. Chir.* **33,** 371–82.

MANGANI, G. (1957). Della relazione esistente tra gruppi sanguigni ed alcune affezioni chirurgiche. *Policlinico*, Sez. prat. **64,** 1049–52.

MANGAT, G. S. & HARRIES, J. R. (1961). ABO groups in Africans with peptic ulcer. *Brit. med. J.* **i,** 589.

MANGIACAPRA, A. (1936). Gruppi sanguigni e malaria. *Rif. med.* **52,** 985–8.

MANITZ, H. (1932). Das humorale Syndrom der Mongoloiden. *Dtsch. Z. Nervenheilk.* **126,** 80–93.

MANLAPAS, F. C., STEIN, A. A., PAGLIARA, A. S., APICELLI, A. A., PORTER, I. H., & PATTERSON, P. R. (1965). Phenylthiocarbamide taste sensitivity in cystic fibrosis. *J. Pediat.* **66,** 8–11.

MANZINI, R. (1960). Correlazioni tra gruppi sanguigni e neoplasie della laringe e del cavo orale. *Arch. ital. Otol.* **71,** 638–44.

MARINE, D., BAUMANN, E. J., SPENCE, A. W., & CIPRA, A. (1932). Further studies on etiology of goiter with particular reference to the action of cyanides. *Proc. Soc. exp. Biol., N. Y.* **29,** 772–5.

MARINE, D. (1935). The pathogenesis and prevention of simple or endemic goiter. *J. Amer. med. Ass.* **104,** 2334–41.

MARKIANOS, I., KARAGEORGOPOULOS, A., MPELEZOS, A., & KOUZOUTZAKOGLOS, R. (1957). Relation of ABO blood groups and Rh factor in leprosy patients. (In Greek.) *Acta microbiol. hellen.* **2,** 35–42.

Marsh, W. L., Øyen, R., Nichols, M. E., & Allen, F. H. (1975). Chronic granulomatous disease and the Kell blood groups. *Brit. J. Haemat.* **29,** 247–62. Marsh *et al.* (1976). *Vox Sang.* **31,** 356–62.

Martella, N. A. (1938). Gruppi sanguigni e neoplasie maligne epiteliali. *Rif. med.* **54,** 1303–4.

Martin, J.-P. (ed.) (1975). *L'alpha-1-antitrypsine et le système Pi.* Paris, INSERM.

Marzi, F. & Turchini, G. (1952). Fattori M, N, P e gruppi sanguigni nelle malattie mentali. *Riv. Biol.* **44,** 527–39.

Masters, A. B. (1967). The distribution of blood groups in psychiatric illness. *Brit. J. Psychiat.* **113,** 1309–15.

Matoušek, M. (1935). Zhoubné nádory ženských rodidel a prsu a krevní skupiny. *Bratisl. lék. Listy* **15,** 334–43.

Matsunaga, E. (1955). Intrauterine selection by the ABO incompatibility of mother and foetus. *Amer. J. hum. Genet.* **7,** 66–71.

Matsunaga, E. (1956). Selektion durch Unverträglichkeit in ABO-Blutgruppensystem zwischen Mutter und Fetus. *Blut* **2,** 188–98.

Matsunaga, E. (1959). Selection in ABO polymorphism in Japanese populations. *J. med. Educ.* **34,** 405–13.

Matsunaga, E. (1962*a*). The dimorphism in human normal cerumen. *Ann. hum. Genet.* **25,** 273–86.

Matsunaga, E. (1962*b*). Selective mechanisms operating on ABO and MN blood groups with special reference to prezygotic selection. *Eugen. Quart.* **9,** 36–43.

Maurer, B., Hickley, N., & Mulcahy, R. (1969). ABO and Rh blood groups in patients with coronary heart disease. *Irish J. med. Sci.* **2,** 105–8.

Mauro, di (1936). Quoted by Marzi & Turchini (1952) and Asaro (1955).

Maxted, G. R. (1940). The incidence of the four main blood groups in rheumatic heart disease. *Arch. Dis. Childh.* **15,** 181–3.

Maxwell, R. D. H. & Maxwell, K. N. (1955). ABO blood group and hypertension. *Brit. med. J.* **ii,** 179–80.

Mayo, C. W. & Fergeson, J. O. (1953). Are certain diseases associated with specific blood groups or Rh antigens? *Arch. Surg., Chicago* **66,** 406–9.

Mayr, E., Diamond, L. K., Levine, R. P., & Mayr, M. (1956). Suspected correlation between blood-groups frequency and pituitary adenomas. *Science* **124,** 932–4.

Mazhdrakov, G. & Grancharov, V. (1960). Blood groups and gastric cancer. *Probl. Oncol.* **6,** 1568–75.

Mazur, J. & Alex. Quoted by Helmbold (1961).

Medalie, J. H., Levene, C., Papier, C., Goldbourt, U., Dreyfuss, F., Oron, D., Neufeld, H., & Riss, E. (1971). Blood groups, myocardial infarction and angina pectoris among 10,000 adult males. *New Engl. J. Med.* **285,** 1348–53.

el-Mehairy, M. M. & el-Tarabishi, N. (1966). The correlation between ABO blood groups and allergic disorders. *Ann. Allergy* **27,** 366–8.

Memória, J. M. Pompeu (1958). Quoted by Araújo *et al.* (1972).

Merikas, G., Christakopoulos, P., & Petropoulos, E. (1966). Distribution of ABO blood group in patients with ulcer disease; its relationship to gastroduodenal bleeding. *Amer. J. dig. Dis.* n.s. **11,** 790–5.

Mertens (1964). Quoted by Vogel & Helmbold (1972).

Meuwissen, H. J., Kaplan, G. T., Frommel, D., & Good, R. A. (1969). Blood-group O in non-lymphopenic hypogammaglobulinaemia. *Lancet* **i,** 374–5.

Meyer, F. (1928). Die Blutgruppenverteilung in der schlesischen Bevölkerung sowie die Beziehung der Blutgruppen zu Geisteskrankheiten. *Dtsch. med. Wschr.* **54,** 1461–2.

Miani, P. (1958). Rapporti tra gruppi sanguigni e glaucoma cronico semplice. *G. ital. Oftal.* **11,** 537–9.

Mikkelsen, O. A. (1967). Dupuytren's disease and blood groups. *Scand. J. plast. Reconstr. Surg.* **1,** 148–9.

Mikolášek, A. & Miluničová, A. (1967). Die Korrelation von Blutgruppenantigenen und -substanzen mit hypertonischer Erkrankung. *Humangenetik* **3,** 295–9.

Mikuchi, T. (1931). Über den Blutgruppentypus bei dem Glaukom. *Acta Soc. ophthal. jap.* **35,** 93–4.

Miller, J. J., Novotny, P., Walker, P. D., Harris, J. R. W., & MacLennan, I. P. B. (1977). *Neisseria gonorrhoeae* and ABO isohemagglutinins. *Infect. Immun.* **15,** 713–19.

Miller, L. H., Mason, S. J., Dvorak, J. A., McGinniss, Mary H., & Rothman, I. K. (1975). Erythrocyte receptors for (*Plasmodium knowlesi*) malaria: Duffy blood group determinants. *Science* **189,** 561–3.

Milošević, B., Stolević, E., & Krajinović, S. (1961). Blood groups in carcinomas of the female genital organs. (In Serbo-Croat.) *Higijena* **13,** 95–100.

Miluničová, A. & Dominec, M. (1966). Blood characteristic and PTC test in young patients suffering from pulmonary tuberculosis or diabetes mellitus. (In Czech.) *Rozhl. Tuberk.* **26,** 545–50.

Miluničová, A. & Hájek, M. (1966). PTC test in patients with malignant goitre. (In Czech.) *Čas. Lék. čes.* **105,** 1227–30.

Miluničová, A., Jandová, A., Laurová, L., Novotná, J., & Škoda, V. (1969*a*). Hereditary blood and serum types, PTC test and level of the fifth fraction of serum lactatedehydrogenase in females with gynecological cancer. (ii. Communication.) *Neoplasma* **16,** 311–16.

Miluničová, A., Jandová, A., & Škoda, V. (1969*b*). Die Ausscheidung von ABH- Blutgruppensubstanzen bei Frauen mit gynäkologischem Karzinom. *Z. ImmunForsch.* **138,** 90–3.

Miluničová, A., Jandová, A., & Škoda, V. (1969*c*). Phenylthiocarbamide tasting ability and malignant tumours. *Hum. Hered.* **19,** 398–401.

Miluničová, A., Jandová, A., & Škoda, V. (1969*d*). Serum haptoglobin type in females with genital cancer. *J. nat. Cancer Inst.* **42,** 749–51.

Minkevich, —. (1925). Isohemagglutination group as a constitutional feature determining the relation of a subject to malarial infection. (In Russian.) *Trud. 3-go vseross. Syezd. Malyarii,* Moskva, 169–72.

Miraglia, M. & Ronaldo, D. (1962). Gruppi sanguigni e leucemie. *Pediatria, Napoli* **70,** 650–5.

Mironesco, T. & Stefanov, G. (1926). Contribution à l'étude du rapport qui existe entre les groupes sanguins et les infections. *C. R. Soc. Biol., Paris* **95,** 140–1.

Misiti, G., Sbuelz, B., & Malatesta, P. (1968). Gruppi sanguigni e orientamento secretorio gastrico nella malattia ulcerosa. *Chir. gastroent.* **2,** 410–23.

Miššík, T. (1962). Relation between ABO blood groups, Rh factor and mental diseases. (In Czech.) *Čes. Psychiat.* **58,** 21–6.

Mital, V. P. & Gupta, S. (1969). The study of ABO blood groups in oral cancer. *Indian J. Cancer* **6,** 34–7.

Mitra, P. N. (1933). The influence of blood group in certain pathological states. *Indian J. med. Res.* **20,** 995–1004.

Mitra, S., Mondal, S., & Basu, A. (1962). The study of ABO blood groups in cancer of the female genital organs and cancer of the breast. *Cancer, Philad.* **15,** 39–41.

Mittman, C. (ed.) (1972). *Pulmonary emphysema and proteolysis.* N. York and London, Academic Press. (Duarte. City of Hope Med. Center symp. series, **2.**)

Mobilio, G. & Torchiana, B. (1960). Considerazioni statistiche fra gli emogruppi del sistema 'ABO' e le principali malattie urologiche. *Riv. Anat. pat. Oncol.* **18,** 861–80.

Mogielnicki, W. & Tarłowska, L. (1964). ABO blood group distribution in patients with cancer of the uterus. (In Polish.) *Nowotwory* **14,** 335–40.

Mollison, P. L. & Hill, L. (1969). ABO groups in hypogammaglobulinaemia. *Lancet* **i,** 467.

Moniwa, H. (1960). Statistical studies on the correlation between ABO-blood groups and some diseases. *Tohoku J. exp. Med.* **72,** 275–89.

Montanari, A. (1929). I gruppi sanguigni in clinica. *Riv. Clin. med.* **30,** 724–54.

Montestrug, E. & Caubet, P. (1948). Les groupes sanguins chez les lépreux. *Arch. Inst. Pasteur Martinique* **1,** 3–8.

Moor-Jankowski, J. K., Holländer, L. P., Huser, H. J., Linder, A., & Schneeberger, M. (1961). Correlation of blood group and disease in a population of known origins. 2nd *Int. Congr. hum. Genet.*, Rome, **2,** 866–8.

MOR, C. & SFORZA, M. (1960). Esiste rapporto fra gruppi sanguigni e malattie chirurgiche? *Arch. Sci. med.* **109,** 528–35.

MORATO, A., GIOVANELLI, E., & SGARBI, M. (1969). Indagine statistica sulla eventuale associazione delle vasculopatie cerebrali acute a focolaio con determinati gruppi sanguigni. *Minerva med., Torino*, pt. sci. **60,** 142–5.

MOROSINI, P., LEE, E. G., JONES, M. N., VESSEY, M. P., HEINONEN, O. P., NEVANLINNA, H. R., & SVINHUFVUD, U. L. M. (1972). Breast cancer and the S blood group system. *Lancet* **i,** 411–12.

MOSBECH, J. (1958). ABO blood groups in stomach cancer. *Acta genet. Stat. med.* **8,** 219–27.

MOSLER, W. Quoted by Helmbold (1961).

MOSLER, W. & WEHLE, F. Quoted by Helmbold (1961).

MOURANT, A. E. (1946). A 'new' human blood group antigen of frequent occurrence. *Nature, Lond.* **158,** 237.

MOURANT, A. E. (1947). The blood groups of the Basques. *Nature, Lond.* **160,** 505.

MOURANT, A. E., KOPEĆ, A. C., & DOMANIEWSKA-SOBCZAK, K. (1958). The ABO blood groups. Comprehensive tables and maps of world distribution. Oxford, Blackwell Scientific Publications (Royal Anthropological Institute, occasional publication no. 13.) Reprinted as Appendix to Mourant *et al.* 1976.

MOURANT, A. E., KOPEĆ, A. C., & DOMANIEWSKA-SOBCZAK, K. (1971). Blood-groups and blood-clotting. *Lancet* **i,** 223–8.

MOURANT, A. E., KOPEĆ, A. C., & DOMANIEWSKA-SOBCZAK, K. (1976). *The distribution of the human blood groups and other polymorphisms*, 2nd ed. London, Oxford University Press. (Appendix: Mourant *et al.* 1958.)

MOURANT, A. E., TILLS, D., & DOMANIEWSKA-SOBCZAK, K. (1976). Sunshine and the geographical distribution of the alleles of the Gc system of plasma proteins. *Hum. Genet.* **33,** 307–14.

MOUREAU, P. & FIRKET, J. (1934). Les groupes sanguins et les maladies. *C. R. Soc. Biol., Paris* **117,** 228–31.

MOUREAU, P. (1935). Contribution à l'étude des facteurs d'individualisation du sang humain et leurs application en médecine légale. *Rev. belge Sci. méd.* **7,** 177–233.

MULLER, O. (1955). Cáncer gástrico y grupos sanguíneos. *Orientación méd.* **4,** 1199–200.

MUNEUCHI, T. (1934). Beiträge zur Kenntnis des Bluttypus bei Leprakranken. *Jap. J. Derm.* **35,** 10.

MUÑOZ-BARATTA, C. (1962). Blood groups and disease. 8th *Congr. int. Soc. Blood Transfus.*, Tokyo, 1960. *Bibl. haemat.* **13,** 260–6.

MURRAY, R. F., ROBINSON, J. C., DUBLIN, T. D., PITT, E. L., & VISNICH, S. (1966). Haptoglobins and rheumatic fever. *Brit. med. J.* **i,** 762–5.

MUSTAKALLIO, E. (1937). Untersuchungen über die M–N, A_1–A_2 und O–A–B Blutgruppen in Finnland. *Acta Soc. Med. 'Duodecim'* s. A, **20,** no. 2, 1–181.

MYRIANTHOPOULOS, N. C. & LEYSHON, W. C. (1967). The relation of blood groups and the secretor factor to amyotrophic lateral sclerosis. *Amer. J. hum. Genet.* **19,** 607–16.

NAIR, C. P., ROY, R. G., & RAGHAVAN, N. G. S. (1959). Blood groups and filariasis. *Bull. Nat. Soc. India Malar.* **7,** 119–21 (quoted by Ayres *et al.* 1976).

NAND, S. & YADAV, M. S. (1964). Blood grouping in osteo-articular tuberculosis. *Indian Practit.* **17,** 727–8.

NARDELLI, L. (1928). I gruppi sanguigne nelle dermatosi. *G. ital. Derm. Sif.* **69,** 943–54.

NARDUCCI, F. (1928). Ricerche sui gruppi sanguigni nei dermopazienti. *G. ital. Derm. Sif.* **69,** 955–7.

NATH, K., JOLLY, J. G., & PARASHAR, S. K. (1963). Blood groups and susceptibility to diseases. *J. Ass. Physicn India* **11,** 667–74.

NAVANI, H. & NARANG, R. K. (1962). A study of ABO blood groups in pulmonary tuberculosis. *Indian J. Chest Dis.* **4,** 109–13.

NAZAROV, K. N. & CHOVDYROVA, G. S. (1972). The distribution of the ABO blood groups in families with Down's disease. (In Russian.) *Vop. Anthrop.* **42,** 153–6.

NEEL, J. V. (1949). The inheritance of sickle cell anemia. *Science* **110,** 64–6.

NEEL, J. V. (1967). Current concepts of the genetic basis of diabetes mellitus and the biological significance of the diabetic predisposition. 6th *Congr. int. Diabet. Fed.*, Stockholm, pp. 68–78. (Excerpta med. int. Congr. Ser. no. 172S.)

NEFZGER, M. D., HRUBEC, Z., & CHALMERS, T. C. (1969). Venous thromboembolism and blood-group. *Lancet* **i,** 887.

NEGRI, M., SERRA, A., & SOINI, A. (1959). Sulle relazioni tra neoplasie della laringe e gruppi sanguigni del sistema ABO. *Tumori* **45,** 201–6.

NERUP, J., PLATZ, P., ORTVED ANDERSEN, O., CHRISTY, M., LYNGSØE, J., POULSEN, J. E., RYDER, L. P., NIELSEN, L. Staub, THOMSEN, M., & SVEJGAARD, A. (1974). HL–A antigens and diabetes mellitus. *Lancet* **ii,** 864–6.

NETTELBLADT, E. & SUNDBLAD, L. (1967). Studies on serum haptoglobins in rheumatoid arthritis. *Opusc. med.* **12,** 233–8.

NEUMAN, J., NOVIZKI, I., BAUERBERG, J., & STEINBERG, J. (1961). Distribución de frecuencias de los grupos sanguíneos del sistema ABO en los enfermos con infarto de miocardio. *Rev. Asoc. méd. argent.* **75,** 534–40.

NEWMAN, E., NAIFEH, G. S., AUER, J. E., & BUCKWALTER, J. A. (1961). Secretion of ABH antigens in peptic ulceration and gastric carcinoma. *Brit. med. J.* **i,** 92–4.

NGUYEN DUONG QUANG, SCHMAUSS, A. K., & NGUYEN NHU BANG (1960). ABO-Blutgruppen und Ulkusleiden in Nordvietnam. *Dtsch. GesundheitsWes.* **15,** 175–80.

NGUYEN DUONG QUANG, SCHMAUSS, A. K., & NGUYEN NHU BANG (1962). ABO-Blutgruppen und Magenkrebs in Nordvietnam. *Dtsch. GesundheitsWes.* **17,** 1758–62.

NICULESCU, N., WEXLER, T., & SCHWARTZENBERG, T. (1969). Some aspects in the distribution of ABO and Rh blood groups in multiple malformations. (In Romanian.) *Viaţa med.* **16,** 307–12.

NIELSEN, L. Staub, JERSILD, C., RYDER, L. P., & SVEJGAARD, A. (1975). HL–A antigen, gene, and haplotype frequencies in Denmark. *Tissue Antigens* **6,** 70–6.

NIELSEN, L. Staub, RYDER, L. P., & SVEJGAARD, A. (1976). The third (AJ) segregant series. In *Histocompatibility testing 1975.* Copenhagen, Munksgaard.

NINNI, M. & BEDARIDA, G. (1959). Rilievi statistici sui rapporti tra gruppi sanguigni e malattie. 7th *Congr. int. Soc. Blood Transfus.*, Rome, 1958. *Bibl. haemat.* **10,** 159–63.

NOWAK, H. (1931–2). Besteht ein Unterschied in den Diphtherieempfänglichkeit bei den Angehörigen der vershiedenen Blutgruppen? *Mschr. Kinderheilk.* **51,** 257–72.

NOWAK, H. (1932). Scharlachempfänglichkeit und Blutgruppen. *Mschr. Kinderheilk.* **54,** 343–58.

ODA, I. (1971). ABO blood groups and their secretor status in patients with uveitis. *Ophtalmologica, Basel* **162,** 298–307.

OGUNBA, E. O. (1970). ABO blood groups, haemoglobin genotypes, and loiasis. *J. med. Genet.* **7,** 56–8.

OHMICHI, N. (1928). Die Bedeutung der Blutgruppen im Gebiete der Dermatologie und der Urologie. *J. Okayama med. Soc.* **40,** 1182–91.

OHNSORGE, — (1927). Blutgruppenuntersuchungen bei Nerven- und Geisteskranken. *Arch. Psychiat. Nervenkr.* **81,** 763.

OIKE, Y., KIKUCHI, Y., & HATAYAMA, S. (1962). ABO blood groups and pulmonary tuberculosis. 8th *Congr. int. Soc. Blood Transfus.*, Tokyo, 1960. *Bibl. haemat.* **13,** 267–9.

OLIVER, M. F. & CUMMING, R. A. (1962). Blood groups and heart disease. *Brit. med. J.* **ii,** 51.

OREL, H. (1927). Zur Klinik der mongoloiden Idiotic. *Z. Kinderheilk.* **44,** 449–72.

ORLANDI, G. & TOSI, C. (1962). Gruppi sanguigni e neoplasie maligne nel polmone. *Arch. ital. Otol.* **73,** 53–65.

OSBORNE, R. H. & DE GEORGE, F. V. (1962). The ABO blood groups in parotid and submaxillary gland tumors. *Amer. J. hum. Genet.* **14,** 199–209.

OSBORNE, R. H. & DE GEORGE, F. V. (1963). The ABO blood groups in neoplastic disease of the ovary. *Amer. J. hum. Genet.* **15,** 380–8.

OSZACKI, J., LEŃCZYK, M., NOSEK, H., & URBAN, A. (1965). Population investigation on carcinoma of the stomach, the appearances of metastases in relation to the age, sex and blood groups of patients. (In Polish.) *Nowotwory* **15,** 227–9.

OTTENBERG, R. (1923). The etiology of eclampsia; historical and critical notes. *J. Amer. med. Ass.* **81,** 295.

OTTO-SERVAIS, M., STAINIER, B., ANDRÉ, A., MOUREAU, P., & BRACQUIER, T. (1959). Groupes sanguins et cancers. Groupes sanguins et diabète. 7th *Congr. int. Soc. Blood Transfus.*, Rome, 1958. *Bibl. haemat.* **10,** 167–73.

PACIORKIEWICZ, M. (1970). The correlation between blood groups and some infectious diseases in children. (In Polish.) *Pediat. pol.* **45,** 943–50.

PALDROCK, A. (1929). Die Blutgruppen der Leprösen in Estland. *Arch. Schiffs.-u. Tropenh.* **33,** 440–6.

PALMARINO, R., AGOSTINO, R., GLORIA, F., LUCARELLI, P., BUSINCO, L., ANTOGNONI, G., MAGGIONI, G., WORKMAN, P. L., & BOTTINI, E. (1975). Red cell acid phosphatase: another polymorphism correlated with malaria? *Amer. J. phys. Anthrop.* **43,** 177–85.

PALMIERI, V. M. (1928). Die Verteilung der morphologisch-konstitutionellen Typen unter den geisteskranken Verbrechern. *Dtsch. Z. ges. gerichtl. Med.* **12,** 592–601.

PAOLI, P. DE (1932). Contributo allo studio dei gruppi sanguigni nelle malatie tubercolari. *Lotta c. Tuberc.* **3,** 494–8.

PAOLUCCI, A. M., FERRO-LUZZI, A., MODIANO, G., MORPURGO, G., & KANASHIRO, V. K. (1971). Taste sensitivity to phenylthiocarbamide (PTC) and endemic goiter in the Indian natives of Peruvian Highlands. *Amer. J. phys. Anthrop.* **34,** 427–30.

PAPAYANNOPOULOS, G. (1958). Duodenal ulcer and the ABO blood-groups. *Lancet* **i,** 1078.

PAPIHA, S. S. & ROBERTS, D. F. (1975). Serum alkaline phosphatase in patients with multiple sclerosis. *Clin. Genet.* **7,** 77–82.

PARKER, G. & WALSH, R. J. (1958). Blood groups and disease: carcinoma of various organs. *Med. J. Austr.* **ii,** 835–6.

PARKER, J. B., THEILIE, A., & SPIELBERGER, C. D. (1961). Frequency of blood types in a homogeneous group of manic-depressive patients. *J. ment. Sci.* **107,** 936–42.

PARR, L. W. (1929). Negative results obtained in the attempt to relate tuberculosis susceptibility or resistance to a particular blood group. *J. prev. Med.* **3,** 237–43.

PAULING, L., ITANO, H. A., SINGER, S. J., & WELLS, I. C. (1949). Sickle cell anemia, a molecular disease. *Science* **110,** 543–8.

PAYNE, R. & ROLFS, M. R. (1958). Fetomaternal leucocyte incompatibility. *J. clin. Invest.* **37,** 1756–63.

PEACOCK, A. C. (1966). Serum haptoglobin type and leukemia: an association with possible etiological significance. *J. nat. Cancer Inst.* **36,** 631–9.

PEACOCK, A. C. & ALEPA, F. P. (1966). Haptoglobin types in patients with juvenile rheumatoid arthritis. *Ann. rheum. Dis.* **25,** 567–9.

PEARCE, K. M. & YATES, P. O. (1965). Blood groups and brain tumors. *J. neurol. Sci.* **2,** 434–41.

PEARSON, M. G. & PINKER, G. D. (1956). ABO blood groups and toxaemia of pregnancy. *Brit. med. J.* **i,** 777–8.

PEARSON, R. J. C. (1964). Blood groups and disease. *Brit. med. J.* **i,** 840–1.

PEEBLES BROWN, D. A., MELROSE, A. G., & WALLACE, J. (1956). The blood groups in peptic ulceration. *Brit. med. J.* **ii,** 135–8.

PEETERS, H. (ed.) (1976). *Protides of the biological fluids. Proceedings of the 23rd colloquium, Brugge 1975.* Oxford, Pergamon Press.

PELL, S., D'ALONZO, C. A., & FLEMING, A. J. (1957). A study of the relation of the ABO blood-groups to peptic ulceration and hypertension. *Ann. intern. Med.* **46,** 1024–30.

PELL, S. & D'ALONZO, C. A. (1961). A three-year study of myocardial infarction in a large employed population. *J. Amer. med. Ass.* **175,** 463–70.

PENNACCHI (1928). Quoted by Marzi & Turchini (1952) and Asaro (1955).

PENROSE, L. S. (1932). The blood grouping of mongolian imbeciles. *Lancet* **i,** 394–5.

PENZIK, A. S. (1930). Die Blutgruppenverhältnisse bei Polyarthritikern. *Ukr. Zbl. Blutgr.* **4,** 250–4.

PERCESEPE, E., SANTORO, E., LUISE, P. DE, & CAJANO, A. (1959). Gruppi sanguigni e carcinoma pulmonare, 7th *Congr. int. Soc. Blood Tranfus.*, Rome, 1958. *Bibl. haemat.* **10,** 174–5.

PERERA, G. A. & ADLER, G. (1960). ABO blood groups in the accelerated form of hypertension. *Ann. intern. Med.* **53,** 84–6.

PERITZ, E. (1967). A statistical study of intrauterine selection factors related to the ABO system. i. The analysis of data on liveborn children. *Ann. hum. Genet.* **30,** 259–71.

PERITZ, E. (1971). A statistical study of the intrauterine selection factors related to the ABO system. ii. The analysis of foetal mortality data. *Ann. hum. Genet.* **34,** 389–94.

PERKEL, J. D. & ISRAELSSON, M. M. (1928). Blutgruppenverteilung bei Syphilis des Zentralnervensystems, der inneren Organe und der Haut. *Derm. Z.* **54,** 261–7.

PERRETTI, F. & PUTIGNANO, A. (1967). Contributo clinico statistico allo studio dei rapporti tra gruppi sanguigni e cancro e fibromiomi dell'utero. *Clin. ostet. ginec.* **69,** 529–35.

PERSSON, I., KØLENDORF, L., & KØLENDORF, K. (1972). PTC taste sensitivity in toxic diffuse goitre. *Hum. Hered.* **22,** 459–65.

PESCE, G. & PONTRANDOLFI, P. (1961). Gruppi sanguigni ed epatocolecistopatie. *Policlinico*, Sez. prat. **68,** 396–9.

PETRAKIS, N. L., DOHERTY, M., LEE, R. E., SMITH, S. C., & PAGE, N. L. (1971). Demonstration and implications of lysozyme and immunoglobins in human ear wax. *Nature, Lond.* **229,** 119–20.

PETRAKIS, N. L., PINGLE, U., PETRAKIS, S. J., & PETRAKIS, S. L. (1971). Evidence for a genetic cline in earwax types in the Middle East and south-east Asia. *Amer. J. phys. Anthrop.* **35,** 141–4.

PETTENKOFER, H. J. & TOMASCHECK, G. Quoted by Helmbold (1961).

PETTENKOFER, H. J., STÖSS, B., HELMBOLD, W., & VOGEL, F. (1962). Alleged causes of the present-day world distribution of the human ABO blood groups. *Nature, Lond.* **193,** 445–6.

PFAHLER, G. E. & WIDMAN, B. P. (1924). The relation of blood groups to malignant disease and the influence of radiotherapy. *Amer. J. Roentgenol.* **12,** 47–50.

PFEIFER, S. & GRÜNWALD, P. (1961). Endemska struma i neka nasljedna svojstva stanovnika otoka Krka. *Drugi jugoslavenski Simpozij o endemskoj gusavosti*, pp. 267–93. Zagreb, KOMNIS.

PHAM-HUU-TRUNG, BESSIS, A., & MOZZICONACCI, P. (1961). Les groupes sanguins et le rheumatisme articulaire aigu. *Sem. Hôp. Paris* **37,** 2763–6.

PIAZZA, A., BELVEDERE, M. C., BERNOCO, D., CONIGHI, C., CONTU, L., CURTONI, E. S., MATTIUZ, P. L., MAYR, W., RICHIARDI, P., SCUDELLER, G., & CEPPELLINI, R. (1973). HL-A variation in four Sardinian villages under differential selective pressure by malaria. In *Histocompatibility testing 1972* (eds. J. Dausset & J. Colombani), pp. 73–84. Copenhagen, Munksgaard.

PIETRANDOLFI, P. & PESCE, G. (1961). Rapporti tra gruppi sanguigni del sistema A.B.O. e gozzo. *Gazz. sanit., Milano* **32,** 430–2.

PIETREK, G. & KINDLER, U. (1971). Haptoglobin-Phänotypen bei Seren mit Geschwulstkrankheiten. *Verh. dtsch. Ges. inn. Med.* **77,** 764–6.

PIKE, L. A. & DICKINS, A. M. (1954). ABO blood groups and toxaemia of pregnancy. *Brit. med. J.* **ii,** 321–3.

PILCZ, A. (1927). Untersuchungen über die Blutgruppenzugehörigkeit bei Geisteskranken. *Jb. Psychiat. Neurol.* **45,** 120–31.

PINETTI, P. (1931). Lo studio del sangue nella lepra. *G. ital. Derm. Sif.* **72,** 1319–35.

PISANI, E. & ACERBI, A. (1960). Correlazioni fra gruppi sanguigni, calcolosi e malformazioni dell'apparato urinario. *Osped. maggiore* **48,** 719–26.

PLOTKIN, S. A. (1958). The ABO blood groups in relation to prematurity and stillbirth. *J. Pediat., St. Louis* **52,** 42–7.

POEHLMANN, A. (1929). Ergebnisse der Blutgruppenforschung und ihre Bedeutung für die Venerologie und Dermatologie. *Zbl. Haut- u. GeschlKr.* **29,** 1–9.

POEHLMANN, A. (1930). Blutgruppe und Syphilis. *Münch. med. Wschr.* **77,** 1007–9.

POLAYES, S. H. (1945). Erythroblastosis fetalis unrelated to the Rh factor: isoimmunization of group O mothers by group A children. *Proc. N. Y. path. Soc.* Nov. 29, 173–7.

POLLARA, C. & MELINA, D. (1957). Gruppi sanguigni e malattie. *Rif. med.* **71,** 929–30.

POPPOFF, N. W. (1927). Isoagglutination und ihre forensische Anwendung in Russland. *Dtsch. Z. ges. gerichtl. Med.* **9,** 411–25.

POST, R. H. & WHITE, P. (1958). Tentative explanation of the high incidence of diabetes. *Diabetes* **7,** 27–32.

POTAPOV, M. I. (1970). Detection of the antigen of the Lewis system, characteristic of the erythrocytes of the secretory group Le (a–b–). (In Russian.) *Probl. Gemat. Pereliv. Krovi* **15,** no. 11, 45–9.

POTTER, C. W. & SCHILD, G. C. (1967). The incidence of HI antibody to influenza virus A2/Singapore/1/57 in individuals of blood groups A and O. *J. Immunol.* **98,** 1320–5.

POVEY, M. S. & HORTON, R. J. (1966). Leprosy and blood groups. *Leprosy Rev.* **37,** 147–50.

PRASAD, K. V. N. & ALI, P. M. (1966). ABO blood groups and leprosy. *Int. J. Leprosy* **34,** 398–404.

PRATT, R. T. C. (1963). Pers. comm. to A. E. Mourant.

PREISLER, O., SIGMOND, I., & STEGMANN, H. (1959). Blutgruppen und Rh-Faktor beim Genitalkarzinom. *Zbl. Gynäk.* **81,** 493–7.

PREISLER, O. & MATTHES, M. Quoted by Helmbold (1961).

PRESTON, A. E. & BARR, A. (1964). The plasma concentration of factor VIII in the normal population. ii. The effects of age, sex and blood group. *Brit. J. Haemat.* **10,** 238–45.

PRINGLE, R., WORT, A. J., & GREEN, C. A. (1964). The significance of ABO groups and secretion status in duodenal ulcer. *Brit. J. Surg.* **51,** 341–3.

PRIOR, C. & VEGNI, L. (1957). I gruppi sanguigni ed i loro rapporti con la patologia dello stomaco (ulcera peptica e cancro). *Atti Accad. fisiocr. Siena*, Sez. med. fis. **4,** 484–90.

PROKOP, J., SKALIČKOVA, O., & ČUPÍK, J. (1938). Contribution aux études biotypologiques dans la schizophrénie. Les groupes sanguins, la constitution et la race. *Encéphale* **33,** 104–8.

PROKOP, O., LANGMANN, H., & PERTZBORN, E. Quoted by Helmbold (1961).

PROMIŃSKA, E. (1967). ABO blood groups in patients with lung tuberculosis. (In Polish.) *Przegl. antrop.* **33,** 3–18.

PROSSER, I. (1957). Rapporti fra i gruppi sanguigni ABO con l'ulcera gastro-duodenale e il carcinoma dello stomaco. *Rass. int. Clin. Terap.* **37,** 218–24.

PROSSER, I. (1959). I gruppi sanguigni ABO e l'ipertrofia della prostata. *Minerva urol.* **11,** 253–5.

PUENTE, J. J. (1927–8). Los grupos sanguíneos en la lepra. *Rev. Asoc. argent. Derm. Sif.* **12,** 125–37.

PUTKONEN, T. (1930). Über die gruppenspezifischen Eigenschaften verschiedener Körperflüssigkeiten. *Acta Soc. Med. 'Duodecim'* **14,** no. 12, 1–113.

RACE, R. R. (1944). An 'incomplete' antibody in human serum. *Nature, Lond.* **153,** 771–2.

RACE, R. R. & SANGER, R. (1975). *Blood groups in man*, 6th ed. Blackwell Scientific Publications, Oxford.

RADIVOIEVICI, A., TOMESCU, N., ZORLEANU, N., SCHAUER, C., & SOCOLOV, M. (1972). Factorii genetici ca factori de risc în reumatismul poliarticular acut. *Med. interna* **24,** 489–96.

RAPHAEL, T., SEARLE, O. M., & HORAN, T. N. (1927). Blood groups in tuberculosis. *Arch. intern. Med.* **40,** 328–31.

REED, H. (1960). The blood groups of cataract patients. *Trans. Canad. ophthal. Soc.* **23,** 77–9.

RENNIE, M. H. & HABER, R. W. (1961). Blood groups and carcinoma of the lung. *Med. J. Aust.* **ii,** 61–2.

RÉVAI, S. & KÖNIG, E. (1968). Vorkommen der Blutgruppen ABO bei an Diabetes mellitus leidenden Kranken. *Z. ärztl. Fortbild.* **62,** 1087–8.

RIBEIRO, E. B. (1963). Os grupos sangüíneos ABO e o câncer de estômago em São Paulo. *Ann. paulist. Med. Cir.* **86,** 87–95.

RICHTER, C. P. & CLISBY, H. (1942). Toxic effects of the bitter tasting phenylthiocarbamide. *Arch. Path.* **33,** 46–57.

RIDDELL, W. J. B. & WYBAR, K. C. (1944). Taste of thiouracil and phenylthiocarbamide. *Nature, Lond.* **154,** 669.

RITTER, H. & HINKELMANN, K. (1966). Zur Balance des Polymorphismus der Haptoglobine. *Humangenetik* **2,** 21–4.

RIZZI, N. (1963). Correlazione tra gruppi sanguigni, fattore Rh e rinite atrofica ozenatosa. *Oto-rino-laring. ital.* **32,** 373–7.

ROBERTS, D. F. (1976*a*). Pers. Comm. to A. E. Mourant.

ROBERTS, D. F. (1976*b*). Sex differences in disease and mortality. In *Equalities and inequalities in health* (eds. C. O. Carter & J. Peel), pp. 13–34.

ROBERTS, J. A. Fraser. The frequencies of the ABO blood-groups in South-Western England. *Ann. Eugen., Lond.* **14,** 109–16.

ROBINSON, M. G., TOLCHIN, D., & HALPERN, C. (1971). Enteric bacterial agents and the ABO blood groups. *Amer. J. hum. Genet.* **23,** 135–45.

ROBSON, E. B. & HARRIS, H. (1967). Further studies on the genetics of placental alkaline phosphatase. *Ann. hum. Genet.* **30,** 219–32.

ROGENTINE, G. N., DELLON, A. L., & CHRETIEN, P. B. (1976). Prolonged disease-free survival in bronchogenic carcinoma associated with HLA Aw19 and B5. A follow-up. In *HLA and disease. 1st int. Symp.*, p. 234. Abstracts, Paris, INSERM.

ROOD, J. J. VAN (1962). *Leucocyte grouping. A method and its application.* Haag, Pasmans.

ROSINSKI, B. (1960). Studies on the patients of the Psychiatric Hospital at Tworki (near Warsaw). 6th *Int. Congr. anthrop. ethnol. Sci.*, Paris **1,** 531–6.

ROSLING, E. (1929). Über den Einfluss der Blutgruppe und des Geschlechts auf das Vorkommen und den Verlauf der Diphterie, nebst einigen Beobachtungen über Altersverschiebung der Blutgruppenverteilung in der normalen Bevölkerung. *Acta path. microbiol. scand.* **6,** 153–91.

ROTELLI, L. & CORIPPO, C. (1959). Rapporti tra alcune malattie e gruppi sanguigni del sistema ABO. *Osped. maggiore* **47,** 70–2.

ROTKIN, I. D. (1965). Are ABO and Rh blood groups associated with cancer of the uterine cervix? *Cancer* **18,** 391–6.

ROYO MARTI, R. (1944–7). Grupos sanguíneos y lepra. *Rev. 'Fontilles'* **1,** 609–16.

RUBASCHKIN, W., MOLDAWSKAJA, W., & PAULI, S. (1927). Blutgruppen und Malaria. *Arch. Schiffs.-u. Tropenh.* **31,** 329–39.

RUDCHENKO, S. N. (1930). Blood groups in lepers. (In Russian.) *Trop. Med. Vet.* **8,** 34–8.

RUNDLE, A. T., SUDELL, B., & QAZI, H. S. (1972). Serum and red-cell phenotypes in epilepsy. *Lancet* **ii,** 1316.

RUNDLE, A. T., SUDELL, B., WOOD, K., & COPPEN, A. (1977). Red cell adenylate kinase phenotypes in the affective disorders. *Hum. Genet.* **36,** 161–6.

RYDER, L. R. & SVEJGAARD, A. (1976). *Associations between HLA and disease.* Report from the HLA and Disease Registry of Copenhagen. [Reprinted on pp. 275–98.]

SADEK, A. M., GUEMEH, N., & FAHIM, M. A. S. (1965*a*). The relationship between ABO blood groups and gastrointestinal diseases. *Alexandria med. J.* **11,** 119–24.

SADEK, A. M., GUEMEH, N., & FAHIM, M. A. S. (1965*b*). The relationship between secretor status of blood group substances and gastro-duodenal diseases and cancer. *Alexandria med. J.* **11,** 274–9.

SAENGUDOM, C. & FLATZ, G. (1967). Zur Verbreitung der ABO-Blutgruppen in der Bevölkerung Nordthailands. *Humangenetik* **3,** 319–27.

SAGAN, Z., ROMEJKO, A., & RZYTKA, J. (1957). Distribution of blood groups in some diseases on the basis of data from clinics in Wrocław. (In Polish.) *Arch. Immun.Terap. dośw.* **5,** 391–9.

SAHA, N. & BANERJEE, B. (1968). Incidence of ABO and Rh blood groups in pulmonary tuberculosis in different ethnic groups. *J. med. Genet.* **5,** 306–7.

SAHA, N. (1969). Incidence of G6PD deficiency in patients of three different ethnic groups suffering from pulmonary tuberculosis. *J. med. Genet.* **6,** 292–3.

SAHA, N. & BANERJEE, B. (1971). ABO blood groups, G6PD deficiency and abnormal haemoglobins in syphilis patients of three ethnic groups. *Acta Genet. med. Gemell.* **20,** 260–3.

SAHA, N., WONG, H. B., BANERJEE, B., & WONG, M. O. (1971). Distribution of ABO blood groups, G6PD deficiency, and abnormal haemoglobins in leprosy. *J. med. Genet.* **8,** 315–16.

SAHA, N. (1973). Distribution of ABO and Le^a blood groups in pulmonary tuberculosis in Chinese. *Clin. Genet.* **4,** 288–90.

SAHA, N., TOH, C. C. S., & GHOSH, M. B. (1973). Genetic association in myocardial infarction. *J. med. Genet.* **10,** 340–5.

SĂHLEANU, V., STOICA, G., & BUTOIANU, E. (1960). Les groupes sanguins ABO et l'hypertension artérielle. (In Romanian.) *Probl. Antrop., Bucureşti* **5**, 245–52.

SAKELLAROPOULOS, S. & COSTEAS, F. (1969). ABO blood groups in relation to myocardial infarction. (In Greek.) *Nosokom Chron.* **31**, 71–6. (Abstract in *Excerpta med. 22*, **8**, no. 1110.)

SAKHAROV, V. V. (1933). Goitre and blood groups. (In Russian.) *Za sots. Zdravookhr. Uzbekist.* no. 3, 56–8.

SALÁZAR MALLÉN, M., AMEZCUA CHAVARRÍA, E., & MITRANI LEVY, D. (1969). Estudios sobre la atopia en Mexico: los grupos eritrocitarios y el serologico Gm (1) en la poblacion normal y en la atopica. *Gac. méd., Méx.* **99**, 730–5.

SALDANHA, P. H. (1956). Apparent pleiotropic effect of genes determining taste thresholds for phenylthiourea. *Lancet* **ii**, 74–6.

SALDANHA, P. H. (1957). Polimorfismo e adaptabilidade diferencial dos grupos sanguíneos ABO. *Rev. brasil. Biol.* **17**, 345–58.

SALECK, W. (1932). Bestehen Beziehungen zwischen Blutgruppen und Geisteskrankheiten? *Z. ImmunForsch.* **74**, 280–97.

SALZANO, F. M., SUÑÉ, M. V., & FERLAUTO, M. (1967). New studies on the relationship between blood groups and leprosy. *Acta genet. Stat. med.* **17**, 530–44.

SAMITIER AZPARREN, J. & CHACON, C. (1958). Grupos sanguíneos y tuberculosis pulmonar. *Rev. esp. Tuberc.* **27**, 129–33.

SAMUEL, S., GUALANDRI, V., & PELLEGRIS, G. (1968). Nota sulle associazioni tra i gruppi sanguigni del sistema ABO e neoplasia dell'endometrio. *Tumori* **54**, 261–4.

SANGER, R. & RACE, R. R. (1947). Subdivisions of the MN blood groups in man. *Nature, Lond.* **160**, 505–6.

SANGER, R. (1955). An association between the P and Jay systems of blood groups. *Nature, Lond.* **176**, 1163–4.

SANGER, R., RACE, R. R., & JACK, J. (1955). The Duffy blood groups of the New York Negroes: the phenotype Fy (a–b–). *Brit. J. Haematol.* **1**, 370–4.

SANGHVI, L. D., BALAKRISHNAN, V., BHATIA, H. M., SUKUMARAN, P. K., & UNDEVIA, J. V. (eds.) (1974). *Human population genetics in India.* New Delhi, Orient Longman Ltd.

SANKALÉ, M., DIVETAIN, C., VESSEREAU, M., & DIOP, B. (1968). Répartition des groupes sanguins chez 120 malades atteints de cancer primitif du foie à Dakar. *Path. biol.* **16**, 1071–3.

SARTOR, V. & FRASER, R. S. (1964). ABO blood groups in patients with congenital and rheumatic valvular heart disease. *Canad. med. Ass. J.* **90**, 428–9.

SASANO, K. T. (1931). A study in blood groups. i. Tuberculosis. *Amer. Rev. Tuberc.* **23**, 207–13.

SAUER, H., MAI, K., & OTTO, H. (1963). Untersuchungen zur Blutgruppenverteilung beim *Diabetes mellitus*. *Klin. Wschr.* **41**, 1052–4.

SCHANFIELD, M. S., GILES, E., & GERSHOWITZ, H. (1975). Genetic studies in the Markham Valley, northeastern Papua New Guinea: gamma globulin (Gm and Inv), group specific component (Gc) and ceruloplasmin (Cp) typing. *Amer. J. phys. Anthrop.* **42**, 1–7.

SCHAPIRO, A. (1929). Die Wassermannsche Reaktion im Zusammenhang mit den Isoagglutinationseigenschaften des Blutes. *Z. ImmunForsch.* **64**, 1–8.

SCHEFFLER, W. Quoted by Helmbold (1961).

SCHERNTHANER, G., LUDWIG, H., & MAYR, W. R. (1976). Juvenile diabetes mellitus: HLA-antigen frequencies dependent on the age of onset of the disease. *J. Immunogenet.* **3**, 117–21.

SCHIFF, F. (1926). Die Blutgruppenverteilung in der Berliner Bevölkerung. ii. Mitteilung. *Klin. Wschr.* **5**, 1660–1.

SCHIFF, F. & SASAKI, H. (1932). Der Ausscheidungstypus, ein auf serologischem Wege nachweisbares mendelndes Merkmal. *Klin. Wschr.* **11**, 1426–9.

SCHIMKE, R. N. & ZIEGLER, D. K. (1970). ABO blood groups and Huntington's chorea. *Lancet* **ii**, 475–6.

SCHMAUSS, A. K., PERLIN, L., & KÜPFERLING, E. (1968). Die Verteilung der ABO-Blutgruppen bei Gallenstein- und Gallenblasenkarzinomkranken. *Dtsch. Z. Verdau.-u. Stoffwechselkr.* **28**, 317–21.

SCHMITT, P. A. (1928). Ueber die Häufikeit der einzelnen Blutgruppen bei Lungentuberkulösen. *Dtsch. med. Wschr.* **54**, 2019–20.

SCHOFIELD, C. B. S. (1966). ABO and Rh blood group distribution among patients attending venereal diseases clinics. *J. med. Genet.* **3**, 101–3.

SCHOLZ (1963). Quoted by Vogel & Helmbold (1972).

SCHOLZ, W. (1968). Untersuchungen über Assoziationen zwischen Carcinomerkrankung und gruppenspezifischen Blutmerkmalen. *Humangenetik* **6**, 88–9.

SCHREIBER, H. W., BARTSCH, W. M., & DAUER, W. (1959). Magenkarzinom und Blutgruppe. *Bruns' Beitr. klin. Chir.* **198**, 193–205.

SCHRÖDER, G. (1955). Bestehen Beziehungen zwischen Blutgruppe und Karzinomerkrankung? *Arch. GeschwulstForsch.* **8**, 230–40.

SCHUBERTH, G. Quoted by Helmbold (1961).

SCHWANTES, A. R., SALZANO, F. M., CASTRO, I. V. DE, & TONDO, C. V. (1967). Haptoglobins and leprosy. *Acta genet. Stat. med.* **17**, 127–36.

SCHWENZER, A. W. Quoted by Helmbold (1961).

SCIALDONE, D. & PANTALONE, T. (1963). Correlazione tra gruppi sanguigni ABO e miopia elevata. Ricerche statistiche. *Ann. Ottalm.* **89**, 375–80.

SCIARRA, D. & MEMEO, S. A. (1957). Rapporti intercorrenti tra gruppi sanguigni e calcolosi renale. *Rev. Anat. pat. Oncol.* **12**, 672–8.

SEGI, M., FUJISAKU, S., KURIHARA, M., & MONIWA, H. (1957*a*). Cancer of cervix uteri and ABO blood groups. *Tohoku J. exp. Med.* **66**, 50.

SEGI, M., FUJISAKU, S., KURIHARA, M., & MONIWA, H. (1957*b*). Stomach cancer and ABO blood groups. *Tohoku J. exp. Med.* **66**, 42.

SEHGAL, V. N., MATHUR, J. S., & RAO, N. S. N. (1966). A.B.O. blood groups in leprosy. *Leprosy Rev.* **37**, 221–2.

SEHGAL, V. N. & DUBE, B. (1967*a*). Secretion of blood group-specific substances in the saliva of leprosy patients. *Int. J. Leprosy* **35**, 375–6.

SEHGAL, V. N. & DUBE, B. (1967*b*). Secretion of blood group specific substances in saliva of vitiligo patients. *Brit. J. Derm.* **79**, 704–5.

SEHGAL, V. N. & DUBE, B. (1968). ABO blood groups and vitiligo. *J. med. Genet.* **5**, 308–9.

SEIFERT, B. (1964). Magenkrebs und ABO-Blutgruppensystem. *Zbl. Chir.* **89**, 1576–80.

SELVERSTONE, B. & COOPER, D. R. (1961). Astrocytomas and ABO blood groups. *J. Neurosurg.* **18**, 602–4.

SEOW, L. J., KWA, S. B., & TEOH, C. K. (1964). A preliminary survey of ABO blood group frequency in nasopharyngeal carcinoma in Chinese patients. *Singapore med. J.* **5**, 93–5.

SERRA, A., KLINGER, R., & GUALANDRI, V. (1963). Sulle differenze di morbilità dei soggetti di fenotipo O, A, B e AB per il diabete mellito. *Minerva med., Torino*, pt. sci. **54**, 3311–15.

SERRA, A., KLINGER, & GUALANDRI, V. (1964). The relation of diabetes mellitus to the blood group phenotypes O, A, B and AB. *Panminerva med.* **6**, 160–4.

SETH, S. (1969). Syphilis in its relation to blood groups. *Anthropologist* special vol., 105–15.

SEYFFERT (1963). Quoted by Vogel & Helmbold (1972).

SHARMA, D. C., JAIN, R. C., & DAVE, S. S. (1969). Relation between duodenal ulcer and blood group in people of the Udaipur region of India. *Gut* **10**, 75.

SHARP, H. L., BRIDGES, R. A., KRIVIT, R. A., & FREIER, E. F. (1969). Cirrhosis associated with alpha$_1$-antitrypsin deficiency: a previously unrecognised inherited disorder. *J. Lab. clin. Med.* **73**, 934–9.

SHAW, E. B., THELANDER, H. E., & KILGARIFF, K. (1932). Blood grouping in poliomyelitis. *J. Pediat.* **1**, 346–8.

SHAW, M. W. & GERSHOWITZ, H. (1962). A search for autosomal linkage in a trisomic population: blood group frequencies in mongols. *Amer. J. hum. Genet.* **14**, 317–34.

SHAW, M. W. & GERSHOWITZ, H. (1963). Blood group frequencies in mongols. *Amer. J. hum. Genet.* **15**, 495–6.

SHENOY, M. A. & DAFTARY, V. G. (1962). ABO blood groups and pulmonary tuberculosis. *Indian J. med. Sci.* **16**, 493–8.

SHEPARD, T. H. & GARTLER, S. M. (1960). Increased incidence of nontasters of phenylthiocarbamide among congenital athyreotic cretins. *Science* **131**, 929.

SHEPPARD, P. M. (1953). Cancer of stomach and ABO blood groups. *Brit. med. J.* **i**, 1220.

SHIRLEY, R. & DESAI, R. G. (1965). Association of leukaemia and blood groups. *J. med. Genet.* **2**, 189–91.

SHREFFLER, D. C. (1965). Genetic studies of blood group-associated variations in human serum alkaline phosphatase. *Amer. J. hum. Genet.* **17**, 71–86.

SIDANA, K. C., SARUP, B. M., KUMAR, R., & JOLLY, J. G. (1970). Study of blood groups in congenital malformations. *Indian J. med. Sci.* **24**, 74–8.

SIEVERS, M. L. (1959). Hereditary aspects of gastric secretory function. *Amer. J. Med.* **27**, 246–55.

SIEVERS, M. L. & CALABRESI, P. (1959). Gastric pepsin secretion and ABO blood groups in polycythemia vera. *Amer. J. dig. Dis.* **4**, 515–21.

SIEVERS, O. (1929). Die Blutgruppenverteilung unter Gesunden und Kranken innerhalb des in Finnland gesammelten Materiales. *Finska LäkSällsk. Handl.* **71**, 836–48.

SIMMONS, R. T., *et al.* (1944). The Rh factor: ethnological aspects. *Med. J. Aust.* **i**, 483–5.

SIMMONS, R. T., GRAYDON, J. J., ZIGAS, V., BAKER, L. L., & GAJDUSEK, D. C. (1961). Studies on kuru. vi. Blood groups in kuru. *Amer. J. trop. Med.* **10**, 665–8.

SIMMONS, R. T., GRAYDON, J. J., CURTAIN, C. C., & BAUMGARTEN, A. (1968). Blood group genetic studies in Laiagam, and Mt. Hagen (lepers), New Guinea. *Archaeol. phys. Anthrop. Oceania* **3**, 49–54.

SIMMONS, R. T., GRAYDON, J. J., GAJDUSEK, D. C., ALPERS, M. P., & HORNABROOK, R. W. (1972). Genetic studies in relation to kuru. ii. Blood-group genetic patterns in kuru patients and populations of the Eastern Highlands of New Guinea. *Amer. J. hum. Genet.* **24**, Suppl., S39–S71.

SIMPSON, C. A., VEJJAJIVA, A., CASPARY, E. A., & MILLER, H. (1965). ABO blood groups in multiple sclerosis. *Lancet* **i**, 1366–7.

SIMPSON, N. E., GUNSON, H. H., & SMITHIES, O. (1962). Frequencies of blood groups, serum haptoglobins and levels of slow alpha$_2$-globulin in diabetics and their relatives. *Diabetes* **11**, 329–33.

SINGH, G. & SHANKER, P. (1966). Vitiligo and blood groups. *Brit. J. Derm.* **78**, 91–2.

SINGH, G. & OJHA, D. (1967). Leprosy and ABO blood groups. *J. med. Genet.* **4**, 107–8.

SINISCALCO, M., BERNINI, L., LATTE, B., & MOTULSKY, A. G. (1961). Favism and thalassaemia in Sardinia and their relationship to malaria. *Nature, Lond.* **190**, 1179–80.

SLONE, D., GAETANO, L. F., LIPWORTH, L., SHAPIRO, S., PARKER LEWIS, G., & JICK, H. (1969). Computer analysis of epidemiologic data on effect of drugs on hospital patients. *Publ. Hlth Rep., Wash.* **84**, 39–52.

SMÅRS, G., BECKMAN, L., & BÖÖK, J. A. (1961). Osteogenesis imperfecta and blood groups. *Acta genet. Stat. med.* **11**, 133–6.

SMELLIE, H. C. (1956). Rhesus (D) factor in sarcoidosis. *Lancet* **i**, 863.

SMITH, R. S. & TRUELOVE, S. C. (1961). Blood groups and secretor in ulcerative colitis. *Brit. med. J.* **1**, 870–1.

SMITHIES, O. (1955). Zone electrophoresis in starch gels: group variations in the serum proteins of normal human adults. *Biochem. J.* **61**, 629–41.

SMITHIES, O. & WALKER, N. F. (1956). Notation for serum protein groups and the genes controlling their inheritance. *Nature, Lond.* **178**, 694–5.

SMITHIES, O., CONNELL, G. E., & DIXON, G. H. (1962). Inheritance of haptoglobin subtypes. *Amer. J. hum. Genet.* **14**, 14–21.

SNYDER, L. H. (1931). Inherited taste deficiency. *Science* **74**, 151–2.

SNYDER, L. H. (1932). Studies in human inheritance. ix. The inheritance of taste deficiency in man. *Ohio J. Sci.* **32**, 436–40.

SOBREVILLA, L. A., GOODMAN, M. L., & KANE, C. A. (1964). Demyelinating central nervous system disease, macular atrophy and acanthocytosis (Bassen–Kornzweig syndrome). *Amer. J. Med.* **37**, 821–8.

SOCHA, W. (1960). Les groupes sanguins A, B, O dans le cancer de l'estomac et dans les ulcères gastro-duodénaux. *Bull. Cancer* **47**, 126–53.

SOCHA, W. (1966). *Problems of serological differentiation of human populations.* (In Polish; English and Russian summaries.) Polish State Medical Publishers, Warsaw.

SOCHA, W., BILIŃSKA, M., KACZERA, Z., PAJDAK, E., & STANKIEWICZ, D. (1969). *Escherichia coli* and ABO blood groups. *Folia biol., Kraków* **17**, 259–69.

SOMOGY, I. & ANGYAL, L. VON (1931). Untersuchungen über Blutgruppenzugehörigkeit bei Geisteskranken. *Arch. Psychiatr. Nervenkr.* **95**, 290–302.

SØRENSEN, K. H. (1957). Peptic ulcer and the ABO blood group system. *Danish med. Bull.* **4**, no. 2, 45–7.

SORIANO LLERAS, A. (1954). Grupos sanguíneos en los tuberculosos. *Ann. Soc. Biol. Bogotá* **6**, 145–6.

SOTTNER, L. (1964). Diabetes mellitus and the taste of phenylthiocarbamide. (In Czech.) *Čas. Lék. čes.* **103**, 1308–13.

SOWA, J. (1970). The distribution of ABO and Rh blood groups in virus hepatitis. (In Polish.) *Wiad. lek.* **23**, 275–7.

SOWIŃSKA, J., STRZELECKA, M., & KUSZYK, T. (1968). ABO blood groups in rheumatic heart disease of children. (In Polish.) *Pol. Tyg. lek.* **23**, 343–6.

SPADA, D. & SARRA, A. (1958). Studio statistico sui tumori maligni dello stomaco in relazione ai gruppi sanguigni ABO. *Clinica, Bologna* **18**, 110–14.

SPANDONARI, A. & REPETTO CARBONESCHI, W. (1957). Correlazioni statistiche dei gruppi sanguigni con l'ulcera gastroduodenale e con il carcinoma dello stomaco. *Rass. ital. Chir. Med.* **6**, 113–17.

SPEISER, P. (1956). Bestehen mathematisch gesicherte Beziehungen der A–B–O-Gruppen, des Rhesusfaktors Rh_0(D) und des Geschlechtes zu Carcinoma ventriculi, Ulsus ventriculi und Ulsus duodeni? *Krebsarzt* **11**, 344–8.

SPEISER, P. (1958*a*). Krankheiten und Blutgruppen. *Krebsarzt* **13**, 208–18.

SPEISER, P. (1958*b*). Krankheiten und Blutgruppen; ueber Beziehung zwischen den Genitalkarzinomen bzw. Mammakarzinomen bei Frauen, Blutgruppen und Rh_0-(D)-Faktor. *Wien. klin. Wschr.* **70**, 315–16.

SPEISER, P. Quoted by Helmbold (1961).

SPENA, A. & GRIPPO, A. (1964). Sulle correlazioni fra neoplasie e gruppi sanguigni del sistema ABO. *Rass. int. Clin. Ter.* **44**, 1064–77.

SPIELMANN, W., TEIXIDOR, D., RENNINGER, W., & MATZNETTER, T. (1970). Blutgruppen und Lepra bei moçambiquanischen Völkerschaften. *Humangenetik* **10**, 304–17.

SPRINGER, G. F. & WIENER, A. S. (1962). Alleged causes of the present-day world distribution of the human *ABO* blood groups. *Nature, Lond.* **193**, 444–5.

SPRUCH, T. & DACKA, E. (1968). ABO blood groups and the incidence of gastric cancer, gastric ulcer and duodenal ulcer. (In Polish.) *Pol. Tyg. lek.* **23**, 979–80.

SRIVASTAVA, D. K., THAKUR, C. P., & DAS, M. (1966). ABO-blood groups in relation to ischaemic heart disease. *Indian Heart J.* **18**, 140–9.

SRIVASTAVA, G. N. & SHUKLA, R. C. (1965). ABO blood groups in vitiligo. *Indian J. med. Res.* **53**, 221–5.

STÄPS, R., BUNDSCHUH, G., & FALK, H. (1961). Über Haptoglobinbefunde an Kranken der Berliner Universitäts-Hautklinik. *Dtsch GesundheitsWes.* **16**, 59–60.

STEINBERG, A. G. (1960). The genetics of acute leukemia in children. *Cancer, Philad.* **13**, 985–99.

STELL, P. M. & KELL, R. A. (1970). Blood groups and hypopharyngeal cancer. *Lancet* **ii**, 819.

STEWART, J. C. & VIDOR, G. I. (1976). Thyrotoxicosis induced by iodine contamination of food—a common unrecognised condition. *Brit. med. J.* **i**, 372–5 and **iii**, 701.

STOIA, I., RÂMNEANȚU, R., & POITAŞ, M. (1969). Blood groups ABO and Rh(D) factor in the rheumatic diseases. *Romanian med. Rev.* **13**, 28–9.

STOUT, T. D. (1976). Pers. comm. to A. E. Mourant.

STRANG, R. R. (1965). ABO blood-groups in Parkinson's disease. *Acta path. microbiol. scand.* **65**, 653.

STRANG, R. R., TOVI, D., & LOPEZ, J. (1966). Astrocytomas and the ABO blood groups. *J. med. Genet.* **3**, 274–5.

STRANG, R. R. (1967). Age, sex, and ABO blood group distributions of 150 patients with cerebral arteriovenous aneurysms. *J. med. Genet.* **4,** 29–30.

STRANG, R. R. (1968). Age, sex and ABO blood distribution of 400 patients with pituitary chromophobe adenoma. *Clin. Med.* **75,** 45–8.

STRASZYŃSKI, A. (1924). Prédisposition aux maladies cutanées chez les sujets appartenant aux divers groupes sérologiques. *C. R. Soc. Biol., Paris* **91,** 1481–2.

STRASZYŃSKI, A. (1925*a*). Susceptibility to certain skin diseases in individuals of different blood groups. (In Polish.) *Przegl. derm.* **20,** 204–12.

STRASZYŃSKI, A. (1925*b*). Über das Ergebnis der Wassermannschen Reaktion innerhalb verschiedener Blutgruppen bei behandelter Lues. *Klin. Wschr.* **4,** 1962–3.

STRENG, O. & RYTI, E. (1927*a*). Die Blutgruppenverteilung bei Gesunden und Kranken in Suomi (Finland). *Acta Soc. Med. 'Duodecim'* **8,** no. 6, 1–57.

STRENG, O. & RYTI, E. (1927*b*). Quoted by Mustakallio (1937).

STRUTHERS, D. (1951). ABO groups of infants and children dying in the West of Scotland (1949–1951). *Brit. J. soc. Med.* **5,** 223–8.

SUJOY, E. & ALLEMAND, H. (1943). El estudio del grupo sanguíneo en 150 casos de poliomielitis anterior aguda. *Arch. argent. Pediat.* **20,** 390–3.

SUK, V. (1931). Cabbage and goitre in Carpathian Ruthenia. A contribution to ethnic pathology. *Anthropologie, Prague* **9,** 1–6.

SUKUMARAN, P. K., MASTER, H. R., UNDEVIA, J. V., BALAKRISHNAN, V., & SANGHVI, L. D. (1966). ABO blood groups in active cases of smallpox. *Indian J. med. Sci.* **20,** 119–22.

SUZUKI, Y., TAKEUCHI, T., & KITAZAWA, Y. (1966). Phenylthiourea taste testing in primary glaucomas. *Acta Soc. ophthal. jap.* **70,** 88–91.

SVEJGAARD, A., JERSILD, C., NIELSEN, L. Staub, & BODMER, W. F. (1974). HL-A antigens and disease statistical and genetical considerations. *Tissue Antigens* **4,** 95–105.

SVEJGAARD, A., HAUGE, M., JERSILD, C., PLATZ, P., RYDER, L. P., NIELSEN, L. Staub, & THOMSEN, M. (1975). *The HLA system. An introductory survey.* S. Karger, Basel.

SWIDER, Z. & KON, N. (1928). Recherches sur les groupes sanguins chez les tuberculeux. *C. R. Soc. Biol., Paris* **98,** 385–6.

SZABOLCS, Z. (1960). Blood groups and gastric cancer. (In Hungarian.) *Orv. Hétil.* **101,** 1351–3.

SZCZEPAŃSKI, L. & JACH, A. (1973). Distribution of ABO and Rh groups in myocardial infarction. (In Polish.) *Pol. Tyg. lek.* **28,** 1262–3.

SZMUNESS, W., GAWRONOWA, H., & HOROCH, C. (1966). Viral hepatitis in blood recipients—a retrospective study. *Epidem. Rev.* **20,** 201–10.

SZMUNESS, W., PRINCE, A. M., & CHERUBIN, C. E. (1971). Serum hepatitis antigen (SH) carrier state: relation to ABO blood groups. *Brit. med. J.* **ii,** 198–9.

SZMYT, J. (1938). Rassen-und Konstitutionselemente bei den an malignen Tumoren leidenden der Lemberger Krankenhaüser. (In Polish.) *Przegl. antrop.* **12,** 223–55.

TAGLIAFERRO, E. (1937*a*). Gruppi sanguigni e carcinoma. *Minerva med., Torino* **28,** 219–20.

TAGLIAFERRO, E. (1937*b*). Gruppi sanguigni e tubercolosi. *Minerva med., Torino* **28,** 391–3.

TAKAHASHI, T. (1969). P.T.C. taste test in eye diseases. *Acta Soc. ophthal. jap.* **73,** 37–45.

TAKANO, K. & MILLER, J. R. (1972). ABO incompatibility as a cause of spontaneous abortion: evidence from abortuses. *J. med. Genet.* **9,** 144–50.

TALBOT, S., WAKLEY, E. J., RYRIE, D., & LANGMAN, M. J. S. (1970). ABO blood-groups and venous thromboembolic disease. *Lancet* **i,** 1257–9.

TALBOT, S., WAKLEY, E. J., & LANGMAN, M. J. S. (1972). A_1, A_2, B, and O blood-groups. Lewis blood-groups, and serum triglyceride and cholesterol concentrations in patients with venous thromboembolic disease. *Lancet* **i,** 1152–4.

TAN, A. L. (1962). The relationship between blood group A and gastric cancer. *Philipp. J. Cancer* **4,** 59–63.

TEDESCHI, G. & CAVAZZUTI, F. (1959). Gruppi sanguigni e diabete mellito. 7th *Congr. int. Soc. Blood Transfus.*, Rome, 1958. *Bibl. haemat.* **10,** 180–4.

TERADA, H. (1929). On the relation between cancer morbidity and the blood types, with reference to the disposition of the cancer. *Gann* **23,** 76–7.

TERASAKI, P. I. & MCCLELLAND, J. D. (1964). Microdroplet assay of human serum cytotoxins. *Nature, Lond.* **204,** 998–1000.

TERRY, M. C. & SEGALL, G. (1947). The association of diabetes and taste-blindness. *J. Hered.* **38,** 135–7.

TERRY, M. C. (1950). Taste-blindness and diabetes in the colored population of Jamaica. *J. Hered.* **41,** 306–7.

THAYER, W. R. & BOVE, J. R. (1965). Blood groups and ulcerative colitis. *Gastroenterology* **48,** 326–30.

THIELER, H., SCHMECHEL, H., & GAERISCH, F. (1966). ABO-Blutgruppenverteilung bei Hepatitis infectiosa. *Z. ges. inn. Med.* **21,** 365–8.

THOMAS, J. C. & HEWITT, E. J. C. (1939). Blood groups in health and in mental disease. *J. ment. Sci.* **85,** 667–88.

THOMAS, K. & HOFMANN, F. (1967). Die Serumgruppen-Systeme Lp(a), Gm(a), Gc und Hp bei Cerebralsklerotikern. *Humangenetik* **4,** 18–22.

THOMPSON, C. E. R., ASHURST, P. M., & BUTLER, T. J. (1968). Survey of haemorrhagic erosive gastritis. *Brit. med. J.* **iii,** 283–5.

THOMPSON, R. (1931). Blood groups and susceptibility to dental caries. *Proc. Soc. exp. Biol., N. Y.* **29,** 106.

THOMSEN, M., JAKOBSEN, B., PLATZ, P., RYDER, L. P., NIELSEN, L. Staub, & SVEJGAARD, A. (1976). LD-typing, polymorphism of MLC determinants. In *Histocompatibility testing 1975*. Copenhagen, Munksgaard.

THOMSEN, O., FRIEDENREICH, V., & WORSAAE, E. (1930). Über die Möglichkeit der Existenz zweier neuer Blutgruppen; auch ein Beitrag zur Beleuchtung sogenannter Untergruppen. *Acta path. microbiol. scand.* **7,** 157–90.

THOMSEN, O. (1931–2). Über mögliche Unterschiede in der Neigung zur Krebsentwicklung bei Individuen verschiedener Blutgruppen. *Krankheitsforschung* **9,** 167–84.

THORSØE, H. (1960). ABO blood groups and fracture of the femoral neck. *Dan. med. Bull.* **7,** 75–7.

THOULD, A. K. & SCOWEN, E. F. (1964). Genetic studies of the syndrome of congenital deafness and simple goitre. *Ann. hum. Genet.* **27,** 283–93.

TIBERA-DUMITRU, M. (1963). La réponse à la PTC dans le goitre thyréopathe. (In Romanian.) *Probl. Antrop. Bücureşti* **7,** 139–44.

TIEDEMANN, H. (1929–30). Blutgruppenverteilung bei Lungentuberkulose. *Z. Tuberk.* **55,** 235–7.

TILLS, D. & LEHMANN, H. (1975). Pers. comm. to A. E. Mourant.

TINNEY, W. S. & WATKINS, C. H. (1941). Blood groups and the blood dyscrasias. *Proc. Mayo Clin.* **16,** 613–14.

TOUSSAINT, J. & MÉRIAUX, J. (1970). Approche statistique des parodontopathies observées en bilan de santé. Leur relation avec le sexe, l'âge et le groupe sanguin. *Concours méd.* **92,** 8745–8.

TRANQUILLI-LEALI, E. (1938). Lussazione congenita dell'anca e gruppo sanguigno. *Arch. Ortop., Milano* **54,** 103–43.

TSUKADA, Y., MOORE, R. H., BROSS, I. D. J., PICKREN, J. W., & COHEN, E. (1964). Blood groups in patients with multiple cancers. *Cancer, Philad.* **17,** 1229–32.

TUROWSKA, B., GAWRZEWSKI, W., & CZAJKOWSKA, L. (1968). Blood group and serum systems in schizophrenia. *Acta med. polon.* **9,** 209–12.

TURUNEN, M. & PASILA, M. (1957). The ABO blood group and carcinoma of the stomach. *Ann. Med. exp. Fenn.* **35,** 100–5.

TYAGI, S. P., PRADHAN, S., & AGARWAL, S. S. (1965). Blood groups in malignant diseases. *J. Indian med. Ass.* **45,** 645–50.

TYAGI, S. P., TIAGI, G. K., & PRADHAN, S. (1967). ABO blood groups in relation to cancer cervix. *Indian J. med. Sci.* **21,** 611–15.

UETAKE, M., TANAKA, T., YOSHIDA, T., HOSHINO, T., TAKAGI, K., SOMEYA, M., & NAKANO, S. (1958). Natural selection among ABO blood groups by gastric carcinoma and peptic ulcer. (In Japanese.) *Jap. J. hum. Genet.* **3,** 156–64.

UGELLI, L. (1936). Distribuzione dei gruppi sanguigni negli individui portatori di ulcere gastroduodenali. *Policlinico*, Sez. prat. **43,** 1591–4.

UNITED KINGDOM, DEPARTMENT OF HEALTH AND SOCIAL SECURITY (1972). *Report on confidential enquiries into maternal deaths in England and Wales 1967–1969*. London, H.M. Stationery Office.

VACHHRAJANI, R. B. & SHENOY, M. A. (1959). A study of ulcer dyspepsia with a note on its relation to A.B.O. blood groups. *J. of J. J. Group Hosp. & Grant med. Coll.* **4,** 83–94.

VAHALA, Z., CHARVÁT, A., & SLEZÁK, Z. (1970). Relation between the blood groups of the A, B, AB, O system and the frequency of ulcers and malignant tumours of the digestive tract. (In Czech.) *Čas. Lék. čes.* **109,** 1057–8.

VALENTINE, W. N. & NEEL, J. V. (1944). Hematologic and genetic study of the transmission of thalassemia (Cooley's anemia; Mediterranean anemia). *Arch. inter. Med.* **74,** 185–96.

VALENTINI, V. (1938). Rapporti tra i gruppi sanguigni e le varie forme di tubercolosi polmonare con particolare riguardo all'appartenenza regionale dei pazienti. *Diagn. Tec. Lab., Napoli* **9,** 81–8.

VALLE, W. W. (1937). Déterminations des groups sanguins chez les lépreux de l'Hospice Prophylactique. *Rev. Méd. Hyg. trop.* **29,** 125.

VANA, L. R. & STEINBERG, A. G. (1975). Haptoglobin—ABO interaction: a possible explanation for the excess of Hp1 among offspring of ABO incompatible matings. *Amer. J. hum. Genet.* **27,** 224–32.

VANARSDEL, P. P. & MOTULSKY, A. G. (1959). Blood groups and secretion of blood group substances. Comparison of allergic with non-allergic persons in a Pacific Northwest college population. *J. Allergy* **30,** 460–3.

VEJJAJIVA, A., FOSTER, J. B., & MILLER, H. (1965). ABO blood-groups in motor-neurone disease. *Lancet* **i,** 87–8.

VELARDE, L. Q. & GONZALES DEL CARPIO, D. (1969). Grupos sanguíneos y carcinoma de cuello uterino; estudio en dos formas histológicas. *Acta cancerol., Lima* **8,** 22–3.

VENTZKE, L. E. & GROSSMAN, M. I. (1962). Response of patients with duodenal ulcer to augmented histamine test as related to blood groups and to secretor status. *Gastroenterology* **42,** 292–4.

VERHAGEN, A. (1951). Rh-Faktor bei Karzinompatienten. *Z. ImmunForsch.* **108,** 355–6.

VERMA, B. S. & DONGRE, A. V. (1965). Leprosy and A.B.O. blood groups. *Leprosy Rev.* **36,** 211–13.

VERMA, B. S. & ACHARYA, P. T. (1966). Tuberculoid leprosy and ABO blood groups. *Brit. J. Derm.* **78,** 552–3.

VESELÝ, K. T. (1969*a*). The distribution of blood groups of the ABO and Rh_o (D) systems amongst patients with epidemic hepatitis, liver cirrhosis and ulcerative colitis. (In Czech.) *Vnitřní Lék.* **15,** 1089–93.

VESELÝ, K. T. (1969*b*). Frequency of blood groups of the ABO and Rh_o (D) systems in patients with lithiasis of the biliary pathways and inflammation of the pancreas. *Čsl. Gastroenter. Výž.* **23,** 130–4.

VESELÝ, K. T. (1969*c*). Relationship between ABO and Rh_o (D) blood groups and urolithiasis. (In Czech.) *Čas. Lék. čes.* **108,** 1049–51.

VESELÝ, K. T. & KUBÍČKOVÁ, Z. (1969). Relationship between blood groups of ABO system and the severity of duodenal ulcers. *Rev. Czech. Med.* **15,** 33–40.

VILARDELL, F. & JORI-SOLÉ, J. (1961). Cancer gástrico y grupos sanguíneos ABO en Barcelona. *Rev. clín. esp.* **80,** 236–8.

VILLANO, P. A. & SANTOIANNI, P. (1972). Psoriasi, gruppo sanguigno M e fattore serico Gm (2). *Minerva dermat.* **47,** 272–5.

VISCONTI, A., TOLIO, A., & CAVA, L. (1961*a*). Correlazione fra neoplasie e gruppi sanguigni del sistema ABO. *Tumori* **47,** 303–16.

VISCONTI, A., TOLIO, A., & PEROTTI, V. (1961*b*). Sulle associazioni fenotipiche dei gruppi sanguigni ABO con il cancro gastrico e l'ulcera gastrica e duodenale. *Tumori* **47,** 378–93.

VISKUM, K. (1973). Respiratory disease and ABO and Rhesus blood groups. *Scand. J. resp. Dis.* **54,** 97–102.

VÖLTER, D., VÖLTER, G., DICK, W., & GRIESSER, G. (1970). ABO-Blutgruppen und Erkrankungen. *Z. Morph. Anthrop.* **62,** 290–322.

VOGEL, F., PETTENKOFER, H. J., & HELMBOLD, W. (1960). Über die Populationsgenetik der ABO-Blutgruppen. 2. Mitteilung. Genhäufigkeit und epidemische Erkrankungen. *Acta genet. Stat. med.* **10,** 267–94.

VOGEL, F. (1963). Neuere Untersuchungen zur Populationsgenetik der ABO-Blutgruppen. 8. *Tag. dtsch Ges. Anthrop.*, Köln, 143–61 (Suppl. to *Homo*).

VOGEL, F., DEHNERT, J., & HELMBOLD, W. (1964). Beziehungen zwischen den ABO-Blutgruppen und der Säuglingsdyspepsie. *Humangenetik* **1,** 31–57.

VOGEL, F. & CHAKRAVARTTI, M. R. (1966*a*). ABO blood groups and smallpox in a rural population of West Bengal and Bihar (India). *Humangenetik* **3,** 166–80.

VOGEL, F. & CHAKRAVARTTI, M. R. (1966*b*). ABO blood groups and the type of leprosy in an Indian population. *Humangenetik* **3,** 186–8.

VOGEL, F., KRÜGER, J., SONG, Y. K., & FLATZ, G. (1969). ABO blood groups, leprosy, and serum proteins. *Humangenetik* **7,** 149–62.

VOGEL, F., KRÜGER, J., CHAKRAVARTTI, M. R., RITTER, H., & FLATZ, G. (1971). ABO blood groups, Inv serum groups, and serum proteins in leprosy patients from West Bengal (India). *Humangenetik* **12,** 284–301.

VOGEL, F. & HELMBOLD, W. (1972). Blutgruppen—Populationsgenetik und Statistik. In *Humangenetik* (ed. B. E. Becker), Vol. I, part 4. Stuttgart, Georg Thieme.

VOS, G. H., CELANO, M. J., FALKOWSKI, F., & LEVINE, P. (1964). Relationship of a hemolysin resembling anti-Tj^a to threatened abortion in Western Australia. *Transfusion, Philad.* **4,** 87–91.

VOS, G. H. & TOVELL, T. (1967). Graph interpretation suggesting understatement of the frequency of spontaneous abortion. *Fertil. Steril.* **18,** 678–84.

VOSSSCHULTE, A. & ZIEGLER, K. (1935). Zur Frage Blutgruppe und Scharlach. *Dtsch. med. Wschr.* **61,** 262–3.

WALLACE, J. (1954). Blood groups and disease. *Brit. med. J.* **ii,** 534.

WALLACE, J., PEEBLES BROWN, D. A., COOK, I. A., & MELROSE, A. G. (1958). The secretor status in duodenal ulcer. *Scottish med. J.* **3,** 105–9.

WALSH, R. J. & MONTGOMERY, C. M. (1947). A new human iso-agglutinin subdividing the MN blood groups. *Nature, Lond.* **160,** 504–5.

WALSH, R. J. & KOOPTZOFF, O. (1956). Blood groups and disease: rheumatic fever. *Australas. Ann. Med.* **5,** 17–19.

WALTER, H., BAJATZADEH, M., KELLERMANN, G., & MATZNETTER, T. (1970). Associations between leprosy and serum protein groups. *Humangenetik* **10,** 298–303.

WALTER, H., KELLERMANN, G., BAJATZADEH, G., KRÜGER, J., & CHAKRAVARTTI, M. R. (1972). Hp, Gc, Cp, Tf, Bg and Pi phenotypes in leprosy patients and healthy controls from West Bengal (India). *Humangenetik* **14,** 314–25.

WALTHER, W. W., RAEBURN, C., & CASE, J. (1956). Blood-groups in relation to malignant diseases. *Lancet* **ii,** 970–2.

WARD, A. M., PICKERING, J. D., & SHORTLAND, J. R. (1975). The renal manifestations of PiZ. In *L'alpha-1-antitrypsine et le système Pi* (ed. J.-P. Martin), pp. 131–4. Paris, INSERM.

WARTENBERG, J. & WĄSIKOWA, R. (1971). Blood groups in children with diabetes and in their families. (In Polish.) *Pediat. pol.* **46,** 457–64.

WATERHOUSE, J. A. H. & HOGBEN, L. (1947). Incompatibility of mother and foetus with respect to the iso-agglutinogen A and its antibody. *Brit. J. soc. Med.* **1,** 1–17.

WATKIN, I. J., TILLS, D., & HEATH, R. B. (1975). Studies of genetic susceptibility of individuals to infection with influenza viruses. *Humangenetik* **30,** 75–9.

WAYJEN, R. G. A. VAN (1960). Verdeling van de ABO-bloedgroepen bij maagkankerpatiënten. *Ned. Tijdsch. Geneesk.* **104,** 2448–55.

WEBSTER, B. & CHESNEY, A. M. (1930). Studies in the etiology of simple goiter. *Amer. J. Path.* **6,** 275–84.

WEHLE (1957). Quoted by Vogel & Helmbold (1972).

WEIDEMANN, M. (1930). Zur Verteilung der Blutgruppen bei den Leprösen Lettlands. *Med. Klinik* **26,** 1155.

WEINBERGER, M. (1943). An investigation on blood groups in tuberculosis. *Brit. J. Tuberc.* **37,** 68–87.

WEINER, W., LEWIS, H. B. M., MOORES, P., SANGER, R., & RACE, R. R. (1957). A gene, y, modifying the blood group antigen A. *Vox Sang.* n.s. **2,** 25–37.

WEISER, F. (1957). Die klassischen Blutgruppen in Beziehung zum Karzinom und peptischen Ulkus. *Wien. med. Wschr.* **107,** 737–8.

WEISS, N. S. (1972). ABO blood type and arteriosclerosis obliterans. *Amer. J. hum. Genet.* **24,** 65–70.

WEITZNER, G. (1925). Hämagglutiningehalt des Blutserums Karzinomkranker. *Med. Klin.* **21,** 1960–1.

WENDE (1965). Quoted by Vogel & Helmbold (1972).

WENDT, G. G. (1968). Blood groups, serum factors and psoriasis vulgaris. *Dermatologica, Basel* **136,** 1–10.

WENDT, G. G., KRÜGER, J., & KINDERMANN, I. (1968). Serumgruppen und Krankheit. *Humangenetik* **6,** 281–99.

WESTERHOLM, B., WIECHEL, B., & EKLUND, G. (1971). Oral contraceptives, venous thromboembolic disease, and ABO blood type. *Lancet* **ii,** 664.

WEWALKA, F. (1960). Die Blutgruppen bei Lebercirrhosen. *Blut* **6,** 261–6.

WHITE, H. & SHOOTER, R. A. (1962). Staphylococcal nasal carriage and wound sepsis in relation to ABO and Rh blood groups of male surgical patients. *Brit. med. J.* **ii,** 307.

WIDSTRÖM, G. & HENSCHEN, A. (1963). The relation between P.T.C. taste response and protein bound iodine in serum. *Scand. J. clin. Lab. Invest.* **15,** Suppl. no. 69, 257–61.

WIECHMANN, E. & PAAL, H. (1926). Ueber die Blutgruppen der Kölner Bevölkerung. *Münch. med. Wschr.* **73,** 606–8.

WIECHMANN, E. & PAAL, H. (1927). Über Hypertonie, insbesondere über die Blutgruppen der Hypertoniker. *Dtsch. Arch. klin. Med.* **154,** 287–95.

WIENER, A. S. & PETERS, H. R. (1940). Hemolytic reactions following transfusions of blood of the homologous group, with three cases in which the same agglutinogen was responsible. *Ann. intern. Med.* **13,** 2306–22.

WIENER, A. S. (1942). The Rh factor and racial origins. *Science* **96,** 407–8.

WIENER, A. S., FREDA, V. J., WEXLER, I. B., & BRANCATO, G. J. (1960*a*). Pathogenesis of ABO hemolytic disease. *Amer. J. Obstet. Gynec.* **79,** 567–92.

WIENER, A. S., UNGER, L. J., & JACK, J. A. (1960*b*). Preuve de l'existence d'un nouveau gène allèle Rh R^{1cd}. *Rev. Hémat.* **15,** 286–90.

WILCZKOWSKI, E. (1927). Blutgruppenuntersuchungen bei Schizophrenie und progressiver Paralyse. *Klin. Wschr.* **6,** 168.

WILK, A., GAJEWSKI, C., & MARCINKIEWICZ, S. (1969). Distribution of blood groups of the system ABO in individuals with different states of refraction of the organ of sight. *Przegl. antrop.* **35,** 311–16.

WILLIAMS, A. O. (1966). Haemoglobin genotypes, ABO blood groups and Burkitts tumor. *J. med. Genet.* **3,** 177–9.

WINSTONE, N. E., HENDERSON, A. J., & BROOKE, B. N. (1960). Blood-groups and secretor status in ulcerative colitis. *Lancet* **ii,** 64–5.

WINTER, H. (1930). Blutgruppen in der Dermatologie; Blutgruppenverteilung in Oberhessen. *Derm. Z.* **57,** 432–41.

WINZELER, M., BRAUN, P., & GROB, P. J. (1974). Familiär gehäufte Bronchiektasen und α_1-Antitrypsin-Mangel. *Schweiz. med. Wschr.* **104,** 1705–11.

WOJTOWICZ, M., PIOCH, E., & CIOK, J. (1960). Blood groups and gastric and duodenal ulcer and gastric cancer. (In Polish.) *Pol. med. Wkly* **15,** 745–7.

WOOD, C. S., HARRISON, G. A., DORÉ, C., & WEINER, J. S. (1972). Selective feeding of *Anopheles gambiae* according to ABO blood group status. *Nature, Lond.* **239,** 165.

WOOD, C. S. (1975). New evidence for a late introduction of malaria into the New World. *Curr. Anthrop.* **16,** 93–104.

WOODROW, J. C. (1974). Pers. comm. to A. E. Mourant.

WOOLF, B. (1954–5). On estimating the relation between blood group and disease. *Ann. hum. Genet.* **19,** 251–3.

WORKMAN, P. L., LUCARELLI, P., AGOSTINO, R., SCARABINO, R., SCACCHI, R., CARAPELLA, E., PALMARINO, R., & BOTTINI, E. (1975). Genetic differentiation among Sardinian villages. *Amer. J. phys. Anthrop.* **43,** 165–76.

WORLD HEALTH ORGANIZATION (1967). *Manual of the international statistical classification of diseases, injuries, and causes of death.* WHO, Geneva.

WORM, M. (1954). Der Rhesusfaktor bei Diabetikerinnen. *Klin. Wschr.* **32,** 892–3.

WOSZCZYK, J. (1966). Distribution of ABO blood groups in patients with gastric ulcer, duodenal ulcer, gastric carcinoma and bile tract calculi. (In Polish.) *Pol. Tyg. lek.* **21,** 1187–90.

WREN, B. G. & VOS, G. H. (1961). Blood group incompatibility as a cause of spontaneous abortion. *J. Obstet. Gynaec. Brit. Cwlth* **68,** 637–47.

WÜRZ, P. (1928). Über die Blutgruppenverteilung bei Schizophrenen. *Schweiz. med. Wschr.* **9,** 353–5.

YANKAH, J. A. K. (1965). Observation on the frequency of ABO and Rh blood groups in leprosy and non-leprosy people in Ghana. *Leprosy Rev.* **36,** 73–4.

YATES, P. O. & PEARCE, K. M. (1960). Recent change in blood-group distribution of astrocytomas. *Lancet* **i,** 194–5.

YEOH, G. S. (1960). Carcinoma of the stomach. A review of 314 cases seen and treated in the surgical professorial unit, General Hospital, Singapore, for the years 1947 to 1959. *Singapore med. J.* **1,** 140–7.

ZERVOPOULOS, G., TSANA, K., & MIHAILIDIS, G. (1967). Relation of mental disease to blood groups. (In Greek.) *Neuropsychiat. Chron.* **6,** 32–47.

ZEYTINOGLU, I. (1957). Relation entre les groupes sanguins ABO et le diabète. *Rev. méd. Suisse romande* **77,** 489–93.

ZIH, S. & THOMA, A. (1967). ABO-Blutgruppen bei rheumatischen Fieber und rheumatischer Karditis. *Humangenetik* **4,** 42–51.

ZOGRAPHOV, D. G. (1962). ABO-Blutgruppen und bösartige Geschwülste. *Oncologia* **15,** 59–64.

ZUBER, E. (1966). ABO and Rh blood groups and diseases. (In Polish.) *Pol. Tyg. lek.* **21,** 101–3.

ZUBER, R. & ANDREAS, H. Quoted by Helmbold (1961).

ZUCKERMAN, A. J. & MCDONALD, J. C. (1963). ABO blood groups and acute hepatitis. *Brit. med. J.* **ii,** 537–8.

ZUCKERMAN, A. J., MILLER, D. L., & MCDONALD, J. C. (1964). ABO blood groups and staphylococcal infection. *Brit. med. J.* **i,** 101.

ZUCKERMAN, A. J. (1966). ABO blood groups and cirrhosis of the liver. *J. med. Genet.* **3,** 33–4.

ZUELZER, W. W. & KAPLAN, E. (1954). ABO heterospecific pregnancy and hemolytic disease: a study of normal and pathologic variants. iv. Pathologic variants. *Amer. J. Dis. Child.* **88,** 319–38.

INDEX

THIS index refers both to the text and the tables. As the bibliography is alphabetically arranged, authors are not otherwise indexed.

Most of the indexed items refer to specific associations between a disease and a polymorphism. In all such cases the primary entry is the name of the disease, with a sub-entry for each polymorphism, abbreviated according to the list below and printed in italics. For neoplasms and certain other localized diseases, the key word is the name of the organ or tissue affected.

Page numbers in roman type refer to the text, and numbers in italics to the tables, including the appendix.

Abbreviation used in index	*Polymorphic system*
ABO	ABO blood groups
Acet	Acetylator (metabolic)
ADA	Adenosine deaminase (red cell enzyme)
AK	Adenylate kinase (red-cell enzyme)
AP	Acid phosphatase (red-cell enzyme)
Ear-wax	Ear-wax types
Fy	Duffy blood groups
Gc	Group-specific component (plasma protein)
G6PD	Glucose-6-phosphate dehydrogenase (red-cell enzyme)
Hb	Haemoglobin (red-cell protein)
HLA	Human leucocyte (histocompatibility) antigens
Hp	Haptoglobin (plasma protein)
Kell	Kell blood groups
MNSs	MNSs blood groups
P	P blood groups
PGM	Phosphoglucomutase (red-cell enzyme)
Pi	Protease inhibitor (trypsin inhibitor) (plasma protein)
PTC	Phenylthiocarbamide taster
Rh	Rhesus blood groups
Se	ABH secretor